Sciatica: Foundations of diagnosis and conservative treatment

Edited by Susan Trager

ISBN 978-1-7341767-0-4

For permissions and/or to contact the publisher, email: integratedclinicsLLC@gmail.com

Cover by Robert Trager. Images from left to right show:

- The erector spinae (solid line) and transversospinalis muscles (dotted line) on an axial lumbar MRI
- An antirotational press, a lumbar stabilization exercise
- Ingrowth of nerves into a lumbar disc
- The sacral thrust test, an orthopedic test for sacroiliac joint pain

Disclaimer:

This book presents the author's interpretation of current research, and first-hand experiences and opinions about sciatica. The author is not your healthcare provider and makes no representations or warranties of any kind with respect to this book or its contents. The author and publisher disclaim all such representations and warranties, including warranties of merchantability and healthcare for a particular purpose. In addition, the author and publisher do not represent or warrant that the information in this book is accurate, complete or current. The information in this book has not been evaluated by the U.S. Food and Drug Administration. This book is not intended to diagnose, treat, cure, or prevent any condition or disease. Please consult with your own health care provider regarding the suggestions and recommendations made in this book. Neither the author nor publisher will be liable for damages arising out of or in connection with the use of this book. You understand that this book is not intended as a substitute for consultation with a licensed healthcare provider, such as your physician. Before you begin any healthcare program, or change your lifestyle in any way, you should consult your physician or another licensed healthcare provider to ensure that you are in good health and that the examples contained in this book will not harm you. As such, use of this book implies your acceptance of this disclaimer.

Table of Contents

Chapter 1 What is sciatica?

Key points

- Sciatica describes symptoms in the sciatic nerve distribution
- Sciatic pain has various patterns corresponding to its nerve roots, nerve trunk, sensory distribution, or referred pain into these distributions
- The broad definition of sciatica reflects the many disorders that cause it

The definition

Sciatica is pain or other sensory symptoms such as numbness or tingling within the **sciatic nerve sensory distribution**. This area includes the sciatic nerve trunk in the thigh and more than half of the territory below the knee. Sciatica is a broad term that describes a set of symptoms rather than a specific diagnosis. While some authors have a restrictive definition of sciatica limited to symptoms below the knee,[1] the term "sciatica" has historically been used to describe pain in the thigh.[2] This book relies on a broad definition: Pain or sensory symptoms spanning the sciatic nerve trunk or distribution can be considered sciatica.

The term *sciatica* stems from the Greek word for the hip, ισχιά "**ischia**," because ancient Greek physicians thought it came from that region. The term **scia** refers to the sinews of the buttocks, thigh, and hip.[2,3] The first terms to describe sciatica were ισχιάς, "ischias", ισχιάδες, "ischiades", and ισχιάδων, "ischiadon" by Hippocrates circa 400 BCE. These described radiating buttocks and thigh pain that could extend further to the leg and ankle.[4] Although ισχιά translates to "hip," it probably referred to the **acetabulofemoral joint** (hip), and the **sacroiliac joint** (the lowest part of the back). This broad definition is found in Isidore's *Etymologiae* (c. 615-630 CE): "The Greeks call the bones of the hip joints, whose tips reach the edge of the pelvis, ισχιά."[5] Caelius Aurelianus (c. 450 CE) explained that the name *ischiadicis* was based on the "painful part" or "the boundary of where [the pain] begins."[1]

Over the course of 1,500 years, the term *ischias* became *sciatica*. The prefix "i" was removed because it was common to pronounce an unaccented vowel lightly before sigma.[7] Pliny the Elder (23-79 CE), a Roman military commander, was the first on record to remove the "i" and form the words sciaticos and sciaticis.[8] As medical terminology developed, the suffix "-ica" was added to indicate a disability of the root word "scia."

The historical focus on the hip may be because low back-related sciatica creates pain in the gluteal region instead of the low back. The **buttocks** is the most commonly painful area in radicular sciatica.[9] Damage to L5 and S1 nerve roots causes upper and lower buttocks pain, respectively.[10] More patients have buttocks pain (90%) than those that have back pain (29%) in radicular sciatica.[9]

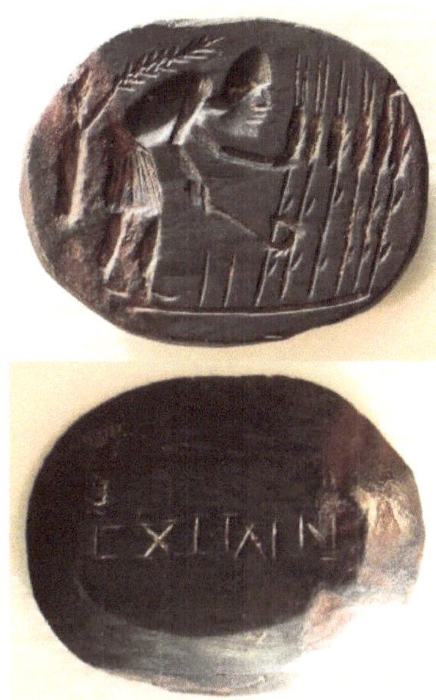

Figure 1: Ancient sciatica amulet. Reaper stooping to cut grain with sickle. Reverse: "for the hips" σχιων or ισχιων "ischion." Other similar gems/amulets used [ι]σχιον for "ischion. Taubman Amulet 115 (Bonner 40), University of Michigan, Creative Commons License.

The classification of sciatica

Sciatica is a **symptom** rather than a specific diagnosis. Multiple classification systems exist for sciatica and are based on its clinical features, pathoanatomy, treatment, screening and prediction tools, and pain mechanisms.[11] The attraction to the term *sciatica* is that it describes a set of symptoms without pointing towards a specific cause. It offers a means for clinicians to communicate with patients and gives a starting point from which to reach a more specific diagnosis.

The broadest classification is **intraspinal** versus **extraspinal**, which describes the cause of symptoms

[1] Author's translation, Aurelianus[6] p. 495

being within or outside of the spine.[13,14] Intraspinal sciatica is typically a radiculopathy, a neuropathic condition of the lumbosacral nerve roots. Extraspinal sciatica can result from diverse pain mechanisms including neuropathic, nociceptive, sensitization, or referred pain, at many anatomical sources outside of the spine.

A patient with sciatica may fit into more than one classification. For example, a patient with back pain and below-knee pain may have a lumbar disc herniation (LDH), with neuropathic pain that centralizes with directional preference exercises. Another patient may have an annular tear (discogenic pain) with low back and above-knee nociceptive pain that does not change with directional preference exercises. Yet another may have extraspinal sciatica caused by chronic hamstring tendinosis and sciatic nerve entrapment.

Table 1: Examples of classification of sciatica. Data adapted from multiple authors[11-14]

Clinical features	• Back and above-knee pain • Back and below-knee pain • Neurogenic claudication • Acute • Chronic
Patho-anatomy	• Intraspinal: Lumbar disc herniation, stenosis, radiculopathy • Extraspinal: Piriformis, sacroiliac joint, hamstring, myofascial
Pain mechanism	• Neuropathic • Nociceptive: Central or peripheral sensitization, somatic or visceral referred
Treatment based	• Mobility deficit • Instability • Postural • Dysfunction • Derangement • Abolition, reduction, or unstable centralization • Peripheralization • No change

Is there a lesion?

Sciatica can occur with varying degrees of nerve injury or "lesion." **Neuropathic** and **radicular** sciatica are at one end of this spectrum. These forms of sciatica result from nerve damage and a block in nerve conduction. **Non-radicular** types of sciatica caused by **somatic referred pain** and **nociceptive pain** are on the other end of this spectrum. In these cases, there is no overt nerve injury or conduction block. There is a gradient or continuum from neuropathic to non-neuropathic forms of sciatica, as many patients do not fit clearly into either category.[15]

Sciatica with or without nerve injury can present with **weakness**. Those with sacroiliitis[16] and greater trochanteric pain syndrome[17] commonly have lower extremity weakness. In these cases, weakness may be mediated by nociceptive signals from damaged or inflamed joints,[18] a concept called **arthrogenic inhibition**.

Sensory loss is most often a sign of neuropathic sciatica, but it can also occur in somatic referred sciatica. One study found that almost half of **non-radicular sciatica** cases verified by imaging or electrodiagnostics had **subclinical sensory loss**.[15] This sensory loss was identified by quantitative sensory testing, an advanced and sensitive tool. Another study found 40% of patients with **sacroiliitis** had lower extremity sensory loss.[16] Sensory loss in non-radicular sciatica could relate to inflammatory changes of the lumbosacral plexus or sciatic nerve trunk, or changes to the central nervous system such as cortical reorganization.

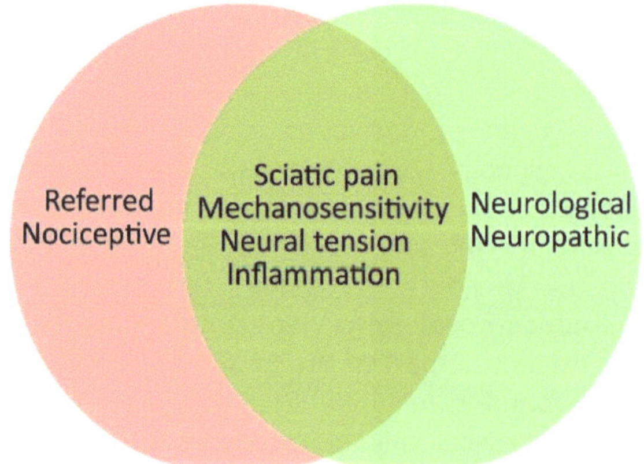

Figure 2: Referred pain from myofascial or nociceptive sources may converge with neurological factors to produce sciatica.

Neurodynamics helps explain how sciatica can occur in the absence of nerve damage. Neurodynamics is the study of the mechanics and physiology of the nervous system and how these components relate to one another. Patients may have multiple contributing factors that increase mechanical sensitivity and tension along the sciatic nerve. For example, one may have a gluteal muscle contracture, hamstring tendinopathy, and anterior head posture.[19] A combination of conditions is more likely produce sciatic pain than any individual factor.

Sciatic pain distribution

The distribution of sciatica is one indicator of its underlying pathology. The pain or symptom pattern can help identify one or more nerve distributions, referred pain from joints, viscera or fascia, or a combination of factors. Pain patterns by themselves are unreliable. Clinicians should interpret the distribution of symptoms in context with other clinical findings for a more accurate diagnosis.

Sciatic nerve sensory distribution

The sensory distribution of the sciatic nerve is distinct from the sensory distributions of the lumbosacral nerve roots. It includes more than half of the area distal to the knee, including the leg and foot, but not the medial leg or arch of the foot. Pain affecting the distribution of the sciatic nerve below the knee may indicate a sciatic nerve trunk lesion. The best example of this pattern is **piriformis syndrome**.[20]

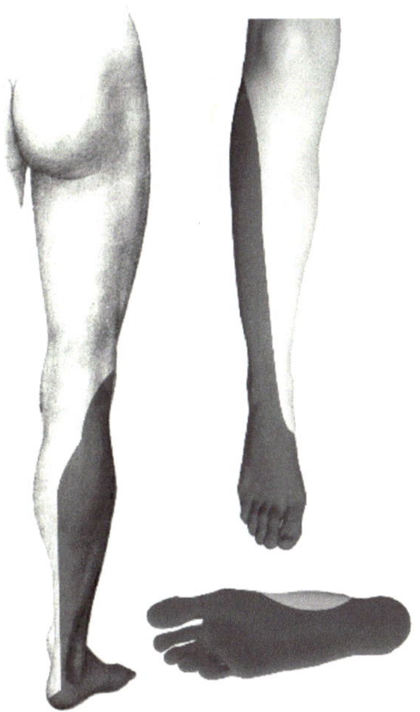

Figure 3: Sciatic nerve sensory distribution. Image by Robert Trager DC. Image of lower extremity modified from Gray's anatomy, public domain, image of leg modified from Andrea Allen (CC by 2.0), and image of foot modified from Pixel AddIct (CC BY 2.0).

The nerve root distributions L4 through S3 overlap with with the sciatic nerve distribution but do not have the same exact territory. These nerve roots branch into other nerves such as the **cluneal nerves** in the gluteal region and perineum, and the posterior, lateral, and anterior **femoral cutaneous nerves** of the thigh. The lumbosacral dermatomes are related to, but different than the sciatic nerve distribution.

Radicular sciatica

Radicular pain follows a **dermatomal distribution**, a pattern of skin corresponding to a single nerve root. An inflamed or compressed nerve root may cause pain, numbness, or other sensations in the skin of the nerve root's sensory distribution. Patients with radicular sciatica seldom have symptoms of an entire single dermatome. More than half of patients with radicular sciatica have pain in a **partial dermatome**.[10]

Radicular sciatica includes lesions of the **L4**, **L5**, **S1**, and **S2** nerve roots, which contribute to the sciatic nerve sensory distribution. Although S3 contributes to the sciatic nerve, its sensory part comes from the perineal nerves which do not connect to the sciatic. The most common forms of radicular sciatica affect either L5 or S1, or both L5 and S1; these make up over 90% of cases of radicular sciatica.[21]

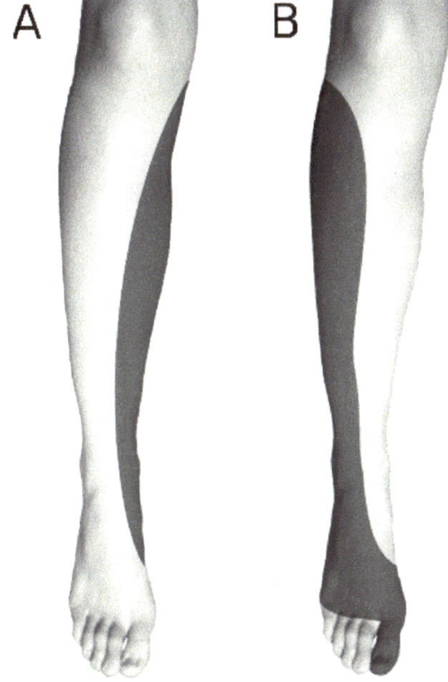

Figure 4: Examples of dermatomal patterns of radicular sciatica of L4 (A) and L5 (B). Image by Robert Trager, DC, using data from Lee's evidence based dermatome map, 2008. Image of leg modified from Andrea Allen (CC by 2.0), and image of foot modified from Pixel AddIct (CC BY 2.0).

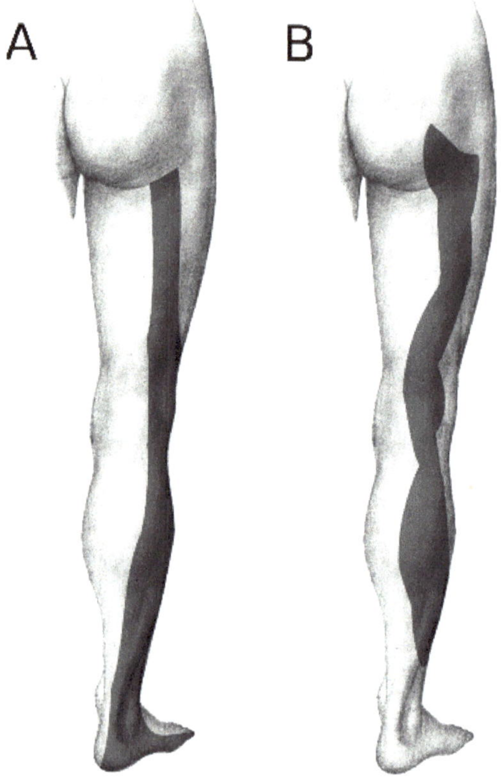

Figure 5: Examples of dermatomal patterns of radicular sciatica of S1 (A) and S2 (B). Image by Robert Trager, DC, using data from Lee's evidence based dermatome map, 2008. Image of lower extremity modified from Gray's anatomy, public domain.

Degenerative spinal conditions may damage more than one nerve root, either on the same side or both sides of the body. Lumbar disc herniations affect one nerve root in 60% of cases and two in 40%.[22] Degenerative lumbar spondylolistheses affect two or more nerve roots in 90% of cases.[23] Involvement of more than one nerve root creates a broader symptom distribution that may span multiple dermatomes.

Sciatic nerve trunk pain

Sciatic nerve trunk pain is deep pain along the trunk of the sciatic nerve that increases with pressure and stretch.[24] This type of pain is thought to arise from the **nervi nervorum**, the small nerves that innervate the sciatic nerve sheath.[24] Injury or inflammation along the sciatic nerve pathway make the nervi nervorum more sensitive to pain.[24]

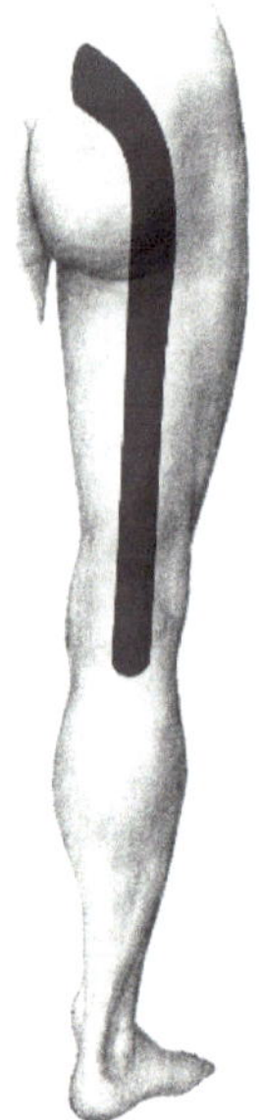

Figure 6: Sciatic nerve trunk pain pattern. Image by Robert Trager, DC, modified from Gray's anatomy, public domain.

Sciatic nerve trunk pain can occur in intraspinal and extraspinal sciatica. For example it is found in 85% of those with **back-related leg pain**,[2] and 45% of those with **piriformis syndrome**.[26] Any injury or inflammation of the L4-S2 nerve roots or sciatic nerve can cause this type of pain.

This type of pain is characterized by deep buttock and thigh pain, and sensitivity of the sciatic nerve to pressure and stretch.[24] It is often described as a deep ache or toothache.[24] Examination findings for this type of pain include pain with pressure over the sciatic trunk and pain with neural tension tests such as the straight leg raise.

Referred pain

The two categories of referred pain are **somatic referred pain** and **visceral referred pain**. This type of pain accounts for nearly one-third (32%) of cases of sciatica.[27] This pain is explained by neurological mechanisms most likely involving the **dorsal horn** of the spinal cord.[28] In referred sciatic pain there is no lumbosacral nerve root or sciatic nerve injury that directly causes sciatica. Referred pain follows a highly variable pattern compared to radicular or intraspinal sciatica.

---

[2] One study found 85% of patients with back-related leg pain had greater sciatic nerve tenderness (via algometry) compared to the asymptomatic leg[25]

Injury and inflammation of joints, soft tissue, and viscera may refer pain into their corresponding segmental level(s). The patient then perceives pain as coming from a healthy area. Pain can refer into part of a single segment or multiple segments of dermatome or sclerotome (bone, joints, and ligaments).

Somatic referred sciatica arises from sensitive structures such as the **hip** and **sacroiliac joints**, gluteal tendons, and even the intervertebral disc.[12] An **annular tear** in the disc may cause referred sciatic pain while leaving the nerve root intact.[29] Hip arthritis may cause sciatic pain because the hip is innervated by the sciatic nerve.[30] Injury to any structure innervated by the nerve roots that make up the sciatic nerve (L4-S3) could cause somatic referred sciatic pain.

Non-sciatic nerve injuries that refer pain into a larger distribution are forms of somatic referred sciatic pain. These include **cluneal nerve entrapment** and **dorsal ramus syndrome**. These nerves have a small distribution, but when entrapped or injured can refer into a much broader area of the thigh and/or leg.

Visceral pathology as a cause of sciatica is less common but may occur when sensory signals converge with those of the sciatic and posterior femoral cutaneous nerve at the spinal segments S1, S2, and S3. In **viscerosomatic convergence** sensory signals interact at the dorsal horn of the spinal cord.

Referred pain may occur in a vague, deep segmental sensory distribution called **sclerotomes**. Sclerotomes are the segments of bone, periosteum, ligaments, tendons, and joint capsules that relate each to a single spinal nerve root. The sclerotomes are analogous to the dermatomes (skin) and myotomes (muscle) but are less distinct and less understood. The few specific regions include the lateral malleolus and dorsal ankle, which relate to L5,[31] and the 5th toe which relates to S1.[32]

The sciatic nerve

The sciatic nerve is the longest, widest, and thickest peripheral nerve in the body. It originates from the **lumbosacral plexus** at the base of the spine then passes through the pelvis into the posterior thigh. The sciatic nerve and its branches innervate about 30 muscles on each side of the body, more than any other nerve.

Authors from the 1400s CE and earlier described the sciatic nerve. It is difficult to determine a precise date of discovery for the sciatic nerve because ancient languages typically equated nerves with connective tissue. The words *nervus* in Latin, *gid* in Hebrew, and *irk* in Arabic all describe nerves, tendons, ligaments and fascia.[33]

The Indian physician Sushruta (c. 600 BCE) may have been the first to anatomically describe the sciatic nerves (Sanskrit: Kandará) and their relationship to the muscles of the legs and feet and their potential to cause Gridhrasi (sciatica).[34] Artwork from the 15th century CE supports the notion that the sciatic nerve was discovered by this time.[33]

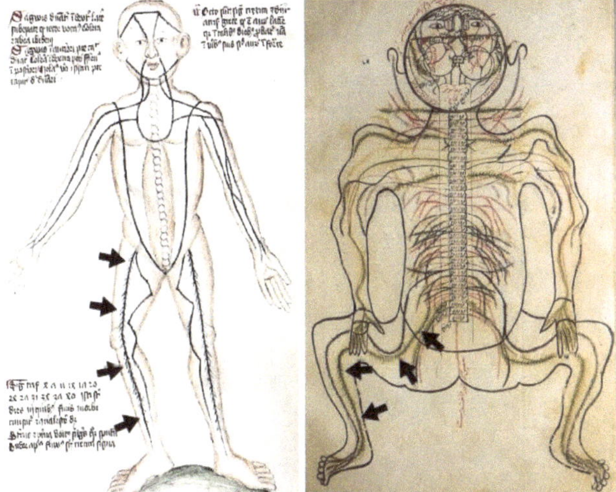

Figure 7: Left - Nerve man, circa 1420-30, MS 49, Wellcome Images. A depiction of the sciatic (outer, lateral) and femoral (inner, medial) nerves in the lower extremities. Right - Illustration of the nervous system, circa 1450, attributed to the Persian physician Mansūr ibn Muhammad ibn Ahmad ibn Yūsuf Ibn Ilyās.[35]

Ancient Judeo-Christian and Native American customs involve **removing the sciatic nerve** from animals before eating the meat. The Judeo-Christian tradition traces to The Book of Genesis,[3] which describes Jacob's limping and possible episode of sciatica after wrestling with an angel.[36] The Talmud also describes the autopsy on a limping ewe to distinguish between spinal cord damage and sciatica.[33] Some Native American tribes also removed the sciatic nerve from the thigh of animals they killed.[37,38]

[3] *Therefore the children of Israel eat not of the sinew which shrank, which is upon the hollow of the thigh, unto this day: because he touched the hollow of Jacob's thigh in the sinew that shrank (King James Bible "Authorized version," Cambridge Edition)*

For example, Cherokees believed if they ate it, they would get a cramp when attempting to run.[38]

Formation and composition

The L4, L5, S1, S2, and S3 nerve roots form the sciatic nerve at the **lumbosacral plexus**. Those with less lumbar vertebrae or sacralization are more likely to have a **prefixed** sacral plexus[39,40] with the sciatic nerve formed from L3 or L4 to S2.[41] Those with an extra thoracic or lumbar vertebra or lumbarization are more likely to have a **postfixed** sacral plexus[39,40] with a sciatic nerve formed from L5 to S4.[41] Prefixed or postfixed variations occur in about 25% of cases.[41]

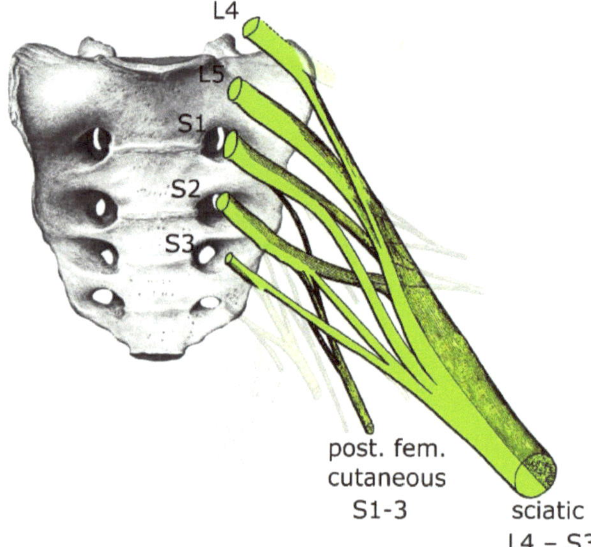

Figure 8: Sciatic nerve originating from the lumbosacral plexus. The posterior femoral cutaneous nerve and sciatic nerve are highlighted whereas other nerves are hidden. Image modified from public domain images of sacrum from Gray's anatomy and sacral plexus from Ely, 1919.

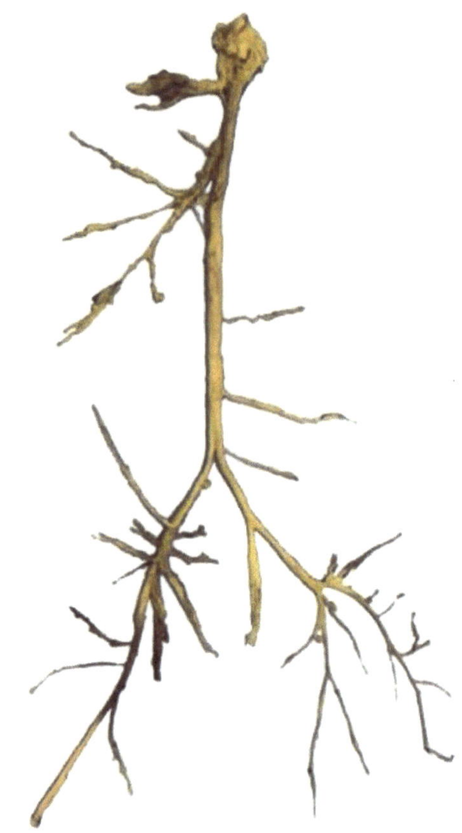

Figure 9: Fully dissected sciatic nerve trunk and branches. Image modified from Gustafson,[44] public domain.

The sciatic nerve has sensory and motor neurons as well as connective tissue, blood vessels, and lymphatic vessels. Its nerve composition is 71% sensory, 23% sympathetic, and 6% motor nerves.[42] A high percentage of **adipose tissue** protects the sciatic nerve in the buttocks and upper thigh.[43] It has more fat and connective tissue in the buttocks, with a ratio of 2:1 fat to tissue, while it is about 1:1 in the mid-thigh and popliteal fossa.[43]

Sympathetic neurons travel with the peroneal and tibial branches of the sciatic nerve.[45] These fibers innervate blood vessels in the lower extremity and affect blood vessel constriction and dilation. Increased sympathetic activity is thought to contribute to sciatic pain by activating trigger points[46] and reducing blood flow.[47]

Early in embryonic development the sciatic nerves each contain a large **sciatic artery** which is the main blood vessel to the lower limb buds.[48] The function of this artery is normally replaced by the femoral artery after the fetal period. Rarely this artery persists into adulthood and predisposes to sciatica.[48]

Small **nervi nervorum** branch from the spinal ganglia, the sciatic nerve and the blood vessels surrounding it.[49] These small nerves innervate the sheath of the sciatic **nerve roots** and **nerve trunk** and sense pressure and stretch.[50] Their innervation of the sciatic nerve and roots may explain sciatic nerve trunk pain and neuropathic sciatic pain.

Course and distribution

The sciatic nerve exits the pelvis through the **greater sciatic foramen**, usually inferior to the piriformis muscle. It continues downwards nearly midway between the **ischial tuberosity** and **greater trochanter** of the femur.[51] It descends through the mid-thigh where it is surrounded by the biceps femoris, adductor muscles, and lateral intermuscular septum.[52]

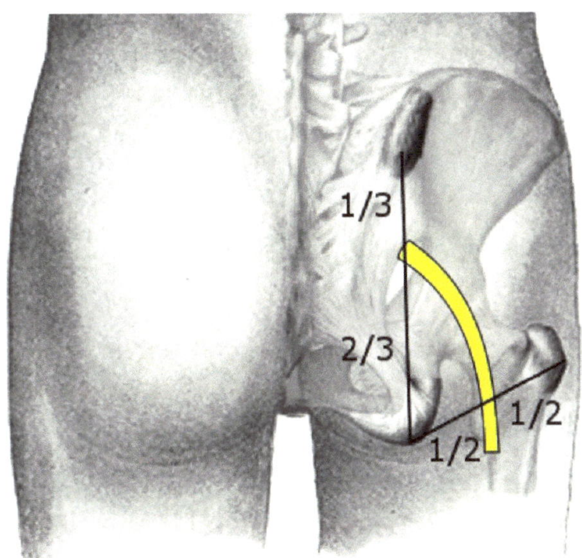

Figure 10: Surface anatomy of the sciatic nerve. The nerve lies about 1/3rd the distance from the PSIS to the ischial tuberosity, and mid-way between the ischial tuberosity and greater trochanter of the femur.[51] Image of buttocks modified from public domain Gray's anatomy, superimposed bone image modified from public domain Sobotta's atlas, by Robert Trager, DC.

The sciatic nerve usually divides internally into the common peroneal and tibial branches which run on a common sheath prior to dividing externally. The **tibial division** is medial, and the **peroneal division** is lateral throughout the course of the sciatic nerve. The sciatic nerve splits into the tibial and common peroneal branches at the lower thigh or popliteal fossa in 75% of people.[53] Occasionally, it separates sooner, within the pelvis, gluteal region, or upper or mid-thigh. Early separation of the sciatic nerve in the pelvis or gluteal region may predispose to nerve compression and cause deep gluteal or piriformis syndromes.

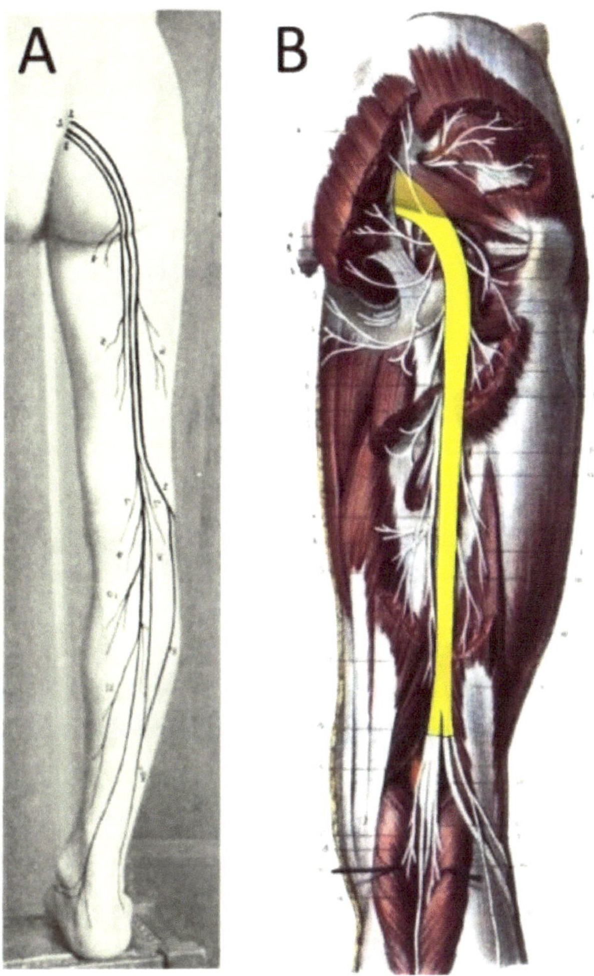

Figure 11: Figure 6:The course of the sciatic nerve. Surface markings (A) and the sciatic nerve trunk (B) in the thigh. Image A from Stookey, 1922, B from public domain Hirschfeld & Léveillé's 1866 atlas.

The sciatic nerve innervates muscles of the posterior thigh and all muscles of the leg and foot. It innervates all lower extremity muscles except for the gluteal muscles, hip flexors, adductors, and quadriceps. Aside from its cutaneous innervation, the sciatic nerve also provides sensory innervation for lower extremity joints including the posterolateral part of the hip capsule,[30] lateral knee joint,[56] and ankle.[57]

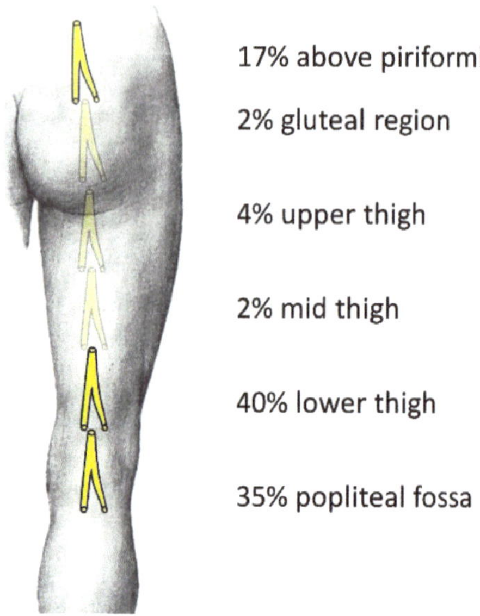

Figure 12: Variability of the division of the sciatic nerve. The sciatic nerve most often divides near the knee with 40% of nerves dividing at the lower thigh and 35% at the popliteal fossa. Data from Prakash.[53] Image modified from Gray's Anatomy, public domain.

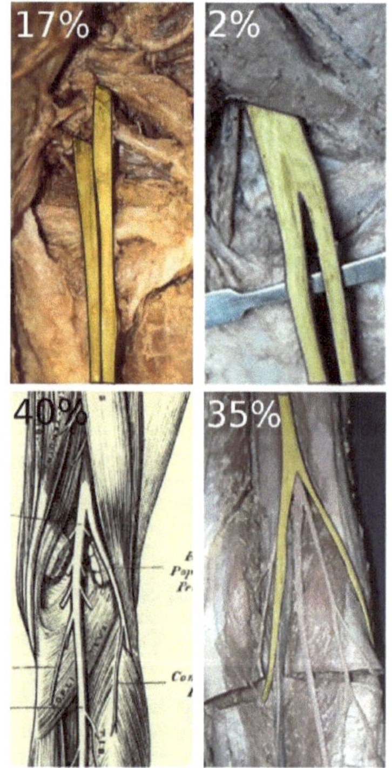

Figure 13: Examples of variable division of the sciatic nerve. Images modified by Robert Trager, DC: Division proximal to piriformis (17%) CC-BY-2.0 from Battaglia,[54] gluteal division (2%) and popliteal fossa (35%) CC-BY-4.0 from Berihu.[55] Division at lower thigh (40%) from Gray's Anatomy, public domain.

The sciatic nerve may supply some sensation of the posterior thigh. Anesthetic block of the sciatic nerve affects the posterior thigh[58] and sciatic nerve lesions produce sensory loss of the posterior thigh.[59] One study in a human and additional studies in mammals have identified a **communicating branch** between the posterior femoral cutaneous nerve and sciatic nerve.[60] The sciatic nerve also occasionally gives cutaneous branches to the thigh.[58,61] The primary innervation of the posterior thigh is provided by the posterior femoral cutaneous nerve.

Posterior femoral cutaneous nerve

The **posterior femoral cutaneous nerve** (PFCN), also called the **small sciatic nerve** or posterior cutaneous nerve of the thigh, innervates skin of the lower buttocks, thigh, and part of the calf. The sensory distribution of this nerve transitions to the sciatic nerve below the knee. The PFCN and its branches have a greater sensory distribution than any other cutaneous nerve.[62] This nerve has much in common with the sciatic including its anatomical origin, related disorders, and symptoms.

Patients diagnosed with sciatica often have symptoms in the posterior thigh in the region of the PFCN. Sciatic pain is thought to be **referred** into the thigh distribution of the PFCN by LDHs that affect the sacral nerve roots.[63] Pain can also occur from PFCN **neuropathy** related to piriformis syndrome,[64,65] deep gluteal syndrome,[66] hamstring injury,[67] and ischiogluteal bursitis.[68]

The PFCN is **anatomically** and **morphologically** related to the sciatic nerve. While it usually arises from the S1, S2, and S3 nerve roots, it also can arise from the sciatic nerve or communicate with it in the thigh. The PFCN frequently arises from the sciatic nerve in other animals, including monkeys.[69,70] However, in humans it arises from the peroneal division of the sciatic nerve trunk in only 5% of cases.[71] Other research shows that the sciatic nerve provides sensory contributions into the PFCN in 10% of cases.[62] The PFCN has similar origins as the sciatic nerve and shares three of the same nerve roots.

The PFCN runs close to the sciatic nerve and shares three of the same nerve roots. The shared origins and route of these nerves explains why their pain syndromes overlap and are difficult to distinguish. The PFCN runs adjacent to the sciatic nerve, sometimes within a common but easily separated sheath.[72] It exits the **infrapiriform foramen** with the sciatic nerve and also can split or pass through the piriformis muscle like the sciatic nerve.[73] It is subject to many of the same injuries in the deep gluteal region as the sciatic.

The PFCN has branches to the gluteal region and perineum. It gives rise to the **inferior cluneal nerves**[74] and **perineal branches** that go to the scrotum and penis or labia.[75] Rarely, in 5% of cases, the PFCN contributes to the **sural nerve** in the leg.[76] The PFCN runs along the **small saphenous vein** in the median of the leg, on the left side of the vein in most patients.[77]

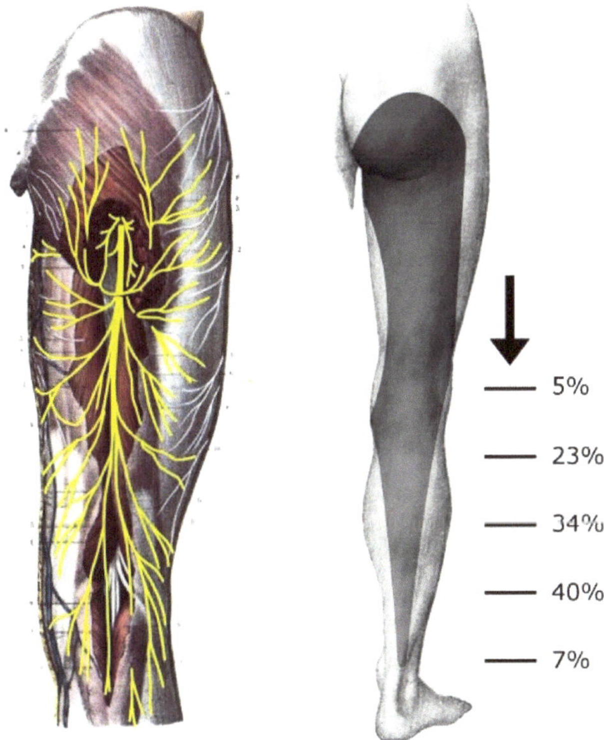

Figure 14: Posterior femoral cutaneous nerve. Left – Image modified by author from Hirschfeld and Leveille's public domain atlas to highlight course of PFCN. Right – Distal limit of the PFCN distribution in percent of the population. Image modified by author from Gray's anatomy public domain atlas. Distribution of PFCN drawn based on research from Kosinski, 1926, Iyer and Shields, 1989, and Darnis et al. 2008

References

1. Valat, J.-P., Genevay, S., Marty, M., Rozenberg, S. & Koes, B. Sciatica. *Best Practice & Research Clinical Rheumatology* **24**, 241–252 (2010).
2. Wulff, W., Library, R. I. A. & Gaddesden, J. of. *Rosa anglica sev Rosa medicinæ Johannis Anglici an early modern Irish translation of a section of the mediaeval medical text-book of John of Gaddesden.* (Published for the Irish Texts Society by Simpkin, Marshall, 1929).
3. Israeli, I. I.-S. al-. *Omnia opera ysaac in hoc volumine contenta: cum quibusdam alijs opusculis: Liber de definitionibus. Liber de elementis. Liber dietaru[m] vniuersaliu[m]: cum co[m]me[n]to petri hispani ...* (Trot, 1515).
4. Byl, S. Rheumatism and Gout in the Corpus Hippocraticum. *antiq* **57**, 89–102 (1988).
5. Barney, S. *The Etymologies of Isidore of Seville*. (Cambridge University Press, 2006).
6. Caelius Aurelianus. *Caelii Aureliani Siccensis, ...De acutis morbis. lib.3. De diuturnis. lib.5. Ad fidem exemplaris manuscripti castigati, & annotationibus illustrati. Cum indice copiosissimo, ac locupletissimo.* (apud Guliel. Rouillium, sub scuto Veneto, 1566).
7. Ameling, W. *et al. Caesarea and the Middle Coast: 1121-2160.* (Walter de Gruyter, 2011).
8. Pliny, the E., Bostock, J. & Riley, H. T. (Henry T. *The natural history of Pliny*. (London, H. G. Bohn, 1856).
9. Rankine, J. J., Fortune, D. G., Hutchinson, C. E., Hughes, D. G. & Main, C. J. Pain drawings in the assessment of nerve root compression: a comparative study with lumbar spine magnetic resonance imaging. *Spine* **23**, 1668–1676 (1998).
10. Kuraishi, K. *et al.* [Study on the area of pain and numbness in cases with lumbosacral radiculopathy]. *No shinkei geka. Neurological surgery* **40**, 877–885 (2012).
11. Stynes, S., Konstantinou, K. & Dunn, K. M. Classification of patients with low back-related leg pain: a systematic review. *BMC Musculoskelet Disord* **17**, 226 (2016).
12. Vulfsons, S., Bar, N. & Eisenberg, E. Back Pain with Leg Pain. *Current pain and headache reports* **21**, 32 (2017).
13. Yoshimoto, M. *et al.* Diagnostic Features of Sciatica Without Lumbar Nerve Root Compression. *Journal of Spinal Disorders & Techniques* **22**, 328–333 (2009).
14. Kulcu, D. G. & Naderi, S. Differential diagnosis of intraspinal and extraspinal non-discogenic sciatica. *Journal of Clinical Neuroscience* **15**, 1246–1252 (2008).
15. Freynhagen, R. *et al.* Pseudoradicular and radicular low-back pain – A disease continuum rather than different entities? Answers from quantitative sensory testing. *PAIN* **135**, 65–74 (2008).
16. Visser, L., Nijssen, P., Tijssen, C., van Middendorp, J. & Schieving, J. Sciatica-like symptoms and the sacroiliac joint: clinical features and differential diagnosis. *European spine journal: official publication of the European Spine Society, the European Spinal Deformity Society, and the European Section of the Cervical Spine Research Society* (2013).
17. Tan, L. A. *et al.* High prevalence of greater trochanteric pain syndrome among patients presenting to spine clinic for evaluation of degenerative lumbar pathologies. *Journal of Clinical Neuroscience* (2018).
18. Freeman, S., Mascia, A. & McGill, S. Arthrogenic neuromusculature inhibition: A foundational investigation of existence in the hip joint. *Clinical Biomechanics* **28**, 171–177 (2013).
19. Moustafa, I. M. & Diab, A. A. The effect of adding forward head posture corrective exercises in the management of lumbosacral radiculopathy: a randomized controlled study. *Journal of manipulative and physiological therapeutics* **38**, 167–178 (2015).
20. Michel, F. *et al.* Piriformis muscle syndrome: Diagnostic criteria and treatment of a monocentric series of 250 patients. *Annals of Physical and Rehabilitation Medicine* **56**, 371–383 (2013).
21. Nafissi, S., Niknam, S. & Hosseini, S. S. Electrophysiological evaluation in lumbosacral radiculopathy. *Iran J Neurol* **11**, 83–86 (2012).
22. Kortelainen, P., Puranen, J., Koivisto, E., Lähde, S. & others. Symptoms and signs of sciatica and their relation to the localization of the lumbar disc herniation. *Spine* **10**, 88 (1985).
23. Epstein, N. E., Epstein, J. A., Carras, R. & Lavine, L. S. Degenerative spondylolisthesis with an intact neural arch: a review of 60 cases with an analysis of clinical findings and the development of surgical management. *Neurosurgery* **13**, 555–561 (1983).
24. Hall, T. M. & Elvey, R. L. Nerve trunk pain: physical diagnosis and treatment. *Manual Therapy* **4**, 63–73 (1999).
25. Walsh, J. & Hall, T. Reliability, validity and diagnostic accuracy of palpation of the sciatic, tibial and common peroneal nerves in the examination of low back related leg pain. *Manual Therapy* **14**, 623–629 (2009).
26. Hopayian, K., Song, F., Riera, R. & Sambandan, S. The clinical features of the piriformis syndrome: a systematic review. *European Spine Journal* **19**, 2095–2109 (2010).
27. Konstantinou, K. *et al.* Characteristics of patients with low back and leg pain seeking treatment in primary care: baseline results from the ATLAS cohort study. *BMC musculoskeletal disorders* **16**, 332 (2015).
28. Randy Jinkins, J. The anatomic and physiologic basis of local, referred and radiating lumbosacral pain syndromes related to disease of the spine. *Journal of Neuroradiology* **31**, 163–180 (2004).
29. Milette, P. C., Fontaine, S., Lepanto, L. & Breton, G. Radiating pain to the lower extremities caused by lumbar disk rupture without spinal nerve root involvement. *American journal of neuroradiology* **16**, 1605–1613 (1995).
30. Birnbaum, K., Prescher, A., Hessler, S. & Heller, K. D. The sensory innervation of the hip joint--an anatomical study. *Surg Radiol Anat* **19**, 371–375 (1997).
31. Takahashi, Y., Ohtori, S. & Takahashi, K. Sclerotomes in the thoracic and lumbar spine, pelvis, and hindlimb bones of rats. *The Journal of Pain* **11**, 652–662 (2010).
32. Takahashi, Y., Ohtori, S. & Takahashi, K. Human map of the segmental sensory structure ("sensoritomes") in the body trunk and lower extremity. *Pain Res* **23**, 133–141 (2008).
33. Preuss, J. *Biblical and Talmudic Medicine*. (Jason Aronson, Incorporated, 2004).
34. Bhishagratna, K. L. & others. *An English translation of the Sushruta Samhita based on original Sanskrit text*. **1**, (Wilkin's Press, 1907).

35. Ilyās, M. Islamic Medical Manuscripts in the NLM - MS P 19. Available at: http://www.nlm.nih.gov/hmd/arabic/p19.html. (Accessed: 15th February 2015)
36. Tubbs, R. S. *et al.* Roots of neuroanatomy, neurology, and neurosurgery as found in the Bible and Talmud. *Neurosurgery* **63**, 156–162; discussion 162-163 (2008).
37. Hodgson, A. *Letters from North America: Written During a Tour in the United States and Canada ...* (Hurst, Robinson, & Company, 1824).
38. Starr, E. *Early History of the Cherokees: Embracing Aboriginal Customs, Religion, Laws, Folk Lore, and Civilization.* (The author, 1917).
39. Horwitz, M. T. The anatomy of (A) the lumbosacral nerve plexus—its relation to variations of vertebral segmentation, and (B), the posterior sacral nerve plexus. *The Anatomical Record* **74**, 91–107 (1939).
40. Quain, J. *Quain's Elements of anatomy.* (London, 1891).
41. Matejčík, V. Anatomical variations of lumbosacral plexus. *Surgical and radiologic anatomy* **32**, 409–414 (2010).
42. Schmalbruch, H. Fiber composition of the rat sciatic nerve. *The Anatomical Record* **215**, 71–81 (1986).
43. Moayeri, N. & Groen, G. J. Differences in Quantitative Architecture of Sciatic Nerve May Explain Differences in Potential Vulnerability to Nerve Injury, Onset Time, and Minimum Effective Anesthetic Volume. *Anesthes* **111**, 1128–1134 (2009).
44. Grinberg, Y. & Joseph, S. Human distal sciatic nerve fascicular anatomy: implications for ankle control using nerve-cuff electrodes. *Journal of rehabilitation research and development* **49**, 309 (2012).
45. Dellon, A. L. *et al.* The sympathetic innervation of the human foot. *Plastic and reconstructive surgery* **129**, 905–909 (2012).
46. Skorupska, E., Rychlik, M., Pawelec, W., Bednarek, A. & Samborski, W. Trigger point-related sympathetic nerve activity in chronic sciatic leg pain: a case study. *Acupuncture in Medicine* **32**, 418–422 (2014).
47. De Weerdt, C., Journee, H., Hogenesch, R. & Beks, J. Sympathetic dysfunction in patients with persistent pain after prolapsed disc surgery. A thermographic study. *Acta neurochirurgica* **89**, 34–36 (1987).
48. Hayashi, S., Nasu, H., Abe, H., Rodríguez-Vázquez, J. & Murakami, G. An artery accompanying the sciatic nerve (arteria comitans nervi ischiadici) and the position of the hip joint: a comparative histological study using chick, mouse, and human foetal specimens. *Folia morphologica* **72**, 41–50 (2013).
49. Hromada, J. ON THE NERVE SUPPLY OF THE CONNECTIVE TISSUE OF SOME PERIPHERAL NERVOUS SYSTEM COMPONENTS. *CTO* **55**, 343–351 (1963).
50. Bove, G. M. & Light, A. R. The nervi nervorum. *Pain Forum* **6**, 181–190 (1997).
51. Currin, S. S., Mirjalili, S. A., Meikle, G. & Stringer, M. D. Revisiting the surface anatomy of the sciatic nerve in the gluteal region. *Clinical Anatomy* **28**, 144–149 (2015).
52. Moayeri, N., van Geffen, G. J., Bruhn, J., Chan, V. W. & Groen, G. J. Correlation among ultrasound, cross-sectional anatomy, and histology of the sciatic nerve: a review. *Regional anesthesia and pain medicine* **35**, 442–449 (2010).
53. Prakash, B. A. *et al.* Sciatic nerve division: a cadaver study in the Indian population and review of the literature. *Singapore Med J* **51**, 721–3 (2010).
54. Battaglia, P. J., Scali, F. & Enix, D. E. Co-presentation of unilateral femoral and bilateral sciatic nerve variants in one cadaver: A case report with clinical implications. *Chiropractic & Manual Therapies* **20**, 34 (2012).
55. Berihu, B. A. & Debeb, Y. G. Anatomical variation in bifurcation and trifurcations of sciatic nerve and its clinical implications: in selected university in Ethiopia. *BMC Research Notes* **8**, 633 (2015).
56. Horner, G. & Dellon, L. Innervation of the human knee joint and implications for surgery. *Clinical orthopaedics and related research* **301**, 221–226 (1994).
57. Tubbs, R. S. *et al.* Sciatic Nerve Intercommunications: New Finding. *World neurosurgery* **98**, 176–181 (2017).
58. Cousins, M. J. *Cousins and Bridenbaugh's Neural Blockade in Clinical Anesthesia and Pain Medicine.* (Lippincott Williams & Wilkins, 2012).
59. Kim, D. H., Murovic, J. A., Tiel, R. & Kline, D. G. Management and outcomes in 353 surgically treated sciatic nerve lesions. *J. Neurosurg.* **101**, 8–17 (2004).
60. Tunali, S., Cankara, N. & Albay, S. A rare case of communicating branch between the posterior femoral cutaneous and the sciatic nerves. *Rom J Morphol Embryol* **52**, 203–205 (2011).
61. Dahlin, L. B. *et al.* Case report: Intraneural perineurioma of the sciatic nerve in an adolescent – strategies for revealing the diagnosis. *Clin Case Rep* **4**, 777–781 (2016).
62. Zenn, M. R. & Millard, J. A. Free inferior gluteal flap harvest with sparing of the posterior femoral cutaneous nerve. *Journal of reconstructive microsurgery* **22**, 509–512 (2006).
63. Falconer, M. A., Glasgow, G. L. & Cole, D. S. Sensory disturbances occurring in sciatica due to intervertebral disc protrusions: some observations on the fifth lumbar and first sacral dermatomes. *Journal of neurology, neurosurgery, and psychiatry* **10**, 72 (1947).
64. Darnis, B. *et al.* Perineal pain and inferior cluneal nerves: anatomy and surgery. *Surg Radiol Anat* **30**, 177–183 (2008).
65. Pecina, M. M., Markiewitz, A. D. & Krmpotic-Nemanic, J. *Tunnel syndromes.* (CRC press, 2001).
66. Hernando, M. F., Cerezal, L., Pérez-Carro, L., Abascal, F. & Canga, A. Deep gluteal syndrome: anatomy, imaging, and management of sciatic nerve entrapments in the subgluteal space. *Skeletal radiology* **44**, 919–934 (2015).
67. Dellon, A. L. Pain with sitting related to injury of the posterior femoral cutaneous nerve. *Microsurgery* **35**, 463–468 (2015).
68. Mieghem, I. M. V., Boets, A., Sciot, R. & Breuseghem, I. V. Ischiogluteal bursitis: an uncommon type of bursitis. *Skeletal Radiol* **33**, 413–416 (2004).
69. Nakanishi, T., Kanno, Y. & others. Comparative morphological remarks on the origin of the posterior femoral cutaneous nerve. *Anatomischer Anzeiger* **139**, 8–23 (1976).
70. da Silva, J. T. *et al.* Neural mobilization promotes nerve regeneration by nerve growth factor and myelin protein zero increased after sciatic nerve injury. *Growth Factors* **33**, 8–13 (2015).
71. Horiguchi, M., Yamada, T. K. & Koizumi, M. Aberrant Cutaneous Nerve of the Thigh Arising from the Sciatic Nerve in the Human. *CTO* **133**, 118–121 (1988).
72. Bardeen, C. R. Development and variation of the nerves and the musculature of the inferior extremity and of the neighboring regions of the trunk in man. *Developmental Dynamics* **6**, 259–390 (1906).
73. Uluutku, M. & Kurtoğlu, Z. Variations of nerves located in deep gluteal region. *Okajimas folia anatomica Japonica* **76**, 273–276 (1999).
74. Ploteau, S., Salaud, C., Hamel, A. & Robert, R. Entrapment of the posterior femoral cutaneous nerve and its inferior cluneal branches: anatomical basis of surgery for inferior cluneal neuralgia. *Surgical and radiologic anatomy: SRA* (2017).
75. Tubbs, R. S. *et al.* Surgical and anatomical landmarks for the perineal branch of the posterior femoral cutaneous nerve: implications in perineal pain syndromes. *Journal of neurosurgery* **111**, 332–335 (2009).
76. Uluutku, H., Can, M. & Kurtoglu, Z. Formation and location of the sural nerve in the newborn. *Surgical and Radiologic Anatomy* **22**, 97–100 (2000).
77. Kosinski, C. The course, mutual relations and distribution of the cutaneous nerves of the metazonal region of leg and foot. *Journal of anatomy* **60**, 274 (1926).

Chapter 2 The pathophysiology of sciatica

Key points

- Common features of sciatica include mechanosensitivity, inflammation, and swelling along the sciatic nerve pathway
- These occur in sciatic pain originating from within or outside the spine
- Central or peripheral sensitization may explain these common features

Mechanosensitivity

Those with sciatica often have sciatic nerve mechanosensitivity, an excessive **tenderness to pressure**, or pain with **neural tension** (nerve elongation). These findings are common in most types of sciatica, including the intraspinal, extraspinal, and neuropathic and nociceptive forms. Stimuli like light pressure or small movements that would normally not be painful become painful. Mechanosensitivity may occur due to sensitization of the central nervous system as well as the peripheral nervous system, in which case there is a heightened response to non-noxious (not actually or potentially damaging) stimuli.

Mechanosensitivity to pressure

Tenderness of the sciatic nerve and its branches is a common feature of sciatica.[1–3] The regions of tenderness may help localize the cause of sciatica but are not diagnostic of specific pathology. The sciatic nerve trunk and its branches, to the small nerves in the feet, may be tender.

The French pediatrician François Valleix (1807-1855 CE) identified points along the sciatic trunk and its branches that were tender to palpation in those with sciatica.[4] These tender became known as **Valleix points**.[4] They include the lumbar spine superior to the sacrum, sacroiliac joint (SIJ), mid-iliac crest, greater sciatic notch, superior greater trochanter, the superior, middle, and inferior part of the sciatic nerve trunk, popliteal space, patella, common peroneal nerve, sural nerve, calcaneus, and foot dorsum.

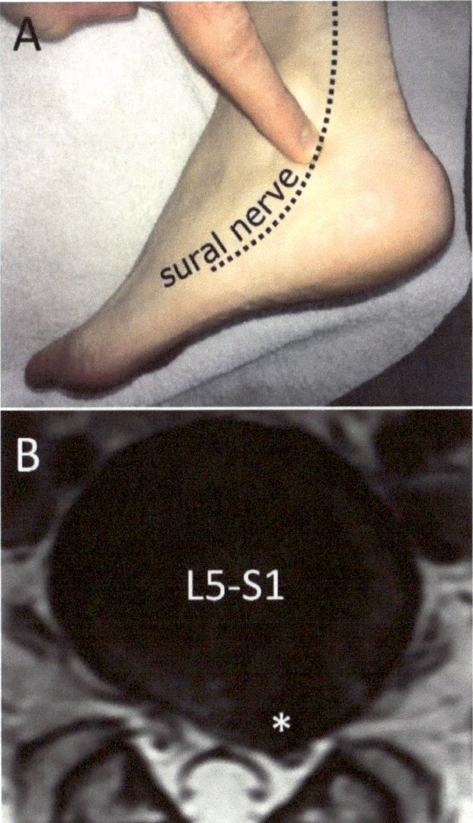

Figure 15: Sural nerve mechanosensitivity. This 59-year-old woman presented with severe LBP with stabbing L ankle pain in the location shown and numbness L S1 dermatome. In the region of pain, the sural nerve was tender and the area around appeared swollen. MRI revealed a left sided L5-S1 LDH (*) compressing the left S1 nerve root. Case shared with permission from patient by Robert Trager, DC.

Most patients with **intraspinal sciatica** have tenderness of the sciatic nerve or its branches. In those with **back-related leg pain**, 90% of patients have tenderness of at least one of three areas: (1) The sciatic nerve, (2) tibial nerve, or (3) common peroneal nerve.[3] One study found over 90% of those with an L5 radiculopathy had tenderness of the lateral branch of the deep peroneal nerve, and 100% of those with S1 radiculopathy had tenderness of the sural nerve.[2] Another study found sciatic nerve tenderness in 89% of patients with acute lumbar disc herniation (LDH).[5]

Extraspinal sciatica may cause sciatic nerve tenderness. Sciatic nerve entrapments such as piriformis syndrome, and inflammatory conditions such as **sacroiliitis** can cause the nerve trunk to be tender.[6] Over half of patients with **piriformis syndrome** have sciatic nerve tenderness at the greater sciatic notch.[7] Less common examples include compression of the L5 spinal nerve,[8] disorder of the lumbosacral plexus,[9] and vascular conditions including ruptured aortic aneurysms[10] and endometriosis.[11]

Those with chronic sciatica are more likely to develop **allodynia** throughout the sciatic distribution, in which non-painful touch stimuli become painful. One study found that about 60% of patients with radicular sciatica had allodynia over the course of the sciatic nerve.[12]

Table 2: Sciatic nerve mechanosensitivity to deep palpation: Examples

Intraspinal	Extraspinal
• Lumbar disc herniation[5] • Lumbar stenosis[13]	• Deep gluteal syndromes,[14] e.g. piriformis syndrome,[7] and internal obturator muscle[14] • Sacroiliitis[6] • Extraforaminal entrapment of the L5 spinal nerve[8] • Lumbosacral plexus disorders,[9] e.g. lumbopelvic tumor[15] • Extrapelvic endometriosis[11] • Ruptured abdominal aortic aneurysm[10]

Mechanosensitivity to stretch

Most cases of sciatica involve neural **mechanosensitivity**, a reduction in tolerance to neurodynamic tests or the provocation of sciatic pain by such tests. These tests include the straight leg raise, femoral nerve stretch test, seated piriformis stretch test, and other variations of these tests. Abnormal pressure, inflammation, tension, or movement restriction at any point in the sciatic nerve pathway can lead to stretch sensitivity.

Intraspinal and extraspinal conditions can cause mechanosensitivity of the sciatic nerve to stretch. Spinal pathology such as LDHs compress or inflame the nerve roots and increase neural tension. Anomalies and injuries of the deep gluteal region entrap the sciatic nerve trunk and restrict its ability to stretch and slide. Inflammatory disorders such as sacroiliitis may sensitize the sciatic nerve to stretch. Nerve entrapments further distal in the leg restrict movement of the sciatic nerve branches.

Mechanical changes to the sciatic nerve in those with sciatica may explain its sensitivity and resistance to stretch. Researchers are using shear wave elastography (a variation of ultrasonography) to study the properties of the sciatic nerve. This imaging modality has shown that the sciatic nerve is stiffer on the side of sciatica,[16,17] including those with LDHs[17] and deep gluteal syndrome.[18] **Stiffness** of the sciatic nerve may explain its inability to stretch during movement.

Table 3: Sciatic nerve mechanosensitivity to stretch: Examples

Intraspinal	Extraspinal
• Lumbar disc herniation • Lumbar stenosis (in 17%),[19] e.g. those with foraminal stenosis[20] • Epidural varicosis[21,22]	• Deep gluteal syndrome[23] and piriformis syndrome[7] • Sacroiliitis (in 16%)[24] • Common peroneal,[25] saphenous,[25] or tibial nerve entrapment or lesion[25]

Central sensitization

Central sensitization is an increased responsiveness of **nociceptive neurons** in the central nervous system to their normal or subthreshold afferent input.[4] In sciatica this can occur following nociceptive signals from LDH as well as from non-discogenic pathology such as myofascial pain syndromes.[26] Repetitive noxious neurological signals may lead to prolonged excitation of the **dorsal horn** and chronic sciatic pain.

Central sensitization may be responsible for **allodynia** throughout the sciatic nerve distribution in those with sciatica.[12,27] Over half of those with radicular sciatica have hypersensitivity to low-intensity

[4] According to the International Association for the Study of Pain (IASP)

stimulation of the skin.[12] It is thought that this is because low level mechanoreceptive input is amplified in the dorsal horn and perceived as painful.[12]

The sensation of **shooting pain** from the back to the leg or foot in radicular sciatica is thought to result from a sweeping wave of neural activity in the **sensitized dorsal horn** of the spinal cord.[12] Sensory neurons from the lower back synapse more laterally in the dorsal horn compared to the leg neurons which synapse more medially. In the most common type of sciatica, discogenic radicular pain, stimulation of the lower back neurons occurs first, which can secondarily stimulate those of the leg. It has been proposed that the further distal the pain radiates in the lower extremity, the more central sensitization is present.[12]

Peripheral sensitization

Peripheral sensitization is defined as an increased responsiveness and reduced threshold of nociceptive neurons in the periphery to the stimulation of their receptive fields.[5] Injury along the sciatic nerve pathway is thought to trigger **nociceptor activation** throughout the sciatic nerve distribution.[28] This hypersensitivity is thought to create mechanical hypersensitivity of the sciatic nerve and its branches and account for much of sciatic pain.

Sciatic nerve mechanosensitivity may result from sensitization of **nervi nervorum**,[29,30] which innervate the sciatic nerve sheath. The nervi nervorum have nociceptive nerve endings that sense mechanical, chemical, and thermal stimuli including pressure and stretch.[30] It is thought that patients with sciatica have tender sciatic nerves that hurt when stretched due to a heightened sensitivity of these nociceptors. One researcher described nervi nervorum as the main cause of sciatic nerve trunk pain:[29]

> *If one asks a patient with sciatica to point to his pain, one will often see the patient press his finger into the sciatic notch, drag it across the buttock... press it between the [hamstrings]... and run the finger down between the muscles to the popliteal [fossa]. His nerve is sore... his epineurium is sore... (Bennet)*

Nerve injuries along the sciatic pathway may sensitize the sciatic nervi nervorum. **Sciatic trunk injury**, for example in piriformis syndrome, directly affects the nervi nervorum.[31] Lumbosacral **nerve root injury** may generate neurological impulses that propagate into the sciatic nerve trunk and sensitize nociceptors of the nervi nervorum.[28] Tears in the **annulus fibrosus**, the outer layers of the lumbar discs, may generate inflammation that sensitizes the small nerves innervating them.[32]

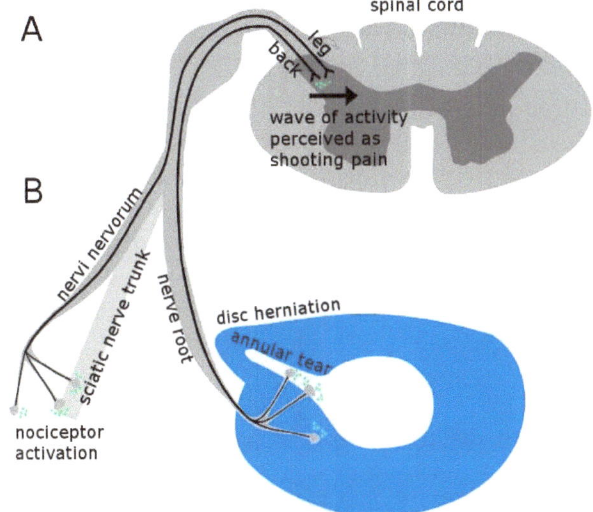

Robert Trager

Figure 16: Central and peripheral sensitization in sciatica. In peripheral sensitization nerve endings including those in the annulus of the disc and the nervi nervorum on the sciatic nerve trunk become sensitized to stimuli. In central sensitization the repetitive noxious stimulus triggers ongoing waves of pain perceived as radiating sciatic pain in the lower extremity.

The evidence for peripheral sensitization in sciatica is supported by studies that show anesthetic injections of branches of the sciatic nerve reduce discogenic radicular pain within minutes.[2,28,33] These studies show that in cases of intra-spinal pathology relief can be obtained by treating the peripheral area of pain.

Inflammation

Sciatica is an inflammatory condition involving the roots, trunk, and/or branches of the sciatic nerve. The symptoms of sciatic nerve mechanosensitivity and trunk pain, allodynia, and other symptoms relate to inflammation. The Italian physician Donato (early 1500s-1566 CE) was the first to describe sciatica as an inflammatory disease:[6]

> *... the fluxion of the articulation of the hip joint is completed on account of any such bordering ligament being stretched, and it is inevitable,*

[5] According to the International Association for the Study of Pain (IASP)

[6] Author's translation, d'Altomare,[34] p. 676

nevertheless, that similar nerves and cords become inflamed

In 1883 the British surgeon John Marshall proposed that inflamed nervi nervorum were responsible for sciatic nerve tenderness and pain:[35] "In an inflamed state... the swollen part of the nerve... the irritating fluids... must excite these nerves."

Neurogenic inflammation

Neurogenic inflammation is tissue inflammation caused by the release of inflammatory mediators from nociceptive **peripheral neuron terminals**. This type of inflammation may create many of the common symptoms of sciatica including tenderness and swelling of the sciatic nerve trunk and its branches and mechanosensitivity to stretch. Neurogenic inflammation also plays a role in pathology of the intervertebral disc and SIJ.

The **axon reflex** is one mechanism by which neurogenic inflammation may occur along the sciatic nerve branches.[36] In this reflex, stimulation of a sensory nerve triggers a release of inflammatory mediators at another branch of the same nerve. The axon reflex may account for inflammation in distant parts of the body in those with sciatica.

Mid-axonal activation may explain the spreading of neurogenic inflammation along the sciatic nerve branches.[37] In theory, an action potential (electric impulse) along one axon can stimulate a neighboring axon. This creates an antidromic action potential (towards the periphery) followed by an inflammatory response. Studies have shown that experimental inflammation of the sciatic nerve triggers activity in the sural nerve.[38]

The sciatic **nervi nervorum** contribute to neurogenic inflammation and may be responsible for nerve trunk hypersensitivity and allodynia.[30] One study found that electrical stimulation of the proximal part of the sciatic nerve caused the release of inflammatory mediators from its nervi nervorum.[39] Another study showed that experimental inflammation of the peroneal nerve led to mechanosensitivity of the sciatic nerve trunk.[40] Inflammatory responses of the nervi nervorum are caused by injuries along the sciatic trunk and branches and contribute to sciatic nerve trunk pain.

Substance P is a major **inflammatory neurotransmitter** involved in the neurogenic inflammation of sciatica. This substance travels via axonal transport along the course of the sciatic nerve and its branches.[41] Substance P is found in the sciatic trunk, tibial nerve, common peroneal nerve, and sural nerve.[36] Electrical stimulation of the sciatic nerve causes release of substance P from nerve terminals in the skin.[42] Injuries along the sciatic pathway may trigger substance P release at nerve terminals in the periphery, causing pain and tenderness.

Hip-spine syndrome and **sacroiliac-joint** related sciatica may involve neurogenic inflammation. One study identified the inflammatory neurotransmitter substance P in the subarticular tissues of those with SIJ and sciatic pain, which was thought to inflame nearby nerves.[43] Mediators of neurogenic inflammation have also been identified in the hip joint in those with hip arthritis.[44] In both cases the inflammation may cause sciatica by affecting affect nearby nerves, by convergence at the dorsal horn, or by the axon reflex. Alternatively, an intraspinal radicular sciatica may trigger the release of neurogenic inflammatory mediators in the hip and SIJ.

Mast cells

Mast cells are immune cells found in the sheathes of the sciatic nerve and its branches.[45] These cells respond to injury of the sciatic nerve by degranulating, meaning they release inflammatory mediators such as **histamine**.[46] Mast cells also increase in number distal to the site of sciatic nerve injury.[45]

Mast cells and the substances they release contribute to mechanosensitivity along the sciatic trunk and distribution. One study using an animal model of sciatic nerve injury found that histamine-suppressing medication reduced signs of mechanosensitivity of the sciatic nerve.[47] Histamine most likely increases sensitivity by activating peripheral nociceptors[47] including the nervi nervorum in the sciatic nerve sheath.

Sciatic nerve edema may be caused by histamine-induced **vascular permeability**.[46] Histamine increases the permeability of the sciatic blood vessels. This allows for an influx of serum albumin, which builds up between sciatic nerve fibers.[48] Experiments of sciatic nerve injury in animals histamine-producing mast cells accumulate in the sciatic nerve **endoneurial compartment**.[45]

Sciatic nerve swelling

Radicular **intraspinal** and non-radicular **extraspinal** forms of sciatica may cause sciatic nerve swelling.[1] Studies have reported sciatic nerve edema in radicular and discogenic sciatica,[1,49–51] in 94% of patients with **piriformis syndrome**,[31] and in 79% of those with hamstring syndrome.[52] Sciatic nerve edema has also been reported in traumatic sciatic neuropathy,[53] aortoiliac occlusive disease,[54] sacroiliitis,[55] endometriosis,[56] tumors of the sciatic nerve,[57] Herpes Zoster-related sciatica,[59] and following hip and gynecologic surgery.[60]

Research using **ultrasonography** (US) has shown that the sciatic nerve enlarges in those with sciatica. Studies have shown increased cross-sectional area (CSA) of the symptomatic sciatic nerve at the mid-thigh level by about 10 mm^2 compared to the asymptomatic side,[1,51,61] an increase of 19%.[49] Studies have also shown that those with sciatica have greater amounts of **hypoechoic** (darker) areas within the sciatic nerve that represent edema and/or inflammation.[51,61] In one study, all patients with unilateral radicular sciatica had increased CSA and/or hypoechoic areas on the side of symptoms.[49]

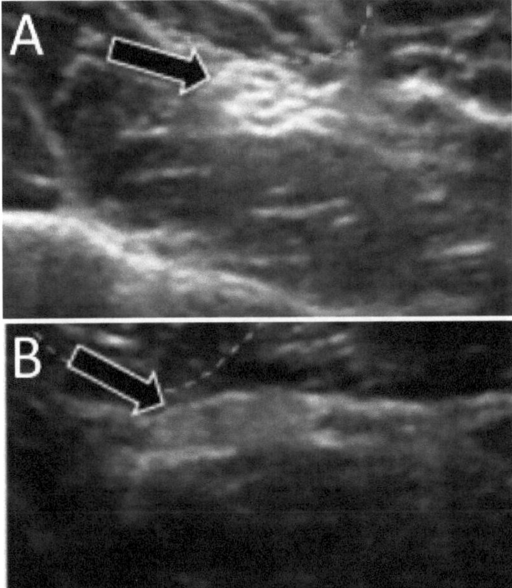

Figure 17: Sciatic nerve swelling in radiculopathy seen using axial diagnostic ultrasound. (A) Normal, hyperechoic and small sciatic nerve (arrow). (B) Low back pain and radiculopathy causing darker signal and increased size of sciatic nerve, signs of edema. The dashed line marks the biceps femoris border. Images CC-BY-2.5 CA from Frost.[49]

Magnetic resonance imaging (MRI) may show sciatic nerve edema. Sequences of T2-weighted or short tau inversion recovery (STIR) show **hyperintensity** and **thickening** of sciatic nerve.[55,60,62] In these images, the bright white signal represents fluid. Other variations of MRI including T1-weighted MRI with a contrast agent such as gadolinium,[55] or magnetic resonance neurography (MRN) may show sciatic nerve edema more clearly.[53,57,63]

Sciatic nerve swelling may be more prominent in **acute sciatica**. Swelling is more prominent in those with a shorter duration of symptoms compared to those with chronic symptoms.[1] This could explain why there is a lack of cases of sciatic nerve swelling in those with LSS. Most research on sciatic nerve swelling is in those with discogenic or extraspinal sciatica. Sciatic nerve swelling does not appear to correlate with clinical variables such as low back or leg pain severity, or disability index.[51,61]

Sciatic neuritis

Modern clinicians and researchers reserve the term sciatic neuritis for inflammatory disorders of the sciatic nerve trunk that are seen on imaging studies. Common examples include deep gluteal or piriformis syndromes,[64] and less common examples include sciatic nerve damage following hip[60] or low back surgery,[65] and tumors of the sciatic nerve.[66] Historically, the diagnosis of sciatic neuritis was much more common.

Clinicians believed that sciatica was an idiopathic (self-originating) inflammatory **neuritis** from the mid-1800s to mid-1900s. The Italian physician Domenico Cotugno was the first to discover swelling of the sciatic nerve in 1764 and the first to publish a textbook devoted to sciatica. He found that the affected nerve sheath was "more thick than usual" and "had a greater quantity of fluid from the head of the fibula to the bottom of the foot" in a patient who died with sciatica.[67] Cotugno claimed that sciatica was caused by an overabundance or abnormality of **cerebrospinal fluid** in the sciatic nerve sheath:[67]

> *For it seems to be an acrid and irritating matter, which lying on the nerve, preys on the stamina, and gives rise to the pain... they are full of a humor which they receive from the brain. (Wilkie, p. 12, p. 90)*

In 1791 the Italian physician and discoverer of electrical muscle contraction Luigi Galvani proposed that an electrical arc formed when the sciatic nerve was swollen, which triggered pain and muscle spasms.[68] In 1826 the Frenchman Gendrin published two autopsies of patients who had sciatica in which he identified redness and **serous infiltration** of the sciatic nerve.[69] In each case the patient suffered from sciatica but died of an additional infectious disease.[69] In 1878 the Frenchman Fernet published the autopsy of a 56-year-old male patient who died from Tuberculosis while also suffering from sciatica.[70] He found reddening and swelling, and a "stiff and retained cylindrical shape" of the sciatic nerve.[70]

In 1905 Hunt of New York reviewed 11 autopsies of sciatica sufferers and found that the majority had swelling of the affected sciatic nerve.[71] He included a new case of a 59 year old man who had sciatica but died from pneumonia, in which he found swelling of the affected sciatic nerve with a firm gelatinous deposit.[71]

Clinicians nearly stopped using the term sciatic neuritis in the 1940s when they accepted LDH as the most common cause of sciatica.[72] Newer research shows that those diagnosing sciatic neuritis were on the right track. Sciatic nerve trunk inflammation is present in disorders such as piriformis syndrome[64] and may be present in many more forms of sciatica.[1,61] Sciatic neuritis is not a disease on its own, but occurs secondary to other pathology.

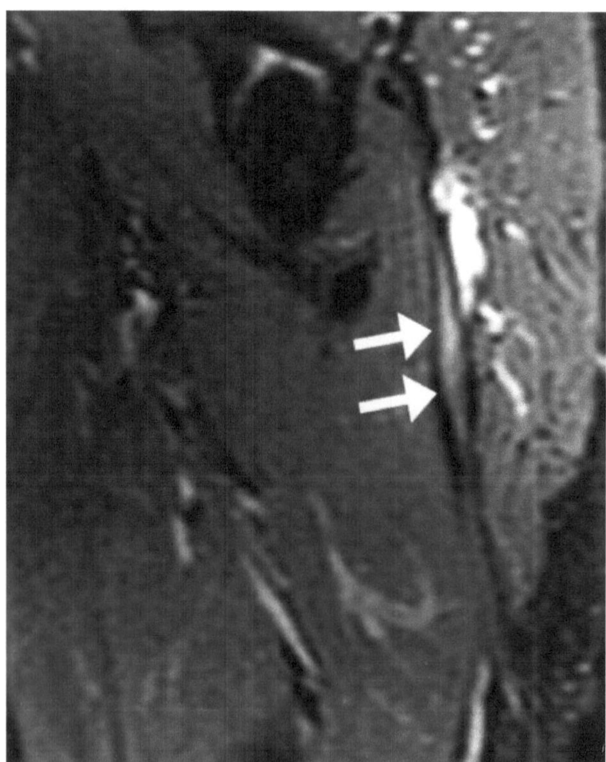

Figure 18: Sciatic nerve swelling in hamstring syndrome. Nerve enlargement and hyperintensity (arrows) are seen on this T2-weighted MRI of the hip. Creative Commons License from Dong.[62]

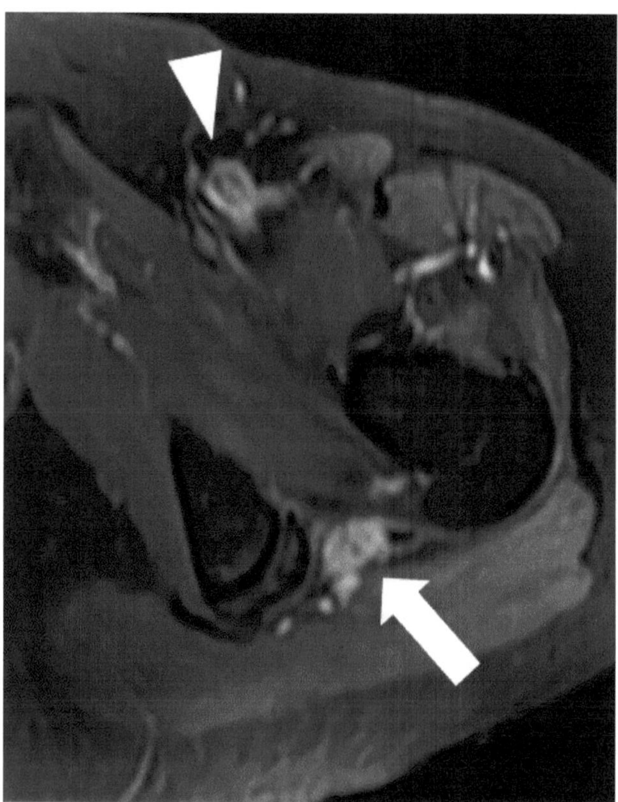

Figure 19: Sciatic nerve (arrow) and femoral nerve (arrowhead) hyperintensity and edema on T2-weighted MRI in herpes zoster infection.[59]

Spread of swelling

Swelling can spread longitudinally along the spaces between the layers of the sciatic nerve sheath. Studies have demonstrated that anesthesia and dye can spread along the sciatic **subparaneural** and **subepimyseal spaces**.[73,74] The sciatic sheath spaces are passageways for fluid to accumulate or travel from one part of the nerve to another.

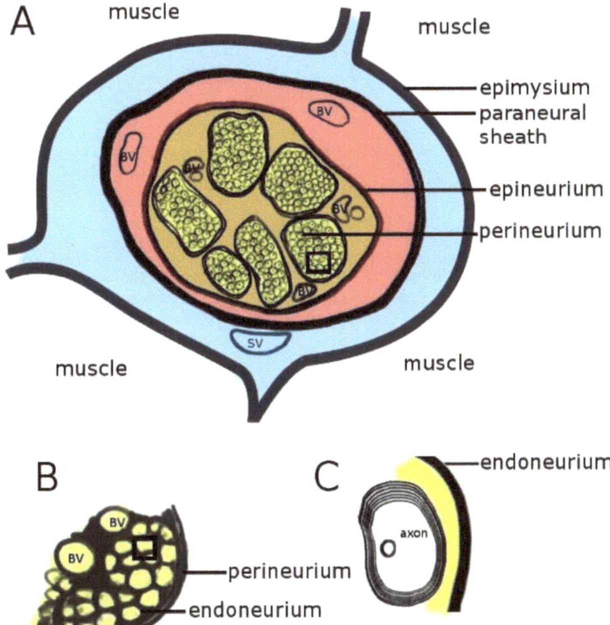

Figure 20: Sciatic nerve, axial section (A), nerve fascicle (B) and axon (C). Spaces are exaggerated to show potential expansion due to swelling. The subepimyseal space (blue) surrounds the sciatic nerve and is a space between it and the muscles. The subparaneural space (red) is the largest potential space within the sciatic nerve. The subepineural (orange) and subendoneural (yellow) spaces, blood vessels (BV) and the sciatic vein (SV) are indicated. Image by Robert Trager, DC.

One study using cadavers found that 10 mL of blue dye injected into the sciatic subparaneural space spread 10-15 cm.[73] These spaces can also be used to inject medications that anesthetize the sciatic nerve. Studies in rats have shown that injected substances diffuse along the sciatic nerve compartments.[75] Rarely, cancer will metastasize along the sciatic sheath.

Direct injury to the main sciatic nerve trunk can cause swelling along the nerve course. Animal studies have also shown that constriction of the proximal sciatic nerve will cause edema to form distally within the nerve over a course of 24-48 hours.[76] When the sciatic nerve is injured its **endoneural space** enlarges to accommodate swelling.[77] At the injury site the nerve may be compressed, but outside of this zone the nerve enlarges.[57]

Central nervous system changes

Brain changes

Growing evidence suggests that areas of the brain become altered in those with low back pain (LBP) and sciatica.[78,79] These changes occur in parts of the brain involved in emotion and cognition.[80] Brain changes correlate with chronicity of pain,[81,82] further radiation of pain,[81] and are thought to relate to changes in proprioception[83] and tactile acuity.[84]

Somatotopy describes the topographical relationship of the body's nerve fibers in the cerebral cortex of the brain. Studies using functional MRI (fMRI) of the brain have identified that sensory signals from the sciatic nerve localize to the contralateral **secondary somatosensory cortex**.[80,85] This topographic map is not static and may change both functionally and structurally in chronic LBP and sciatica.[80]

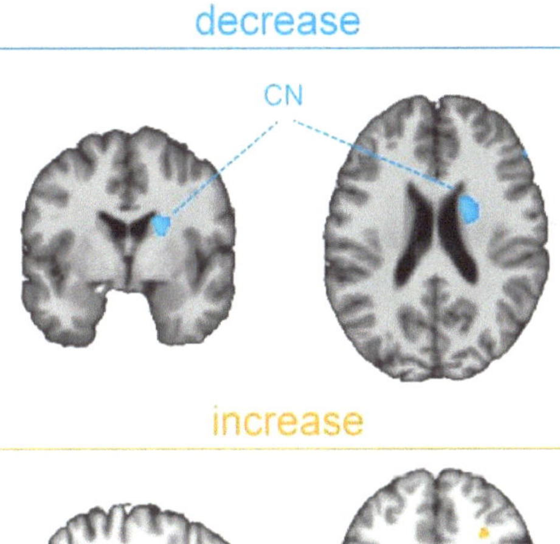

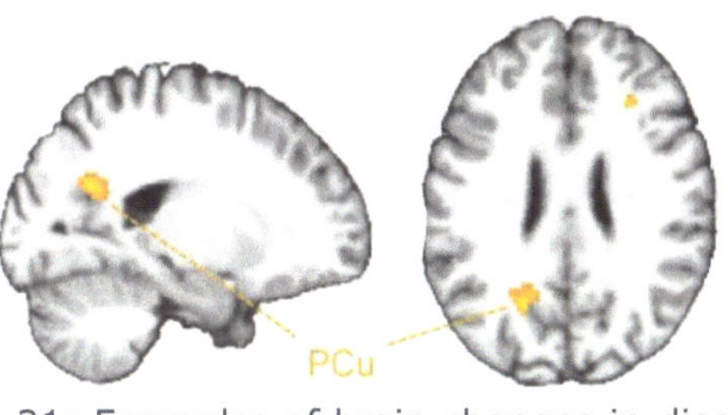

Figure 21: Examples of brain changes in discogenic sciatica. There is typically a decrease (blue) in the volume of the right caudate nucleus, and increase (orange) in the left lateral precuneal region (PCu). Image Creative Commons Attribution License from Luchtmann[79]

A systematic review of fMRI in patients with chronic LBP and/or sciatica found that the most consistent brain changes occurred in areas involved in **emotion** and **cognition**.[86] These brain changes involve the **default mode network**, a network of brain regions that are active at rest.[86] Patients with discogenic sciatica may have multiple brain alterations including areas with reduced or increased gray matter volume.[79]

Studies of tactile acuity in patients with LBP support the concept of blurring of the brain. Patients with chronic LBP may have a **sensory dissociation**, a discrepancy between the actual size and their perception.[84] The typical pattern may be **macrosomatognosia**, an enlargement of the body part in pain, rather than a shrinkage.[84] It is thought that a perceived body part enlargement correlates with expansion of the back region of the brain.[84]

One fMRI imaging study found that those with chronic LBP with or without sciatica had a **blurred representation** of the lumbar spine in the somatosensory cortex.[78] One study found an **expanded back representation** which pushed into neighboring leg and foot areas.[82] Blurred and expanded brain changes may account for chronicity of pain[82] as well as deficits of proprioception.[83]

Neural drive

Weakness in those with sciatica may be indirectly due to changes in the central nervous system (CNS) rather than directly from damage to a nerve root or local muscle atrophy. Both neuropathic radicular sciatica and non-radicular non-neuropathic sciatica can present with weakness. It is thought that weakness may result from a reorganization of the brain cortex[87] or by the brain prioritizing pain avoidance more than muscle contraction.[88]

Those with non-neuropathic extraspinal or myofascial sciatica may have lower extremity weakness despite the absence of nerve compression on imaging studies. Weakness occurs in nearly two thirds of those with **greater trochanteric pain syndrome**,[89] and one third of patients with **SIJ pain** radiating distal to the buttocks.[24] Weakness in non-neuropathic sciatica may be explained by mechanisms involving the spinal cord or brain. One such phenomenon, called **arthrogenic inhibition** or **neuromuscular inhibition**, describes the reflexive inhibition of muscles following a joint injury or effusion.[90] It is suspected that this reflexive non-neuropathic weakness involves a central mechanism.[90]

Studies of LBP and/or intraspinal radicular sciatica have found that patients have a reduced **corticospinal drive**,[87,88,91] meaning there is a reduced ability to recruit motor units. These studies typically use a combination of transcranial magnetic stimulation and electromyography to compare a neurological response to normal controls. One such study found that patients with discogenic sciatica had a higher threshold for generating motor evoked potentials of the gastrocnemius and tibialis anterior leg muscles.[91] Another similar study found that reduced corticospinal drive in sciatica correlated positively with the level of disability as measured by outcome assessment tests.[87]

The mind-body connection

Mental stress, anxiety about health, and **kinesiophobia** (fear of movement) are known to contribute to or prolong sciatica. These influences help explain the lack of correlation between lumbar spine pathology and symptoms.

The English physician Anstie was the first to relate sciatica to psychosomatic influences in 1871. He stated that "hysteric" sciatica was "produced by some fatigue, or mental distress," and compared this scenario to headaches.[92] In 1896 the French neurologist Joseph Babinski related certain cases of sciatica to psychosomatic causes, which he called hysteric pseudosciatica.[93] He believed that a normal Achilles reflex would identify this psychosomatic form,[93] a diagnostic that is no longer used.

Stress influences the development of sciatica as well as the time it takes to recover. Those with high levels of mental stress have three times the odds of having sciatica compared to those without it.[94] Kinesophobia,[95,96] other health complaints in addition to sciatica,[95] **fear avoidance** beliefs,[97] worrying and health anxiety,[97] and **psychosomatic problems**[98] all increase the time it takes to recover from sciatica. Those with emotional distress have 3.4 times the odds of continuing to suffer from sciatica and LDH after 1 year, and 3.3 times the odds at 2 years.[96]

One modern author has suggested that most cases of sciatica are not caused by LDH but instead are psychosomatic in origin.[99] He describes a cyclical relationship between pain syndromes and diagnostic imaging results, leading to increased pain:[99]

> *[S]ciatica... raises the spectre of the herniated disc and the possibility of surgery. In this media-dominated age very few people have not heard of herniated discs and the idea arouses great anxiety, resulting in greater pain. If... imaging studies show a herniation, the apprehension is multiplied even further... (Sarno, 2010)*

Certain cases of sciatica may fit into the category of **tension myositis syndrome**.[99] In this syndrome, factors such as stress and anxiety affect the autonomic nervous system in such a way that reduces blood flow to certain muscles, nerves and tendons. It is possible that the ancient beliefs of worrying about demons or spirits relate to modern notions about health anxiety and worrying about LDHs. Luckily, if this is the case, there are ways to desensitize one's self to kinesiophobia and to reduce unwanted stress.

Sympathetically mediated pain

Sympathetic nervous system (SNS) activity could be the link between psychological and physical components of sciatica. The balance of SNS and parasympathetic nervous system (PNS) activity supports the homeostatic balance of the body. The SNS acts as the "fight or flight" system, and acts to increase heart rate, constrict blood vessels in the skin and visceral organs to promote blood flow to the muscles, and in general promote survival in response to danger. In addition to danger, mental stress may activate the SNS.

Sympatheticotonia or sympathicotonia, an over-activation of the SNS, may lead to **central sensitization**, which is an increased sensitivity of the central nervous system to pain. Although some authors have placed sciatica and radiculopathy in the category of **sympathetically maintained pain** or over-activation of the SNS, the proportion of patients in which the SNS is involved remains in question.

The British surgeon John Hilton was one of the first to describe sciatic pain referral from the hip and SIJs, and in 1879 ascribed this phenomenon to the sympathetic nervous system:[100]

> *Pain in any part, when not associated with increase of temperature (the local symptom of local inflammation) must be looked upon as sympathetic pain, caused by an exalted sensitiveness of the nerves of the part, and it is to be regarded as a pain depending upon a cause situated remotely from the part where it is felt (Hilton, p. 40)*

A study of patients with persistent sciatica after lumbar discectomy concluded that the continued sciatic pain represented a form of reflex sympathetic dystrophy or what is now called **complex regional pain syndrome** (CRPS).[101] The authors based this on their finding of a correlation between the patient's pain level and reduced temperature in the legs and feet as seen on thermography.

Some studies have found that sympathetic or autonomic symptoms reduce following treatment for sciatica. One study identified that burning pain, sweating, edema in the extremity, and disturbances of circulation were reduced significantly after treatment for CRPS using sympathetic blocks and ketamine.[102] This suggested that the sciatic symptoms were due to CRPS.[102] Another study found that dry needling reduced sciatic pain and improved skin temperature, suggesting that needling influenced the sympathetic nervous system.[103]

The sympathetic nervous system is both anatomically and clinically related to long-standing cases of sciatica. In animal and some human studies, sympathetic nerve fibers have been found to innervate the **posterior longitudinal ligament**, **dura mater**, the **intervertebral disc** and its endplate, and facet joints.[104–107] Rami of the sympathetic nervous system also anastomose with the **lumbosacral plexus** which forms the sciatic nerve.

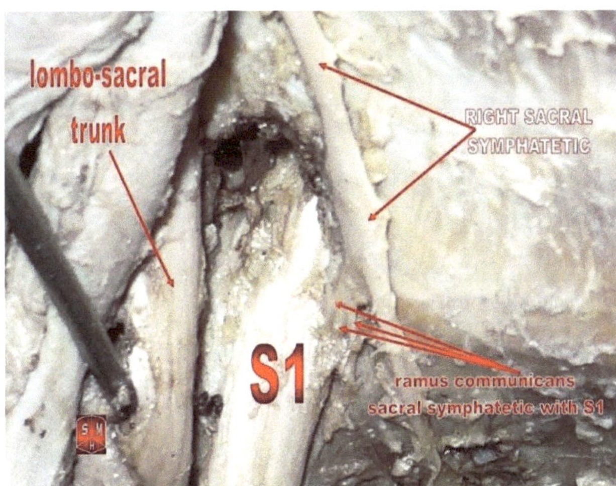

Figure 22: Connection between the sacral sympathetic chain and the S1 spinal nerve (set of three arrows). This connection helps explain the effects of the SNS on the lower extremity in cases of sciatica, as stimulation of one component (S1 or SNS) may affect the other. Image from Adrian Halga, CC BY-SA 3.0 license

References

1. Kara, M. *et al.* Sonographic evaluation of sciatic nerves in patients with unilateral sciatica. *Arch Phys Med Rehabil* **93**, 1598–1602 (2012).
2. Gore, S. & Nadkarni, S. Sciatica: Detection and Confirmation by New Method. *International journal of spine surgery* **8**, 1 (2014).
3. Walsh, J. & Hall, T. Reliability, validity and diagnostic accuracy of palpation of the sciatic, tibial and common peroneal nerves in the examination of low back related leg pain. *Manual Therapy* **14**, 623–629 (2009).
4. Valleix, F. L. I. *Traité des névralgies, ou, Affections douloureuses des nerfs*. (Baillière, 1841).
5. Rocha, Q. M. W., Sakata, R. K. & Issy, A. M. Low back pain: comparison of epidural analgesia with bupivacaine associated to methylprednisolone, fentanyl and methylprednisolone plus fentanyl. *Revista Brasileira de Anestesiologia* **51**, 407–413 (2001).
6. Tüzün, Ç. *et al.* An atypical psoriatic spondylitis case, successfully treated with methotrexate. *Clin Rheumatol* **15**, 403–409 (1996).

7. Hopayian, K., Song, F., Riera, R. & Sambandan, S. The clinical features of the piriformis syndrome: a systematic review. *European Spine Journal* **19**, 2095–2109 (2010).
8. Miyamoto, S. *et al.* A case of L5 radiculopathy caused by far-out syndrome.
9. Evans, B. A., Stevens, J. C. & Dyck, P. J. Lumbosacral plexus neuropathy. *Neurology* **31**, 1327–1327 (1981).
10. Kawamura, K. *et al.* A case of threatened rupture of abdominal aortic aneurysm occurred with intractable low back pain. *Journal of Tokushima National Hospital* **2**, 27–29 (2011).
11. Floyd, J. R., Keeler, E. R., Euscher, E. D. & McCutcheon, I. E. Cyclic sciatica from extrapelvic endometriosis affecting the sciatic nerve: Case report. *Journal of Neurosurgery: Spine* **14**, 281–289 (2011).
12. Defrin, R., Devor, M. & Brill, S. Tactile allodynia in patients with lumbar radicular pain (sciatica). *PAIN®* **155**, 2551–2559 (2014).
13. Adachi, S. *et al.* The tibial nerve compression test for the diagnosis of lumbar spinal canal stenosis—A simple and reliable physical examination for use by primary care physicians. *Acta orthopaedica et traumatologica turcica* (2017).
14. Meknas, K., Christensen, A. & Johansen, O. The internal obturator muscle may cause sciatic pain. *Pain* **104**, 375–380 (2003).
15. Sim, F., Dahlin, D., Stauffer, R. & Edward, L. Primary bone tumors simulating lumbar disc syndrome. *Spine* **2**, 65–74 (1977).
16. Neto, T. *et al.* Noninvasive Measurement of Sciatic Nerve Stiffness in Patients With Chronic Low Back Related Leg Pain Using Shear Wave Elastography. *J Ultrasound Med* (2018). doi:10.1002/jum.14679
17. Çelebi, U. O., Burulday, V., Özveren, M. F., Doğan, A. & Akgül, M. H. Sonoelastographic evaluation of the sciatic nerve in patients with unilateral lumbar disc herniation. *Skeletal Radiol* **48**, 129–136 (2019).
18. Stajic, S. *et al.* Role of sciatic nerve stiffness in surgical decision making and follow up in patients with deep gluteal syndrome. *bioRxiv* 390120 (2018).
19. Konno, S. *et al.* Development of a clinical diagnosis support tool to identify patients with lumbar spinal stenosis. *European Spine Journal* **16**, 1951–1957 (2007).
20. Yamada, H. *et al.* Development of a support tool for the clinical diagnosis of symptomatic lumbar intra-and/or extra-foraminal stenosis. *Journal of Orthopaedic Science* **20**, 811–817 (2015).
21. Paksoy, Y. & Gormus, N. Epidural venous plexus enlargements presenting with radiculopathy and back pain in patients with inferior vena cava obstruction or occlusion. *Spine* **29**, 2419–2424 (2004).
22. Hammer, A., Knight, I. & Agarwal, A. Localized venous plexi in the spine simulating prolapse of an intervertebral disc: a report of six cases. *Spine* **28**, E5–E12 (2003).
23. Martin, H. D., Kivlan, B. R., Palmer, I. J. & Martin, R. L. Diagnostic accuracy of clinical tests for sciatic nerve entrapment in the gluteal region. *Knee Surgery, Sports Traumatology, Arthroscopy* **22**, 882–888 (2014).
24. Visser, L., Nijssen, P., Tijssen, C., van Middendorp, J. & Schieving, J. Sciatica-like symptoms and the sacroiliac joint: clinical features and differential diagnosis. *European spine journal: official publication of the European Spine Society, the European Spinal Deformity Society, and the European Section of the Cervical Spine Research Society* (2013).
25. Saal, J. A., Dillingham, M. F., Gamburd, R. S. & Fanton, G. S. The pseudoradicular syndrome. Lower extremity peripheral nerve entrapment masquerading as lumbar radiculopathy. *Spine* **13**, 926–930 (1988).
26. Fernández-de-las-Peñas, C. & Dommerholt, J. Myofascial trigger points: peripheral or central phenomenon? *Current rheumatology reports* **16**, 395 (2014).
27. Smart, K. M., Blake, C., Staines, A. & Doody, C. The Discriminative validity of 'nociceptive,' 'peripheral neuropathic,' and 'central sensitization' as mechanisms-based classifications of musculoskeletal pain. *Clin J Pain* **27**, 655–663 (2011).
28. Xavier, A. V., Farrell, C. E., McDanal, J. & Kissin, I. Does antidromic activation of nociceptors play a role in sciatic radicular pain? *Pain* **40**, 77–79 (1990).
29. Bennett, G. J. Can we distinguish between inflammatory and neuropathic pain. *Pain Research & Management* (2006).
30. Hall, T. M. & Elvey, R. L. Nerve trunk pain: physical diagnosis and treatment. *Manual Therapy* **4**, 63–73 (1999).
31. Filler, A. G. *et al.* Sciatica of nondisc origin and piriformis syndrome: diagnosis by magnetic resonance neurography and interventional magnetic resonance imaging with outcome study of resulting treatment. *Journal of Neurosurgery: Spine* **2**, 99–115 (2005).
32. Stefanakis, M. *et al.* Annulus fissures are mechanically and chemically conducive to the ingrowth of nerves and blood vessels. *Spine* **37**, 1883–1891 (2012).
33. Tajiri, K., Takahashi, K., Ikeda, K. & Tomita, K. Common peroneal nerve block for sciatica. *Clin. Orthop. Relat. Res.* 203–207 (1998).
34. Altomare, D. A. d'. *Donati Antonii ab Altomari ... Omnia, quae hucusque in lucem prodierunt, Opera, nunc primùm in unum collecta, & ab eodem auctore diligentissimè recognita & aucta: cum locis omnibus in margine additis, horum omnium elenchum sexta pagina commonstrabit.* (apud Gulielmum Rouillium, 1565).
35. Marshall, J. Bradshaw lecture on nerve-stretching for the relief or cure of pain. *British Medical Journal* **2**, 1173 (1883).
36. Gundersen, K., Øktedalen, O. & Fonnum, F. Substance P in subdivisions of the sciatic nerve, and in red and white skeletal muscles. *Brain research* **329**, 97–103 (1985).
37. Sorkin, L. S., Eddinger, K. A., Woller, S. A. & Yaksh, T. L. Origins of antidromic activity in sensory afferent fibers and neurogenic inflammation. *Semin Immunopathol* 1–11 (2018). doi:10.1007/s00281-017-0669-2
38. Sorkin, L. S., Xiao, W.-H., Wagner, R. & Myers, R. R. Tumour necrosis factor-α induces ectopic activity in nociceptive primary afferent fibres. *Neuroscience* **81**, 255–262 (1997).
39. Sauer, S. K., Bove, G. M., Averbeck, B. & Reeh, P. W. Rat peripheral nerve components release calcitonin gene-related peptide and prostaglandin E2 in response to noxious stimuli: evidence that nervi nervorum are nociceptors*S. K. Sauer and G. M. Bove contributed equally to this study.*. *Neuroscience* **92**, 319–325 (1999).
40. Dilley, A., Lynn, B. & Pang, S. J. Pressure and stretch mechanosensitivity of peripheral nerve fibres following local inflammation of the nerve trunk. *Pain* **117**, 462–472 (2005).
41. Brimijoin, S., Lundberg, J. M., Brodin, E., Ho, T. & others. Axonal transport of substance P in the vagus and sciatic nerves of the guinea pig. *Brain research* **191**, 443–457 (1980).
42. White, D. M. & Helme, R. D. Release of substance P from peripheral nerve terminals following electrical stimulation of the sciatic nerve. *Brain Research* **336**, 27–31 (1985).
43. Fortin, J. D., Vilensky, J. A. & Merkel, G. J. Can the sacroiliac joint cause sciatica? *Pain Physician* **6**, 269–271 (2003).
44. Takeshita, M. *et al.* Sensory innervation and inflammatory cytokines in hypertrophic synovia associated with pain transmission in osteoarthritis of the hip: a case–control study. *Rheumatology (Oxford)* **51**, 1790–1795 (2012).
45. Enerbäck, L., Olsson, Y. & Sourander, P. Mast cells in normal and sectioned peripheral nerve. *Z.Zellforsch* **66**, 596–608 (1965).
46. Olsson, Y. Degranulation of mast cells in peripheral nerve injuries. *Acta Neurologica Scandinavica* **43**, 365–374 (1967).
47. Zuo, Y., Perkins, N. M., Tracey, D. J. & Geczy, C. L. Inflammation and hyperalgesia induced by nerve injury in the rat: a key role of mast cells. *Pain* **105**, 467–479 (2003).
48. Olsson, Y. Studies on vascular permeability in peripheral nerves. *Acta Neuropathol* **7**, 1–15 (1966).
49. Frost, L. Lower Back and Lower Limb Neuromuscular Structure and Function in Chronic Low Back Pain Patients with Associated Radiculopathy. (University of Guelph, 2014).
50. Frost, L. R. & Brown, S. H. Muscle activation timing and balance response in chronic lower back pain patients with associated radiculopathy. *Clinical Biomechanics* **32**, 124–130 (2016).
51. Sarafraz, H. *et al.* Neuromuscular morphometric characteristics in low back pain with unilateral radiculopathy caused by disc herniation: An ultrasound imaging evaluation. *Musculoskeletal Science and Practice* **40**, 80–86 (2019).
52. Bucknor, M. D., Steinbach, L. S., Saloner, D. & Chin, C. T. Magnetic resonance neurography evaluation of chronic extraspinal sciatica after remote proximal hamstring injury: a preliminary retrospective analysis. *J. Neurosurg.* 1–7 (2014). doi:10.3171/2014.4.JNS13940
53. Agnollitto, P. M. *et al.* Sciatic neuropathy: findings on magnetic resonance neurography. *Radiologia Brasileira* **50**, 190–196 (2017).
54. Ciftci, S., Ekinci, A. S., TABAKOGLU, A. Y. & Bademkiran, F. Bilateral Ischemic Lumbosacral Plexopathy Presenting as Acute Paraparesia Due to Vascular Graft Occlusion in a Patient With Leriche Syndrome. *Journal of Neurological Sciences (Turkish)* **34**, (2017).
55. Neufeld, E. A. *et al.* MR imaging of the lumbosacral plexus: a review of techniques and pathologies. *Journal of Neuroimaging* **25**, 691–703 (2015).
56. Siquara De Sousa, A. C., Capek, S., Amrami, K. K. & Spinner, R. J. Neural involvement in endometriosis: Review of anatomic distribution and mechanisms. *Clin Anat* **28**, 1029–1038 (2015).
57. Moore, K. R., Tsuruda, J. S. & Dailey, A. T. The Value of MR Neurography for Evaluating Extraspinal Neuropathic Leg Pain: A Pictorial Essay. *AJNR Am J Neuroradiol* **22**, 786–794 (2001).
58. Byun, J. H., Hong, J. T., Son, B. C. & Lee, S. W. Schwannoma of the superficial peroneal nerve presenting as sciatica. *J Korean Neurosurg Soc* **38**, 306–308 (2005).
59. Choi, Y. R., Oh, C. H. & Choi, W. A Case of Herpes Zoster Presented with Lower Limb Paresis. *Cureus* **10**, (2018).
60. Flug, J. A., Burge, A., Melisaratos, D., Miller, T. T. & Carrino, J. A. Post-operative extra-spinal etiologies of sciatic nerve impingement. *Skeletal radiology* 1–9 (2018).
61. Frost, L. R. & Brown, S. H. M. Neuromuscular ultrasound imaging in low back pain patients with radiculopathy. *Man Ther* (2015). doi:10.1016/j.math.2015.05.003
62. Dong, Q. *et al.* Entrapment Neuropathies in the Upper and Lower Limbs: Anatomy and MRI Features. *Radiol Res Pract* **2012**, (2012).
63. Burge, A. J., Gold, S. L., Kuong, S. & Potter, H. G. High-resolution magnetic resonance imaging of the lower extremity nerves. *Neuroimaging Clinics* **24**, 151–170 (2014).
64. Hernando, M. F., Cerezal, L., Pérez-Carro, L., Abascal, F. & Canga, A. Deep gluteal syndrome: anatomy, imaging, and management of sciatic nerve entrapments in the subgluteal space. *Skeletal radiology* **44**, 919–934 (2015).
65. Elahi, F., Hitchon, P. & Reddy, C. G. Acute sciatic neuritis following lumbar laminectomy. *Case reports in medicine* **2014**, (2014).

66. Wadhwa, V. *et al.* Sciatic nerve tumor and tumor-like lesions—uncommon pathologies. *Skeletal radiology* **41**, 763–774 (2012).
67. Cotugno, D. *A Treatise on the Nervous Sciatica: Or, Nervous Hip Gout* ... (J. Wilkie, 1775).
68. Galvani, L. *De viribus electricitatis in motu musculari*. (1791).
69. Gendrin, A. N. (Augustin N. *Histoire anatomique des inflammations*. (Paris : Béchet ;, 1826).
70. Fernet. De la sciatique et de sa nature. *Archives Gènèrales de Mèdicine* (1878).
71. Hunt, R. A contribution to the pathology of sciatica. *American Medicine* **9**, (1905).
72. Holmes, J. M. & Sworn, B. Sciatic neuritis. *British Medical Journal* **2**, 350 (1945).
73. Andersen, H. L., Andersen, S. L. & Tranum-Jensen, J. Injection Inside the Paraneural Sheath of the Sciatic Nerve: Direct Comparison Among Ultrasound Imaging, Macroscopic Anatomy, and Histologic Analysis. *Regional Anesthesia and Pain Medicine* **37**, 410 (2012).
74. Reina, M. A. *et al.* Electron microscopy of human peripheral nerves of clinical relevance to the practice of nerve blocks. A structural and ultrastructural review based on original experimental and laboratory data. *Revista Española de Anestesiología y Reanimación* **60**, 552–562 (2013).
75. Seo, Y., Shinar, H., Morita, Y. & Navon, G. Anisotropic and restricted diffusion of water in the sciatic nerve: A 2 H double-quantum-filtered NMR study. *Magnetic resonance in medicine* **42**, 461–466 (1999).
76. Bendszus, M., Wessig, C., Solymosi, L., Reiners, K. & Koltzenburg, M. MRI of peripheral nerve degeneration and regeneration: correlation with electrophysiology and histology. *Experimental neurology* **188**, 171–177 (2004).
77. Gocmen, S. & Sirin, S. The effects of low-dose radiation in the treatment of sciatic nerve injury in rats. *Turkish neurosurgery* **22**, 167–173 (2012).
78. Hotz-Boendermaker, S., Marcar, V. L., Meier, M. L., Boendermaker, B. & Humphreys, B. K. Reorganization in secondary somatosensory cortex in chronic low back pain patients. *Spine* **41**, E667–E673 (2016).
79. Luchtmann, M. *et al.* Structural brain alterations in patients with lumbar disc herniation: a preliminary study. *PLoS One* **9**, e90816 (2014).
80. Chang, C. & Shyu, B.-C. A fMRI study of brain activations during non-noxious and noxious electrical stimulation of the sciatic nerve of rats. *Brain research* **897**, 71–81 (2001).
81. Apkarian, A. V. *et al.* Chronic Back Pain Is Associated with Decreased Prefrontal and Thalamic Gray Matter Density. *J. Neurosci.* **24**, 10410–10415 (2004).
82. Flor, H., Braun, C., Elbert, T. & Birbaumer, N. Extensive reorganization of primary somatosensory cortex in chronic back pain patients. *Neuroscience letters* **224**, 5–8 (1997).
83. Ung, H. *et al.* Multivariate classification of structural MRI data detects chronic low back pain. *Cerebral cortex* **24**, 1037–1044 (2012).
84. Adamczyk, W. M., Luedtke, K., Saulicz, O. & Saulicz, E. Sensory dissociation in chronic low back pain: Two case reports. *Physiotherapy theory and practice* 1–9 (2018).
85. Koefman, A. J., Licari, M., Bynevelt, M. & Lind, C. R. Functional magnetic resonance imaging evaluation of lumbosacral radiculopathic pain. *Journal of Neurosurgery: Spine* **25**, 517–522 (2016).
86. Ng, S. K. *et al.* The Relationship Between Structural and Functional Brain Changes and Altered Emotion and Cognition in Chronic Low Back Pain Brain Changes. *The Clinical journal of pain* **34**, 237–261 (2018).
87. Strutton, P. H., Theodorou, S., Catley, M., McGregor, A. H. & Davey, N. J. Corticospinal excitability in patients with chronic low back pain. *Clinical Spine Surgery* **18**, 420–424 (2005).
88. Chiou, S. Y., Shih, Y. F., Chou, L. W., McGregor, A. H. & Strutton, P. H. Impaired neural drive in patients with low back pain. *European Journal of Pain* **18**, 794–802
89. Tan, L. A. *et al.* High prevalence of greater trochanteric pain syndrome among patients presenting to spine clinic for evaluation of degenerative lumbar pathologies. *Journal of Clinical Neuroscience* (2018).
90. Freeman, S., Mascia, A. & McGill, S. Arthrogenic neuromusculature inhibition: A foundational investigation of existence in the hip joint. *Clinical Biomechanics* **28**, 171–177 (2013).
91. Strutton, P. H., Catley, M., McGregor, A. H. & Davey, N. J. Corticospinal excitability in patients with unilateral sciatica. *Neuroscience letters* **353**, 33–36 (2003).
92. Anstie, F. E. *Neuralgia and the Diseases that Resemble it*. (Appleton, 1872).
93. Kakitani, F. T., Collares, D., Kurozawa, A. Y., Lima, P. M. G. de & Teive, H. A. G. How many Babinski's signs are there? *Arquivos de Neuro-Psiquiatria* **68**, 662–665 (2010).
94. Miranda, H., Viikari-Juntura, E., Martikainen, R., Takala, E.-P. & Riihimäki, H. Individual factors, occupational loading, and physical exercise as predictors of sciatic pain. *Spine* **27**, 1102–1108 (2002).
95. Haugen, A. J. *et al.* Estimates of success in patients with sciatica due to lumbar disc herniation depend upon outcome measure. *European Spine Journal* **20**, 1669–1675 (2011).
96. Haugen, A. J. *et al.* Prognostic factors for non-success in patients with sciatica and disc herniation. *BMC musculoskeletal disorders* **13**, 183 (2012).
97. Jensen, O. K., Nielsen, C. V. & Stengaard-Pedersen, K. One-year prognosis in sick-listed low back pain patients with and without radiculopathy. Prognostic factors influencing pain and disability. *The Spine Journal* **10**, 659–675 (2010).
98. Tubach, F., Beauté, J. & Leclerc, A. Natural history and prognostic indicators of sciatica. *Journal of Clinical Epidemiology* **57**, 174–179 (2004).
99. Sarno, J. E. *Healing Back Pain: The Mind-Body Connection.* (Grand Central Life & Style, 2010).
100. Hilton, J. *On Rest and Pain: A Course of Lectures on the Influence of Mechanical and Physiological Rest in the Treatment of Accidents and Surgical Diseases, and the Diagnostic Value of Pain.* (Wood, 1879).
101. De Weerdt, C., Journee, H., Hogenesch, R. & Beks, J. Sympathetic dysfunction in patients with persistent pain after prolapsed disc surgery. A thermographic study. *Acta neurochirurgica* **89**, 34–36 (1987).
102. Ochoa, G. & Abella, P. Disk Herniation-Related Sciatica Radicular Pain: An Expression of a CRPS ? *Global Spine Journal* **02**, (2012).
103. Skorupska, E., Rychlik, M. & Samborski, W. Intensive vasodilatation in the sciatic pain area after dry needling. *BMC Complementary and Alternative Medicine* **15**, 72 (2015).
104. Konnai, Y., Honda, T., Sekiguchi, Y., Kikuchi, S. & Sugiura, Y. Sensory innervation of the lumbar dura mater passing through the sympathetic trunk in rats. *Spine* **25**, 776–782 (2000).
105. Takebayashi, T., Cavanaugh, J. M., Kallakuri, S., Chen, C. & Yamashita, T. Sympathetic afferent units from lumbar intervertebral discs. *Bone & Joint Journal* **88-B**, 554–557 (2006).
106. Suseki, K. *et al.* CGRP-immunoreactive nerve fibers projecting to lumbar facet joints through the paravertebral sympathetic trunk in rats. *Neuroscience Letters* **221**, 41–44 (1996).
107. Brown, M. *et al.* Sensory and sympathetic innervation of the vertebral endplate in patients with degenerative disc disease. *Journal of Bone & Joint Surgery, British Volume* **79**, 147–153 (1997).

Chapter 3 The causes of sciatica

Key points

- Low back disorders are the most common cause of sciatica
- Gluteal region disorders are the second most common cause of sciatica
- Systemic illness such as autoimmune or vascular disease may contribute to sciatica
- Patients may have more than one source of pain

A changing paradigm

The two most common causes of sciatica are **lumbar disc herniations (LDH)** and **lumbar stenosis (LSS)**. Lumbar disc herniation is a condition in which intervertebral disc material extends beyond its normal boundary and into the spinal canal or intervertebral foramen. Lumbar spinal stenosis is a disorder of the lumbosacral nerve roots caused by narrowing of the spinal canal or foramina. The pain resulting from both LDH and LSS is thought to arise due from compression, degeneration, swelling, and inflammation of lumbar and sacral nerve roots.[1]

Physicians have held various ideas about the cause of sciatica for thousands of years. The earliest concepts in the BCE era involved the notion that fluids within the body were out of balance. Later theories focused on the hip joint and finally the sciatic nerve itself. Until at least 1917 sciatica was mostly considered a neuritis, "a disease in itself, a distinct entity."[2]

Some early physicians recognized the **multifactorial** nature of sciatica. In 1864 Henry William Fuller, a medical doctor in London, was the first on record to state "sciatica is not itself a disease, but rather is a symptom of many diseases."[3] Around 1930 the discovery of LDH brought major attention, which allowed systemic and non-spinal causes to be overlooked. A similar trend occurred with the diagnosis of LSS.

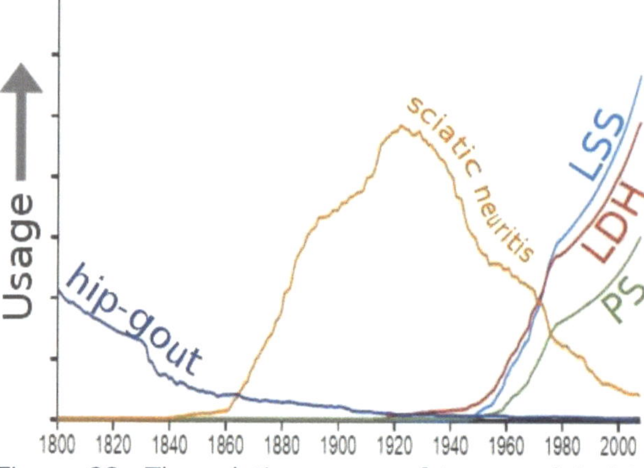

Figure 23: The relative usage of terms related to select popular sciatica diagnoses in books. Information obtained from Google's ngram service. Abbreviations include: lumbar disc herniation (LDH), lumbar spinal stenosis (LSS), piriformis syndrome (PS). The popularity of hip-gout faded in the late 1800s, and popularity of sciatic neuritis faded after about 1920.

Lumbar disc pathology is not always painful. **Degenerative disc changes** are common in people that do not suffer from back pain or sciatica. For example, over half of patients age 30 have signs of disc degeneration, and over half of those age 50 will have at least one lumbar disc bulge.[4] Asymptomatic disc protrusions also increase with age, in contrast to disc extrusions and sequestrations which are rare, and occur in less than 5% of asymptomatic people.[5] Changes to the lumbar discs are not necessarily painful and may be a part of **normal aging**.[4]

Lumbar spinal stenosis (LSS) is the second most common cause of sciatica. There is a poor correlation between severity of LSS on imaging studies and the severity of symptoms. One systematic review in 2016 was unable to prove any correlation between MRI findings of LSS and the severity of the patient's pain.[6]

Although LDH is the most common cause of sciatica, it accounts for only about half of all cases.[7] Some authors estimate that 90% of cases of sciatica are caused by LDHs.[8,9] However, this number is probably an overestimate, due in part to research studies that fail to include mild cases of sciatica, exclude rare causes of sciatica, or rely on lumbar MRI which misses pelvic, sacroiliac, or lower extremity causes of sciatica.

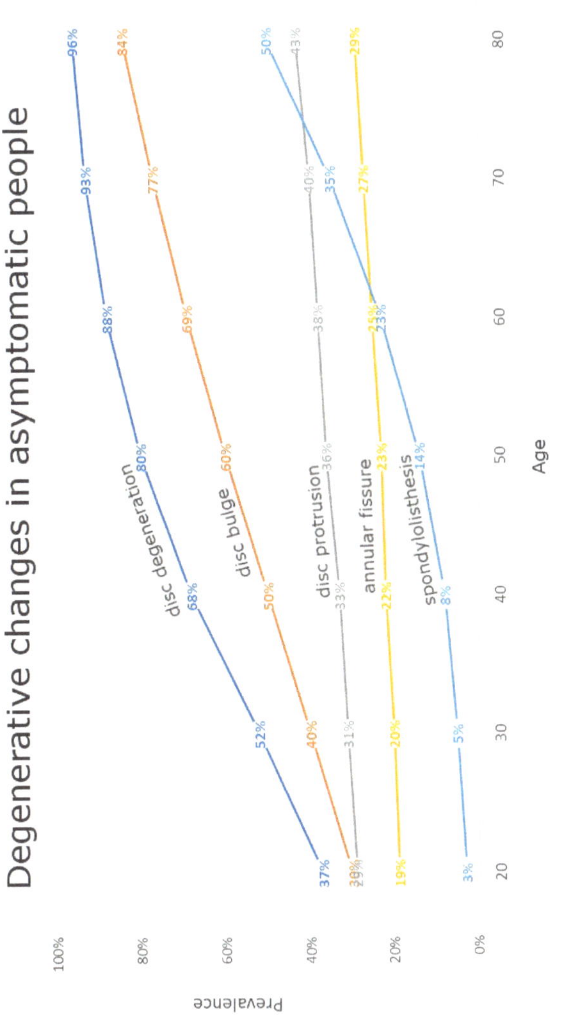

Figure 24: Asymptomatic disc changes are common and increase with age. Data adapted from Brinjikji.[4] Disc extrusions and sequestrations are not common even with aging.

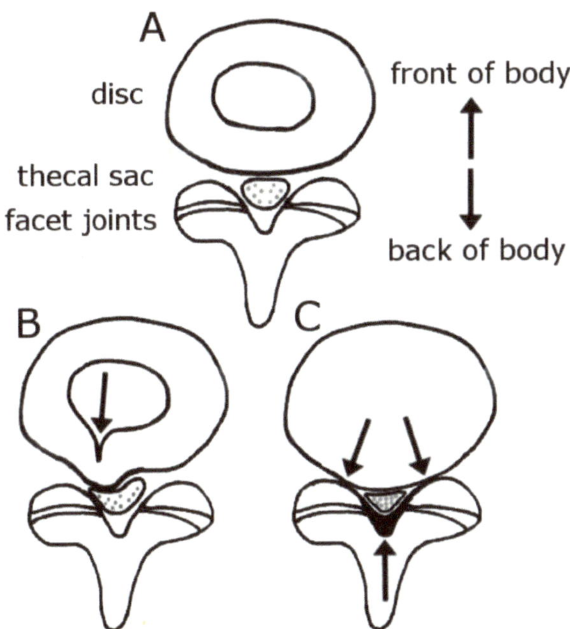

Figure 25: The two most common causes of sciatica. A: Normal IVD, thecal sac with its cauda equina (lumbar, sacral, and coccygeal nerve roots), and facet joints. B: Lumbar disc herniation causing a compression of the nerve roots within the thecal sac. C: Lumbar stenosis with a broad-based disc bulge and enlargement of the facet joints and spinal ligaments that narrows of the spinal canal and compresses the nerve roots.

Extraspinal or **non-radicular** causes of sciatica do not involve the nerve roots of the low back. One study of 452 patients with sciatica found that only 61% had nerve root compression caused by lumbar LDH or LSS.[7] The other 39% of patients with sciatica had no evidence of nerve root involvement.[7] Another study, a surgical series of patients undergoing lumbar spine surgery for sciatica, found no nerve root compression in 18% of cases.[10] Extraspinal and non-radicular causes of sciatica make up a surprising 18-39% of cases of sciatic pain.

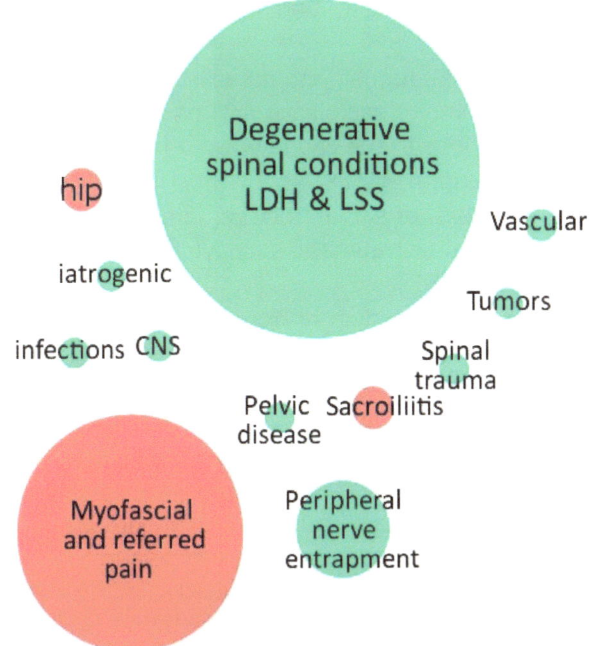

Figure 26: Causes of sciatica visual cluster. Circle size is proportional to the % cause of sciatica. Smallest circles are <1%. Sacroiliac and hip are each 1%. Peripheral nerve entrapment is 5%. Green indicates neurogenic pain while red indicates referred somatic pain

Table 4: Causes of sciatica by percentage

Degenerative spinal conditions: 61%[7] • LDH, LSS, lumbar disc bulge, instability, annular fissure
Myofascial & referred pain: >32%[7] • Myofascial pain or trigger points with referred sciatic pain (~20%),[11] greater trochanteric pain syndrome (18%)[11]
Peripheral nerve entrapments/injuries: >5% • Deep gluteal or piriformis syndromes (5%),[12] all other (1%):[13] Sciatic n. in the thigh, common peroneal nerve, tibial nerve, posterior femoral cutaneous nerve, superior cluneal nerve
Inflammatory conditions & arthritides: 1%[12,14] • Sacroiliitis; ankylosing spondylitis, calcium pyrophosphate deposition disease, gout, tumoral calcinosis, vasculitic neuropathy, inflammatory radiculitis
Hip joint diseases: 1%[14] • Hip joint cysts, acetabulofemoral joint arthritis, osteonecrosis
Pelvic diseases: <1%[15] to 8%[12] • Nerve compression by fetus, endometriosis, hematoma, pelvic tumor, uterine fibroid, ovarian cyst, retroverted uterus
Tumors: <1%[16,17] • Tumors of the spine and sacrum, cauda equina, sciatic n., and vascular malformations
Infections: <1%[16] • Bacterial, fungal, and parasitic infections of the spine or sacroiliac joint; bacterial or viral infections of the cauda equina
Spinal trauma: <1%[14,15,18] • Vertebral or sacral fracture, lumbosacral dislocation or traumatic spondylolisthesis
Iatrogenic: <1% • Fibrosis, scarring, or nerve trauma related to surgery, spinal injection, or radiation
Neurologic diseases: <1% • Amyotrophic lateral sclerosis, multiple sclerosis, hereditary motor and sensory neuropathy
Vascular diseases: <1% • Rare as primary cause including aortoiliac occlusive disease & epidural varices. Arterial stenosis may be a contributing factor in a larger percentage of patients (8%)[19]

One study using electromyography (EMG) in patients with suspected lumbosacral radiculopathy (a low back nerve root disorder) found that 30% of patients suspected of having radicular sciatica actually had a myofascial disorder.[11] The most common diagnoses aside from radiculopathy (60%) were **myofascial pain syndrome** (20%) and **trochanteric bursitis** or iliotibial band syndrome (18%).[11] The study also found that 24% of those with radiculopathy also had an overlapping myofascial disorder. The advantage of this study was that it relied on the functional information provided by EMG rather than MRI which may show asymptomatic disc pathology.

Each case of sciatica may result from a combination of factors. For example, a patient may have a disc bulge with a secondary piriformis syndrome, with components of both intraspinal and extraspinal sciatica. A patient may have lumbar stenosis complicated by trochanteric bursitis. Any combination of degenerative spinal conditions, infectious diseases, vascular compromise, nerve entrapment, or other disease may combine to produce the symptom of sciatica.

The development of advanced imaging techniques in the 20th century made it easier to diagnose LDH and, as a side effect, ignore the less common causes of sciatica. Advanced imaging does not easily distinguish **symptomatic** from **asymptomatic** LDHs. It is only part of the diagnostic puzzle and must be correlated with a good history and physical examination. Over-reliance on diagnostic imaging combined with the high prevalence of disc degeneration may lead to over-diagnosis of discogenic sciatica.

Although the diagnosis of LDH and LSS has increased in recent years, these disorders only cause 6 out of 10 cases of sciatica. This should force us to re-examine forgotten concepts about sciatica such as hip and sacroiliac arthritis, myofascial disorders of the gluteal region, and sciatic nerve entrapment. Every hundred years the focus has shifted to a new condition as the primary cause of sciatica. Clinicians need to break this cycle by reframing sciatica as a symptom with many causes.

Abnormal neurodynamics

Fibrosis and adhesions

Fibrous adhesions, also called **periradicular fibrosis**, **perineural adhesions**, **epidural fibrosis**, **granulation tissue**, or **scar tissue**, may adhere nerve roots to the spine. Fibroblasts produce this fibrotic tissue in response to inflammation, for example in response to an LDH. Fibrosis tethers nerve roots and restricts movement along the sciatic nerve pathway.

One study in 1965 reported fibrous adhesions as a cause of sciatica. The researchers found nerve root adhesions in autopsies of people who suffered from sciatica.[20] The investigators hypothesized that these adhesions could increase sciatic nerve tension:[20]

> *The tethering effect of innumerable filmy fibrous adhesions, and particularly those in the region of the foramina, makes the nerve root a relatively fixed point from which downward stretch occurs... in those cases where downward movement is less, tension in the nerve and pressure over the bony prominences are correspondingly increased.*

In a healthy person the **conus medullaris** (the end of the spinal cord) slides up and down with body movements. The conus medullaris normally slides inferiorly 3.5 mm when the leg is raised.[21] This movement can be limited by spinal pathology such as fibrous adhesions and LDHs, which reduce this sliding to about 0.8 mm.[22] Normal sliding of the conus is thought to protect against adverse neural tension.[23]

The lumbosacral **nerve roots** slide through the intervertebral foramina with leg movements. The roots normally slide **3-4 millimeters** when the leg is raised.[24] Intraspinal pathology such as LDHs reduce this nerve root sliding to 1 millimeter or less.[24] Limitations of nerve root sliding limits blood flow and causes damage when the sciatic nerve is placed under tension.[25]

A 5-10% increase in neural tension can limit **blood flow** to the nerve, **axoplasmic flow**, and **nerve conduction**.[26] In sciatica, these factors may already be limited, so that when stretch is applied they are further restricted. Neural tension applied to an already-inflamed nerve causes neural discharges that can be painful.

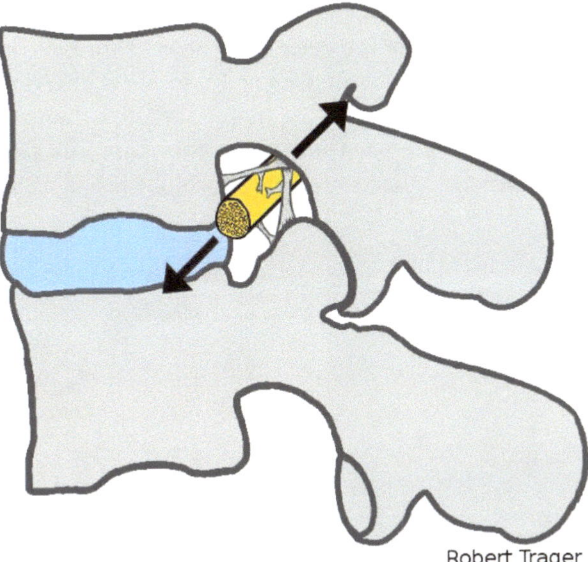

Robert Trager

Figure 27: Nerve root within the intervertebral foramen (IVF). Ligaments normally protect the nerve roots from friction by centering them within the IVF and protecting them from friction and excessive traction (arrows). Any abnormal increase or decrease in connective tissue will adversely affect the movement of the nerve root. Image by Robert Trager, DC.

Layers of sheathes surround the sciatic nerve trunk while multiple membranes and ligaments surround the sciatic nerve roots. Pathology or binding of this connective tissue restricts movement of the sciatic nerve pathway or directly compresses the neural structures. Excessive tethering at any point will increase tension along the rest of the pathway and increase the likelihood of sciatica.

Foraminal ligaments hold the nerve roots in the center of the intervertebral foramina. This protects the nerve roots from compression, friction, and excessive traction. Injury to the foraminal ligaments disturbs the delicate balance of nerve root mechanics. An increase or thickening of ligamentous tissue restricts nerve movement while a decrease or weakening leads to excessive movement and friction.[27]

Foraminal ligaments are involved in nerve root compression in cases of LDH and LSS.[28] These conditions cause inflammation that results in an increase in fibrosis around the affected nerve roots and a decrease in blood flow to them.[29] While the foraminal ligaments normally protect the nerve roots, as they degenerate and calcify they may impinge upon the nerves in a **guillotine effect**.[30] Calcification of the ligaments around the nerve roots leads to nerve root compression and lack of blood flow.

In patients with discogenic sciatica, fibrous adhesions restrict **nerve root gliding** through the intervertebral foramina. One study found that sugical removal of LDH and fibrotic material restored normal nerve root gliding.[25] The nerve roots can only slide fully when they are free of abnormal fibrous adhesions.

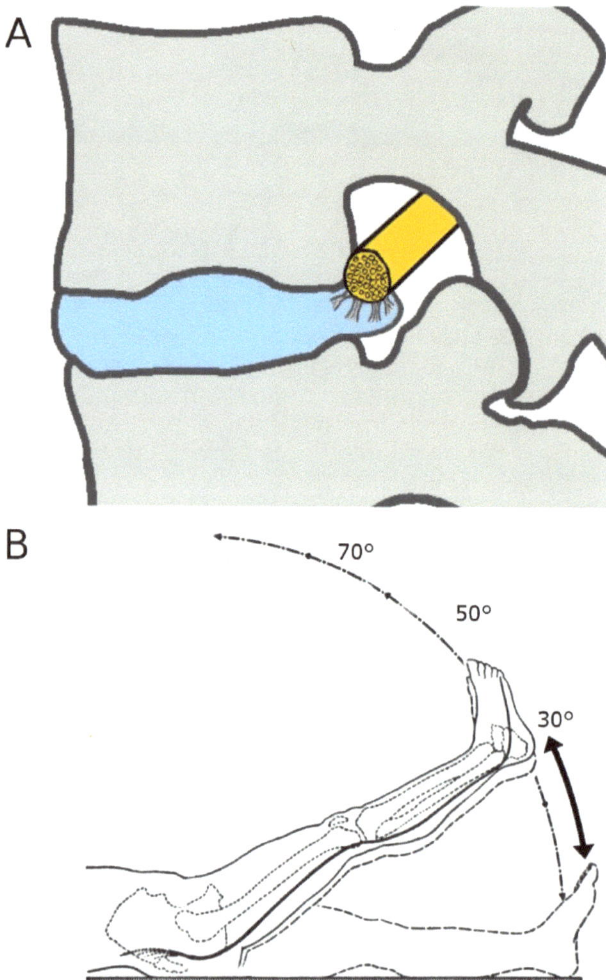

Figure 28: Fibrotic adhesions between the disc and nerve root limit nerve root mobility (A) and as a result also restrict sciatic nerve mobility, for example causing pain at a reduced angle of the straight leg raise test (B). Right image modified by author from public domain image from Ver Brugghen's Neurosurgery in general practice, 1952.

Fibrosis around the nerve roots is one of the most common reasons for back surgery to fail in treating radicular pain. Studies using epiduroscopy (a fiber optic scope) of the lower back of patients with chronic nerve root pain often show an "angry red swollen nerve" root surrounded by adhesions.[29] One study of patients diagnosed with **failed back surgery syndrome** identified adhesions in over 90% of patients.[31]

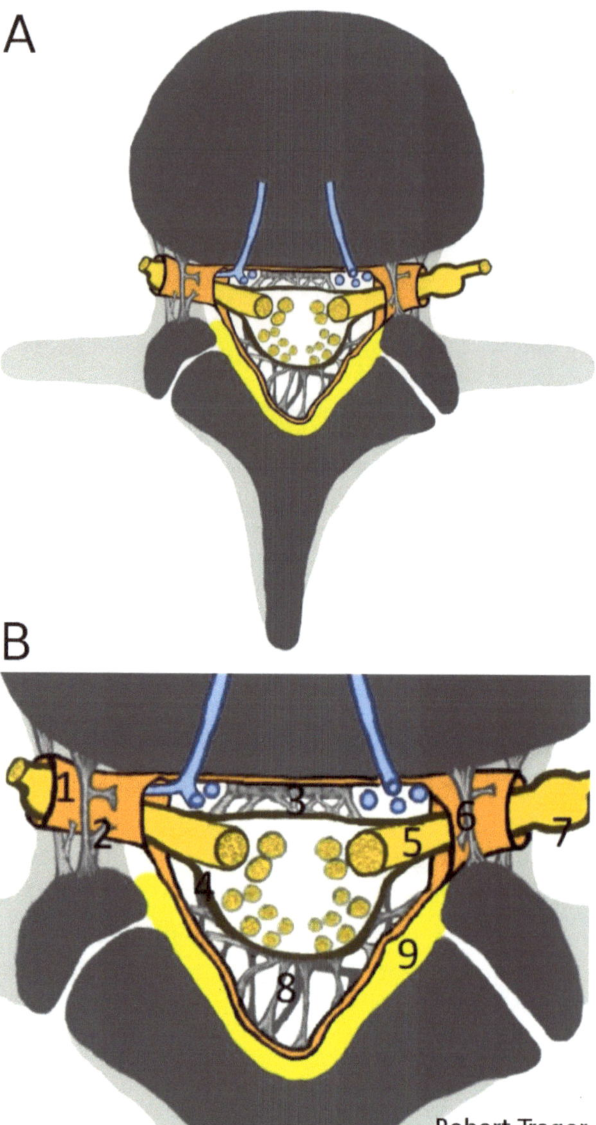

Figure 29: Ligaments connecting the lumbosacral nerve roots to the spine, in an axial section of a lumbar vertebrae (A) spinal segment, and (B) close-up of spinal canal. Peridural membrane (1), intraforaminal ligament (2), ventromedian ligaments of Trolard (3), which attach to the posterior longitudinal ligament (not labeled), thecal sac dura mater (4), nerve root (5), transforaminal ligament (6), dural sheath (7), dorsolateral ligaments of Hoffman (8), and ligamentum flavum (9). Image by Robert Trager, DC.

Myofascial tension

Myofascial (muscle and fascia) tension and increased neural tension are interwoven problems in sciatica. While each condition can occur separately, there is overlap between these two factors. Contracted or injured gluteal muscles and hamstrings can entrap or compress the sciatic nerve. Leg muscles such as the soleus in soleal sling syndrome can entrap branches of the sciatic nerve.

Those with tight or injured **hamstrings** are more likely to have sciatic nerve tension symptoms. One study found that lower extremity pain during the slump test was more common in people that felt they had tight hamstrings.[32] Nearly half of these symptoms were completely relieved by neck extension, indicating a neural component of the lower extremity symptoms.[32] Another study found a painful slump test was more common in athletes with a history of hamstring strain.[33]

Adhesions between the **epimysium** (outer sheath) of the thigh muscles and the **paraneural sheath** (outer sheath) of the sciatic nerve may limit sciatic mobility following hamstring injury. The sciatic nerve passes through a tunnel formed by the epimysium of the biceps femoris, semimembranosus, and adductor magnus (hamstring muscles). Surgical studies have shown that scarring of the biceps femoris tendon related to injury may adhere to the sciatic nerve.[34,35] Chronic injury of these muscles may restrict movement of the traversing sciatic nerve.

Tethered cord

Tethered cord syndrome is a painful condition of increased spinal cord tension caused by an abnormal attachment of spinal connective tissue. Thickened or tight tissue at the end of the cord called the **filum terminale** pulls the spinal cord downward. Normally the spinal cord ends at L1 but in tethered cord syndrome the cord extends below L2. Over 50% of those with tethered cord syndrome have sciatica or some kind of leg pain.[36] Tethered cord syndrome is an extreme example of increased neural tension.

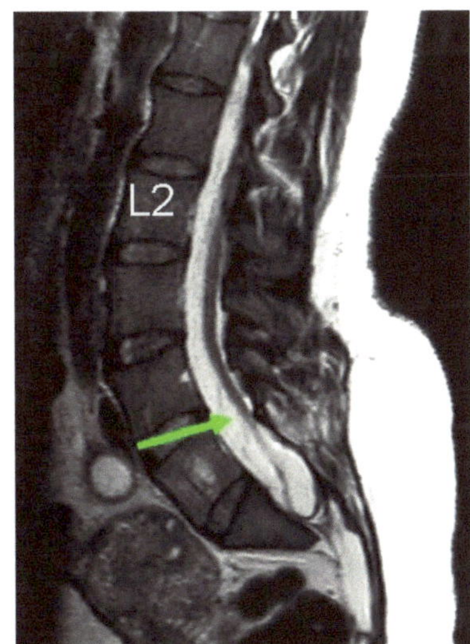

Figure 30: Patient with tethered cord syndrome causing back and leg pain. The spinal cord ends much lower in the spine (arrow) than normal. Right image CC-BY-2.0 license from Moens et al.[37]

Spiraling

The sciatic nerve derives some of its normal **elasticity** from a coiling mechanism called **Fontana's spiral bands**. These bands are formed from coiling or spiraling of perineurium and endoneurium.[38] When movements stretch the sciatic nerve, the distance between bands increases and the nerve uncoils. When movements lessen this stretch, the nerve recoils, and the bands become closer. One study using human cadavers observed this spiraling during a straight leg raise.[39] Sciatic nerve coiling may enable the nerve to stretch properly.[38] Adhesions or damage to the perineurium may interfere with sciatic nerve mobility by interfering with spiraling.

Neural ischemia

Prolonged excessive stretching of the sciatic nerve restricts blood flow within the nerve and can cause sciatica. This type of injury is rare but can occur following surgery under anesthesia if the patient is placed in a flexed position such as the jack-knife.[40] This can also occur when one falls asleep in a fully flexed position, for example while inebriated.[41] People that develop an injury in this manner may have severe sciatica at first, but typically have a good recovery.

Discogenic sciatica

Discogenic sciatica is sciatic pain that originates from a disorder of the lumbar IVD. It may result from IVD bulges, herniations, or annular tears that cause nerve root compression or inflammation.[42,43] Disc herniations are the most common cause of sciatica.

Epidemiology

Up to 14% of the population develops disc-related sciatica each year.[44] The peak incidence is at age 39, and 68% of LDH occur between the ages of 33 and 45.[45] The most common segment for LDH and nerve root compression in the intervertebral foramen is L4-5, followed by L5-S1 and L3-4.[46] LDHs and nerve root compression at L1-2 and L2-3 are rare.

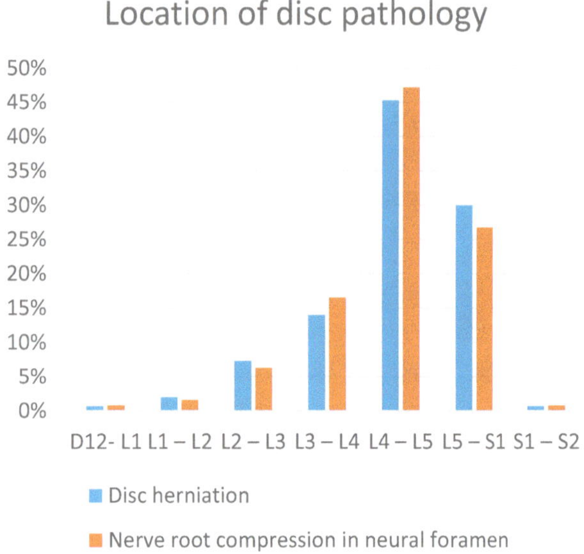

Figure 31: Location of LDHs and nerve root compression in the intervertebral foramen. Data adapted from Suthar et al.[46]

Aging paradox

Disc herniations most often occur in young and middle-aged adults, even though discs degenerate with increasing age. Disc degeneration may be associated with some forms of LDH; however, disc degeneration and herniation are not equivalent. Disc herniations occur more often in healthy discs than degenerated ones.[47] Disc degeneration is not a prerequisite for LDH.[48]

The nucleus pulposus (NP) of a younger, healthier, disc is more likely to herniate than an older, degenerated disc. Younger discs have more **proteoglycans** which gives them a greater potential to absorb water[49] and a higher **intra-discal pressure**. Older discs contain less water, have more collagen, are more **fibrotic** and stiffer,[50,51] and have a lower intra-discal pressure.[52]

Disc pressure is part of the mechanism of LDH. **High intra-discal pressure** coupled with **mechanical failure** of the endplate or annulus, forces NP material out of the disc. This problem is illustrated by astronauts who experience above-normal swelling and pressure of the NP in the low-gravity environment of outer space, and are at a greater risk of LDH.[47]

Table 5: Phases of the lumbar IVD, adapted from Antoniou[53]

Phase and age	Major processes
Age 0-15 Growth	• Synthesis of aggrecan and procollagens I and II • Denaturation of type II collagen
Age 15-40 Aging and maturation	• Reduction in synthesis of cartilage molecules except for type I procollagen
Age 40-80 Degeneration and fibrosis	• Increase in denatured type II collagen

It is not entirely clear what **normal aging** of the lumbar disc consists of,[51] although it begins in the teenage years.[53] All discs lose their blood supply in the first half of the second decade of life, which contributes to disc aging.[54] Discs gradually dehydrate with age, which appears as a darkening of the NP on a T2-weighted MRI. In addition, the NP becomes less homogenous and the boundary between the NP and annulus fibrosus (AF) disappears.[55] At a molecular level, collagen fibers cross-link (bundle) together which makes the disc more fibrotic and stiffer.[51,56] Chondrocytes (disc cells) have a limited lifespan and gradually become **senescent**, a period in which they are inactive. Factors that damage the disc such as trauma, smoking, and diabetes often accelerate chondrocyte senescence.[57] Healthy discs have more living chondrocytes than herniated discs.[58] Chondrocytes in degenerated or herniated discs proliferate quickly in areas of damage, possibly to help with repair, then become senescent.[59]

Disc degeneration is any detrimental change of the lumbar IVD that is inconsistent with normal aging.[51] Some authors consider disc degeneration to be a form of accelerated aging.[60] However, one study found that disc degeneration was distinct from normal aging in that there was a chronic low-grade inflammation.[60]

Discovery of the disc herniation

Hippocrates may have been the first to describe the IVD when he described a "mucus and ligamentous connection extending from the cartilages right to the spinal cord" around 400 BCE.[61] In 1838 Key, Aspland, and King reported autopsy findings of an "intervertebral substance, projected into the canal" at T12 and L2 as the cause of a patient's paralysis.[62] In 1858 Luschka illustrated the "extension" of the nucleus of the IVD at L2-3, based on autopsy.[63] Henry Gray's first iconic anatomy text was published this same year, illustrating the "pulpy center" and surrounding fibers of the disc.[64]

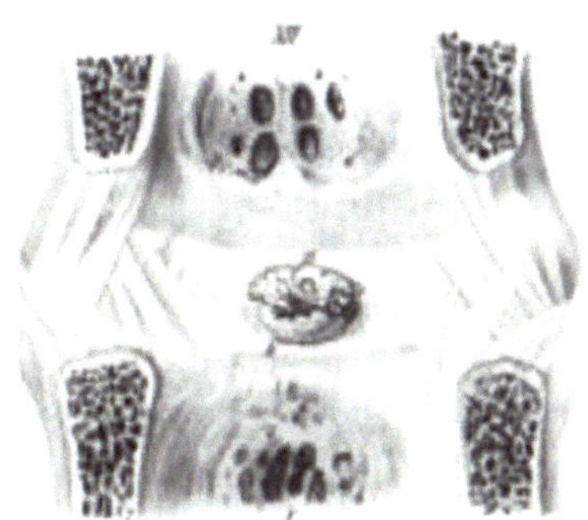

Figure 32: Hubert Luschka's illustration of an "extension" of the nucleus from Die Halbgelenke des menschlichen Körpers, 1858, public domain.

In 1879 Vulpian identified an LDH in a dog.[65] In 1896 Kocher identified a disc "dislocation" at L1-2 in an autopsy of a 26-year-old man who had fallen 100 feet.[66] In 1908 Krause and Oppenheim performed the first discectomy when they surgically removed a cartilaginous "tumor-mass" to resolve a patient's sciatic pain.[67]

In 1911 Middleton identified displaced disc material in the vertebral canal at T12-L1 on autopsy of a man who was lifting a heavy object, felt a "crack" in his low back, and developed paraplegia.[68] That same year Goldthwait was the first to suggest a "possible displacement of the intervertebral disk" in a patient suffering from sciatica who did not respond to conservative treatment.[69]

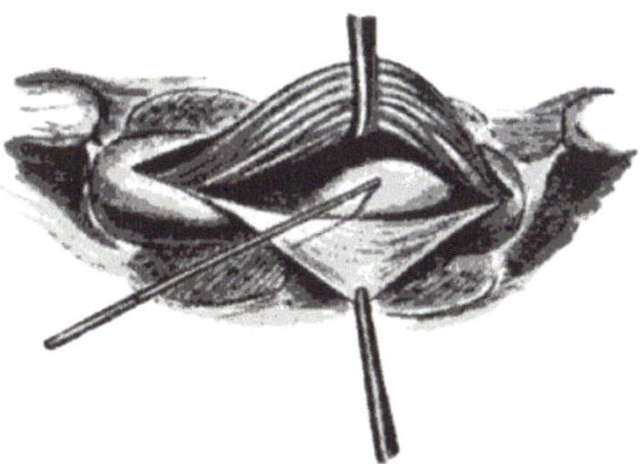

Figure 33: Extradural enchondroma, Krause, 1911, public domain. The excised tissue was probably an LDH but was mistaken for a cartilaginous tumor.

From 1922-1934 multiple authors (e.g. Adson, Bucy, Alpers) described "chondromas" of the IVD, and a consensus built that this lesion was more common than previously thought.[70,71] In 1928 Alajouanine & Petit-dutaillis of Paris realized that these common spinal masses were a "herniation of the central pulp of the disc."[72] In 1929 Dandy surgically removed "loose vertebral cartilage" to alleviate two cases of sciatica.[73] In 1934 Mixter and Barr published a series of nineteen discectomies which conclusively linked rupture of the disc to sciatica.[74]

Disc anatomy & physiology

There are five IVDs that make up the large joints on the front part of the lower back. Each disc has a fibrous outer ring called the **annulus fibrosus (AF)** and an inner gelatinous core called the **nucleus pulposus (NP)**. Hard but porous **cartilaginous endplates (CEPs)** sandwich the top and bottom of the disc. The endplates enable nutrients to diffuse into the disc from the surrounding vasculature. The health of the IVD depends on mechanical, metabolic, nutritional, and genetic factors, and age.

Table 6: Makeup of a healthy disc

	NP	AF	CEP
Cells/mm³	5,000[75]	9,000[75]	4,000[76]
ECM (main)	PGs (aggrecan), COL II [77]	COL I,[77] PGs	COL II, [78] PGs[78]
Water content %	77-81[79]	64-77[79]	46-64[79]
Collagens dry wt %	20-30[56]	58-74[56]	41-71[80]
Proteo-glycans dry wt %	35-65[81]	20[81]	10[78]
Elastin dry wt %	2[82]	2[81]	NA
PG:COL ratio	27:1[83]	2:1[83]	2:1[83]
Collagen (COL), Proteoglycans (PGs), weight (wt)			

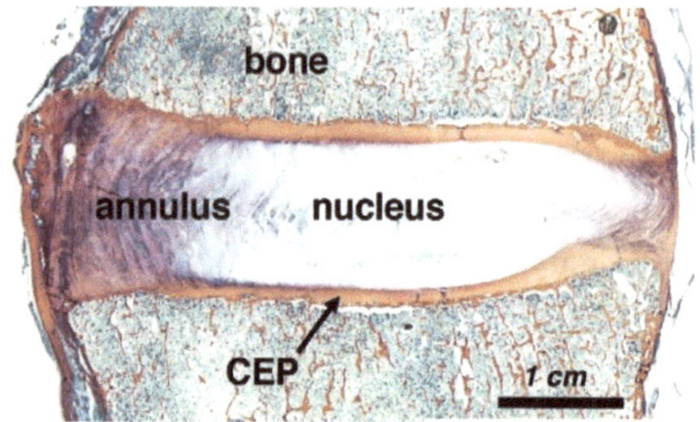

Figure 34: Mid-sagittal section of a human lumbar disc, showing the annulus fibrosis, nucleus pulposus, and cartilaginous endplate (CEP). Image Creative Commons License from Berg-Johansen[47]

Chondrocytes

Chondrocytes are the cells that live in and support the health of IVD structure. Cells of the NP, AF, and CEP produce different types of **extracellular matrix** (**ECM**) such as collagen and proteoglycans.[84] These cells have specialized functions and mechanical properties that help reinforce the structure and environment of their resident part of the disc.

Stem cells exist within the AF, CEP, and NP of the lumbar discs.[85] These cells form clusters around fissures in the annulus which help heal disc damage.[59] Disc stem cells migrate from niches (specific zones) towards damaged areas of the disc to help with repair.[86]

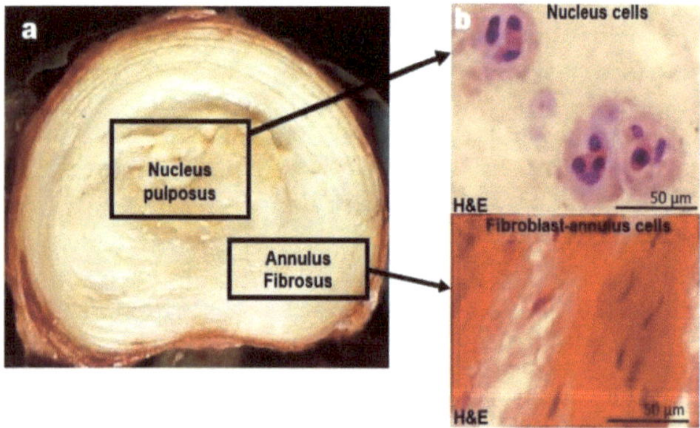

Figure 35: Macroscopic (a) and microscopic (b) view of the lumbar disc. The NP is sparsely populated by round cells that mainly produce proteoglygans, while the AF is densely populated by long fibroblast-like cells that mainly produce collagen. Image Creative Commons 3.0 License from Lama.[48]

Water content

Water makes up the greatest mass of the IVDs. Its relative weight is highest in the NP (77-81%), followed by the AF (64-77%), and CEP (46-64%).[79] Water is responsible for the biomechanical properties of the disc including shock-absorption and mobility.

Water content correlates with the amount of **glycosaminoglycans (GAGs)**, which are highest in the NP.[53] These molecules have a strong negative charge which attracts water.

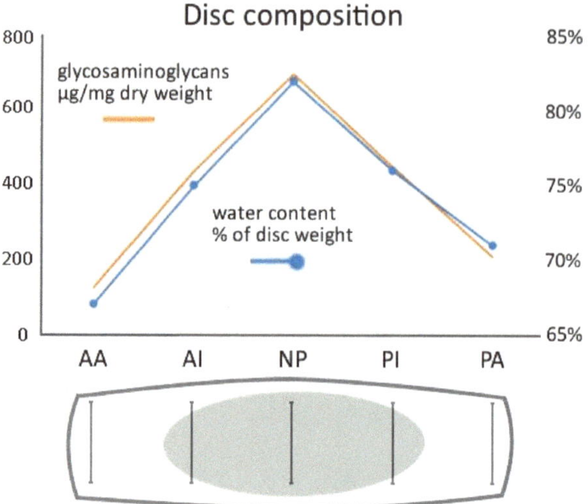

Figure 36: Glycosaminoglycan and water content of the lumbar IVDs. Data adapted from Antoniou et al,[53] using discs from age 15-25. Abbreviations: Anterior annulus (AA), anterior intermediate (AI), nucleus pulposus (NP), posterior intermediate (PI), and posterior annulus (PA). Image by Robert Trager, DC.

Nucleus pulposus

The nucleus pulposus is the gelatinous core of the IVD, which acts as a shock absorber[87] or hydrostatic ball-bearing.[88] The NP has the greatest amount of proteoglycans by dry weight percentage of any part of the disc. The NP normally has a high amount of pressure which helps support loads through the spine.

The most abundant ECM components of the NP are **proteoglycans**, the most common of which is **aggrecan**. Aggrecans are proteins that look like a bottlebrush, with the bristles being smaller molecules called glycosaminoglycans. Over 90% of the NP glycosaminoglycans consist of chondroitin sulfate and keratan sulfate.[56] These sulfated molecules have a negative charge which generates an **osmotic force** that attracts water into the NP.[89,90]

The **high proteoglycan to collagen ratio** of the NP gives it gel-like qualities.[83] For this reason, the NP is the only part of the disc that behaves more like a fluid than a solid structure. The NP also has greater amounts of proteoglycans than other types of cartilage in the body.[83] These gelatinous characteristics enable the NP to move in three planes of motion in response to loads.[83]

The NP generates high pressures that other parts of the disc must hold. The **intradiscal pressure** varies from 0.1 megapascal (MPa) to 1.1 megapascal during normal activities of daily living such as lying down to standing (not including lifting).[91] In comparison, a basketball with pressure of 9 pound-force per square inch (psi) is 0.06 Mpa. A typical car tire has a pressure of 32 psi or 0.22 MPa. This means that the normal pressure in the disc ranges from half to five times higher than the pressure in a car tire.

The NP chondrocytes have **aquaporins**, specialized water channels that help actively transport water into these cells. The intensity of the NP on T2 weighted MRI correlates directly with the amount of aquaporins.[92] Herniated and degenerated discs have less aquaporins than healthy ones.[93]

Annulus fibrosus

The AF is a structure made of rings of lamella, parallel bundles of **collagen proteins** that hold the NP. There are about 20 concentric rings of lamella that alternate each row at an oblique angle between upwards or downwards.[94] These fibers anchor into the vertebral bone, like steel-reinforced concrete, which increases their ability to withstand mechanical pressure from the NP.[95,96]

The most abundant ECM component in the AF is a protein called **type I collagen.**[77] Collagen makes up between 58-74% of the dry weight of the AF.[56] Collagen fibers make up strong barriers that resist large amounts of outward stresses from the NP when it is under pressure.[89]

Proteoglycans make up about 20% of the dry weight of the AF.[81] Proteoglycans are dispersed between bundles of collagen fibers[56] where they are the major component of the **interlamellar matrix**.[97] These proteins help absorb water and lubricate between lamellae.[97]

The AF contains about 2% (dry weight) of **elastin**, which helps the AF return to its normal shape, after the disc is deformed.[81] These fibers, along with other proteins, make up **cross-bridges** between AF lamina that help keep the lamina from separating.[98]

Lipids make up about 0.5 to 2% of the wet weight of the lumbar IVD.[99] The lipids in the IVD include triglycerides, phospholipids, and free fatty acids. These mostly exist in the AF, where they may act to lubricate the concentric lamellar rings of collagen fibers.[100]

The **disco-vertebral junction** is the area where the annulus anchors into the vertebral endplate. Collagen fibers from the AF branch out and integrate into the vertebral bone which increases the strength of this juncture. Disc herniations are less likely to occur at this site; instead, they tend to occur in the AF or around these junctions by separating a fragment of bone or endplate.[95]

Cartilaginous endplate

The cartilaginous endplates (CEPs) are thin, porous structures that confine the superior and inferior aspect of the NP and part of the AF. The CEP is the main route for **nutrient diffusion** into the NP.[84] The endplate is at most 1 millimeter thick, and porous, which allows nutrients to pass through into the avascular NP.[78] On the side of the vertebral bodies the CEP parallels another thin layer called the bony endplate.

Aside from water, the greatest mass of the CEP consists of type II **collagen**. Collagens make up 41-71% of the dry weight of the CEP,[80] followed by proteoglycans which make up 10%[78] Cartilaginous endplates have a **high collagen to proteoglycan ratio** which makes them strong and resistant to damage.[101]

The CEP transmits and **distributes loads** from the NP to the surrounding vertebra. It resists swelling pressure from the NP and prevents it from herniating into the vertebrae on either side. During this process, the CEP stretches like a drumhead as it retains the NP.[102]

The CEP allows solutes to exchange between the surrounding blood supply and IVD. This exchange occurs more rapidly in discs that are loaded and unloaded slowly as opposed to not at all.[103] **Nutrients** such as glucose, oxygen, and amino acids enter the disc while **metabolic wastes** such as lactate and degraded disc materials exit.[104]

Disc metabolism

Glycolysis is the main metabolic pathway used by healthy IVD cells.[105] Glycolysis uses glucose to produce energy in the form of adenosine triphosphate (ATP). This pathway typically runs anaerobically (without oxygen) because the oxygen concentration of the IVD is low (1-5%) and produces lactate as a byproduct.[106,107] Disc cells may have the ability to produce ATP from the citric acid cycle through fatty acid oxidation, but do not rely on this pathway for energy.[89]

The byproduct of glycolysis, **lactate**, can accumulate and damage the lumbar IVD. Lactate causes a drop in pH in the disc, making it more acidic. The optimal pH for disc chondrocytes is 6.7, and anything less than 6.5 may be detrimental to these cells.[108]

Research suggests that lactate causes inflammation, sensitizes nociceptors to stimulation, and breaks down disc proteoglycans.[109] One study showed that higher lactate levels in the cerebrospinal fluid correlated with a longer symptom duration in those with radicular sciatica.[110]

Carbonic anhydrase enzymes help counterbalance the negative byproducts of disc metabolism. These enzymes protect the disc against oxidative damage[108] and prevent the cellular pH from getting too low (too acidic).[111] Carbonic anhydrases help get rid of excess protons (related to acidity) from the disc cells, including those generated by glycolysis.[111]

Degenerated disc cells are more metabolically active than healthy disc cells.[112] They use a greater proportion of **aerobic metabolism**, using oxygen and oxidative phosphorylation to produce ATP.[105] These changes could represent a beneficial adaptation to disc damage.[112] The greater use of oxygen could relate to the vascular ingrowth seen in damaged discs which would increase oxygen supply.[105] Some research indicates that a conversion from glycolytic to aerobic metabolism could shorten the duration of symptoms in those with discogenic radiculopathy.[110]

Disc herniation fragments

Fragments of herniated discs contain varying amounts of NP, CEP, and AF material. The percentage of the predominant component of LDHs, e.g. either NP, CEP, or AF, varies between patients. Studies report a wide variability in the major component of LDH fragments, of mainly NP in 16-54% of cases, CEP in 6-44%, and AF in 2-78%.[113-115]

The percentage of each component depends on age and other variables. Nucleus pulposus material is less common with increasing age,[116] and is most commonly found in those age 30 or less.[115] Annular material is more common with increasing age.[115,116] Cartilaginous endplate material is more often found in middle-aged patients.[114] The larger the LDH, the greater the likelihood of CEP material being present.[114]

Disc innervation

Nerves innervate the lumbar discs in a **multisegmental** (from many levels) and bilateral manner.[118] Two types of nerves innervate the lumbar discs, the gray **rami communicans** from the lumbar sympathetic ganglia, and the **sinuvertebral nerve**, also called the recurrent meningeal nerve.[119] Branches of these nerves that enter the outer layer of the disc are called the **peridiscal nerves**.

Mechanoreceptors

Mechanoreceptors are specialized sensory organs at nerve endings that sense tension, pressure, and movement. Healthy discs have only a small number of mechanoreceptors in the outer AF.[120] The two most abundant mechanoreceptors are the **Ruffini receptors** and **Golgi tendon organs**, with Pacinian corpuscles being the least abundant[121] or absent altogether.[120] These mechanoreceptors occupy the outer third of the AF and anterior and posterior longitudinal ligaments.[120-122]

Nerve ingrowth

The excess growth of nerves into lumbar discs, also called **hyperinnervation**,[109] may account for **discogenic pain** (pain arising from the lumbar disc).[123] While a healthy disc only contains nerves in its outermost layer of AF, a damaged disc has nerves that penetrate much deeper.[77] **Annular fissures** enable nerve endings to grow into the disc by reducing the physical pressure and **proteoglycans**, which both normally obstruct nerve ingrowth.[124]

Nerve fibers may reach the **nucleus pulposus**[117,122,125] or central part[126] of the disc. Studies have shown that nerve fibers grow abnormally deep into **herniated discs** (with or without sciatica)[125,126] and **degenerated discs**.[117,122] One study found that non-herniated discs in patients with scoliosis and degenerative spondylolisthesis did not have nerve ingrowth.[126]

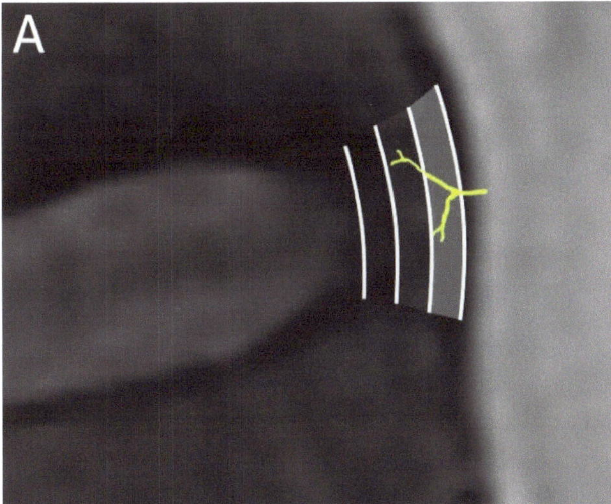

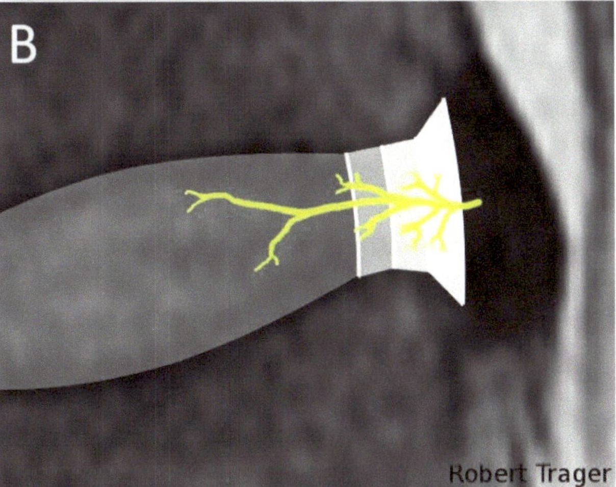

Figure 37: Nerve ingrowth into the disc. Healthy discs (A) only have nerve fibers in the outer annulus, in contrast to pathologic discs (B) which may have nerves deep into the nucleus. Healthy discs: 26% have nerve fibers in the outer third of the annulus, 6% in the middle third, 0% in the inner third, and 0% in the NP. Pathological discs: 83% have nerves in the outer annulus, 77% in the middle third, 57% in the inner third, and 30% in the nucleus. Shading corresponds to frequency of nerve fibers. Data from Freemont.[117]

Research suggests that most of the nociceptive (pain) sensation passes either directly into the **sympathetic chain** or through the **sinuvertebral nerve** towards the sympathetic chain. These neurons then ascend the spine and enter the spinal cord at **L1 or L2**.[127] The blending and ascending of nerve fibers into higher levels may explain why discogenic pain is diffuse and does not match the pattern of a single nerve root.[119]

Nerve ingrowth into damaged lumbar discs may account for **referred sciatic pain** as well as reflex **muscle spasms**. Some of these nerves act as mechanoreceptors, which can stimulate muscles to contract.[121] Discs of those with low back pain (LBP) have a greater amount of mechanoreceptors,[121] which could indicate they are more sensitive to changes in pressure, tension, or movement. One study found that an anesthetic sympathetic block alleviated lumbar spasms in those with LBP and sciatica.[128] Another study found that anesthetic injection into lumbar discs could alleviate radiating lower extremity symptoms.[129]

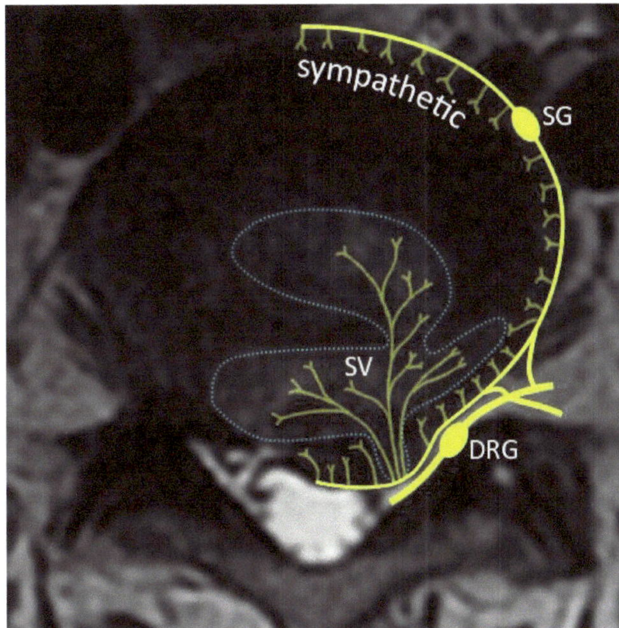

Figure 38: Ingrowth of nerves into an area of disc herniation. Nerve fibers from the sinuvertebral nerve (SV) invade an area of disc herniation (dotted area). Other nerves such as the sympathetic branches from the sympathetic ganglia (SG) which are in this case further from the site of disc herniation innervate the outer layer of AF as normal.

Vascular ingrowth accompanies nerve ingrowth. The lumbar IVD becomes mostly avascular (without blood vessels) around age 10-15, when the blood vessels atrophy and regress.[54] In adults, blood vessels normally enter the outer third of the AF, and rarely, in 6% of people, enter the middle third.[31] Blood vessels grow into damaged discs and may account for some of the symptoms of discogenic pain.[77]

Disc adaptation and repair

In a healthy and active individual, the disc continually repairs broken-down connective tissue. Connective tissue proteins such as collagen and elastin are stable for years and have a slow turnover rate.[82,130] Disc chondrocytes slowly produce these proteins to replace those that have become damaged.[82] In a healthy disc, the process of **anabolism** (building) is in balance with the **catabolism** (breakdown) of disc proteins.

Certain **hormones**, substances, and nutrients keep disc anabolism and catabolism in balance. Catabolism is stimulated by inflammation, glycation (sugar),[94] leptin (obesity),[131] and an acidic disc pH.[109] Hormones such as melatonin,[132] testosterone,[133] estrogen[134] and IGF-1[57] stimulate anabolism of the IVD.

Mechanical stress influences the anabolism/catabolism balance. Ideally, the nuclear chondrocytes produce a high amount of proteoglycans which helps absorb water. Shear stress can be harmful as it increases production of collagen and reduces production of proteoglycans in the NP.[135] High (≥ 30 atm) or low (≤ 1 atm) pressure also reduces the amount of proteoglycans produced by the NP cells.[136] Conversely, a low or physiological level of pressure (3 atm) is beneficial as it stimulates the production of proteoglycans by the nuclear chondrocytes.[136]

Mechanical factors

Mechanical stresses may damage the disc if applied in specific directions, repetitions, and amounts. Specific locations within the disc are more likely to fail with certain types or combinations of loading. Typically, **single-plane movements** are safer for the disc than **combined movements** in more than one plane.

Degeneration of the IVD often begins with damage to the annulus or endplates with repetitive mechanical stresses related to bending, lifting, and twisting. Damage can accumulate in a wear-and-tear process in which the disc **fatigues** after repetitive loading.

Acute injury is also a cause of damage. When the IVD is suddenly loaded with the lumbar spine in a flexed position, the junction between the annulus and endplate may tear.[137] Lumbar flexion combined with rotation is another position that puts the annulus at risk of fissuring.[138]

Ancient people suspected repetitive overuse of the low back to be a cause of sciatica. Amulets found in the Near East dating from 100 BCE to 500 CE show a person bending (and likely twisting) to cut grain with the word *sciatica* on the reverse side.[139] Caelius Aurelianus (c. 450 CE) described "...a violent snatching during exercise... digging in the earth when unused to this activity, or attempting to lift certain weights" as causes of sciatica.[140] (Author's translation p. 495)

Complex movements

Single-plane movements place a safe amount of stress on the lumbar disc while **complex postures**, also called **combined movements**, can be more harmful. Stress levels spike when movements such as flexion, rotation, lateral bending, and axial compression are combined.[141–143] A combination of axial compression, flexion, lateral bending, and axial rotation gives the highest risk for caudal endplate junction failure.[141]

Axial rotation

Repetitive or extreme axial torsion (twisting) of the IVD can damage the AF and make it easier for NP material to herniate through the AF. One study found that repeated axial torsion of a cow spinal unit (disc and vertebrae) damaged bundles of ECM (collagen and elastin) in the AF.[144] These areas of damage in the AF can accumulate and eventually allow the NP to progress outwards and herniate. Axial rotation is less likely to damage the endplate junction.[145]

Axial torsion by itself places a safe level of axial and circumferential stress on the AF. Axial torsion combined with flexion can increase these stresses to an unsafe level that the AF may not support.[142] Axial torsion with either axial compression or lateral bending is unlikely to cause failure of the AF.[142]

Axial compression

The lumbar IVD can withstand and may even benefit from substantial axial compression. Low level loading and unloading enhances **nutrient and waste exchange** to and from the disc.[103] Loading also stimulates NP cells **heat-shock response**, an adaptive response to stress.[146] The gelatinous NP disperses load into the CEP and AF.[94,102] Axial compression of the disc generates the lowest axial and circumferential stress on the AF of any single-plane movement.[142]

Flexion

The lumbar IVD is susceptible to damage when flexed, when flexion coincides with compression or another plane of movement. Complex movements that incorporate flexion, lateral bending, axial rotation, and compression are the most likely to injure the **endplate junction** (**EPJ**), followed by the AF.[141] Although flexion may place the greatest stress on the endplate junction,[147] by itself (without axial compression) it is unlikely to injure the endplate junction.[141]

The **EPJ** is the most susceptible to tearing when the disc is under tension, which occurs when the lumbar spine flexes.[148] One experimental study found that complex loading led to **EPJ** failure in 75% and **annulus fibrosus** failure in 25% of cow spinal units.[141] High bending loads may avulse the CEP rather than tearing the annular fibers.[148]

Flexion of the disc generates the greatest axial and circumferential stress on the AF of any single-plane movement.[142] Flexion combined with axial rotation generates the greatest stress of any two planes of motion, and reaches levels that may damage the AF.[142] The posterolateral part of the AF experiences the greatest stress during these movements.[142]

Lateral bending

Lateral bending, by itself, places a low amount of axial and circumferential stress on the AF.[142] Pure lateral bending is also unlikely to injure the endplate junction.[141] Lateral bending may only reach unsafe levels of stress when combined with lumbar flexion.[142]

Extension

Repetitive extension of the lumbar spine is more harmful to the vertebrae and facet joints than to the disc. One study using animal spinal units found that repeated extension disrupted the growth zones of the vertebrae.[149] Extension also caused the NP to migrate anteriorly rather than posteriorly,[149] which is the opposite direction of a typical radiculopathy-causing LDH.

Surprise loading

Surprise loading is any sudden load placed on the IVD more rapidly than the muscular or motor system can react or accommodate for. The spinal muscles need up to **one second** to respond to a surprise load.[143] Surprise loading is most likely to damage the EPJ, followed by the mid-span fibers of the AF.[137]

Herniation pathway

There are two general pathways for a disc to herniate, either (1) by a failure of the endplate junction with the AF, or (2) through a tear in the AF. Endplate-junction failures (EPJF) account for 65% of LDHs, while AF tears account for up to 25%.[150] Often, disc material may begin to herniate at the EPJ, then progress secondarily through the AF.

Endplate junction injuries

Endplate junction injuries, also called **endplate junction failures**, or injuries of the **endplate-bone interface** or **disc-vertebra interface**,[151] are the most common mechanism underlying LDH.[150] In an endplate junction injury, annular fibers avulse (pull off) a piece of calcified or cartilaginous endplate from the vertebra, which provides a path for the NP to migrate through.[151,152]

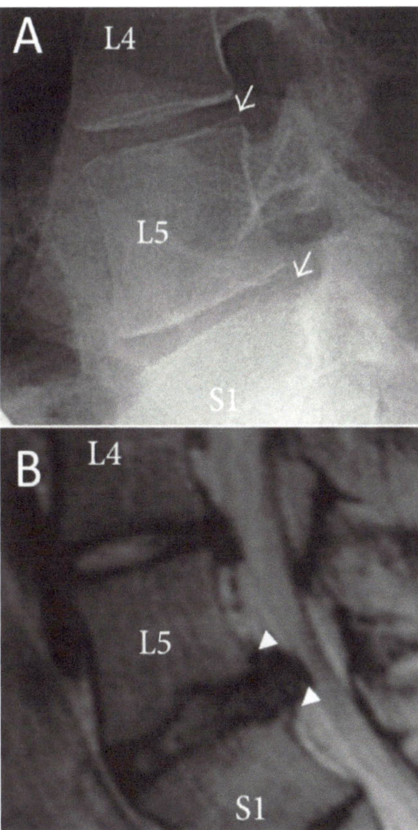

Figure 39: Endplate lesions seen on radiograph (A, arrows), and MRI (B, arrowheads) in a 14-year-old. Case from Morimoto[153] under CC-BY-4.0 license.

Endplate junction failures are due to **bony failure** in 71% of cases and isolated **cartilaginous endplate failures** in 26%.[152] Tidemark avulsions are another name for injuries at the mineralized region connecting the outer AF and calcified cartilage layer of CEP.[47] These two areas of injury may stem from different mechanisms and have different clinical pictures. Cartilaginous endplate avulsions may stem from trauma and result in LDH, whereas the more common tidemark avulsions may occur with repetitive loading, and do not necessarily cause herniation.[151]

Endplate junction failures are due to **bony failure** in 71% of cases and isolated **cartilaginous endplate failures** in 26%.[152] Tidemark avulsions are another name for injuries at the mineralized region connecting the outer AF and calcified cartilage layer of CEP.[47] These two areas of injury may stem from different mechanisms and have different clinical pictures. Cartilaginous endplate avulsions may stem from trauma and result in LDH, whereas the more common tidemark avulsions may occur with repetitive loading, and do not necessarily cause herniation.[151]

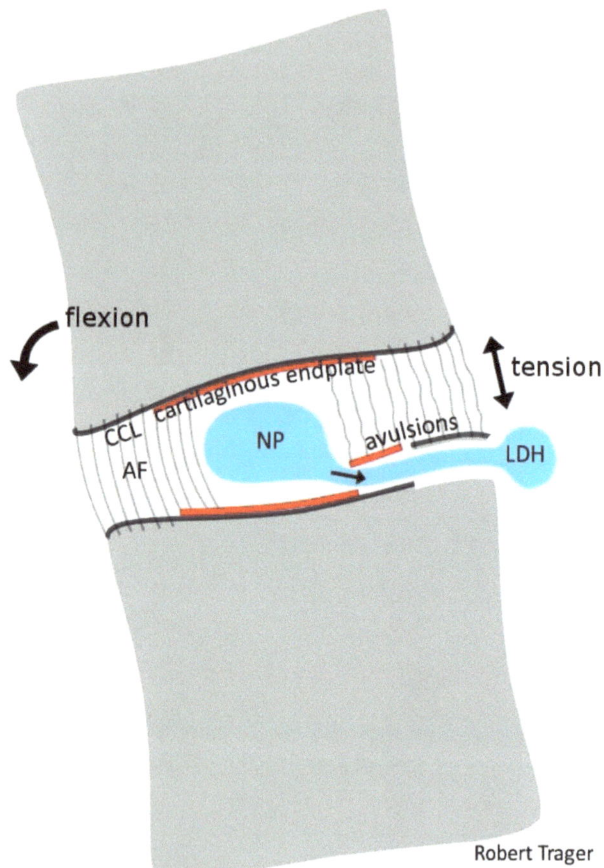

Figure 40: Endplate junction injuries. Lumbar flexion tenses the AF, which may avulse the CEP and calcified cartilage layer of the endplate (CCL), and create a pathway (arrow) for the nucleus pulposus (NP) to migrate and form a lumbar disc herniation (LDH). Image by Robert Trager, DC.

The endplate junction is prone to injury because it is a sharp transition from soft (disc material) to hard (bone) material.[148] In addition, the AF has a stronger connection to the cartilaginous and bony endplate than the endplate has to the vertebra.[147,152] The endplate junction is the weakest part of the disc in tension (lumbar flexion),[145,147] and is less affected by torsion (rotation).[145] Surprise loading also increases the risk of endplate junction injuries.[137] Signs of endplate lesions may be visible on plain radiographs, computed tomography, and standard MRI,[47,150,154] although specialized MRI techniques are used to see them more accurately for research purposes.[152] Standard MRI does not usually show endplate injuries involving the CEP, however those in the bony endplate may appear.[47]

Annular pathway

Tears in the AF interfere with its ability to hold the pressurized NP, allowing NP material to migrate out of the center of the disc and form a herniation. However, LDHs seldom penetrate solely through the AF. Nucleus pulposus material typically only breaches the AF secondary to an endplate injury, which provides the initial pathway for LDH.[148] A surgical study found that only 11% of cases of LDH resulted from the annular pathway. These cases had imaging signs of a disrupted AF but had an intact endplate.[150]

Nucleus pulposus material follows a **convoluted path** to herniate.[155] Typically, tears in the mid-annular fibers allow for pockets of NP material to form, which then connect and enlarge, forming a pathway for NP material to herniate.[155] This pathway is not usually linear, as NP material may **track circumferentially** along the annular lamella before entering the outer layers of AF.[156,157]

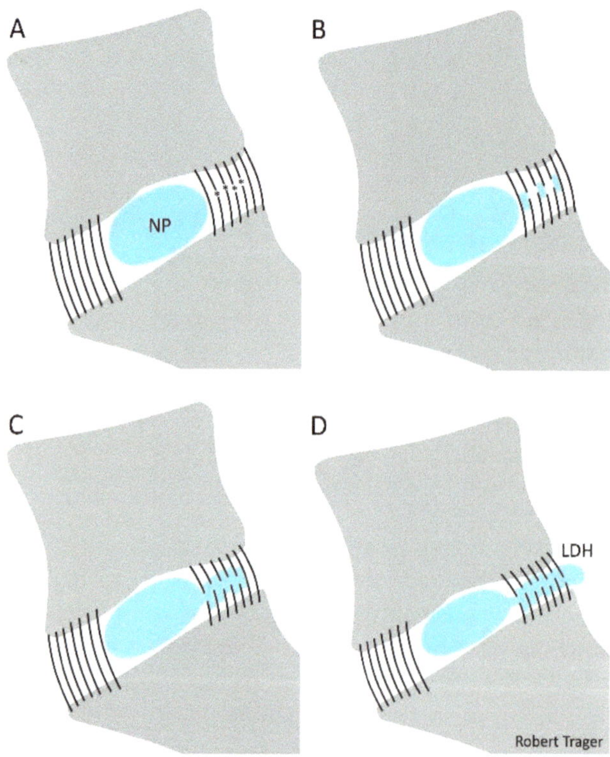

Figure 41: Annular pathway of herniation. A: Tears in the mid-annular fibers (*). B: These tears allow pockets of nucleus pulposus (NP) material to accumulate. C: Pockets of NP enlarge and connect. D: This forms a direct pathway for lumbar disc herniation (LDH). Image by Robert Trager, DC, based on the research of Wade et al.[155]

Provocative discography studies may show tracking of NP material in damaged discs. Physicians perform these studies by injecting a contrast agent into the NP, then performing imaging which may show migration of the contrast agent. These studies may show fluid migrating from the center of the IVD outwards and circumferentially along the path of the AF lamina.[156] Further migration of contrast into outer disc or leakage into the spinal canal indicates greater damage to the AF.

Herniation of NP material through the AF occurs via a sequence of events. Initially, posterior lamellae of the AF develop **circumferential** tears (along the direction of the lamellae). Next these tears fill with nuclear material, forming pockets. Finally, these pockets connect to form a direct **radial** tear (path leading outwards) for NP to migrate into an LDH.[155]

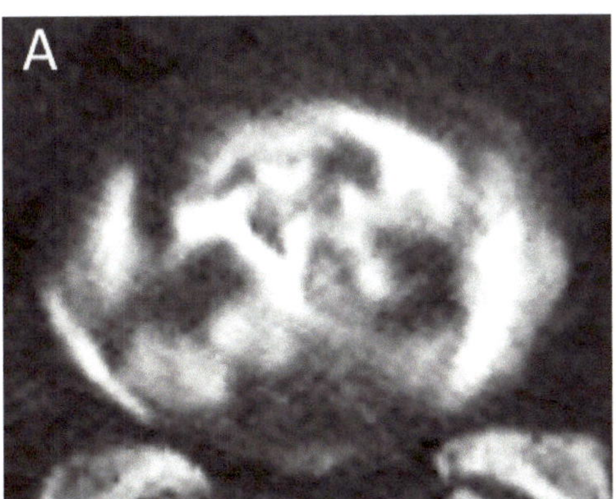

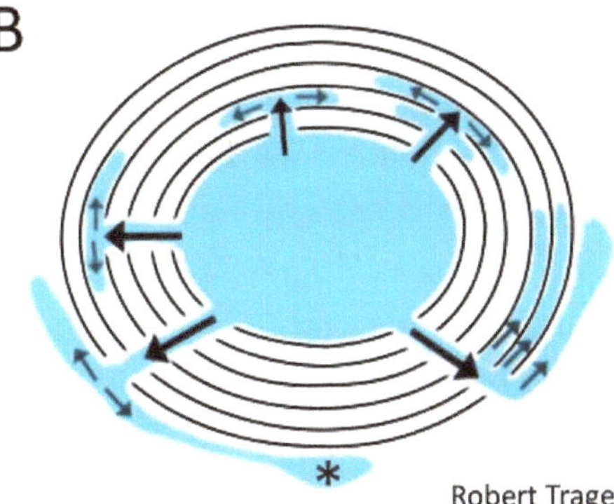

Figure 42: Circumferential tracking of NP material. This 30-year-old woman presented with chronic LBP radiating to the left gluteal region, posterior thigh, and calf. MRI showed a central disc protrusion at L5-S1 and provocative discography showed a grade 5-disc disruption. Image A shows an axial section at the L5-S1 disc on a CT scan, with the injected contrast agent migrating peripherally and circumferentialy. Image B is a schematic of the same image, showing the peripheral (large dark arrows) and circumferential (small lighter arrows) migration of nuclear material resulting in the disc protrusion. Image shared with permission of patient by Robert Trager, DC.

Lifestyle factors

The IVD contains living cells that rely on diffusion of nutrients such as glucose and oxygen from the outer parts of the disc. Any factor that reduces blood flow to the disc limits the disc cells' ability to receive nutrients, get rid of waste products, and to maintain a neutral pH (acid-base balance).[158] **Smoking** and **atherosclerosis** increase the risk for disc degeneration and herniation through adverse effects on the circulatory system.[138,158]

Glycation

Prolonged elevation in blood **glucose** damages the lumbar discs. There is some evidence that those with type II **diabetes** mellitus are at greater risk of LDH.[159] Excess sugar harms the lumbar discs by binding to and weakening the structural proteins.

Glycation is the process in which a sugar molecule attaches to a protein or lipid. In the IVD, this occurs to disc structural proteins having lysine such as proteoglycans and glycosaminoglycans.[130,160] The result is the formation of **advanced glycation end products** (AGEs) which interfere with normal disc function.[130] The formation of AGEs from structural disc proteins makes the disc more brittle, stiff, and prone to damage.[130]

Minerals and electrolytes

Discs with herniations have altered levels of minerals and electrolytes compared to healthy discs. An altered trace element status disrupts the normal **viscoelastic qualities** of the disc and impairs its ability to absorb water and support loads. An imbalance of electrolytes and minerals may make the disc dehydrated, brittle, and prone to damage.

Healthy discs have greater levels of **potassium**. One study found that healthy discs had over 2 times the amount of potassium (0.3 vs. 0.13 mg/kg).[161] Potassium is an electrolyte that helps maintain the water content of the lumbar IVD, in particular the NP where it is in the highest concentration.[162]

Compression of a disc causes it to lose water but not potassium. After water loss, potassium is at a high concentration, which increases the **osmotic force** of the disc and helps draw water back into the disc.[162] A loss of disc potassium may reduce the ability of the NP to hydrate and lead to disc damage.

Sodium is an important electrolyte that is five[161] to ten[162] times more abundant than potassium in the lumbar IVD. Its concentration does not differ significantly between healthy and herniated discs, however it does reduce with age.[161] Research using a special type of MRI called a sodium (Na) MRI has shown that the level of sodium correlates with the amount of proteoglycans in the lumbar IVD.[163] Discs with less sodium on MRI have less proteoglycans and are more degenerated.[163]

Healthy lumbar discs have elevated levels of **copper** (Cu) compared to other body tissues and degenerated discs. One study found that healthy discs had about five times greater copper than herniated disc material (5.9 vs. 1.2 mg/kg).[161] Healthy discs also have three times greater levels of Cu than bone and cartilage.[164] Copper is the only trace mineral found in a higher concentration in the disc than in bone and cartilage.

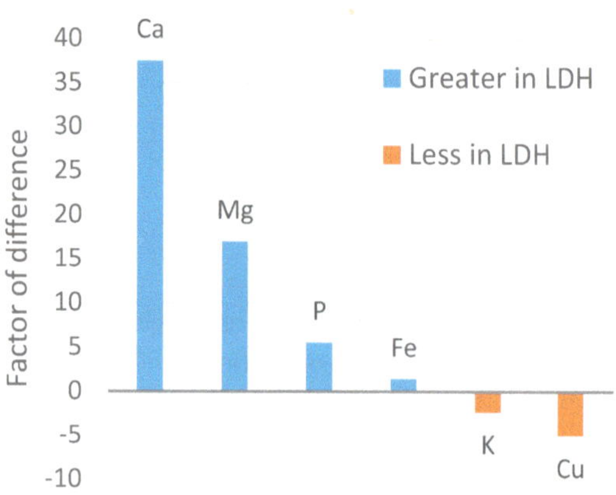

Figure 43: Relative difference of trace elements in a herniated versus healthy lumbar disc. A herniated disc has 38 times greater calcium and five times less copper than a healthy disc. Data from Staszkiewicz et al.[161]

Enzymes that build and sustain disc structure and metabolism require Cu. Copper is a cofactor for **lysyl oxidase**, an enzyme that catalyzes the cross-linking of collagen and elastin, both important structural components of the disc. The enzyme **cytochrome oxidase** that produces cellular energy in the mitochondria of chondrocytes also requires Cu.

Herniated discs have higher amounts of **calcium** and **phosphorus**. One study found that herniated disc material had 38 times the amount of calcium compared to healthy discs (1.5 vs. 0.04 mg/kg), making it the greatest difference of any trace element from healthy to unhealthy discs.[161] The study also found that the amount of calcium in herniated discs correlated strongly with the amount of phosphorus.[161] This may be because high calcium levels combine with phosphorus to form **calcium pyrophosphate** in the IVD. Other research has shown that microscopic calcifications occur in over half (54%) of herniated lumbar discs compared with less than 10% of normal discs (8%).[165]

Herniated[161] and degenerated discs[164] have greater amounts of **magnesium** (Mg). Some research shows that this may be part of the natural healing response to disc injury. Macrophages and fibroblasts that migrate to the disc to help repair it may raise the Mg content of degenerated discs.[164]

Herniated discs have higher amounts of **iron** (Fe).[161] Iron is necessary for certain proteins and oxygen transport, but can be harmful in too high of a concentration. Those with hemochromatosis (iron overload) may develop calcifications in the lumbar discs, but it is unclear if iron causes the same effect in those without hemochromatosis.

Toxin accumulation

Environmental toxicants can accumulate in the lumbar IVD. Examples include **lead** (Pb),[161,164,166,167] **cadmium** (Cd),[161,164,166,167] and **aluminum** (Al).[164,166–168]

The concentration of these toxicants is influenced by environmental factors, genetics, and blood flow to the disc.[161] Certain substances such as Aluminum (Al) and Lead (Pb) increase with age.[167] Toxicants have complex associations, such as a positive correlation between Al and Mg but a negative correlation between Cd and Mg.[164,167]

Toxicants may have a detrimental effect on lumbar disc tissue. One study using animals found that Pb exposure lead to death of disc chondrocytes and reduced the disc height.[169] Cadmium may damage disc proteins by disturbing the function of enzymes.[166] Fortunately, the disc is not the main reservoir for these toxicants, as they tend to accumulate in other body tissues at greater concentrations.[164,167]

Types of discogenic sciatica

Diverse types of disc pathology may cause sciatica. The most common cause, an LDH, is a **focal displacement** of disc material beyond the normal limits of the IVD.[170] Annular fissures (tears in the AF) and disc bulges (a generalized extension of the disc) are less likely to cause sciatica. The most common classification of LDH is by shape, distinguishing three types of LDH: **protrusions**, **extrusions**, and **sequestrations**.[170]

Disc bulges involve more than 25% of the disc circumference.[170] Disc protrusions involve less than 25% of the disc circumference and their base is wider than the displaced herniated material.[170] Disc extrusions involve less than 25% of the disc circumference and their base is narrower than the displaced herniated material.[170] In disc sequestrations, the herniated material has no connection to the disc.[170]

The size and location of LDHs predict the likelihood that they will cause sciatica. Larger LDHs have a stronger relationship to sciatic pain. Those with at least **6.8 millimeters** of anterior to posterior dimension predict the presence of sciatica with 98% probability.[172] Conversely, LDHs of less than 3 millimeters do not have a strong correlation with sciatic symptoms.[172] Lumbar discs that compress a nerve root have 2.6 times greater odds of causing leg pain.[173] Discs can herniate and not compress a nerve root, for example, with small LDHs in the central part of the spinal column.

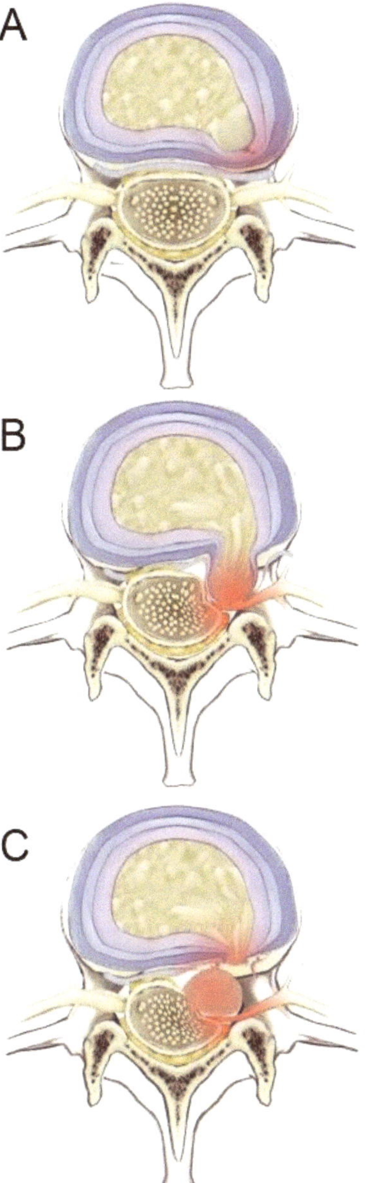

Figure 44: Disc herniation types. Protrusion (A), extrusion (B), and sequestration (C). Image from Weiner,[171] CC-BY-2.0 License.

Disc extrusions have the strongest association with sciatic pain and increase the odds of having radicular pain by a factor of 5.4.[174] **Nerve root impingement** by any material including any type of disc bulge or herniation also increases the odds of sciatic pain.[174]

Table 7: Classification of lumbar disc herniations.

Morphology[170]	• Protrusion • Extrusion • Sequestration
Location in the axial plane[170]	• Central • Subarticular • Foraminal • Extraforaminal • Anterior
Location in the sagittal plane[170]	• Discal • Infrapedicular • Pedicular • Suprapedicular
Relation to the posterior longitudinal ligament[170]	• Subligamentous • Transligamentous
Segment	• Upper (L1-2, L2-3) • Mid lumbar (L3-4) • Low lumbar (L4-5, L5-S1) • Sacral (S1-S2)
Symptoms	• Symptomatic • Asymptomatic
Degree of nerve root compression[175]	• None • Abutment • Displacement • Entrapment
Degree of spinal canal or foraminal compromise[170]	• Mild (<1/3) • Moderate (between 1/3 and 2/3) • Severe (> 2/3)
Consistency [115,176]	• Soft (mostly NP) • Hard (CEP, AF, bone, or calcification)
Histology	• CEP • NP • AF

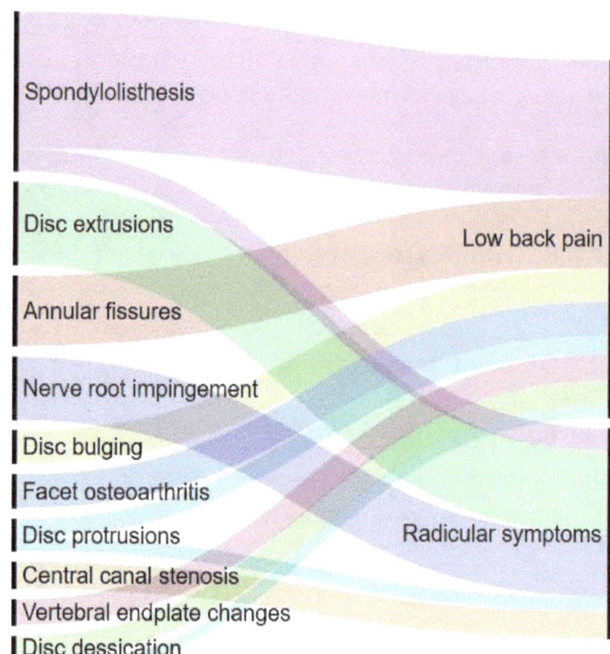

Figure 45: The relationship between imaging findings and symptoms. Data adapted from Suri et al.[174] The width of each row corresponds to the magnitude of the Diagnostic Odds Ratio (DOR). For example, spondylolisthesis has a large odds ratio of 8.9 for low back pain, and a small odds ratio of 1.5 for radicular symptoms.

Annular fissures

Annular fissures, also called annular tears, occasionally cause sciatica by allowing the NP to leak and inflame the lumbosacral nerve roots.[43,123,177] This condition is also called a **chemical radiculopathy** or **painful disc** andx is seen on MRI as a **high intensity zone**. However, annular fissures do not often cause sciatica and instead have a greater association with chronic lower back pain.[174]

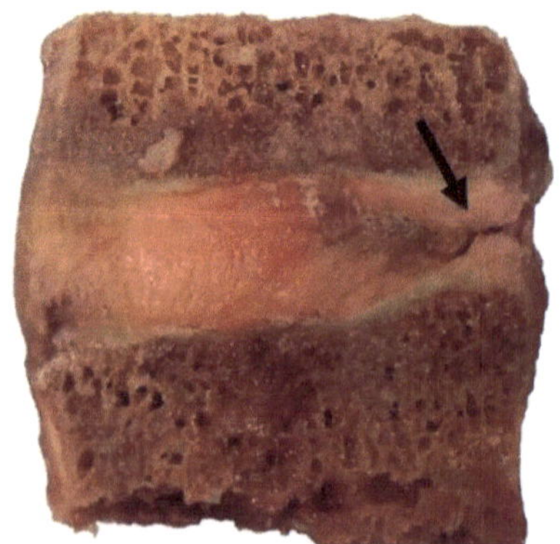

Figure 46: Annular fissure in a cadaveric disc (arrow). Image Creative Commons Attribution License from Berg-Johansen[47]

Disc degeneration refers to disc desiccation (loss of fluid), disc narrowing, changes to the endplate, and presence of osteophytes at the edge of the vertebrae. These findings are related to lower back pain but by themselves do not have a significant association with sciatica.[174]

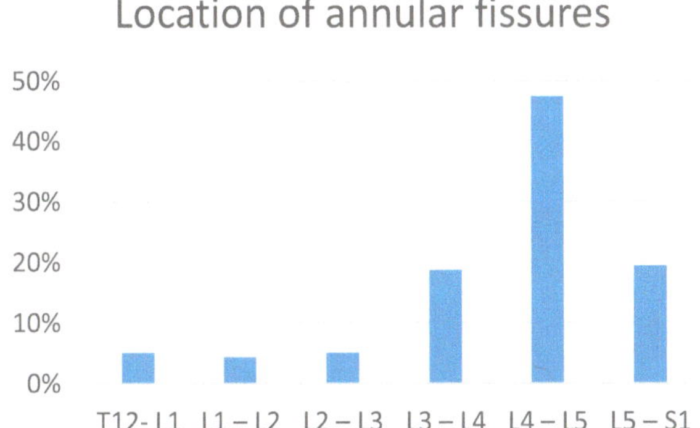

Figure 47: Location of annular fissures. The most annular fissures occur at L4-5. Data adapted from Suthar et al.[46]

Symptoms

The classic symptom of discogenic sciatica is **radicular pain**, pain that radiates from the lower back into the lower extremity in the distribution of a nerve root. In over 90% of cases of discogenic sciatica this pain is only on one side[178] and only one or two nerve roots are affected.[179] In over 90% of cases either the L5 or S1 nerve root or both are affected.[180]

Cauda equina syndrome is a severe surgical emergency and rare outcome of LDH involving compression of multiple nerve roots in the lower back. This condition is recognized by rapidly progressing sensory and motor deficits,[182] an area of involvement greater than the typical LDH, symptoms in the saddle or groin region, and bladder involvement. Discogenic sciatica rarely progresses into cauda equina syndrome.

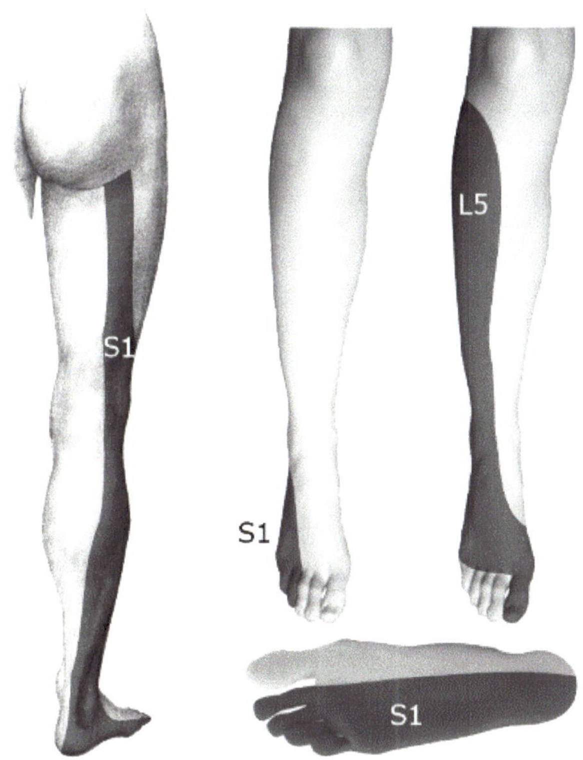

Figure 48: L5 and S1 dermatomes (shaded). Non-shaded regions indicate areas of major variability and overlap. Drawing based on Lee's 2008 evidence based dermatome map.[181] Image by Robert Trager, DC, by modification of public domain Gray's anatomy images (left), image of leg by Andrea Allen (CC by 2.0), and image of foot by Pixel AddIct (CC BY 2.0).

Spinal stenosis

Lumbar spinal stenosis (LSS) is a degenerative condition of the lumbar spine that narrows the lumbar vertebral canal or neural foramina. Lower extremity pain related to these changes is called neurogenic claudication. Some authors use the term **symptomatic lumbar stenosis** to describe this scenario.[183] Disc degeneration, ligament thickening, and bony growth around the facet joints are the most common causes of LSS. The presence of claudication or sciatic symptoms in those with LSS depends on many factors including the lumbar canal size, lumbar instability, inflammation, and metabolic and cardiovascular health. A narrowed lumbar canal is only one risk factor for sciatica and does not necessarily cause symptoms by itself.

Table 8: Classification of lumbar stenosis.

Cause[198]	• Congenital • Developmental • Acquired • Combined
Location[194,198,199]	• Central • Lateral recess • Foraminal • Extraforaminal • Mixed (Central, lateral recess, and/or foraminal)
Distribution[194]	• Single level • Multi-level
Kinematic[199]	• Stable • Unstable
Symptoms[186]	• Symptomatic • Asymptomatic
Structures involved[200,201]	• Soft stenosis / ligamentous • Hard stenosis / nonligamentous

Around 450 CE, Caelius Aurelianus described a type of LBP that forced people to sit or bend forwards to obtain relief.[184] Today, clinicians would recognize these symptoms as neurogenic claudication. In 1918, the French neurologist and radiologist Sicard believed the main cause of sciatica was compression and inflammation of the nerve roots and their vessels in the intervertebral foramina.[185] In 1950 the Dutch physician Verbiest published cases linking lower extremity pain with walking to a narrowed spinal canal.[187]

Although the prevalence of radiographic LSS increases with age, only a fraction of those with a narrowed canal develops symptoms. The prevalence also varies depending on which criteria are used to diagnose LSS on imaging studies.[188] One study in Japan found that 77% of people of an average age of 66 had imaging findings of LSS, but only 9% of these had symptoms of LSS.[189] Symptomatic LSS increases with age starting from around age 60.[190]

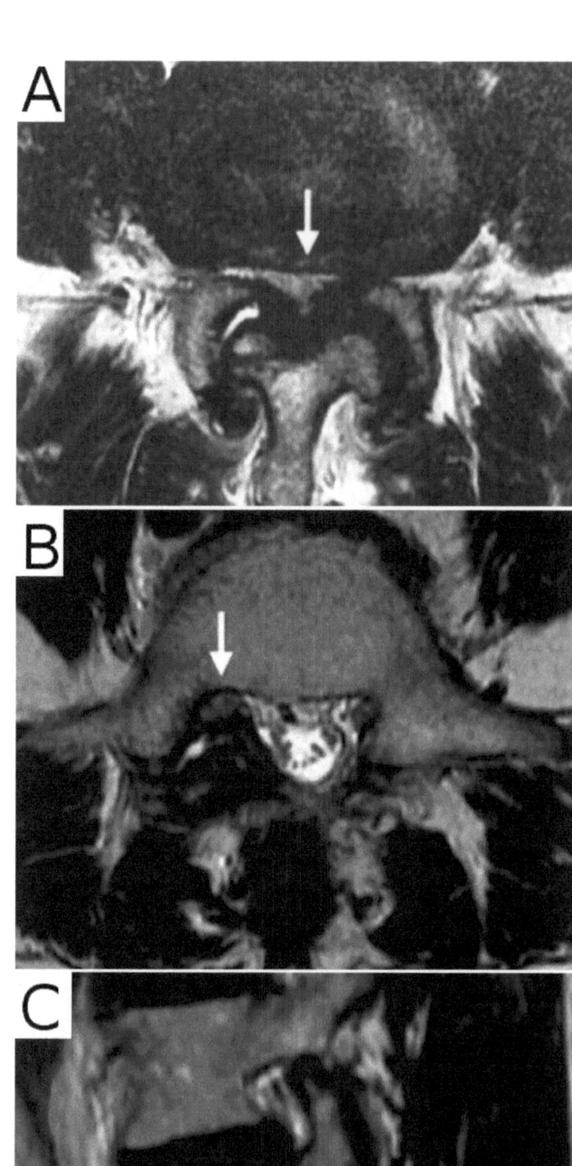

Figure 49: Locations of lumbar stenosis. Central canal (A), lateral recess (B), and foraminal (C). Cropped from Jiann-Her Lin, CC-BY-4.0 license.[186]

The timing of the closure of the **neurocentral synchondrosis** (NCS), a growth plate between the vertebral body and **pedicles**, is the major factor that determines size of the lumbar spinal canal.[191,192] The mid-sagittal diameter of the lumbar canal increases until age 5 when the NCS begins to close[192] although it remains open until age 10.[193] The coronal dimension of the spinal canal, as measured by the **interpedicular distance**, increases until age 17.[192] Early NCS closure may be caused by genetic, prenatal, and environmental factors in childhood and thus relates to both congenital LSS (born with LSS) and developmental LSS (begins in childhood).

Acquired stenosis is the most common type of LSS. One study found that absolute (≤ 10 mm spinal canal) acquired stenosis occurred in 7.3% of people while the sum of congenital and developmental occurred in 2.6% of a population with an average age of 53.[188] When less restrictive criteria are used to diagnose LSS (≤ 12 mm spinal canal), the prevalence of acquired stenosis is even greater (23.6%) than that of congenital and developmental stenosis (4.7%).[188]

Most patients with LSS have **mixed stenosis** involving the central canal, lateral recess and/or intervertebral foramen (about 68%).[194] Only a fraction of these patients have isolated stenosis of the central canal or lateral regions.[194] Considering only moderate-to-severe imaging findings, the most common pattern of LSS is **single-level** involvement, occurring in about 60% of patients.[194] The most commonly involved lumbar segment is **L4-5**, which is stenotic in 61% of those with LSS.[194]

Those with LSS may have a **clinically silent** spinal narrowing that becomes symptomatic abruptly. The lumbosacral nerve roots may be damaged by inflammation related to disc pathology, ischemia due to vascular pathology, or repetitive stretch due to lumbar instability.[195] Other research has shown that LSS may convert from asymptomatic to symptomatic following a hip[196] or cervical spine surgery.[197] Vascular pathology, inflammation, and/or lumbar instability are the most common reasons for someone with LSS may suddenly develop symptoms.[195]

Radiographic features of LSS do not correlate well with symptoms. In general, research has shown that imaging findings of LSS correlate with the level of **disability** but not pain severity. Imaging features of LSS correlate with walking distance,[202] disability index scores,[202,203] and the amount of neurological impairment.[204] Newer imaging techniques such as dynamic or loaded imaging may identify parameters that correlate better with symptoms.

A smaller lumbar canal worsens the clinical features of LDH. Lumbar stenosis increases the likelihood of motor deficit in those with LDH. Lumbar stenosis also predisposes patients with concurrent LDH to develop **cauda equina syndrome**.[205] According to one author, inflammatory conditions such as LDHs are one reason why asymptomatic cases of LSS become symptomatic.[195]

Congenital stenosis

Genes affecting the structure and development of bone affect the size of the lumbar spinal canal. This includes genes regulating **collagen** production,[207-209] regulatory glycoproteins,[210] and signaling proteins.[211] One study found that signaling molecules ERK1 and ERK2 in chondrocytes (cartilage cells) control the timing of the closure of the neurocentral synchondrosis. If these genes become activated too soon the synchondrosis closes and the spinal canal is smaller.[212]

Genes affecting long bone length affect the **vertebral pedicles** and the size of the spinal canal. Achondroplasia, a type of dwarfism, is a classic example of congenital stenosis with shortened pedicles. Those with achondroplasia have smaller spinal canals due to early closure of the neurocentral synchondrosis.[213] This is caused by increased activation of genes that encode bone growth signaling molecules (ERK1 and ERK2).[212] People of average height with short arm length also have short pedicles, which suggests that long bone growth is a general indicator of spinal canal size.[214]

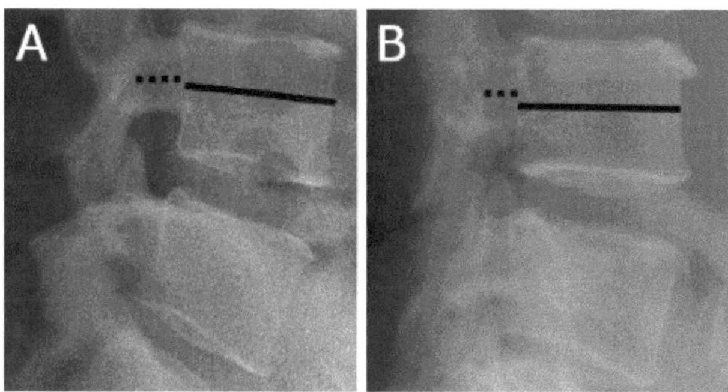

Figure 50: Normal (A) and short pedicles (B) in a sagittal plain-film radiograph. In patient A the value of the vertebral body (normal line) divided by the pedicle (dashed line) is less than 2.8, in patient B the value is greater than 2.8. Lines added to CC-BY-4.0 license image from Cheung.[206]

Patients with **short pedicles** have a greater risk of symptomatic LSS. One study found that the anterior-to-posterior (AP) dimension of the vertebral body divided by the AP dimension of the pedicle should be less than a factor of 2.8 at all levels on a plain-film sagittal radiograph. A factor over 2.8 was predictive of symptomatic LSS.[206]

Some people have a genetic predisposition for larger spinal canals. Taller people are more likely to have a larger spinal canal.[215] Those with connective tissue hypermobility syndromes including Marfan's, Ehlers-Danlos, and Loeys-Dietz syndromes may develop a widening of the spinal canal called dural ectasia, however these patients may develop other unwanted spinal problems such as scoliosis and spondylolisthesis.[216] In general, those with longer limbs compared to trunk length have a larger spinal canal.[214]

Developmental stenosis

Most of the development of the spinal canal size occurs **in utero**. Prenatal factors including a low birthweight,[217] shortened gestational age,[218] low placental weight,[217,218] maternal smoking during pregnancy,[217] and greater maternal age are associated with a narrowed spinal canal.[218] These limitations are not totally permanent, as the canal has some potential for catch-up growth, but do predispose to LSS.[217]

Malnutrition during early growth reduces the lumbar canal size. One archeological study found a smaller lumbar canal in the spines of native Americans eating a low-protein corn-based diet with those eating a high protein hunter-gatherer diet.[219] Another study identified a positive correlation between early-life malnutrition and developmental LSS.[220] Another study identified a positive correlation of dental hypoplasia, a sign of poor nutrition, with reduced lumbar canal size.[221]

Physiological stress or poor general health may stop the final phase of development of the lumbar spinal canal during childhood.[221] One longitudinal study found a positive association between the number of childhood **infections** and the presence of LSS.[222] Another study found a correlation between growth arrest lines (Harris lines) in long bones which occur in disease and malnutrition and the presence of LSS.[221]

Instability in LSS

Spinal instability, the loss of the ability of the spine under physiologic loads to maintain its pattern of displacement,[223] may account for the lack of correlation between imaging findings and symptoms of LSS. Imaging centers may perform radiographs or MRIs with the patient lying down, which is usually painless, rather than upright, which increases pain and displacement in LSS. Some cases of LSS may go undiagnosed due to imaging parameters.[224]

Weight-bearing MRIs or **standing radiographs** may correlate better with symptoms of LSS because they show the spine under load and in a position that provokes symptoms. Weight-bearing exacerbates spondylolistheses, slippage of vertebrae on one another, as well as ligament buckling and disc bulging. Some studies have found a better correlation between LSS symptoms and upright or axial loaded MRIs (rather than supine).[225,226] Other studies have found that standing radiographs showed a greater frequency of spondylolisthesis compared to supine MRI.[227] One study estimated that supine MRI missed one in three cases of LSS.[228]

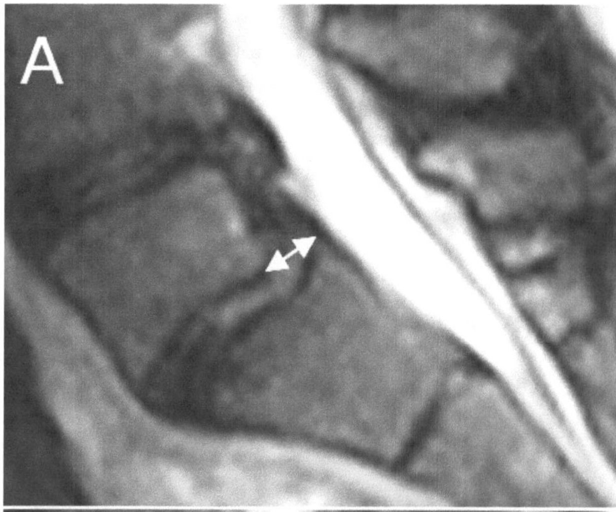

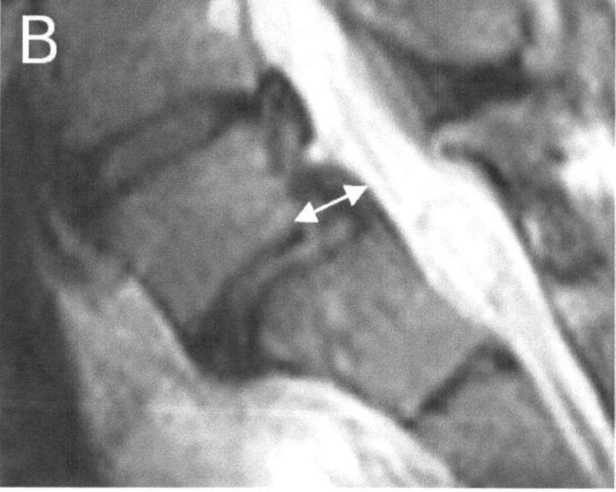

Figure 51: Lying supine (a) vs. standing (b). Standing exacerbates L5 anterolisthesis and disc protrusion. Images CC BY 2.0 license from Tarantino et al: Lumbar spine MRI in upright position for diagnosing acute and chronic low back pain: statistical analysis of morphological changes, 2012

Dynamic imaging such as **flexion/extension** radiographs or positional MRI can show changes in position of vertebrae with movement. Radiologists compare static with dynamic imaging determine if vertebrae move with the trunk flexed, extended, or loaded by gravity. More than **3 millimeters of motion** of a lumbar vertebra between standing flexion and extension images correlates with back and/or leg pain.[229]

Static radiographs and supine MRIs can show indirect signs of instability. Those with a degenerative **anterolisthesis** (forward slippage) on neutral-posture standing radiograph have 16.9 times greater odds of having instability with spinal bending.[230] Retrolisthesis, traction spurs, and spondyloarthrosis are additional signs of instability on plain-film radiographs.[230] The presence of a **facet joint effusion** greater than **1.5 millimeters** on non-weight bearing MRIs is another sign of instability.[231] **Synovial cysts** and **annular fissures** are additional signs of instability on MRI.[232]

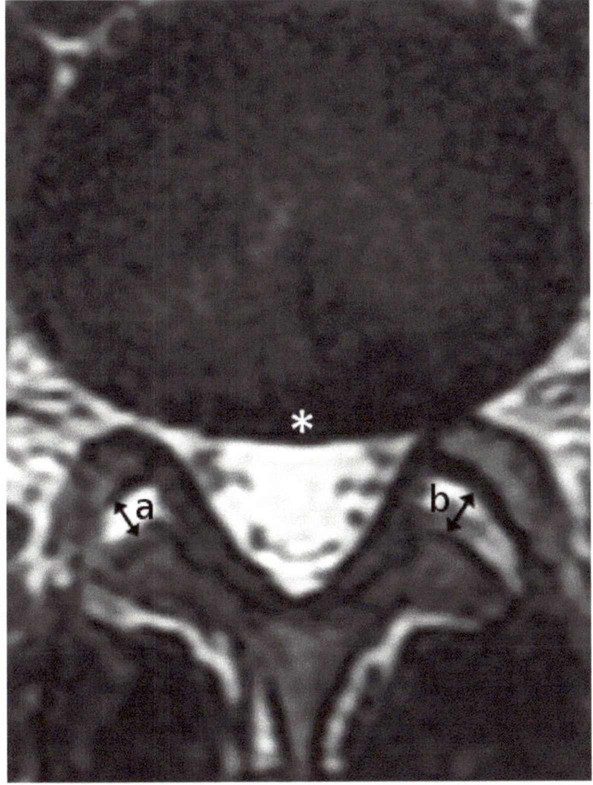

Figure 52: A facet joint effusion over 1.5 mm seen on MRI (supine MRI shown) may be a significant finding when the IVD changes are mild, such as this 4 mm disc bulge (*). Facet effusion 3.5 mm on R (a) and 4.5 mm on L (b). This 47-year-old male patient with chronic L sided sciatic pain involving the posterior/lateral glute, thigh, and leg responded well to a lumbar stabilization exercise program. Case shared with permission of patient by Robert Trager, DC.

Spondylolisthesis

The term spondylolisthesis describes slippage or displacement of a vertebra. It most commonly refers to **anterolisthesis**, a forward slippage of a vertebra, although it may also refer to lateral or retrolistheses.[233] This chapter will utilize the conventional definition of spondylolisthesis as an anterolisthesis. Spondylolisthesis is a common cause of sciatic pain and may be the most common cause of LSS in the elderly.[234] Spondylolisthesis is not always symptomatic, and the presence of symptoms depends on many factors including the type of pathology, degree of slippage, spino-pelvic posture, presence of stability, and inflammation.

The most common types of spondylolisthesis are **isthmic** and **degenerative**. An isthmic spondylolisthesis is a separation of the **pars interarticularis** (pars), the connection point of the facet joints. This can occur due to a stress fracture, repeated microfractures, or acute trauma. The most common causes of pars separation are repetitive trauma, spinal hyperextension with or without rotation, and impact caused by landing forces in sports.[235] A degenerative spondylolisthesis (**DSPL**) is a listhesis that does not have a pars defect and does not result from acute trauma or other pathology.

Table 9: Classification of lumbar spondylolisthesis.

Type (Wiltse)[233,236]	• Dysplastic • Isthmic (ISPL) • Degenerative (DSPL) • Traumatic • Pathologic • Iatrogenic
Etiology[237]	• Developmental • Acquired
Direction[233,238]	• Anterolisthesis • Retrolisthesis • Lateral listhesis
Degree of slip	• 1 (0-25%), 2 (25-50%), 3 (50-75%), 4 (75-100%)(Meyerding) [239] • Percentage slip of sacral base (1-100%)(Taillard)[240]
Disc height[241,242]	• Normal or slightly reduced • Reduced • Grossly reduced
Degree of dysplasia[237]	• Low-dysplastic • High-dysplastic
Spino-pelvic balance[243]	• Balanced (C7 ≤ hip axis) • Unbalanced (C7 > hip axis)
Pelvic incidence [243]	• Nutcracker (low pelvic incidence <45°) • Normal • Shear (high pelvic incidence ≥60°)
Symptoms	• Symptomatic • Asymptomatic
Kinematic[244]	• Dynamic (unstable) • Static (stable)

Isthmic spondylolisthesis is more common in those under age 50[245] while DSPL is more common in those over age 50. Degenerative spondylolistheses are slightly more common in women than men (1.3:1 ratio).[235] Degenerative spondylolisthesis is most common at L4,[235] while isthmic[246,247] and traumatic spondylolisthesis are most common at L5.[248] Retrolisthesis is most common at L3 and L4.[249]

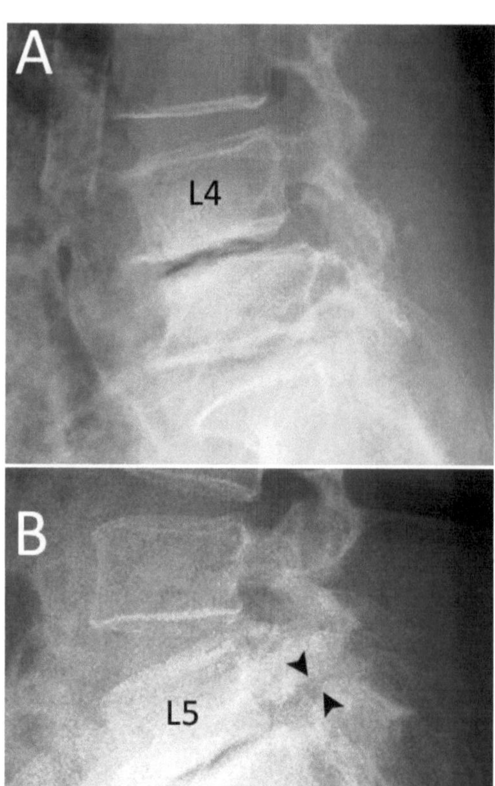

Figure 53: Degenerative (A) spondylolisthesis at L4 and isthmic (B) spondylolisthesis at L5. In degenerative spondylolisthesis the pars interarticularis is intact while in isthmic the pars has a defect (arrowheads). Both examples also show a vacuum sign (lucency) in the IVD inferior to the listhesis. CC-by-2.0 license from Lin et al.[256]

Spondylolistheses, especially mild ones, are often **asymptomatic** or an incidental imaging finding.[234] About 1/3rd of those with spondylolisthesis have signs and/or symptoms of radiculopathy.[250] The frequency of neurological symptoms correlates with degree of slippage.[250] Symptoms may be on one or both sides.

Conditions causing **ligament laxity** are associated with lumbar spondylolisthesis. This includes Ehlers-Danlos syndrome,[233] Loeys-Dietz syndrome,[251] Marfan syndrome,[251] and ligament laxity during pregnancy.[252] One study found that people with a genetic variation in collagen type IX were more likely to have lumbar spondylolisthesis with LSS.[253]

Abnormal orientation of the zygapophyseal (facet) joints influences the likelihood of spondylolisthesis by allowing for greater anterior shearing of the superior vertebral segment. **Facet tropism**, an asymmetry of the facet joint angles, is associated with degenerative and isthmic spondylolistheses.[254,255] **Sagittally oriented** (running in a front-to-back direction) facet joints increase the likelihood of developing degenerative spondylolisthesis.[255]

Facet joint **inflammation** may cause sciatic pain in degenerative spondylolisthesis. Studies have found elevated inflammatory mediators including interleukins and TNF-α in the facet joints of those with degenerative spondylolisthesis.[257,258] Inflammation may also arise from damaged collagen proteins found in the spinal connective tissue. Those with a genetic variant of collagen that includes tryptophan which may become oxidized and inflamed.[253] Inflammation from these regions affects the nearby nerve roots and causes radicular sciatic pain.

Hypertrophy of the **facet joints** and spinal **ligaments** are a common feature of spondylolisthesis. These occur in both isthmic[259] and degenerative[252] spondylolistheses. Hypertrophy of the superior articular process and ligamentum flavum create LSS. However, these changes may be a natural compensation for instability and help stabilize the spine.[246]

Isthmic spondylolistheses widen the lumbar canal[247] but can still cause nerve root compression. These types of spondylolistheses can lead to formation of a **fibrocartilaginous mass** or **bony callus** around the pars interarticularis that compresses or deviates the nerve root.[260] The nerve root can also become caught between the disc and intervertebral foramen in a **pincer** type mechanism.[261]

Sagittal spinopelvic alignment

The sagittal spinopelvic alignment, **spinopelvic balance**, or **spinopelvic posture** refers to the normal range of alignment between the spine and pelvis.[243] This alignment can be measured in many ways, most commonly using the sagittal vertical axis (SVA), pelvic incidence (PI), pelvic tilt (PT), and sacral slope (SS). The measurement of these variables and normal ranges vary depending on age and are beyond the scope of this chapter. Those with degenerative and isthmic spondylolistheses have a worse spinopelvic alignment including increased pelvic incidence, sacral slope, and pelvic tilt compared to asymptomatic people.[262]

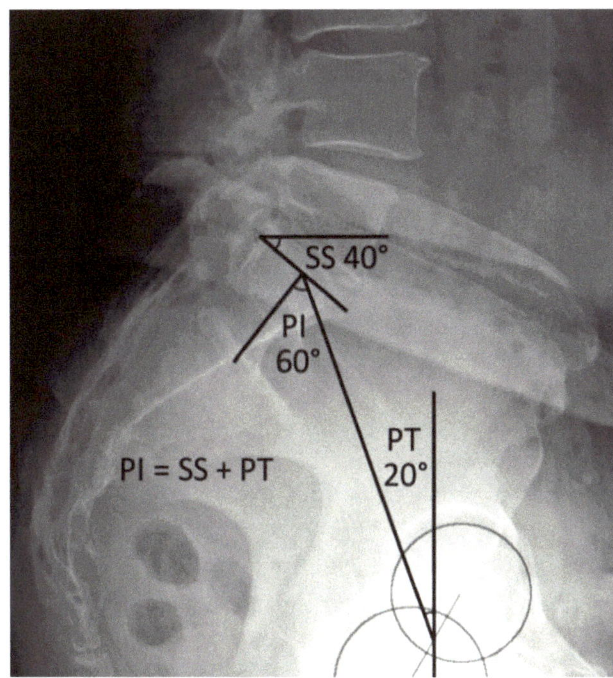

Figure 54: Spinopelvic alignment measurements. The degrees of pelvic incidence (PI) equals the sum of sacral slope (SS) and pelvic tilt (PT). Image shows a 4-millimeter degenerative spondylolisthesis at L4, shared with permission of patient by Robert Trager, DC.

The **sagittal vertical axis** (SVA) is the distance between the **C7 plumb line** (a vertical line from the body of the 7th cervical vertebrae) and the posterior superior corner of the **sacral base**. As C7 moves anterior to the sacrum (worse sagittal alignment), the lumbosacral and hip muscles must work harder to keep the torso upright.[263] Those with degenerative spondylolisthesis typically have an increased SVA (C7 anterior to sacrum) while those with isthmic may have a normal SVA.[262]

Pelvic incidence (PI) is the angle formed between a line perpendicular to the mid-sacral plate and another line from the mid-sacral plate to the axis of the femoral heads, and equals the sum of SS and PT. The pelvic incidence varies slightly depending on posture and may depend on movement at the sacroiliac joints (SIJs).[264] Pelvic incidence correlates with PT, lumbar lordosis (LL) and SS. Those with a high PI have a high PT, LL, and SS and those with a low PI have a low PT, LL, and SS.

A high pelvic incidence and high sacral slope increase **shear stress** at the lumbosacral junction.[243] One study found a positive correlation between SS and PI and the degree of slippage of L5 in those with degenerative spondylolisthesis.[265] This posture increases the anterior shear force on L5,[265] which pulls L5 anteriorly during flexion and posteriorly during extension.[266]

Pelvic incidence is higher in those with degenerative and isthmic spondylolisthesis compared with asymptomatic people.[262] A greater degree of PI correlates with a greater degree of slippage in isthmic spondylolisthesis.[267] A high PI may increase lumbar lordosis, which increases shear stress the lumbar vertebrae.[262,268]

In young people, a low sacral slope and pelvic incidence may create a **nutcracker effect** on L5 and increase the risk of isthmic spondylolisthesis.[243,263] This posture creates a hyperextension between L4 and the sacrum[263] which impinges the posterior elements (facet joint and pars interarticularis) of L4 and L5.[236] This effect may displace L5 anteriorly during spinal extension if a fracture develops.[266]

Low bone density is associated with the presence of degenerative spondylolisthesis and increased pain levels in those with LSS.[270] Normally the body compensates for instability by remodeling bone around the facet joints and generating bony osteophytes, which stabilizes the vertebrae and prevents slippage. Low bone density may limit the body's ability to generate **stabilizing osteophytes** that keep the spondylolisthesis in check.[270]

Ligamentum flavum hypertrophy

The ligamentum flavum (LF) appears yellow due to its rich content of **elastic fibers**. The LF is connected to the epidural fat anteriorly and vertebral lamina posteriorly[271] It has connections to the **multifidus** muscle infero-laterally.[271–273] The LF becomes tense during lumbar flexion[274] and relaxed and thickened during lumbar extension.[271]

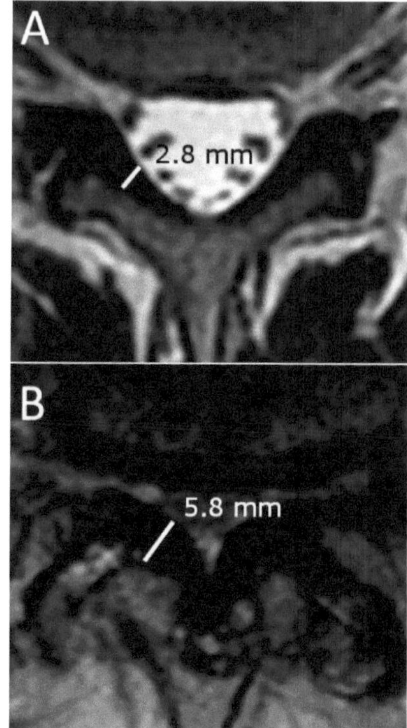

Figure 55: Ligamentum flavum thickness. (A) A 28-year-old man without LSS, (B) a 69-year-old woman with LSS and neurogenic claudication. Measurements are taken perpendicular to the long axis of the LF, at the midpoint from medial-to-lateral, as described by Chokshi.[269]

The LF is thinner and more elastic in younger healthy people but thickens with aging and LSS. The LF is up to **70% elastic fibers** in a young, healthy person. Aging and LSS causes a replacement of these elastic fibers with a greater proportion of **fibrosis** and **collagen** fibers, which can make up over 75% of the LF.[275] The LF should generally be less than **4 millimeters** thick,[276] however because it thickens with age, a value slightly greater may be normal in elderly patients.[277]

Repetitive **mechanical stress** creates inflammation within the LF, which leads to scar formation, fibrosis, and LF hypertrophy.[278] One study found a correlation between radiographic instability signs including the vacuum sign, spondylolisthesis, disc degeneration, facet joint osteoarthritis, and traction spurs.[279] Other studies found a positive correlation between angular **segmental motion** on flexion-extension radiographs and LF thickness.[276,278]

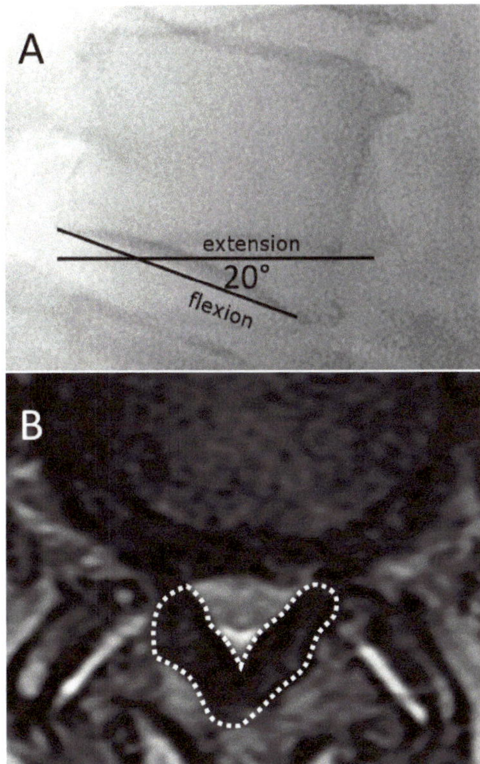

Figure 56: Mechanical stress model of ligamentum flavum hypertrophy. Image A shows increased angular motion from extension to flexion (images superimposed) at L4, while image B shows thickened ligamentum flavum at L4-5. Images are of a 66-year-old woman with neur

The LF may thicken secondary to facet joint **inflammation**.[269,276,280] Studies have found a positive correlation between **facet joint osteoarthritis** and LF thickness.[276,280] Inflammatory mediators that leak from the facet joint may trigger the LF to thicken and scar.[269] Ligamentum flavum thickening may occur due to facet joint degeneration in the absence of disc space narrowing.[269]

Some research shows that disc degeneration causes the LF to **buckle** into the spinal canal. One imaging study found a correlation of disc degeneration with LF thickness.[281] Other histological research found that thicker LFs had less elastic fibers.[282] Reduced elasticity would cause the LF to become lax and buckle and appear thickened on imaging studies. Buckling would also explain why the LF thickens up to 2 mm during extension,[271] a position that exacerbates LSS symptoms.

Diabetes mellitus damages and thickens the LF. There is a negative correlation between blood glucose and amount of elastic fibers of the ligamentum flavum.[283] Diabetics have less elastic fibers in their LF[283] and thicker LF[284] compared to non-diabetics. Elevated glucose and other sugar metabolites such as sorbitol may stimulate fibroblasts within the LF to produce inflammatory mediators and cause fibrosis.[284] Another hypothesis is that increased sugar content in the LF attracts water via **osmosis** causing the LF to enlarge.[284]

Cardiovascular and metabolic factors

Lifestyle factors help explain why those with LSS can develop symptoms. Cardiovascular diseases and diabetes mellitus (DM) damage the small blood vessels that supply the lumbosacral nerve roots and IVDs and lead to other degenerative changes within the spine. Increased weight may worsen pre-existing lumbar instability and discogenic pain.

Blood vessel diseases may increase the likelihood of symptomatic LSS. Studies have found a correlation of **hypertension** with symptomatic LSS.[285,286] Another study found a strong association between **atherosclerosis** (plaque buildup) of the aorta and lumbar arteries with LSS, in particular in younger people.[287] Hypertension may damage these vessels causing them to harden, which reduces blood flow to the lumbosacral nerve roots and accelerates lumbar disc degeneration.[286,288]

Heart disease may exacerbate LSS symptoms and is more common in those with symptomatic LSS than the general population.[285] Those with heart disease may develop retrograde engorgement of the vertebral veins, which connect indirectly to the inferior vena cava.[289] This **venous stasis** increases in pressure and compresses the lumbosacral nerve roots and small blood vessels that supply them. This exacerbates symptoms of LSS, in particular when lying flat at night.[289]

Those with DM are more likely to have symptomatic LSS.[183,285,286,290] One study found that those with DM had 3.9 times the odds of developing symptomatic LSS.[183] Elevated glucose levels causes the ligamentum flavum to **thicken**, **fibrose**,[291] and lose elasticity.[283] Elevated blood sugar also accelerates disc degeneration and damages peripheral nerves and the small blood vessels around the lumbosacral nerve roots.[286]

Other studies have found a correlation between weight and symptomatic LSS. Studies have correlated **obesity** with LSS,[292,293] and one study also found an association of increased **waist circumference.**[292] Increased weight increases loading on the spine[293] and could exacerbate lumbar instability.

Spinal instability

Strength of the core muscles, including the **low back** muscles, deep **abdominal** muscles, and **diaphragm** helps protect against lower back injuries. Weakness or lack of coordination of the core muscles causes instability under load and a greater risk for tearing the AF. Lumbar instability correlates significantly with sciatic pain.[229] Instability is thought to create **torsional stress** and **shear stress** on the disc, leading to disc degeneration, bulging, or herniation over time.[294] The core muscles contribute to spinal stability which may reduce the risk of discogenic sciatica.

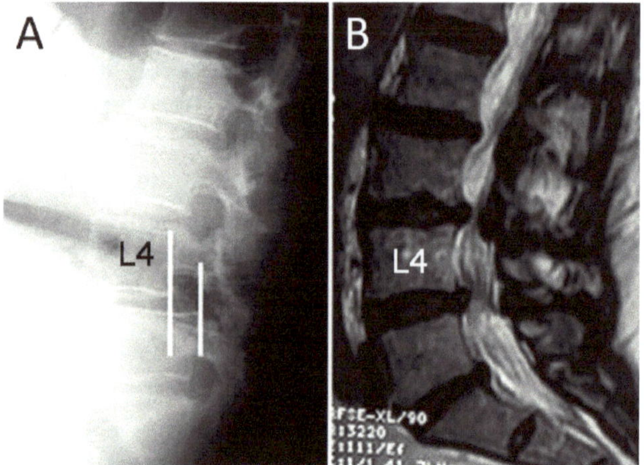

Figure 57: Lumbar instability seen on a standing flexion radiograph but not visible in a supine sagittal MRI, in the same patient. Images Creative Commons License from Caterini.[295]

Multifidus

The lumbar multifidus is a **deep spinal stabilizer** on the posterior aspect of the spine. This muscle often is weak, fatty, and atrophied in those with LBP and sciatica. When the multifidus is weak the discs are more susceptible to pathological translation and rotation that damages the discs and other structures of the spine.

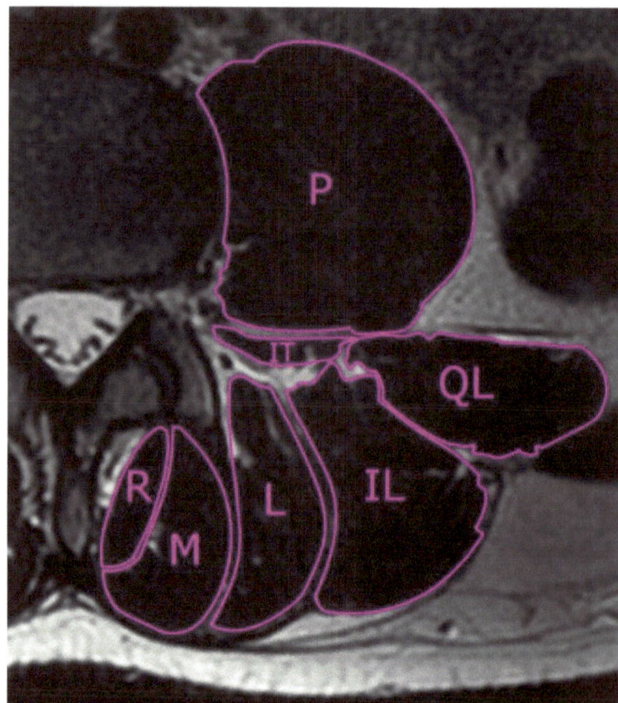

Figure 58: Lumbar muscles shown in an axial MRI at L3-4. (R) Rotatores, (M) Multifidus, (L) Longissimus, (IL) Iliocostalis, (QL) Quadratus lumborum, (P) Psoas, (IT) intertransversarii. Image by Robert Trager, DC

There is a strong correlation between multifidus dysfunction and atrophy and spine-related sciatica. Those with discogenic radiculopathy have a significantly reduced multifidus cross-sectional area[296] and less multifidus endurance.[297] Lumbar stenosis symptoms of lower extremity weakness are worse when the multifidus is atrophied.[298] Multifidus **fat deposition** and **infiltration** correlate with discogenic radicular sciatica.[299] Fat deposition can be seen on MRI as an increased **multifidus-lamina distance.**

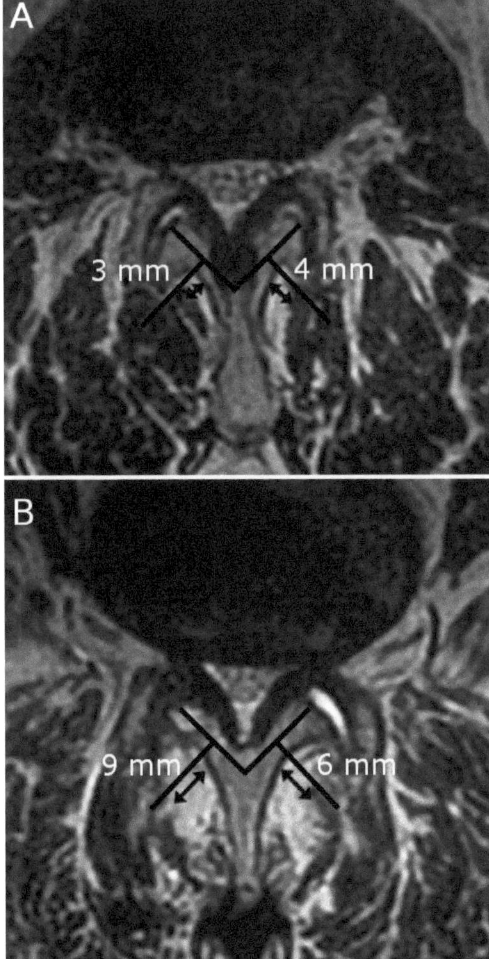

Figure 59: Multifidus-lamina distance. Two axial sections in a 63-year-old woman with an L4-5 degenerative anterolisthesis. Image A at L2-3 shows a normal distance and image B at L4-5 shows an increased distance. The measurement is taken along a line perpendicular to the midpoint of the lamina (lines), with the distance (arrows) being the gap between bone and muscle. Image shared with permission from patient by Robert Trager, DC.

Weakness of the multifidus has far-reaching consequences. Atrophy of this muscle may lead to damage of the medial branch of the dorsal ramus nerve and, in turn, lead to an ongoing cycle of weakness and pain called **dorsal ramus syndrome**. Multifidus atrophy and dorsal ramus nerve damage has a unique set of symptoms and pain referral pattern.

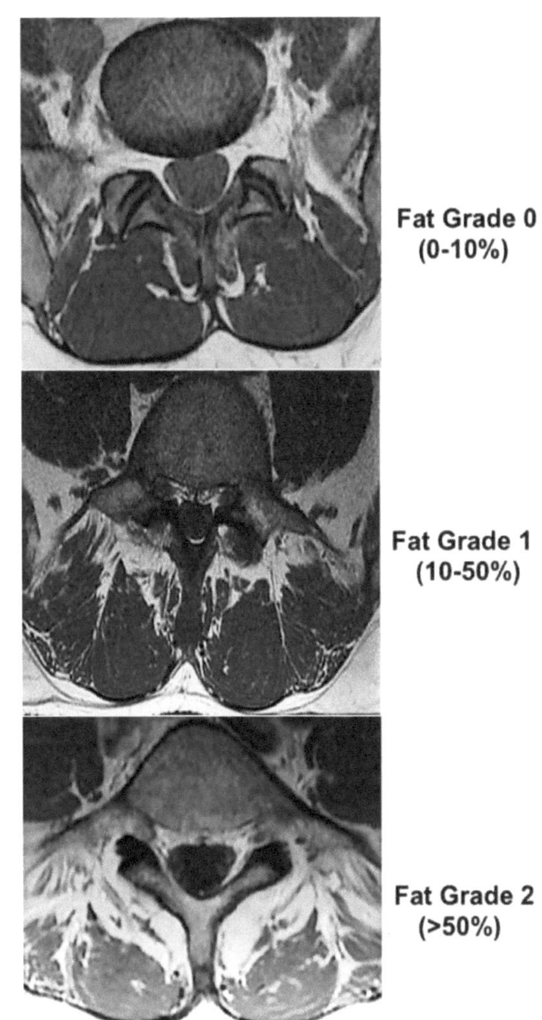

Figure 60: Grades of fat infiltration of the lumbar multifidus. Image CC-BY 4.0 License from Hildebrandt.[300]

Psoas

The psoas are large muscles that run between the low back and proximal femurs. These muscles flex the hips and help stabilize the lumbar spine. The psoas helps maintain a neutral **lumbar lordosis** while standing and while under load.[301] Those with psoas atrophy have less ability to stabilize the spine against loads, making it more susceptible to injury. The spine-stabilizing functions of the psoas helps prevent symptoms of discogenic sciatica and LSS.

Psoas atrophy is associated with spine-related sciatica. Same-side psoas atrophy has a significant correlation with nerve root compression in people with LBP.[302] Those with psoas atrophy on the side of LDH have longer lasting sciatic symptoms.[303] Lumbar stenosis symptoms are also worse when the psoas muscle is atrophied. Those with a large psoas cross-sectional area have significantly less leg pain and tingling and improved performance with activities of daily living.[298]

Transversus abdominis

The transversus abdominis (TA) is a muscle of the anterior and lateral abdominal wall that helps stabilize the spine. The TA contracts with the diaphragm and pelvic floor muscles to brace the spine when it is loaded.[304] Along with these muscles and the paraspinal muscles, it forms the front part of the **abdominal canister**.[304] This canister system gives internal **pneumatic support** to stabilize the spine and protect it against injury when bearing loads.

Weakness or dysfunction of the transversus abdominus predisposes the lumbar spine to injury. Healthy **co-contraction** of the abdominal canister muscles during lifting takes loads off the spine.[305] Those with LDH have decreased ability to contract the transversus abdominus muscle.[297]

There are two main pathological postural patterns for core muscle dysfunction. Those with a **central posterior cinch** have a reflexively hyperactive erector spinae and underactive anterior and lateral abdominal muscles.[304] Those with a **central anterior cinch** have a chronically overactive transversus abdominus which causes the lower abdomen to be drawn inwards.[304] Both patterns cause diaphragm dysfunction and interfere with lumbosacral stability.

Breathing mechanics

Abnormal breathing mechanics are associated with low back disorders. Those with back pain and sciatica have a higher resting position of the diaphragm and less ability to fully contract the diaphragm. The diaphragm works with other core muscles to maintain **intra-abdominal pressure** and stabilize and protect the spine. Those that cannot fully use the diaphragm are at a greater risk for low back and disc injuries.

Intra-abdominal pressure stabilizes the spine from the front,[306] whereas the erector spinae and transversospinalis group stabilize the spine from the back. Co-contraction of the diaphragm with the other core muscles (transversus abdominis, pelvic floor) increases the pressure within the abdomen. This pressure helps to stabilize the spine and prevent unwanted shearing or torsional forces when lifting or under load.

Those with low back disorders such as LDHs and LSS have a higher **resting position** of the diaphragm.[306] They also have significantly less **diaphragmatic excursion** compared to those with healthy lower backs.[306] Excursion is reduced on average by 18 mm while breathing at rest and by 25 mm while resisting loads with the lower extremities.[306] Some patients with LBP have a highly positioned **bulging diaphragm** that does not contract well.[306]

Those with lower back pain and sciatica have poor breathing mechanics when resisting loads. They have a smaller diaphragm excursion during postural tasks such as resisted hip and shoulder flexion.[307] This means that the normal intra-abdominal pressure stabilizing function of the diaphragm is compromised.

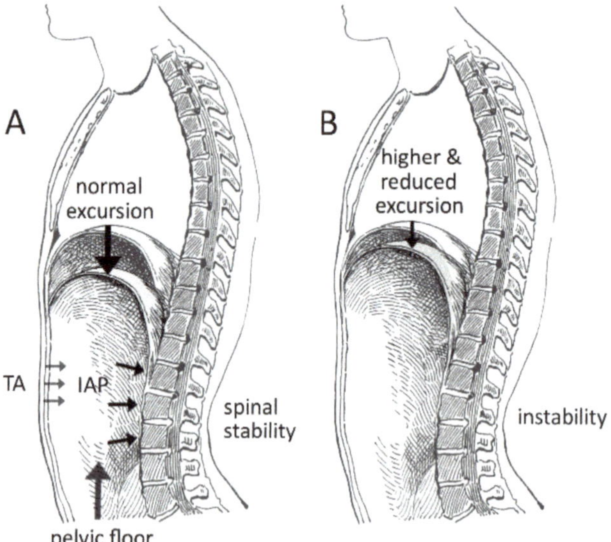

Figure 61: Normal and abnormal diaphragm mechanics. Image A shows normal co-activation of the diaphragm, transversus abdominis (TA), and pelvic floor to generate intra-abdominal pressure (IAP), which stabilizes and protects the lumbar spine. Image B shows a typical low back disorder with a higher resting position less movement of the diaphragm. Images modified from public domain by Robert Trager, DC.

It is unclear if abnormal breathing patterns are a cause or effect of low back conditions. Poor diaphragm activation may be due to **muscle guarding** in response to spine injury. The converse may also be true, that poor breathing mechanics causes spinal instability and predisposes one to low back injury.[307] The lumbar paraspinal erector muscles may be chronically tight to compensate for diaphragm weakness and loss of intra-abdominal pressure. This chronic tension may perpetuate sciatica due to unrelenting tension placed on the lumbar spine.

Table 10. Breathing mechanics in healthy people vs. those with low back conditions

	Healthy person	**LBP +/- leg pain**
Diaphragm position at rest	Lower	Higher
Diaphragm excursion	Greater	Lesser
Diaphragm endurance	Greater	Lesser
Intra-abdominal pressure	Greater	Lesser
Lumbosacral stability	Greater	Lesser

Dorsal ramus syndrome

The dorsal rami or posterior rami are branches of the spinal nerve that innervate the multifidus and skin of the back. Dorsal ramus syndrome is a type of low back or sciatic pain caused by injury or irritation of the **medial branch** of the dorsal ramus. Dorsal ramus syndrome often coincides with multifidus weakness or atrophy. A problem with the dorsal ramus causes problems with the multifidus and vice versa.

Those with dorsal ramus syndrome have denervation of the lumbar multifidus but normal innervation of the lower extremities.[308] The main symptoms are LBP and lumbar multifidus weakness and atrophy, with or without sciatic pain. Some patients have weakness in the legs, which is thought to be caused by nociceptive inhibition of motor signals.[309]

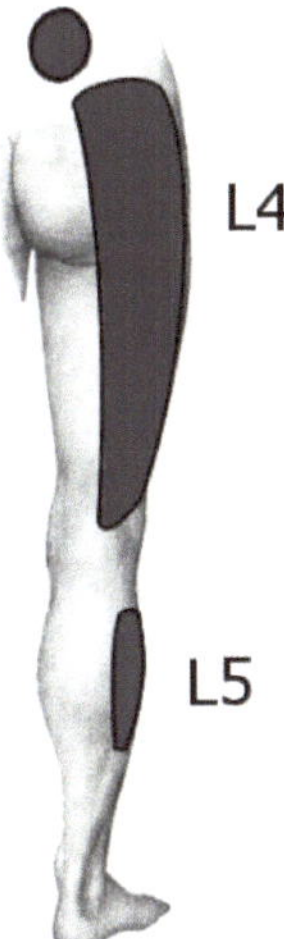

Figure 62: Referred pain pattern from the L4 and L5 multifidus and the dorsal ramus, based on the work of Cornwall[312] and Kellgren.[313] Images modified by Robert Trager from public domain (Gray's Anatomy).

Dorsal ramus syndrome is more common in those with **lumbar instability**, for example a spondylolisthesis.[310,311] Because the medial branch of the dorsal ramus innervates the multifidus, damage to it disables the multifidus from stabilizing the spine. The classic presentation of dorsal ramus syndrome is LBP or sciatic pain with vertebral **listhesis** and normal nerve root function.

The medial branch of the dorsal ramus passes through a small **osteoligamentous tunnel** at the posterior aspect of the lower lumbar vertebrae. The **mamillo-accessory ligament** forms a tunnel called the mamillo-accessory foramen by crossing from the accessory and mammillary bony processes. The medial branch of the dorsal ramus is at risk for compression when the mamillo-accessory ligament ossifies. It is also at risk of entrapment or traction injury if the lumbar spine becomes unstable.

Dorsal ramus syndrome can cause a **vague pattern** of referred sciatic pain which does not necessarily match a dermatome.[310] Each spinal nerve has a dorsal ramus, and irritation of this ramus causes referred pain in any part of the root's segmental pattern. Those with dorsal ramus syndrome should not have any segmental sensory deficit or reflex loss.

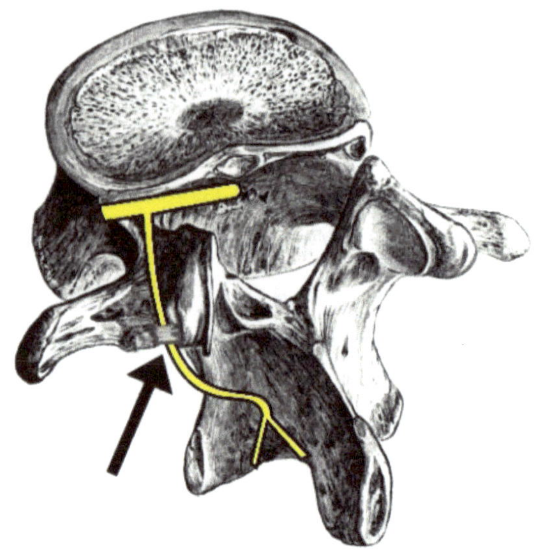

Figure 63: The medial branch of the dorsal ramus passes through the mamillo accessory foramen (arrow) and is at risk of compression and entrapment in this tunnel. Image modified by Robert Trager, DC from public domain (Gray's Anatomy).

Multifidus atrophy may contribute to dorsal ramus syndrome independently from discogenic radiculopathy. In many patients with sciatic pain there is atrophy of the multifidus but no LDH, nerve compression, or lumbar stenosis.[310,314] It is thought that the lumbar instability induced by multifidus atrophy over-stretches or irritates this nerve, which then causes pain referral into the sciatic nerve distribution.[314]

Table 11: Comparison of the classic presentation of lumbosacral radiculopathy (LSR) and dorsal ramus syndrome (DRS)

	LSR	**DRS**
Pain pattern	Dermatomal	Vaguely delineated, radiates into buttocks or lower extremity
Examination	Weakness, sensory, and/or motor deficit	Paraspinal motor loss or atrophy, lower extremities usually normal
MRI	Abnormalities around nerve root including disc pathology, stenosis	Multifidus atrophy, otherwise normal

Adipose within the lumbar multifidus increases the odds of leg pain being present. Those below age 45 with severe lumbar multifidus **intramuscular adipose** have about double the odds of developing sciatica (OR 2.08).[315] There is also a significant correlation between multifidus atrophy and leg pain, independent of LDH or nerve root compression.[314] Multifidus atrophy can either damage the discs and spine by causing instability or cause a separate dorsal ramus syndrome.

Multifidus weakness may propagate a cycle of low back and sciatic pain that continues unless intervened upon. Weakness predisposes the lumbar spine to instability and dorsal ramus to injury. Dorsal ramus injury can cause referred sciatic pain which leads to further guarding and disuse of the lower back, causing more weakness.

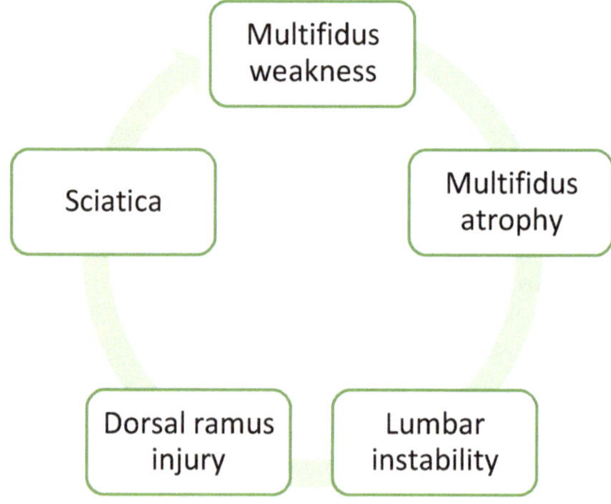

Figure 64: Dorsal ramus syndrome pathogenesis

Myofascial sciatica

Myofascial disorders can contribute to or cause sciatica independently yet also can result from radicular sciatica. Myofascial conditions may lead to peripheral or central sensitization, a reduction in threshold needed to stimulate nociceptors (pain receptors) along the sciatic nerve pathway. Conversely, those with radicular sciatica may secondarily develop myofascial pain.

There is much overlap between myofascial disorders and radicular sciatica. Patients with lumbosacral radiculopathy have an increased prevalence of lumbar and gluteal **myofascial trigger point** pain, **plantar fasciitis**, **iliotibial band syndrome** and **trochanteric bursitis**.[11] Women suffering with **chronic pelvic pain** after giving birth may develop referred pain into the lower extremities. In these patients the pressure on the coccyx can refer pain into the sciatic nerve pathway.[316]

Inflammation within and outside of the spine can sensitize the sciatic nerve pathway and predispose one to develop sciatica. Inflammation and tissue damage cause production of hydrogen ions, histamine, and other **inflammatory mediators** that lead to painful sensations. Over time these factors can make nociceptors more sensitive to stimuli, leading to more pain.

Trigger points and referred pain

Trigger points **(TrPs)** are hyper-irritable spots within taut bands of skeletal muscle. Trigger points become more painful with compression, contraction, stretching, or overload.[317] **Referred pain** is the main characteristic of a trigger point and is the perception of pain at a distant site when the trigger point is stimulated. Myofascial TrPs can exist either independently or can arise subsequent to discogenic or nerve root pain. In other words, they can be a cause or effect of sciatica.

Trigger points can arise following an injury along the sciatic nerve pathway or act as a source of sensitization to create sciatica. One study using EMG found that about 20% of patients suspected of having lumbar or sacral radiculopathy had lower limb pain caused by TrPs instead of a nerve lesion.[11] Trigger points are also found in the majority of those with radicular sciatica. One study found 76% of those with radiculopathy had at least one gluteal trigger point.[318]

Denervation supersensitivity

When a nerve is partially denervated (damaged) its innervated structures become extremely sensitive to stimulation. This process is called **denervation supersensitivity**.[319] In contrast, more severe nerve root damage causes nearly opposite symptoms such as numbness and weakness. In denervation supersensitivity the muscles develop a compensatory upregulation in acetylcholine receptors followed by increased resting muscle tone and spasms.[319]

Denervation supersensitivity caused by partial damage of a nerve root increases sensitivity and muscle activity. Symptoms include hypertonicity (tightness) of muscles, hyperesthesia (skin sensitivity), hyperalgesia (sensitivity of deep tissues), and myofascial pain within the nerve root distribution. This category of sciatica can be described as the **partial denervation** or **irritation** group.

Conversely, a complete lesion of a nerve root decreases sensitivity and muscle activity. Symptoms include muscle hypotonia (weakness), hypoesthesia (numbness), and hyporeflexia (loss of reflexes). This category of sciatica can be described as the **total denervation** or **neural compression** group and includes patients with neurological deficits.

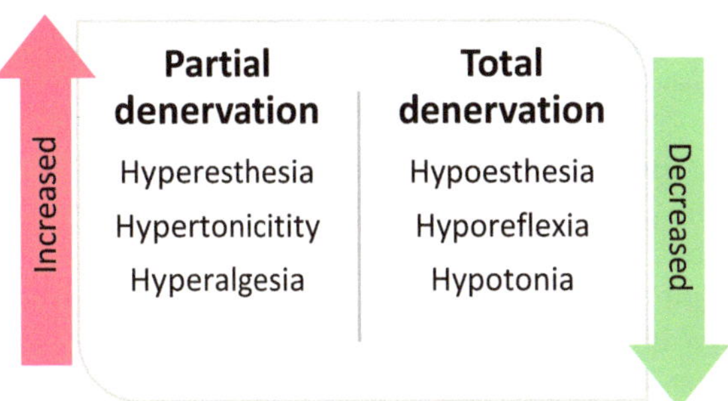

Figure 65: Partial versus total denervation. Clinical signs and symptoms vary depending on the degree of nerve injury. Clinical features are hyper- or increased with partial denervation and hypo- or decreased with denervation. Data adapted from Gunn.[319]

Patients with radicular sciatica often have signs of denervation supersensitivity such as tenderness of the muscles and their connective tissue and bones.[320] Some authors describe these symptoms as **sclerotomal** (bone and periosteum) or **myotomal** (muscle) pain to contrast with dermatomal (skin) pain.[319,321,322] In radicular sciatica myotomal tenderness corresponds with **motor points**, the area of nerve stimulation at the neurovascular bundle of the muscle. These points are similar between individuals, and often coincide with trigger points,[323] which may also arise from denervation supersensitivity.

Myofascial disorders in radicular sciatica

Certain myofascial disorders are more common in those with radicular sciatica. This group of conditions is called **myofascial pain of radiculopathic origin**[324] or **neuropathic myofascial pain syndromes**[325] and includes include tendinitis, trigger points, recurrent strains, camping, and fibrosis of the muscles and fascia innervated by the sciatic nerve. Myofascial pain syndromes in the lower extremities may arise as a prodrome or a sequela of radicular sciatica.

Research suggests that myofascial disorders are more common in those with radicular sciatica.[318,322,326] One study reported coexisting myofascial trigger points in up to a third of patients with lumbar radiculopathy.[322] Another study reported gluteal trigger points in 76% of those with lumbosacral radiculopathy.[318]

Myofascial pain may be a **precursor** to LDH or stenosis.[327,328] At first, compression of a healthy nerve root may not produce back pain, but rather myofascial pain or trigger points in the nerve's distribution.[328] **Prespondylosis** refers to the subtle neurological and myofascial symptoms that may be precursors to a radiculopathy.[328]

Myofascial pain may persist long after the initiation and resolution of radicular sciatica. Persistent muscle disorders may explain why some patients do not improve with treatment of the spine-related causes of sciatica.[329] One study found that patients with persistent symptoms after **lumbar fusion surgery** often had pain related to the gluteus medius muscle.[330] One author described myofascial pain related to radicular sciatica as "an **organic memory circuit** for the initiating event," which when treated could quickly alleviate the patient's symptoms.[331]

Myofascial disorders coexisting with radicular sciatica may be a common reason for **misdiagnosis**[332] and treatment failure.[322] One study found that sciatic patients who did not improve often had coexisting disorders such as myofascial pain.[322] Abnormalities seen on lumbar imaging such as LDHs may explain how sciatic pain initiated but, in instances of myofascial pain, fail to explain how it is perpetuated.[329]

Table 12: Myofascial disorders associated with radicular sciatica

Segment	Myofascial syndromes
L4	GTPS,[333] TrPs of quadriceps and extensor hallucis longus[334]
L5	GTPS,[333] iliotibial band syndrome, plantar fasciitis,[335] recurrent hamstring strains,[336,337] TrPs of the extensor hallucis longus, hamstring, and gastrocnemius[334]
S1	GTPS,[333] plantar fasciitis,[335] TrPs of the gastrocnemius, extensor hallucis longus, hamstring, and tibialis posterior[334]
Greater trochanteric pain syndrome (GTPS), trigger points (TrPs)	

Recurrent strains of the thigh and leg muscles in athletes may relate to damage to the lumbosacral nerve roots.[336,337] Nerve injury may cause motor deficits that make these muscles more susceptible to injury. One study found that cricket pace bowlers with a history of lumbar stress fractures had increased odds of calf, quadriceps, and hamstring strains.[336] Other conditions such as greater trochanteric pain syndrome (GTPS) are associated with gluteal muscle weakness[338] and by the same logic could also relate to lumbosacral radiculopathy.

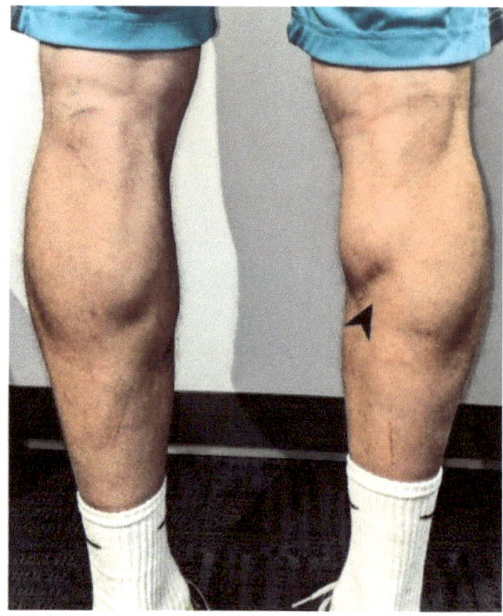

Figure 66: Disc-related calf strain. This 53-year-old man developed acute radiating LBP with right lower extremity numbness and weakness after bending over. MRI revealed an LDH and annular fissure at L5-S1. He suffered from calf cramps and developed this deformity (arrowhead) of the R calf within 1 week, which did not subside even with improvement of the other symptoms after 1 month.

Greater trochanteric pain syndrome is a condition of pain and tenderness in the region around the greater trochanter of the femur. Research has identified a correlation between GTPS and low back conditions.[333,339,340] One study reported an incidence of 12% of this condition in those with lumbosacral radiculopathy.[11] Another study found 76% of those with lumbosacral radiculopathy had gluteal trigger points, compared with 2% of healthy volunteers.[318] Still another study found that about half of patients with degenerative lumbar spine conditions also suffered from GTPS.[333]

Plantar fasciitis (PF), a condition involving plantar heel pain and tenderness at the insertion of the plantar fascia on the calcaneus, is more common in those with lumbosacral radiculopathy. Some authors describe low back-related plantar fasciitis as **neuropathic heel pain**.[335] One study found that those with three-quarters of those PF suffered from LBP.[341] Another study found that 57% of those with plantar fasciitis had symptoms of radiculopathy.[335] In these patients, symptoms seemed to relate to nerve compression at L4-5 or L5-S1 disc lesions causing L5 or S1 radiculopathy.[335] According to Gunn, radiculopathy may trigger PF by causing a shortening of the flexor digitorum brevis and lumbricals.[342]

Greater trochanteric pain syndrome

Greater trochanteric pain syndrome (GTPS) is a generic term that describes pain and tenderness around the greater trochanter of the femur and radiating pain into the buttocks or lateral thigh.[340] This syndrome includes **gluteal muscle tendinosis**, tendinitis, tears, trigger points, iliotibial band disorders, and bursitis.[343] This condition was formerly called **trochanteric bursitis**, but its name was changed to GTPS because edema is not always present. Greater trochanteric pain syndrome has been called a **great mimicker** due to its frequent confusion with lumbar disc conditions and radiculopathy.[344]

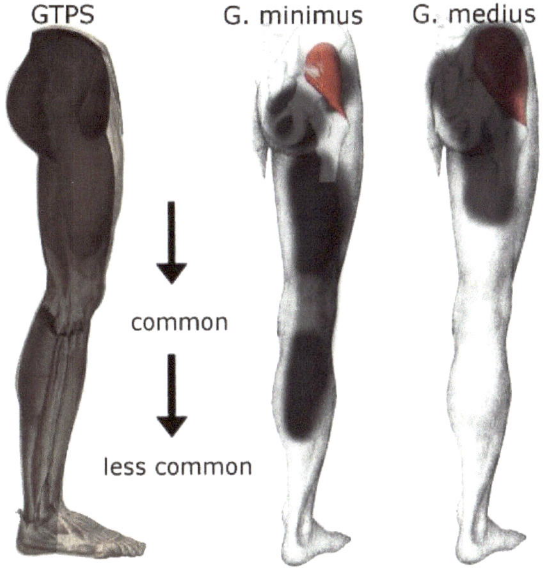

Figure 67: Left: GTPS pain referral, modified from Jean Baptiste Marc Bourgery, public domain, based on data from Tortolani[340] and Williams.[343] Middle and right - Gluteus minimus and medius trigger point pain referral, based on Travell & Simons. Images from Gray's anatomy image of lower extremity, public domain, and modified from Anatomography gluteal muscle images CC 2.1 attribution share-alike Japan license

Many ancient physicians believed that sciatica originated in the muscles and sinews around the hip joint. The North African physician Constantinus Africanus (c.?-1098) wrote:[345]

> *The disease sciatica originates because of the humors in the sinews of the deep muscles that descend [into the thigh] ... Most [cases] also happen because of viscous phlegmatic humors in the concavity of the hip joint... Sometimes, pain descends to the leg, the heel, and all the way to the smallest toe of the foot. (Author's translation, p. 185-6)*

Jonas Kellgren was a pioneer diagnosing referred pain from ligaments and tendons and, in the 1930s, was the first to formally identify sciatica originating from the trochanteric region.[346] He diagnosed myofascial gluteal sciatica by excluding spinal pathology, palpating the area around the hip, and performing a diagnostic injection.[347]

In 1976, Swezey presented 70 cases of patients who had radiating pain in the lower extremity originating from the trochanteric region.[348] He popularized the term **pseudoradiculopathy** to define myofascial pain from the trochanteric muscles or bursa that mimicked nerve root pathology. Travell and Simons' classic text the *Trigger Point Manual,* published in 1992, presented their findings of muscle trigger point referral maps. They identified the ability of the gluteus medius and minimus muscles to cause referred sciatic pain.[349]

Greater trochanteric pain syndrome may be the most common cause of sciatica that does not involve a nerve injury. One study found that 20% of patients referred to a spinal surgery center for LBP had GTPS based on signs and symptoms and improvement with anesthetic injection.[340] In another study of patients with suspected lumbosacral radiculopathy, GTPS was identified in 18% of patients based on physical examination and electromyography.[11]

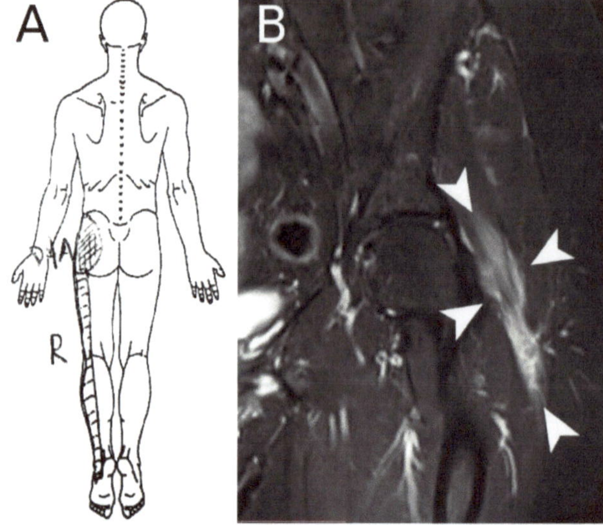

Figure 68: A 59-year-old house cleaner presented with a 2-year history of left sided gluteal & sciatic radiating pain (left image). Examination showed normal strength, sensation, and reflexes, but pain with manual gluteal muscle testing. Straight leg raising was limited with local gluteal and hip pain on the left side. MRI revealed T2 hyperintensity in the left gluteus minimus muscle and the trochanteric bursa (arrowheads) indicating tendinitis or tear and trochanteric bursitis. The patient improved with myofascial release & trigger point injections in the gluteal and trochanteric region. Case shared with patient's permission by Robert Trager, DC.

The **gluteal tendons**, **tensor fascia lata**, and **iliotibial band** are thought to be responsible for radiating pain in GTPS.[340] While GTPS typically causes radiating pain into the buttocks and lateral thigh, stopping at the knee, it occasionally causes pain distal to the knee.[343] In contrast to deep gluteal or piriformis syndromes, there is no sciatic nerve lesion in GTPS. Pain beyond the knee may be related to a central neurological pain referral, or caused by fascial connections of the **lateral line**, a continuous band of fascia including the iliotibial band and the peroneal muscles of the outer leg.

Peripheral nerve entrapment

There is an overlap between myofascial causes of sciatica and peripheral nerve entrapments. Chronically **contracted muscles** can compress small nerves or even the large sciatic nerve. Cases thought to represent myofascial sciatica may also involve components of nerve entrapment. Myofascial and peripheral nerve syndromes account for most non-radicular cases of sciatica.

Physicians who performed sciatic nerve stretching to treat sciatica in the late 1800s were the first to theorize that nerve entrapments caused sciatica. Their hypothesis for the relief obtained by stretching was a release of the sciatic nerve from adhesions to its surrounding nerve sheath.[350]

Muscle contractures in the lower back, hip, and lower extremity can entrap or compress peripheral nerves and even the exiting spinal nerves. There are many entrapment syndromes of the sciatic nerve and its branches. It is thought that trauma, fibrosis, anomalies, avulsions, tendinosis, strains, calcifications, or spasms of these muscles or their tendons contributes to the compression of the nerves.[351]

Connective tissue of muscles forms an added sheath around the sciatic nerve. This fascial sheath around the sciatic nerve is called the **epimysium** and exists in the buttocks, for example between the gluteus maximus and quadratus femoris, and also lower in the thigh, between the hamstring muscles.[352]

Table 13: Myofascial sources of peripheral nerve entrapment that can cause sciatica

Myofascial structure	Peripheral nerve compressed
Gemelli and obturator internus muscles	Sciatic[351]
Gluteus maximus	Sciatic[351]
Hamstring tendons (proximal)	Sciatic[353]
Iliolumbar ligament (part of quadratus lumborum)	L5 spinal nerve[354]
Piriformis muscle	PFCN,[355] sciatic[351]
Quadratus femoris	Sciatic[351]
Soleal sling at the popliteal fossa	Tibial[356,357]
Tarsal tunnel at the ankle	Tibial
Tensor fascia lata	PFCN[358]
Thoracolumbar fascia & latissimus dorsi at the iliac crest	Superior cluneal[359,360]
Posterior femoral cutaneous (PFCN)	

Deep gluteal syndrome

Deep gluteal syndrome (DGS) is a condition of buttocks and/or sciatic nerve distribution pain arising from entrapment of the sciatic nerve in the buttocks.

Piriformis syndrome is the best-known form of DGS and involves entrapment of the sciatic nerve by the piriformis muscle. Other types of DGS include anomalous **fibrous bands** within the buttocks that compress or attach to the sciatic nerve, anomalies of the sciatic nerve, **trauma** to the gluteal region, **ischiofemoral impingement**, and disorders of other muscles including the quadratus femoris, hamstrings, and gemellus and obturator internus.[351]

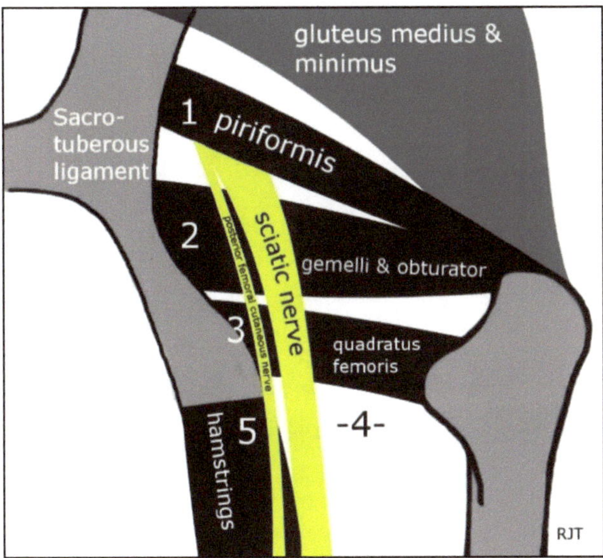

Figure 69: Deep gluteal space. View from the posterior of the right gluteal region. Major causes of compression of the sciatic nerve and the smaller posterior femoral cutaneous nerve are (1) pathology or anatomical variations of the sciatic nerve and piriformis muscle, (2) scissoring type of entrapment between the piriformis and gemelli and obturator internus, (3) injuries to quadratus femoris, (4) narrowing of the space between the hip and ischium, (5) hamstring tendinosis, and (6) contracture of the overlying gluteus maximus (not shown). Image by Robert Trager, DC.

Piriformis syndrome

Piriformis syndrome (PS) is a subset of DGS that involves compression of the sciatic nerve by the piriformis muscle. Piriformis syndrome causes about 5% of cases of sciatica.[12] The causes of sciatic nerve entrapment in piriformis syndrome include anatomical variations, hypertrophy of the piriformis muscle, and trauma to the buttocks.[362]

Clinicians began to diagnose PS in the early to mid-1900s. In 1908 Petrén suggested sciatica could be caused by inflammation of the gluteus medius and piriformis.[363] In 1938 Beaton and Anson identified anomalies in cadavers including division of the sciatic nerve that passed through the piriformis muscle.[364] They suggested that spasm of the piriformis muscle could compress the sciatic nerve and result in pain.

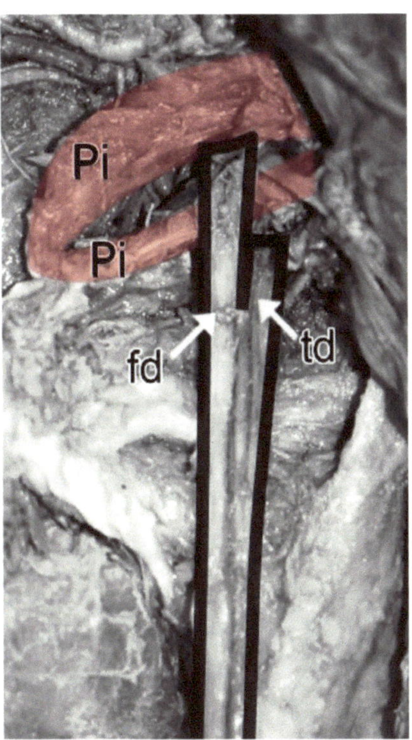

Figure 70: The most common anatomical variation of the sciatic nerve, in a left gluteal region. The fibular division (fd) of the sciatic nerve pierces the piriformis muscle (Pi) while the tibial division (td) passes inferior to it. Image modified from Battaglia et al,[370] CC-BY-2.0 license.

Half of patients with PS experience radiating sciatic pain. Most patients have local buttocks pain,[362] 33% have pain in the anterior leg and foot dorsum, 22% have pain in the lateral leg and foot, and 45% have fluctuating symptoms throughout the entire sciatic nerve distribution.[365] The two most common areas of leg symptoms correspond to the distributions of the **superficial peroneal nerve** and **sural nerve**, which are cutaneous branches of the common peroneal nerve. An anatomic variant in which the common peroneal nerve pierces the piriformis muscle may account for these leg symptoms.

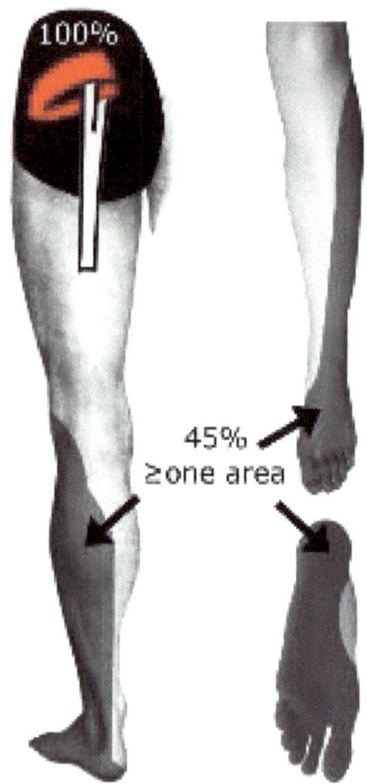

Figure 71: Piriformis syndrome symptom distribution. Data adapted from Hopayian[362] and Michel.[362] Image of leg modified from Andrea Allen (CC by 2.0), thigh public domain from Gray's anatomy.

Those with **anatomical variations** between the sciatic nerve and piriformis muscle have an increased risk of developing piriformis syndrome. In most people, about 88%, the sciatic nerve emerges from the pelvis inferior to the piriformis muscle. Anatomical variations occur in about 12% of patients.[366,367] The most common of these variations is when the sciatic nerve divides in the pelvis, the **common peroneal nerve** pierces the piriformis muscle, and the **tibial nerve** passes inferior to the piriformis.[366]

The piriformis muscle may **hypertrophy** (grow larger) in those who overuse this muscle. Overuse is thought to cause piriformis syndrome in 44% of cases.[368] Hypertrophy of the piriformis muscle can squeeze the sciatic nerve that passes deep to it.[366,369] Hypertrophy may compound upon an anatomical variation to increase the likelihood of piriformis syndrome.

Trauma to the buttocks is a cause of piriformis syndrome in about 20% of patients.[368] Many of these patients report falling from a standing height.[371] Trauma is thought to cause an inflammatory cascade and/or direct sciatic nerve damage that leads to piriformis syndrome.[371] Trauma can also cause a hematoma that reduces space for the sciatic nerve to pass through the buttocks. Microtrauma such as that caused by prolonged sitting is another suspected cause of sciatica.

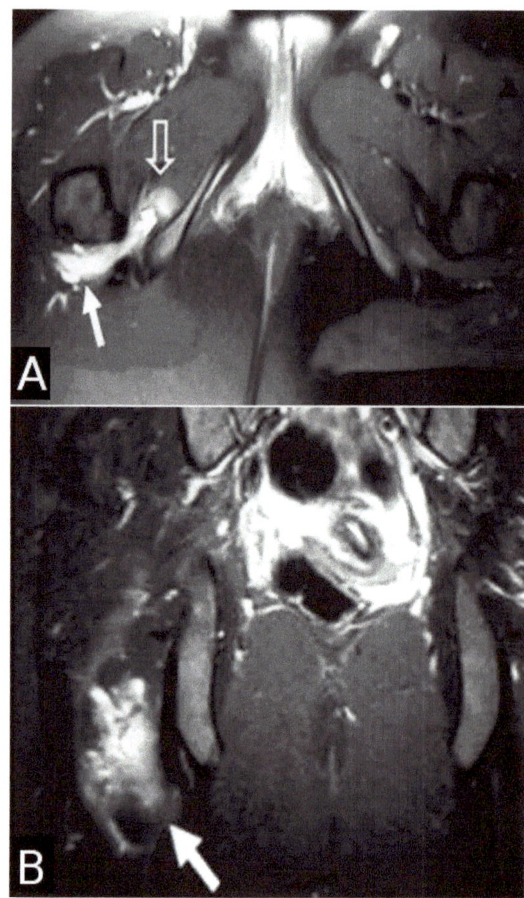

Figure 72: Sciatic pain caused by quadratus femoris tear. The axial fat suppressed proton density turbo spin echo (TSE) (a) and coronal short tau inversion recovery (STIR) images (b), show the hematoma in the quadratus femoris muscle (arrows) extending to the obturator internus muscle (open arrow). Case and images from Bano,[361] CC-BY-2.0 license.

The most common symptoms, occurring in about half of patients, are **buttocks pain** and aggravation of pain with **sitting**.[362] The piriformis muscle or greater sciatic notch are tender in over half of cases.[362] Patients may also have LBP or pain with intercourse.

Posterior femoral cutaneous nerve entrapment

The posterior femoral cutaneous nerve (PFCN) initially runs parallel to the sciatic nerve and is susceptible to many of the same injuries as the sciatic. It lies medial to the sciatic nerve as it emerges from the infrapiriform foramen. The two nerves may travel in a **common sheath** in this region.[373]

The PFCN may be compressed at the **piriformis** muscle in gluteal injuries[374] or in cases of anatomical variation.[375] Part of the PFCN pierces the piriformis in 16% and the entire PFCN pierces the piriformis in 4% of people.[375] Some cases of piriformis syndrome may affect the sciatic and PFCN.

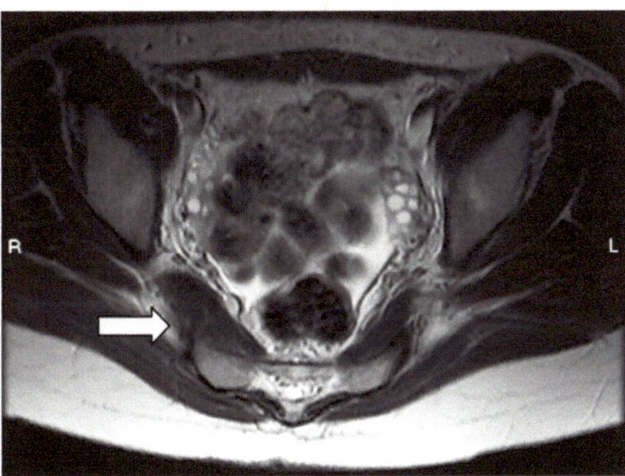

Figure 73: Hypertrophy of the piriformis muscle (arrow) can compress the sciatic nerve and the PFCN. Note the opposite piriformis is much smaller. Image CC BY 4.0 license from Sun et al.[372]

The PFCN courses just lateral to the **ischial tuberosity** where it is at risk for compression.[376] It is susceptible to entrapment related to proximal **hamstring tendinosis** or hamstring injury,[377] and fibrous expansion of the **ischial tuberosity**.[376]

The PFCN is at risk of entrapment within the fascia of the gluteal region and thigh. The PFCN can become entrapped within the **fascia lata** (fascia of the thigh),[358] or scar tissue from hip surgery.[377]

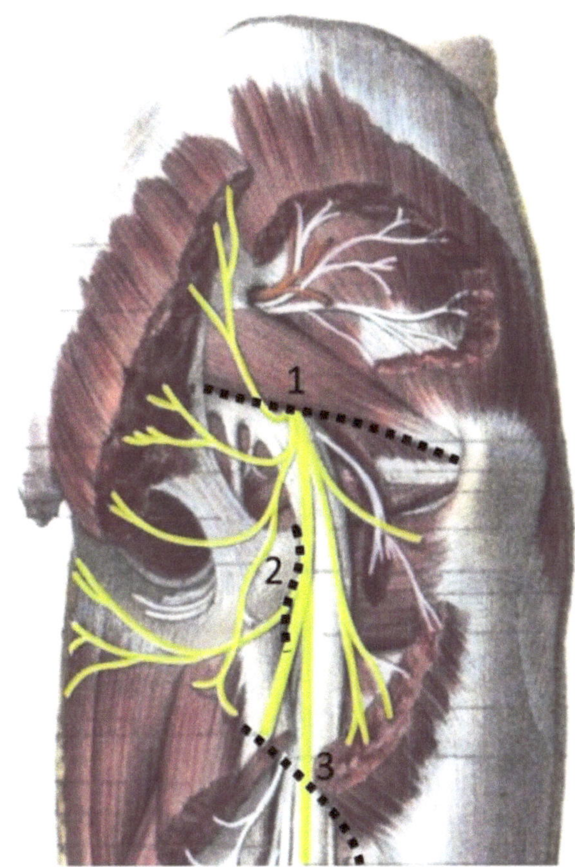

Figure 74: Common entrapment sites of the PFCN (dotted lines): the piriformis muscle (1), ischial tuberosity and proximal hamstring attachment (2), and the fascia of the thigh (3). Image modified from public domain (Hirschfeld and Léveillé) by Robert Trager, DC.

Symptoms of PFCN entrapment include radiating pain down the posterior thigh, popliteal fossa, and sometimes further down the leg, and increased pain with **sitting**. Injury of the PFCN causes **sensory deficits** rather than motor deficits as it has limited or no muscle innervation. A sensory pattern with no motor deficits helps distinguish PFCN from sciatic nerve injuries. Posterior femoral cutaneous nerve injuries may also cause **perineal pain**,[378] involving the penis or labia due to the perineal branches from the PFCN.

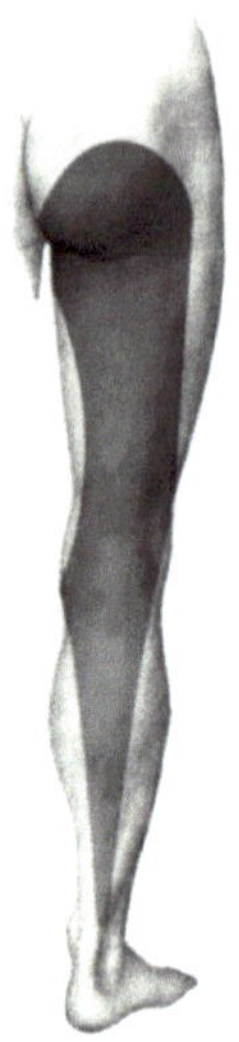

Figure 75: PFCN distribution. This nerve gives off a long third branch which has a variable distribution. The PFCN generally descends mid-thigh but innervates the skin as far distal as the heel.[374] Image modified from public domain (Gray's anatomy), by Robert Trager, DC.

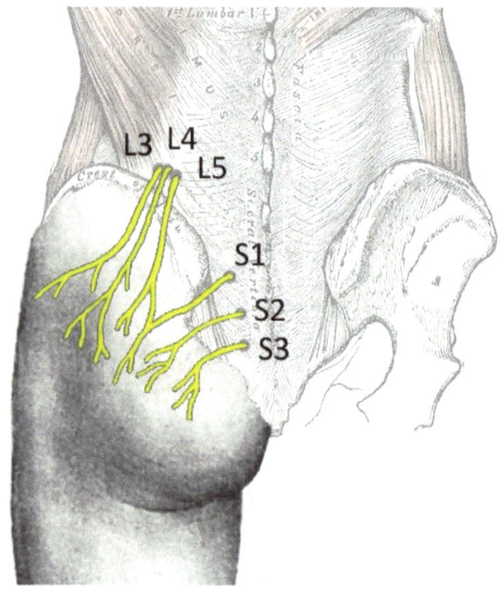

Figure 76: Superior cluneal nerve origin from the lumbosacral nerves and path through the iliolumbar membrane and towards the gluteal region. Image modified from public domain (Gray's Anatomy) by Robert Trager, DC.

Superior cluneal nerve entrapment

The superior cluneal nerves (SCNs) come from the lumbar nerves L3, L4, and L5 and often anastomose with the medial cluneal nerves which come from S1, S2, and S3.[379] Together these nerves innervate the skin of the upper and middle buttocks. Superior cluneal nerve entrapment can cause radiating pain not only along the distribution of the cluneal nerves but also the distribution of the sciatic nerve.[360]

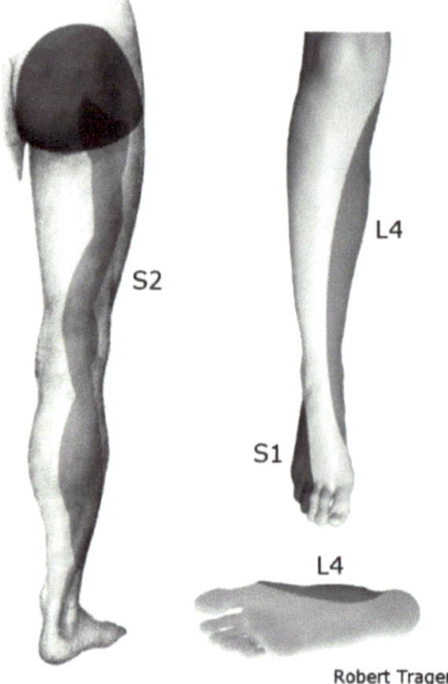

Figure 77: Superior cluneal nerve entrapment. Entrapment or compression of the superior cluneal nerves causes pain in the buttocks and occasionally referred pain in the lumbar and sacral dermatomes. Image by Robert Trager, DC by modification of public domain Gray's Anatomy images. leg modified from Andrea Allen (CC-BY-2.0)

The superior cluneal nerves are at risk for entrapment as they penetrate through connective tissue just above the iliac crest.[380] At this site the thoracolumbar fascia and origin of the latissimus dorsi muscle form an **osteofibrous tunnel**.[381] This passageway is a specialized part of superficial fascia called the **iliolumbar membrane**. It is thought to be a type of retinacula cutis,[380] a skin ligament that anchors the skin to the deep fascia and allows the passage of nerves from the subcutaneous layer to the skin.

When an SCN becomes entrapped it may present as a swollen and tender lump above the iliac crest. It is thought that the shared origin and anastomosis of the superior cluneal nerves from L3-5, and S1-3 accounts for their ability to cause sciatica when compressed.[360]

Palpation findings in this syndrome resemble the **cellulalgia** or tender **crestal point** in patients with lumbosacral radiculopathy. Superior cluneal nerve entrapment is a cause of sciatica but can occur secondary to spinal pathology. Palpation of the iliac crest that triggers radiating sciatic pain can occur in SCN entrapment and myofascial pain secondary to spinal pathology. In sciatica, many trigger points, motor points, cellulalgic points, and peripheral nerves become sources of peripheral sensitization that feed into the sciatic pain pathway.

Hamstring syndrome

Proximal hamstring tendinopathy, also known as **proximal hamstring syndrome,**[382] hamstring syndrome,[35] and **ischial tunnel syndrome**, involves entrapment of the sciatic nerve by adhesions to the hamstring attachment. This condition is most often caused by **tendinosis** or thickening and degeneration of the hamstring tendons at the ischial tuberosity following acute or repetitive injury, blunt force trauma, or hip replacement.[383] The tendons can thicken, become inflamed, and attach to the sciatic nerve. One surgeon who operated on many cases noted:[353]

> *These tendinous structures could be as tense as a violin string and extend to the thigh over the sciatic nerve. When a finger was placed along the sciatic nerve and the hip was flexed with the knee extended one could feel how these tendinous structures compressed the nerve. (Saikku, 2010)*

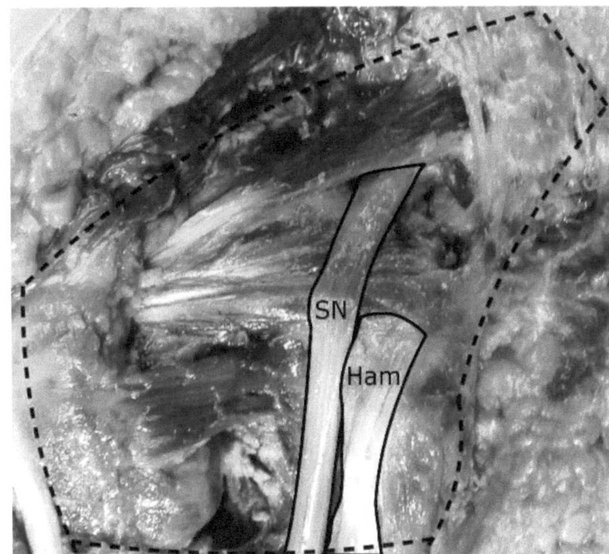

Figure 78: Left deep gluteal space highlighting the sciatic nerve (SN) and hamstring origin (ham). Thickening and inflammation of the hamstring origin can entrap the close-by sciatic nerve. Image modified from Martin et al,[386] CC-BY-4.0 license.

In the 1870s to the early 1900s surgeons investigated the utility of surgically freeing the sciatic nerve from adhesions of the nerve sheath and surrounding muscles, a procedure called neurectasy.[384] One surgeon described adhesions of the sciatic nerve in 1902:[385]

> *Men of sedentary occupations sit all day with the legs in a state of flexion... When they go to bed for sleep they still lie with their thighs drawn up. A good healthy stretching of the legs is never attempted. What wonder then, that the muscles of flexion become contracted, and also the great sciatic nerve itself. Its sheath adheres to it, and literally "grows into its shell."(Chapman, 1902)*

After neurectasy fell out of favor due to iatrogenic injuries, lack of success, and introduction of other therapies, the theory of adhesion was not addressed again until a 1988 publication described hamstring syndrome.[35] Newer research has solidified the clinical entity of entrapment or adhesion of the sciatic nerve to the hamstrings.[353]

Hamstring tears may similarly restrict sciatic **nerve mobility**. The bleeding from the muscle limits the ability of the sciatic nerve to slide through the thigh during movement, and over time can lead to sciatic nerve inflammation and tension.[387] The first published case of hamstring syndrome in 1939 described pain, numbness, and weakness of the leg, ankle, and foot in a former football player who had suffered a torn hamstring.[388] The patient's symptoms were resolved after resection of fibrous tissue from the semitendinosus which was placing pressure on the sciatic nerve.

The pain pattern and clinical findings of hamstring syndrome mimics lumbosacral nerve root pathology. Both conditions produce a similar pain pattern and may have a positive straight leg raise.[35] Not all hamstring tears or tendinopathies cause sciatica, and it is unclear what percentage of these will lead to sciatica.

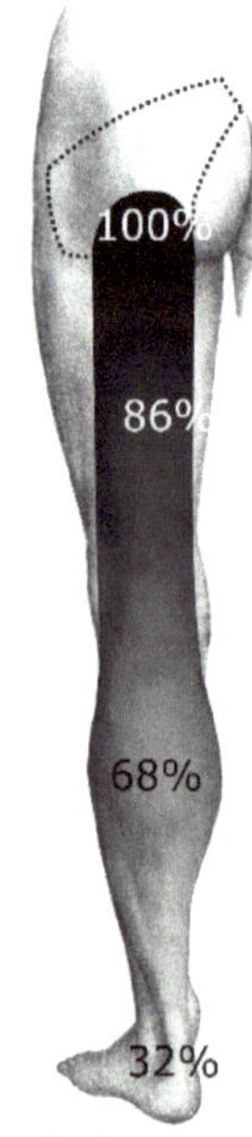

Figure 79: Proximal hamstring syndrome pain pattern. Image modified from Gray's anatomy by Robert Trager, DC, based on data from Saikku et al.[353]

Soleal sling syndrome

Soleal sling syndrome is entrapment of the **tibial nerve** under the **tendinous arch of the soleus** in the upper calf with pain and numbness in the leg and foot.[389] The tibial nerve is at risk of compression as it passes through the arch, also called the soleal sling. The most common cause of soleal sling syndrome is trauma to the knee.[389] Overuse of the calf muscles, surgeries, knee cysts and tumors can also cause nerve entrapment at the soleal sling.[389]

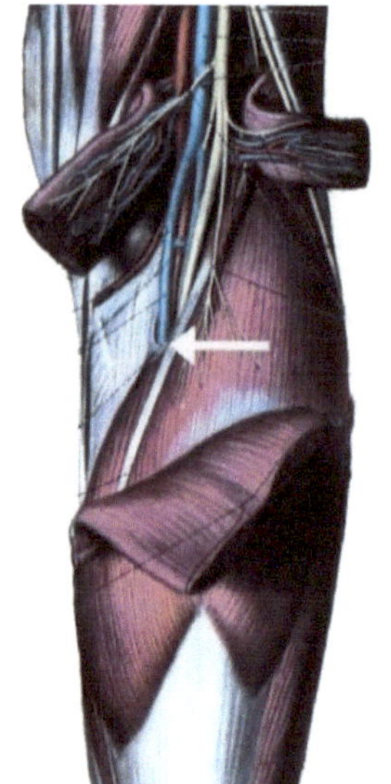
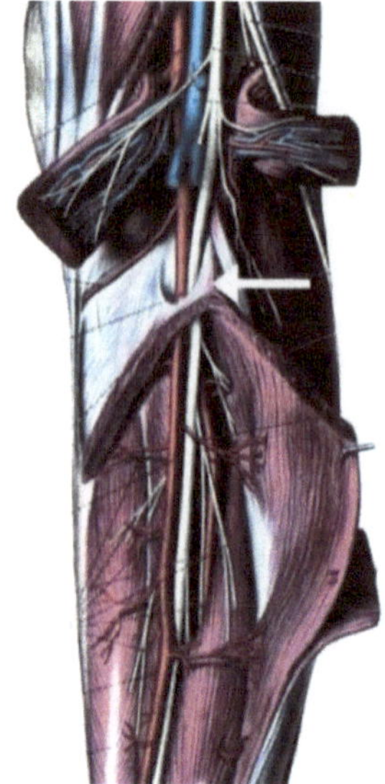

Figure 80: Soleal sling. The tibial nerve passes through the sling (white arrow) with the popliteal artery and vein (not labeled). The left image shows the overlying gastrocnemius muscle resected away. The right image shows the soleus opened, to see the tibial nerve passing deep to it. Image modified from Sobotta's anatomy 1908, public domain

Soleal sling syndrome symptoms mimic those of S1 radiculopathy.[389] There is pain in the popliteal fossa or upper calf that is increased with weight bearing.[389] Pain may radiate down the leg to the foot.[356] The most reliable symptom is numbness or pain in the **sole of the foot**.[357,389] The toe muscles are often weak.[357,389]

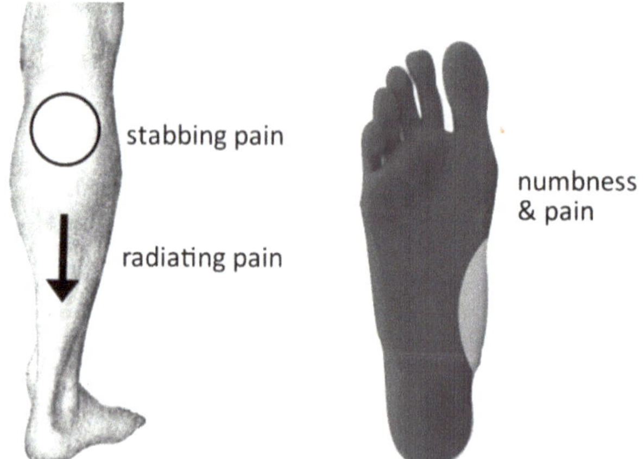

Figure 81: Symptoms of soleal sling syndrome. Image by Robert Trager, DC, by modification of public domain Gray's anatomy image of leg and image of foot by Pixel AddIct (CC-BY-2.0).

Peroneal tunnel syndrome

The common peroneal nerve (CPN) is at risk of entrapment at the **fibular head** as it passes deep to the **peroneus longus** muscle in the peroneal tunnel. Most patients with CPN entrapment have pain in the superficial peroneal nerve distribution, and about half have symptoms in the deep peroneal nerve distribution (between the 1st and 2nd toes).[390] Common peroneal entrapment is most often caused by trauma, including **ankle inversion sprains**.[391] The second leading cause is prolonged compression, for example habitual leg crossing or squatting.[391]

The pain distribution of CPN entrapment mimics that of L5 radiculopathy.[393,394] Common peroneal entrapment can be distinguished from radiculopathy by examination findings in the leg and foot. In CPN entrapment, passive or resisted **ankle inversion** provokes symptoms. Also, the ankle dorsiflexors may be weak, while ankle plantar flexion, toe plantar flexion[395] and hip strength are normal.[396] Deep tendon reflexes are normal.[395]

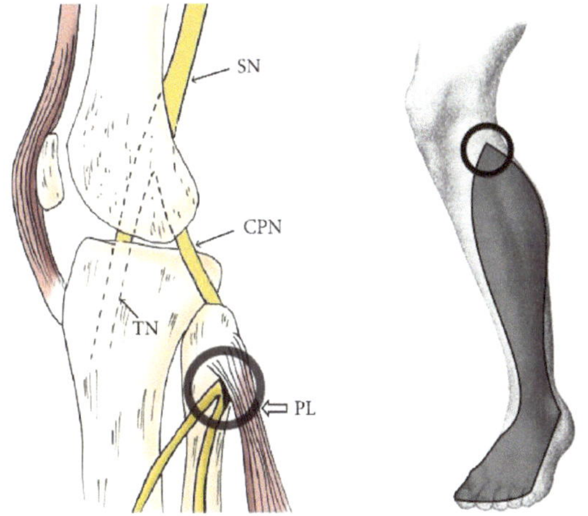

Figure 82: Common peroneal nerve entrapment. Left - entrapment of the common peroneal nerve (CPN) at the peroneus longus (PL) peroneal tunnel (circle) near the fibular neck (circle). Right - sensory distribution of common peroneal nerve entrapment. Other labels are SN, sciatic nerve, TN, tibial nerve. Left image from Dong,[392] creative commons attribution license. Right image by Robert Trager, DC.

Lumbosacral extraforaminal stenosis

Lumbosacral extraforaminal stenosis refers to nerve entrapment between the lowest lumbar segment and the sacrum. This condition typically affects the **L5 spinal nerve** or ventral ramus, which is at risk of compression from surrounding ligaments, osteophytes, disc pathology, and anomalous **transitional vertebrae**. Lumbosacral extraforaminal stenosis has the clinical features of a radiculopathy but is technically not one because it affects just distal to the nerve root. The largest studies of this condition reported its prevalence in 9-11% of cadavers.[397,398] One surgical series reported the most common cause of this condition to be lumbosacral osteophytes, followed by disc bulges, then LDHs.[354] Another study reported that 27% of patients with failed back surgery syndrome had ongoing L5 symptoms caused by extraforaminal stenosis.[399]

Lumbosacral tunnel syndrome

Lumbosacral tunnel syndrome is an entrapment of the L5 ventral root as it exits the spinal canal in the lumbosacral tunnel. This is an **osteofibrous tunnel** bounded by the lowest lumbar vertebra, sacral ala, and lumbosacral ligament. This condition refers to pathology of the ligaments connecting the lumbar spine with the sacrum and ilium causing a reduced function and/or size of the lumbosacral tunnel. Lumbosacral tunnel syndrome is associated with lumbar instability and discogenic pathology but may occur in isolation.

In 1925, Danforth described lumbosacral tunnel syndrome in an autopsy of two individuals who suffered from sciatica. In one patient the L5 ventral ramus was entrapped by a "sickle shaped ligament" and in another, by an osteophytic outgrowth.[400] In 1944 one investigator found the L5 ventral ramus "bent sharply" and compressed by "ligamentous strands" connecting L5 and the sacrum.[401]

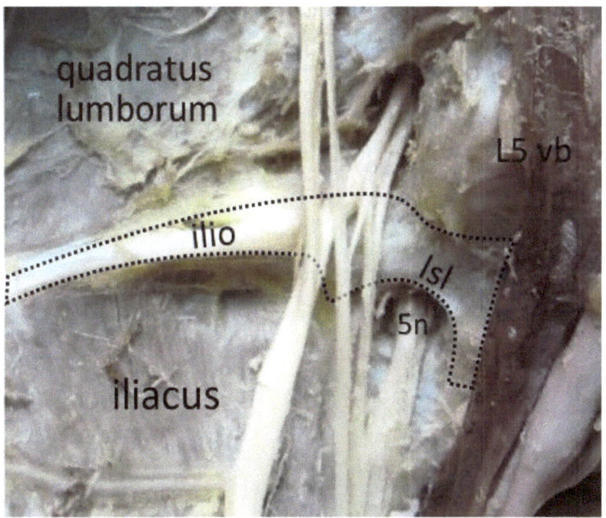

Figure 83: The lumbosacral tunnel. The lumbosacral ligament (lsl) forms a hood from which the L5 ventral ramus (5n) emerges. The lumbosacral ligament connects to the iliolumbar ligament (ilio), quadratus lumborum, and iliacus in addition to the L5 vertebral body (vb). Image CC-BY-2.0 license, modified from Lu et al.[415]

Abnormalities of the lumbosacral ligament may compress the L5 ventral ramus as it traverses the lumbosacral tunnel. Autopsy studies have suggested that a **tight lumbosacral ligament** may flatten or damage the L5 ventral ramus.[397,398,402] In these studies, the investigators were unable to pass a probe freely under the ligament. Other studies identified lumbosacral ligament **calcification** as a cause of the syndrome.[403,404] Still other studies suggested that **fibrous bands**[397] and **rami communicants**[405] could tether the nerve to the lumbosacral tunnel.

Lumbosacral tunnel syndrome damages the L5 ventral ramus. Studies have shown that abnormal tightness, calcification, or adhesions of the lumbosacral ligament thins the L5 **myelin sheath**,[398] causes **neural fibrosis**,[397,398] and **flattens** the nerve.[397,398,402]

Ligaments of the lumbosacral tunnel

The iliolumbar and lumbosacral ligaments do not exist early in life. One study found that they form from muscle between the 2nd and 4th decades and become completely ligamentous by the 5th decade.[403] One study concluded that they derived from the **quadratus lumborum**,[403] while another concluded the **iliacus muscle**.[406]

Stress may induce the change from muscle to ligament. Investigations into the anatomy of these ligaments have concluded this is a **stress-induced metaplasia**.[398,403] The iliolumbar and lumbosacral ligaments **stabilize** the lumbosacral junction. These ligaments resist rotation, flexion, extension, and lateral bending of L5 on the sacrum.[407] Repeated stress of movement may cause muscular fibers to transform in to the lumbo-ilio-sacral ligaments.

Some research suggests that lumbar instability and degenerative changes cause lumbosacral tunnel syndrome. One autopsy study found that all specimens with a tight lumbosacral ligament had **degenerated discs** and **facet joints**.[397] The investigators hypothesized that instability increased the amount of **fibrous bands** surrounding the L5 ventral ramus.[397] One surgical series reported lumbosacral ligament hypertrophy in extraforaminal L5-S1 LDHs.[408]

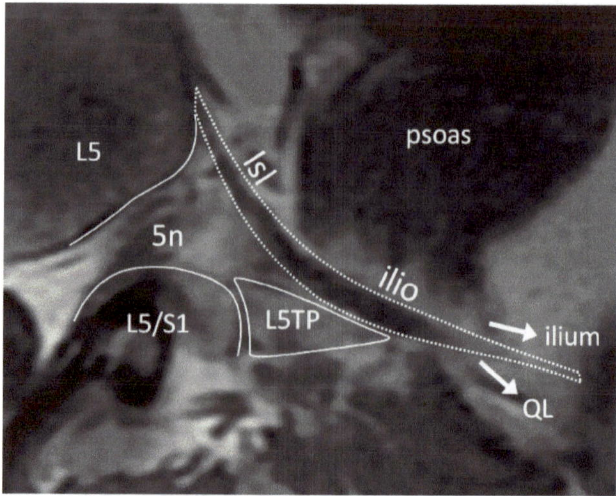

Figure 84: Anatomy of the lumbosacral tunnel. The L5 ventral ramus (5n) enters a prism-shaped passageway bordered by the lumbosacral ligament (lsl), L5, and the sacrum, deep to the psoas. The lumbosacral ligament continues into the iliolumbar (ilio) ligament (dotted line). Also shown is the L5/S1 facet joint, transverse process of L5 (L5TP), and continuation of the ligament to the ilium and quadratus lumborum (QL). Image by Robert Trager, DC

The **iliolumbar ligament** (ILL) runs laterally from the lowest transverse process, usually L5, to the iliac crest. The ILL also connects to the QL fascia.[404] The **lumbosacral ligament** (LSL) attaches between the L5 TP and VB and the sacrum.[409] Some anatomy texts consider it an inferior band of the iliolumbar ligament.[403] The LSL forms the roof of the lumbosacral tunnel.[405,409,410] The LSL attaches anteriorly to the psoas muscle.[403]

The **lumbosacral hood** or **sickle-shaped ligament**[400,411] is a segment of the lumbosacral and iliolumbar ligaments.[412] It forms a crescent-shaped **canopy** from which the L5 ventral ramus appears at the distal part of the lumbosacral tunnel.[409]

Far-out syndrome

Far-out syndrome is a compression of the L5 spinal nerve between the **L5 transverse process** and **sacral ala**.[413] Degenerative scoliosis, spondylolisthesis, transitional vertebrae, osteophytes at L5 or sacral ala, or a combination of these factors may cause this condition.

The space between the L5 transverse process (TP) and sacral ala is normally at least 2-3 centimeters from superior to inferior.[414] If the space is limited to less than **2 centimeters**, the surrounding bony structures may compress the L5 nerve. One autopsy study found that a narrow space between the TP and ala had signs of L5 ventral ramus injury including **fibrosis** and vascular hyalinization.[414]

A lumbar scoliosis may cause the **L5 transverse process** on the **convex side** to be closer to sacral ala and compress the L5 spinal nerve.[416] One study of patients with far-out syndrome found many patients had a **lumbar scoliosis** of least 5° and/or **L5-S1 disc wedging** of at least 3°.[416] These positional changes can compress the L5 spinal nerve which has an already-narrow extraforaminal space.[414] A lumbar convexity on the same side as L5-distribution sciatic symptoms is a sign of far-out syndrome.

Younger patients with an **isthmic spondylolisthesis** may develop far-out syndrome. As the L5 vertebra slip forwards, it also moves **inferiorly**, which brings the transverse processes closer to the sacral alae.[413] Researchers estimate that 20-30% of anterolisthesis (forward slippage) is necessary to produce far-out syndrome.[413]

Osteophytes on the anterolateral aspect of the L5 vertebral body or **sacral ala**[417] may entrap the L5 spinal nerve. Clinical[354] and autopsy[416] studies have identified osteophytes as the most common cause of L5 extraforaminal impingement. These can exist as an isolated finding, but typically occur in conjunction with a lumbosacral **disc bulge**.[354]

Transitional vertebrae with an **enlarged transverse process** or accessory articulation may entrap the L5 spinal nerve.[418–421] These transitional vertebrae may develop osteophytes that further reduce the space available for the L5 nerve.[419,420] Bertolotti's syndrome is another term to describe extraforaminal entrapment of the L5 spinal nerve.

Bertolotti's syndrome

Bertolotti's syndrome is the combination of sciatica with a **lumbosacral transitional vertebra** (LSTV). These vertebrae have an enlarged transverse process, extra joint, or fusion with the sacrum on one or both sides. These vertebrae may compress the L5 spinal nerve after it exits the spine and increase the likelihood of disc pathology at the disc above.

Goldthwait first made the association between the presence of a transitional segment and sciatica in 1909.[69] He believed that these segments could press against the lumbosacral trunk and cause leg pain, weakness, and numbness. In 1917 the Italian physician Bertolotti further established a link between transitional vertebrae and LBP.[422] He also correctly predicted that an enlarged transverse process was unlikely to cause symptoms, while other types of LSTVs were more likely to do so.[423]

The Castellvi classification of transitional segments describes their radiographic appearance. Type I LSTVs have a dysplastic (enlarged) **transverse process** (TP) with height > 19mm. Type II have an enlarged TP with a **pseudoarthrosis** (joint) with the sacral ala. Type III have an enlarged TP **fused** to the sacral ala. Type I, II, and III may be unilateral (A) or bilateral (B). Type IV are **mixed**, with type II on one side and type III on the other.[424]

Transitional segments that form a joint with the sacrum increase the odds of developing **radiating LBP**.[425,426] Types with pseudoarthroses (Types II and IV) are the most likely to cause radiating pain, while types I and III are unlikely to do so.[425,426] One study found up to 70% of patients with type II LSTV had symptoms related to compression of the nerve exiting the transitional foramen.[427]

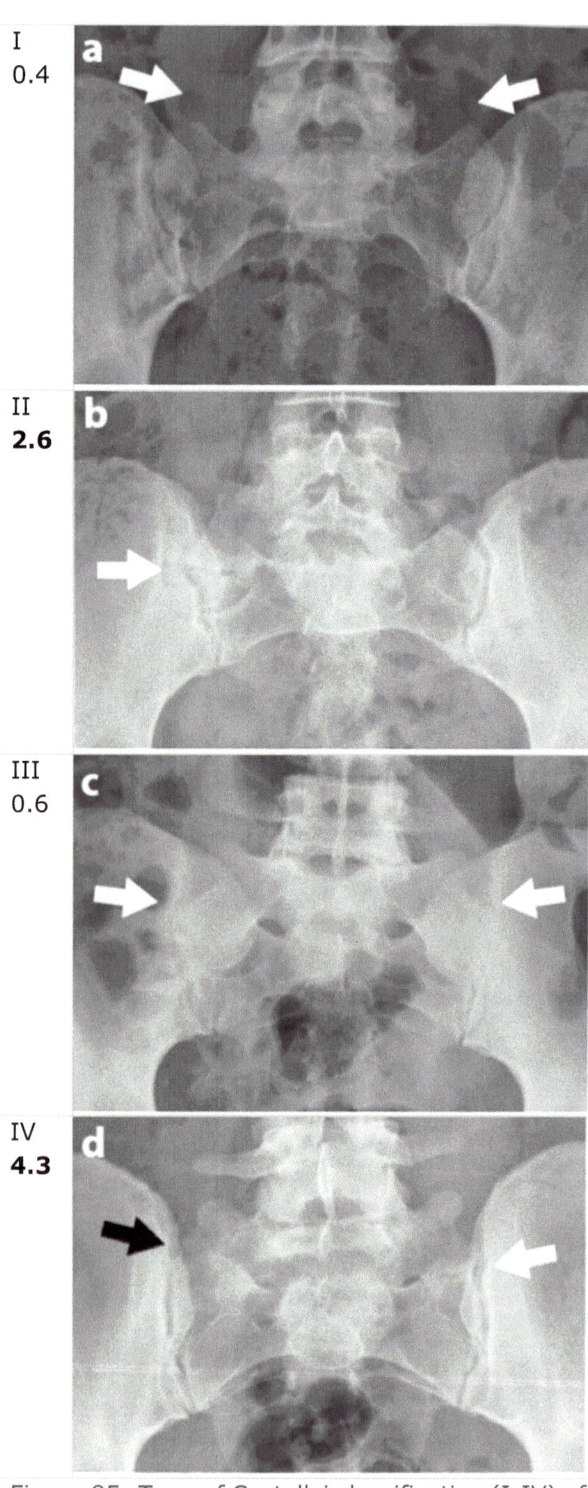

Figure 85: Type of Castellvi classification (I-IV) of lumbosacral transitional vertebrae and odds (OR)[426] of radiating gluteal pain. Images CC-BY-4.0 from de Bruin[430]

Transitional segments protect the transitional disc but predispose the disc above to damage. One study found that the types II, III, and IV transitional segment level discs had lower rates of LDH, annular tears, and disc degeneration, while the disc above had increased rates of these findings.[428] The increase in disc pathology cephalad to LSTVs may be due to **hypermobility** at this level.[429] This type of adjacent segment pathology also occurs to discs above lumbar fusion surgeries.

The sacroiliac joint

The sacroiliac joint (SIJ) can cause sciatica either by referral of pain or from leakage of **inflammatory mediators** into the nearby sensitive nerves that pass over it. One study that performed both lumbar and pelvic MRI on 209 patients with sciatica found that symptoms were due to **sacroiliitis** (inflammation of the SIJ) in only 1% of the patients.[14]

In the early 1900s, prior to the popularization of LDH as a diagnosis, clinicians believed the SIJ was a major cause of sciatica. The first medical doctor to give attention to the SIJ as a cause of sciatica was the British surgeon John Hilton in 1879.[431] Joel Ernest Goldthwait, who founded the Orthopaedic Service at Massachusetts General Hospital in 1899, believed that sciatica was most often caused by a displacement of the sacrum or pelvis and subsequent irritation of the nearby nerves.[69] In 1899 the British neurologist Gowers linked rheumatic disease at the lumbosacral region to inflammation of the lumbosacral trunk, but he believed that disease began in the sacral plexus and spread to the SIJ:[432]

> *...there are cases with a strong disposition for fibrous rheumatism to fix itself in the tissues of the pelvis, sacral and lumbar regions... The mass of the "sacral plexus" is prolonged into it, and the membranes covering this, and its branches, including the lumbo-sacral cord, are very liable to be the seat of such inflammation... (Gowers, p 126)*

In 1909 Fred Albee concluded that "close proximity" of the lumbosacral trunk to the SIJ explained the persistent symptoms of sciatica.[433] In 1928 Yeoman correlated sciatica with arthritic changes of the **anterior sacroiliac ligament** and inflammation of the piriformis muscle.[434] He attributed 36% of cases of sciatica to arthritis of the SIJ based on radiographic findings.[434] During this time period doctors frequently treated the SIJ in patients with sciatica using injections, SIJ manipulation, and bracing.

The discovery of LDH as a cause of sciatica in 1934 and mistaken notion that the SIJ was a synchondrosis overshadowed the diagnosis and treatment of the SIJ. In the 1990s the SIJ re-appeared into focus as studies showed that inflammatory changes within the joint could cause sciatica. In 1999 Joseph Fortin discovered that inflammatory mediators could leak from the SIJ into the nearby nerves, which explained the appearance of sciatica in cases of sacroiliitis:[435]

> *...in a traumatized and inflamed [sacroiliac] joint, extravasation of synovial fluid containing inflammatory mediators including substance P could traverse any of the three pathways [from the sacroiliac joint to surrounding neural structures] described and irritate one or more of the neural elements that compose the sciatic nerve (L4-S2).(Fortin)*

Fortin discovered pathways of movement of fluid from the SIJ into the neighboring nerves by using arthrography and injecting a contrast agent into the SIJ. Fortin discovered migration of fluid out of the SIJ into three nearby structures: (1) The **L5 root canal**, (2) the **dorsal sacral foramina**, and (3) the **sacral plexus.**

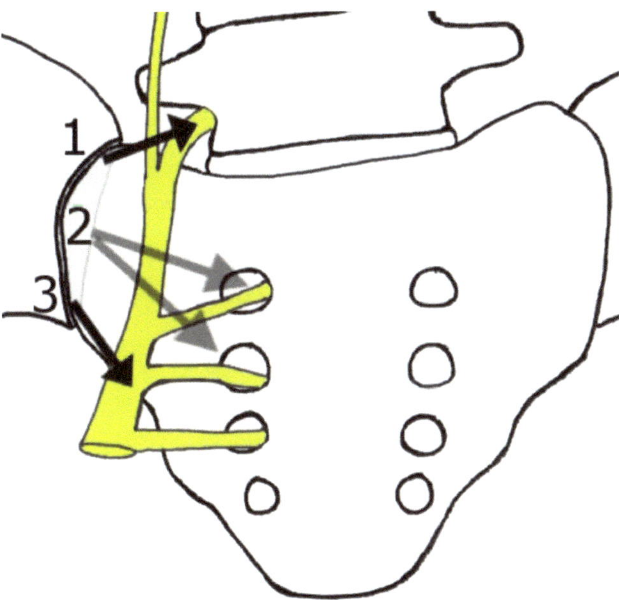

Figure 86: Three routes of spread of inflammatory mediators from the SIJ to nearby structures: (1) To the L5 nerve sheath, (2) Posteriorly to the sacral foramina (posteriorly), and (3) anteriorly to the lumbosacral plexus. Image by Robert Trager, DC.

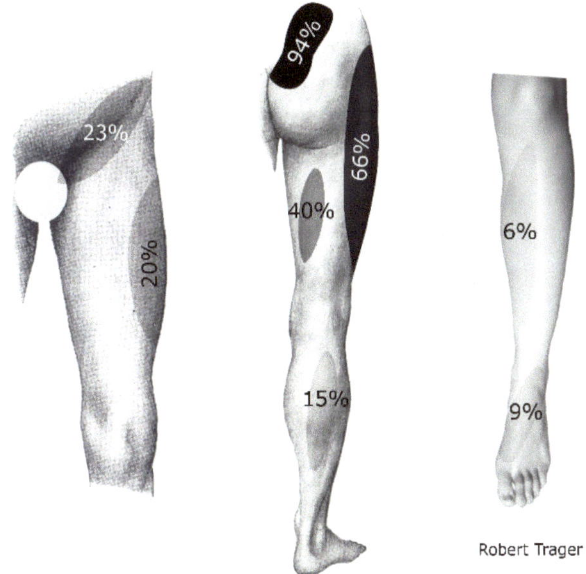

Figure 87: Sacroiliac joint pain referral zones. Inflammation of the SIJ can cause radiating pain along the sciatic nerve distribution. Percentages indicate the proportion of patients with SIJ pain and pain in that body part. Opacity levels of pain referral corresponds to symptom frequency. Data adapted from Murakami.[437] Image of thigh and lower extremity from public domain Grey's Anatomy, leg (right) modified from Andrea Allen (CC-BY-2.0). Image by Robert Trager, DC.

Studies using anesthetic SIJ injections have mapped its pain referral patterns. These studies have found that the most common symptoms are **PSIS** or **buttocks pain**, occurring in 94% of patients, followed by posterior and/or lateral thigh pain in about a third of patients.[436,437] The further inferior in the extremity, the less frequently patients experience symptoms. Symptoms are distinguished from radicular syndromes in that they are **non-dermatomal**,[437] and radiating pain is **proximal to the knee** in about two-thirds of patients.[436] Only about 10% of patients experience symptoms in the foot,[436,437] which are usually described as numbness or tingling.[437]

Sacroiliitis can cause sciatica in cases of inflammatory arthritides including **psoriatic arthritis**,[438] **reactive sacroiliitis**,[438] **Crohn's disease**,[439] and other **seronegative spondyloarthropathies**.[439–441] These cases probably cause sciatica through leakage of inflammation to the nearby nerves as identified by Fortin.

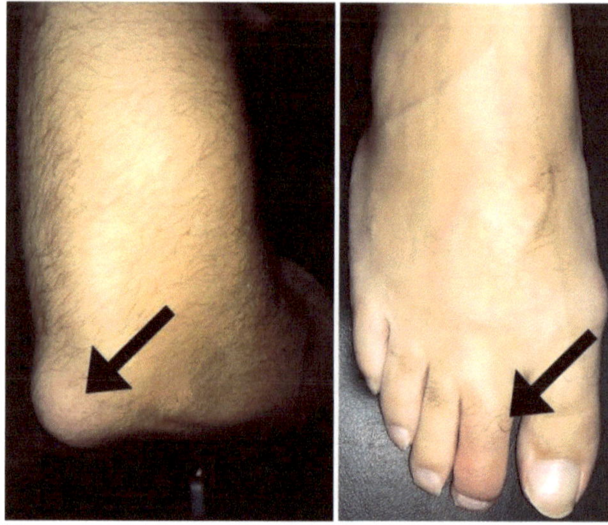

Figure 88: Case of sciatica related to gout and suspected sacroiliitis. An otherwise healthy 45-year-old man presented with a 3-day history of acute severe R SIJ pain with radiation into the gluteal region, thigh, and calf, that began the day after eating a dinner of crab and asparagus (both have purines that can precipitate gout attacks in those predisposed). He also developed painful swelling in the ankles, elbows, and one toe (arrows). He had no prior episodes but had a family history of gout. Symptoms subsided with medication to treat gout. Image shared with patient's permission by Robert Trager, DC.

Leakage of inflammatory substances may not the only mechanism responsible for pain. Because the sciatic nerve is innervated from the dorsal rami of S1-4, sciatica could be caused by local irritation of the joint itself, with pain being **referred** into the S1 or S2 segments in the lower extremity.[442]

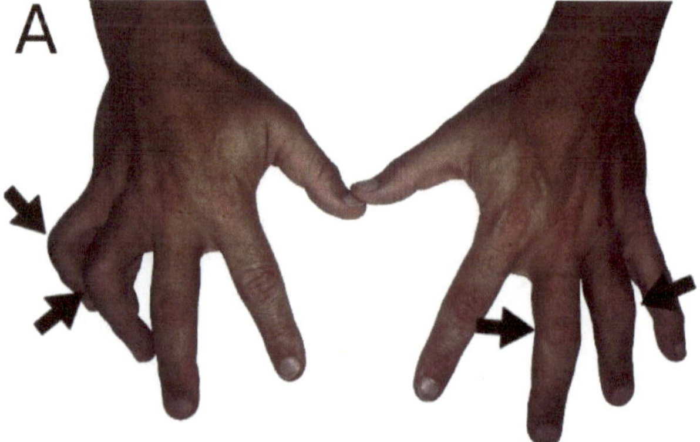

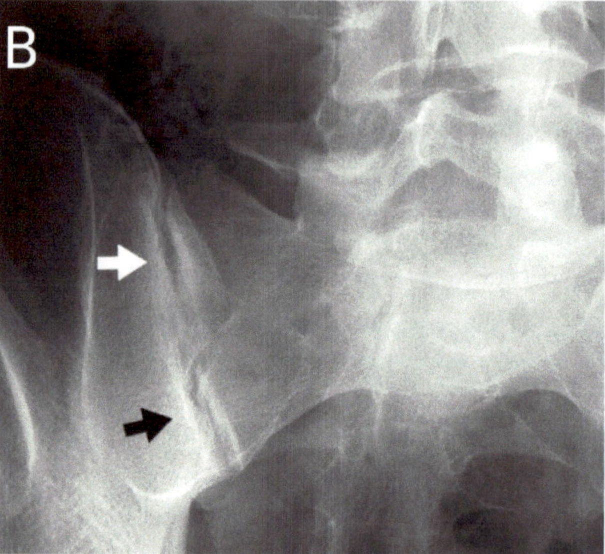

Figure 89: Sacroiliitis with sciatica. A 42 year-old-man with a history of Crohn's disease presented with a 3-week history of severe aching, stabbing R SIJ pain with radiation to R leg, tingling in R posterior thigh, and soreness and tightness in R calf. He also had arthritis of the PIP joints of both hands (A, arrows) and could not fully extend the fingers. Examination revealed 4/5 strength R calf mm. Imaging revealed sclerosis of R SIJ (B). Patient responded well to soft-tissue manipulation, SIJ HVLA manipulation, and diagnostic/therapeutic injection into the SIJ.

Double-crush syndrome

Sciatic pain may result from a combination of nerve lesions involving the nerve roots, trunk, or branches. Double-crush syndrome is a collection of symptoms related to the additive effect of more than one nerve lesion, one being central and another being more peripheral. In sciatica, double-crush syndrome occurs with the combination of an ipsilateral spinal and extraspinal nerve lesion. Peripheral neuropathies and nerve entrapments along the sciatic nerve course and branches may be more common in those with sciatica.

One in ten of those with sciatic pain may have more than one nerve lesion. One study that used both MRI and electrodiagnostic testing on 165 patients with sciatica found that 8.5% had both **radiculopathy** and **peripheral neuropathy**.[443] An EMG study reported that 9% of those with LSS had slowed nerve conduction velocity.[444] Another EMG study identified **polyneuropathy** in 12% of patients with LSS.[445] Each of these studies excluded patients with systemic causes of neuropathy including diabetes.

Specific types of **nerve entrapments** are associated with lumbosacral radiculopathy. These include **tarsal tunnel syndrome**, which occurs in nearly 5% of those with radiculopathy,[446] and **cluneal nerve entrapment**, which is associated with thoracolumbar or lumbar fracture.[360] Other lesions involving the superficial peroneal nerve,[447] sural nerve,[448] and lateral femoral cutaneous nerve[449] may occur but appear to be less common.

Double-crush lesions may be underdiagnosed in sciatic patients. Clinicians may identify double-crush lesions, especially in patients with chronic symptoms.[448,450,451] In other cases they are only identified by a clinician or surgeon following lumbar spine surgery.[330,449,452] The most common double-crush lesions include the **superior cluneal nerve** (SCN), **posterior tibial nerve**, and **common peroneal nerve**.[330,449,452]

Double-crush lesions in sciatica may relate to impaired **axoplasmic flow**.[448,451,453] In this model, lesions along the course of a nerve have an additive effect in disrupting the flow of nutrients along the nerve. Metabolic disorders such as **diabetes** may predispose patients to double-crush lesions in sciatica.[451] It is also possible that altered gait or biomechanics play a role in the simultaneous involvement of spinal and extraspinal nerves.[446]

Studies have shown a correspondence between the side of spinal involvement and side of nerve entrapment. One study found that 89% of tarsal tunnel syndrome cases occurred only on the side of radiculopathy, when present, and another 7% of cases were bilateral.[446] Another study found that 75% of cluneal nerve entrapments occurred on the same side of a symptomatic LDH, when present.[449] Peripheral nerve lesions on the same side as radicular sciatica provide additional evidence that these conditions are causally linked.

Circulation

Lack of blood flow to the sciatic nerve or its roots, trunk, or branches can predispose one to develop sciatica, cause sciatica, or arise secondarily to longstanding sciatica. As an individual factor, circulatory disturbances rarely cause sciatica.

Hippocrates was the first on record to relate sciatica to the circulatory system circa 400 BCE. He introduced a system of health involving the balance of the four humors: Blood, yellow bile, black bile, and phlegm. Hippocrates' believed that sciatica arose when excess bile and phlegm caused the blood to congeal and stop circulating, and described symptoms associated with sciatica such as coldness of the loins and erectile dysfunction.[454] The Ayurvedic text Charaka Saṃhitā (c. 300 BCE) had a similar description of how sciatica developed. Aggravated vayu was thought to bring pitta (bilious humour) and kapha (mucus) to the wrong places, causing obstructions and drying up the *rasa* (blood).[455]

Patients with sciatica often experience a cold sensation in the affected lower extremity and foot. This phenomenon, called the **cold foot syndrome** of sciatica,[456] may be related to reduced blood flow in the distribution of the sciatic nerve. Many studies have identified that the leg affected by sciatica have at least a 1°C lower temperature compared to the unaffected side.[457–459] Patients with discogenic sciatica have, on average, a 12.5% reduction in leg blood flow as measured by angiography.[460]

Those with sciatic pain may have reduced blood flow in the affected limb through due to increased activity of the **sympathetic nervous system** (SNS).[460] The SNS may activate in cases of pain and inflammation and cause vasoconstriction, a narrowing of blood vessels. Sympathetic nerves run into the lumbosacral nerve roots[461] and along the sciatic nerve and its branches.[462] Because of their close anatomic relationship, the two pathways (SNS nerves and sciatic nerve) may become stimulated together. Some researchers suspect, based on temperature differences that are abolished following therapy, that those with sciatic pain have SNS-mediated vasoconstriction.[326,463]

Regardless of the cause of sciatica the result can be a lack of blood flow and a corresponding reduction in temperature. Conversely, the lack of blood flow may be a predisposing factor to any other major cause of sciatica. Macnab describes the lack of blood flow as a risk factor for nerve root pathology:[464]

> *It is most likely that one of the significant events in the pathogenesis of sciatica is the primary upset in vascular supply to a nerve root, with the secondary phenomenon of interference with nerve root nutrition... (Macnab, p. 85)*

Vascular diseases adversely affect both the spine itself and the nerve roots that make up the sciatic nerve. Reduced blood flow through the **lumbar arteries** leads to reduced nutrition to the IVDs and eventual **disc degeneration**.[288] A study using magnetic resonance angiography found that patients with occlusion of two or more lumbar arteries had a greater odds of having sciatica.[19]

Disorders of the abdominal aorta can cause sciatica due to lack of blood flow to the cauda equina (lumbar and sacral nerve roots), such as in **aortoiliac occlusive disease**[465] and aortic aneurysms.[466] Lack of proper blood flow can directly cause sciatica due to lack of perfusion into the cauda equina, or indirectly through gradual degeneration of the spine.

Leriche Syndrome and aortic aneurysms

Leriche or **small aorta syndrome** is a condition involving stenosis of the aorta or iliac arteries which results in lower extremity pain, typically exacerbated by physical exertion.[465] Sciatica is a possible outcome of having this condition. Any cause of vascular blockages including **atherosclerosis** and risk factors such as **smoking** can contribute to the development of Leriche syndrome. The symptoms are diverse and can range from pain with exercise in the buttocks, thigh, and calves, paresthesia, to radiating leg pain.

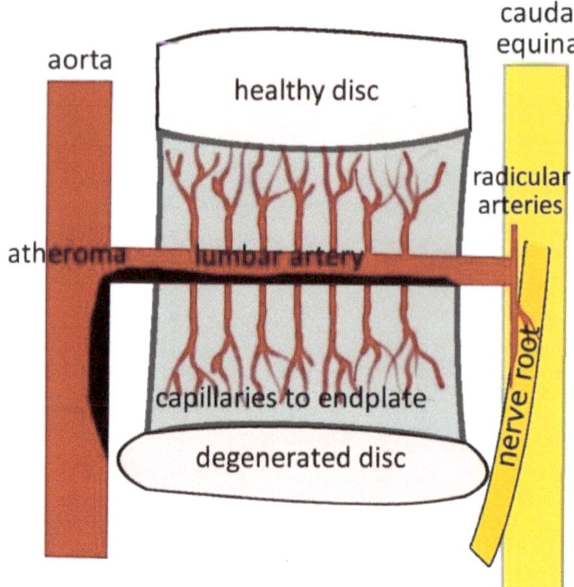

Figure 90: Blood supply to the IVD and cauda equina. An arterial blockage is shown here as an atheroma, indicated by a dark deposit in the aorta and lumbar artery. Blockage of these arteries reduce blood supply to the discs as well as the lumbosacral nerve roots and predispose one to disc degeneration and radiculopathy. Image by Robert Trager, DC.

Suboptimal blood flow to the nerve roots of the lower back could predispose one to spinal pathology and nerve root injury. Poor blood flow could increase risk of developing sciatica given any other insult or injury to the nerve roots or sciatic nerve. The effects of atherosclerosis and **spinal stenosis** can compound upon one another, as they both contribute to leg pain during exertion.[195]

Vascular occlusion in Leriche syndrome deprives the lower extremity muscles and the cauda equina of blood flow. The long-term loss of circulation is enough to damage the nerves to the point where there is neuropathic pain. Physical examination can show loss of sensation and reflexes, while electromyography can show denervation of the affected nerve roots.[467]

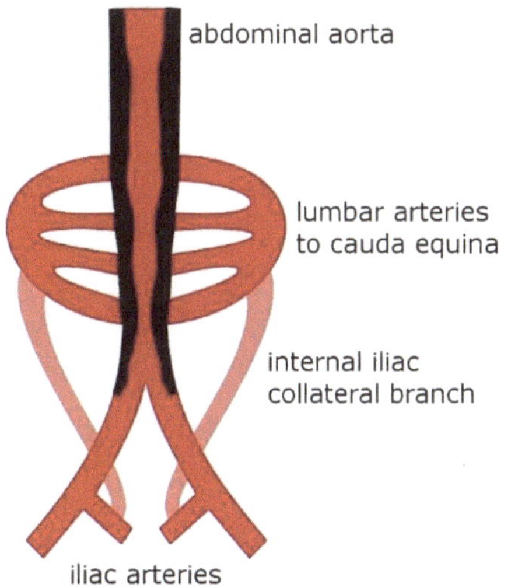

Figure 91: Blood supply of the cauda equina and effect of an atheroma (dark wavy buildup) at the juncture of the abdominal aorta and common iliac arteries. Image by Robert Trager, DC.

Lumbar **aorta calcification** is associated with LBP[288] but may also indicate a diminished blood flow to the nerve roots of the lower back. The cauda equina derive their blood supply primarily from branches of the abdominal aorta and partially from the internal iliac artery.[465] If these branches become blocked or if the aorta itself becomes blocked, the cauda equina do not have sufficient blood flow.

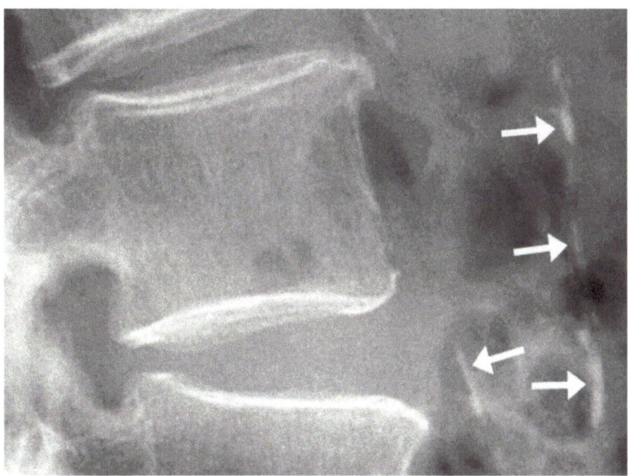

Figure 92: Aortic calcification (arrows) seen on a lateral lumbar radiograph, in a 76-year-old man with LSS and neurogenic claudication. Image shared with patient's permission by Robert Trager, DC.

Aortic aneurysms can deprive blood flow to the cauda equina just as in Leriche syndrome, but they can also directly compress the nerves that descend through the pelvis due to their space-occupying nature.[466,468]

The hip

There is a correlation and a causal relationship between hip joint arthritis and sciatic pain. The two conditions occur more often together than chance occurrence would explain. There is also evidence that pathology of one adversely affects the other. Biomechanical limitations of the hip restrict spinal and sciatic nerve mobility, and inflammatory conditions of the spine can affect the hip. The **shared sensory innervation** of the hip and sciatic nerve allows for pain referral from one area to the other.

One of the first theories of sciatica was disease of the hip joint. The modern word *sciatica* has its root in the Greek word for hip, ισχιά or "ischia. Hippocrates was the first to relate the hip joint to sciatica circa 400 BCE.[7] Many other ancient authors equated sciatica with arthritis of the hip joint, including Aëtius (5th-6th century CE), a Greek Byzantine physician who wrote "[arthritis] in anyone's hip joint, is called sciatica, *coxendicu morbus.*"[8] The term **hip-gout** was used as a synonym for sciatica in the 1600s, 1700s and 1800s CE, as it was thought to have a similar mechanism as gout.[471]

Some ancient clinicians attempted to differentiate hip and sciatic pain. Aretaeus of Cappadocia remarked in 50 CE that radiating pain from the hip to the heel or great toe "has the appearance of anything rather than an affection of the hip-joint."[472] Later, Domenicus Cotugno of Italy described an "anterior sciatica" relating to the femoral nerve and "fore part of the hip", and **posterior sciatica** or **true sciatica** related to the sciatic nerve.[473] He correctly observed that hip pain rarely radiated pain distal to the knee.[473]

Hip joint pain referral

The L4 and L5 spinal cord segments allow for pain referral from the hip into the lower extremity in the distribution of the sciatic nerve. This pain pattern may involve or mimic the **L4** or **L5** nerve root sensory distributions. The earliest theories to explain pain referral are based on **convergence**, in which painful stimuli from different body parts synapse with the same second-order neuron in the central nervous

[7] *After protracted attacks of sciatica, when the head of the bone alternately escapes from and returns to the cavity, an accumulation of synovia occurs. (Coar, p. 187)* [469]

[8] Author's translation, Aëtius, p. 716[470]

system. In the case of the hip, the sciatic nerve innervates the hip and parts of the lower extremity. The convergence of neural signals from the hip and sciatic nerve allows for referral of hip pain to the lower extremity.

In 1785 the British surgeon Sir Frederick Treves described referred pain involving the sciatic nerve, using the example of hip pain referred to the knee.[474] In 1879 the British surgeon John Hilton also described sciatic pain referral and pointed out that the hip joint capsule shares the same innervation as the heel and foot.[431]

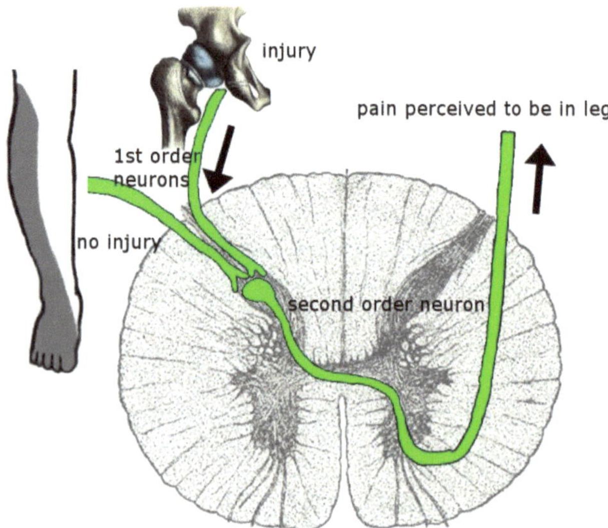

Figure 93: Mechanism of referred pain from the hip joint into the leg based on the model of convergence. Sensory branches of the sciatic nerve innervate both the posterior hip joint and the leg and foot. Patients may interpret pain as coming from the leg and foot even if it originates from the hip, because sensory information from the two regions converges upon a shared second order neuron in the spinal cord.

These early observations have been validated by research that shows the sciatic nerve innervates the **posterolateral hip capsule**.[475] The posterior hip is variably innervated by multiple sciatic nerve branches including a **direct articular branch** from the sciatic, the nerve to the quadratus femoris and the superior gluteal nerve.[475] Conversely, the anterior hip joint is innervated by the femoral nerve.[475]

In the early 1900s, some physicians theorized that hip joint arthritis referred pain from the **articular nerves** to the lumbosacral segments. In 1916 professor Robert Reid theorized the sensory innervation of the hip joint from L4, L5, and S1 could refer pain to the leg.[476] This same year Dr. William Bruce presented 691 cases of sciatica in which he claimed that most cases were caused by referred pain from hip joint arthritis. He based his theory on the observations that hip arthritis, tenderness, and loss of range of motion were common findings on the same side of sciatic pain.[476]

Hip joint pain referral may relate to its **sclerotomes**. The acetabulum is innervated mostly by L4, but also L3, L5, and S1.[477–479] Damage and inflammation to these segmental areas of the acetabulum could refer pain into the corresponding dermatome(s).Pain referral from the hip joint can occur in the **sciatic nerve distribution**. One study that mapped hip pain referral patterns with therapeutic injections found that symptoms referred most often into the buttocks, in 71% of cases, followed by the lateral thigh (27%), posterior thigh (24%), lateral leg (8%), posterior leg (8%), and foot (6%).[480] Referral also frequently involved non-sciatic regions, most often the groin, in 55% of cases.[480] This study has corroborated by others that confirm hip pain can refer into the distal lower extremities.[481,482]

Groin pain is the most specific region of pain corresponding to **hip osteoarthritis** (specificity of 70%).[482] While thigh and leg pain does not by itself distinguish hip from spine symptoms, spine-related sciatica is more likely to radiate distal to the knee. Hip pain radiates distal to the knee in only 22% of cases of hip pain[480] compared to 77% of radicular sciatic pain.[7]

Hip spine syndrome

Hip-spine syndrome describes the common coexistence, overlap, and interplay between hip and spine pathology and pain. It includes a tetrad of (1) **degenerative changes of the hip**, (2) **lumbar stenosis**, (3) **hip flexion contracture**, and (4) **radiculopathy**.[483] The presence of hip arthritis increases the odds of also having degenerative low back conditions. The converse is also true, that those with low back symptoms are more likely to have hip pain and pathology.

Clinicians may misdiagnose the primary source of pathology in hip-spine patients. Radiographic signs of hip or spine arthritis may be misleading as these changes can be **asymptomatic**. For example, LSS symptoms poorly correlate with imaging findings. The pain patterns of hip and spine pathology overlap, especially within the **L4** and **L5 distribution**. In rare cases, misdiagnosed patients have unnecessary spinal surgery when hip arthritis is the main cause of their symptoms.[484,485]

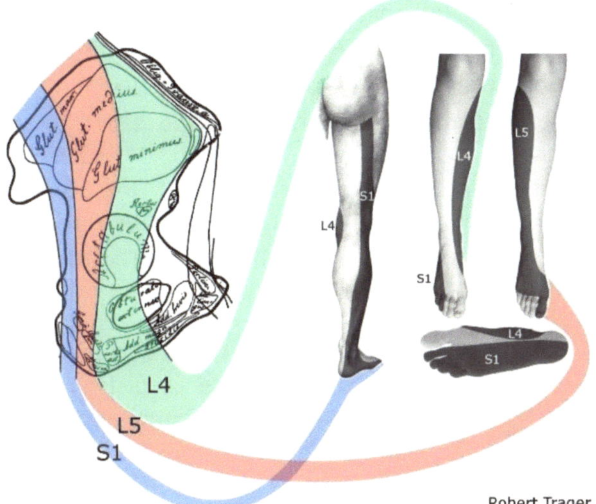

Figure 94: Sclerotomal innervation of the hip and its referral pattern. The acetabulum is mostly innervated by L4 and to a lesser degree by L5 and S1. Pain may refer from these zones into the corresponding dermatome. Image of pelvis from Bolk, 1894, public domain, thigh and lower extremity from public domain Grey's Anatomy, leg modified from Andrea Allen (CC by 2.0).

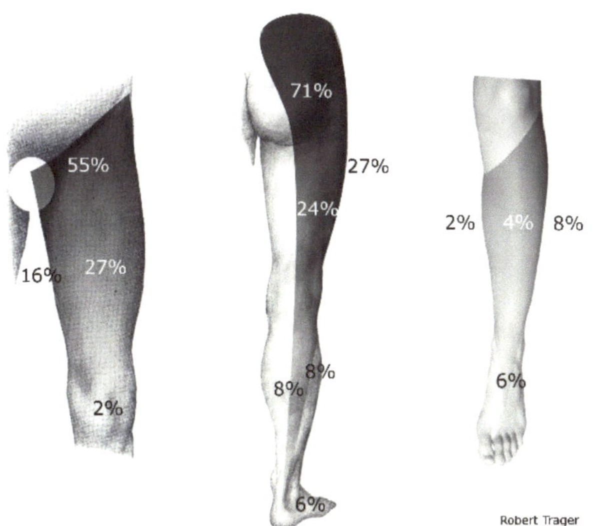

Figure 95: Hip joint pain referral patterns. Image by Robert Trager, DC, based on data from Lesher et al.[480] Image of thigh and lower extremity from public domain Grey's Anatomy, leg (right image) modified from Andrea Allen (CC by 2.0).

Hip pain is common in those with LBP and vice versa. Over 70% of older adults with LBP also have hip pain or stiffness.[486] The majority of those with LBP also have pain with provocative orthopedic testing of the hip.[487] Those with a combination of low back and hip symptoms have more severe LBP and greater disability levels associated with LBP.[487]

Hip abnormalities are more common in those with LBP. About 80% of patients with LBP also have radiographic **hip osteoarthritis**, **femoroacetabular impingement**, or **degenerative dysplasia**.[488] Twenty percent of LBP patients have moderate to severe hip OA.[488] One large osteological study found that presence of hip OA increased the odds of spinal OA being present.[489] Another osteological study showed that hips with **cam deformities** were significantly more likely to have spinal arthritis.[490]

Researchers suggest that abnormal hip biomechanics and transfers load to the spine.[490] Loss of hip range of motion places greater demands and wear-and-tear on the low back. Asymmetry of hip rotation causes **asymmetrical loading** on the lumbar spine. Reduced hip extension, such as is seen in **ischiofemoral impingement**, causes increased facet joint loading.[491] Reduced hip range of motion may cause a compensatory increase in lumbar and pelvic rotation.[492]

Hip OA increases the odds of developing a **degenerative spondylolisthesis** (DS). One study found that **primary hip OA** increases the odds of DS by a factor of 1.9.[493] This study found that DS was present in 22% of those with hip OA, about double that of the general population.[493] This finding was not explained by body mass index, gender, or other variables. Patients that undergo total hip arthroplasty also have an increased risk of degenerative spondylolisthesis and LDH.[494]

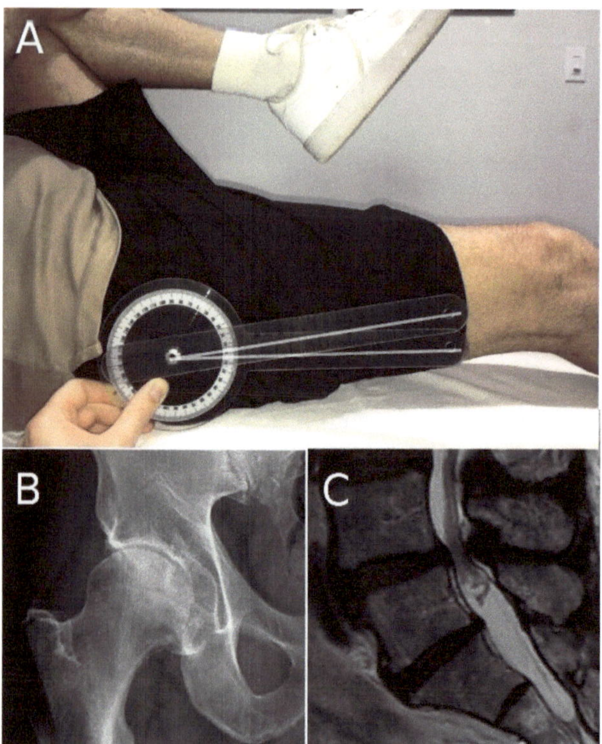

Figure 96: Hip-spine syndrome. This 77-year-old man presented with chronic LBP radiating to BL shins and feet with numbness, had R sided hip flexion contracture of 8 degrees (A), right hip OA (B), and L4 anterolisthesis causing LSS (C). He was diagnosed with L5 radiculopathy. The patient improved with flexion-distraction, hip mobilization exercises, and dry needling of the lumbar paraspinal muscles. Case shared with permission from patient by Robert Trager, DC.

Neurogenic inflammation may explain the relationship between hip and spine pathology. The hip and low back are both innervated by branches of the sciatic nerve. It is possible that damage to one branch of the sciatic nerve pathway causes the release of inflammatory mediators in other branches. Damage to the sciatic pathway has been suggested to increase inflammatory hip joint pain.[495]

Hip flexor contractures

Hip flexion contracture, also called **hip flexion deformity** or **psoas contracture** is a state in which the hip is fixed in flexion with a limited ability or inability to reach a neutral position or extend. Hip and low back disorders can cause this deformity. Hip flexion contractures are thought to place excess stress on the lumbar spine and lead to degenerative lumbar conditions.[483]

Caelius Aurelianus was the first on record to relate the psoas muscle to sciatic pain in his book chapter *Sciatica and Psoitis*.[496] He described that those with severe sciatica developed hardening of the hip and stiffening of the loin muscles of the spine, causing the body to be "drawn and bent forward."[496] Around 1960 Arthur Michel proposed that the common link between hip and spine pathology was a failure of iliopsoas elongation during growth from age five through twelve.[497] He suggested that an increased iliopsoas pulling force would predispose one to degenerative changes in the spine such as **spondylosis** and **spondylolisthesis**. He also hypothesized that shortened iliopsoas would create a shearing force at the acetabulum and predispose to **hip dysplasia**.

The psoas originates from T12 or L1 and L2-4 and descends inferiorly to attach to the lesser trochanter of the femur. The psoas has attachments at the vertebral bodies, IVDs, and small fascicles from the transverse processes. It acts as both a spinal stabilizer and a hip flexor.

Those with LBP have less **passive hip extension**.[498–500] Loss of hip extension correlates with LBP better than any other hip range of motion.[498,499] The correlation between LBP and loss of hip extension is thought to relate to hip flexion contracture involving the psoas.[498]

An increased **lumbar lordosis** may be an adaptation to limited hip extension.[491] While there is a wide range of normal degrees of lumbar lordosis, about 29°±12,[502] those with hip OA have on average an increased lordosis angle of about 39°.[503] Hip flexion contracture may explain the correlation between hip OA and hyperlordosis.

The psoas muscle adds a **compressive force** to the lumbar spine that helps stabilize it. The compressive force increases from L1 to L5 where it is the highest.[501] It has been estimated that in a 99 kilogram adult the psoas adds 40-70 kilograms of compression through the lumbar IVDs during standing and sitting.[504] The compressive force of the psoas accounts for about one-third of the overall load on the IVD.[504] When the psoas is inactive and not stabilizing the spine, for example when reclining supine, compressive loads reduce below 40 kilograms.[504]

The psoas adds an **anterior shearing force** to the lumbar spine. As with the compressive force, the shear force also increases from L1 to L5 where it is the highest.[501] This is opposed by the posterior shearing force of the posterior spinal muscles.[505] A balance between anterior and posterior shear forces is necessary to maintain spinal stability. The psoas anterior shear force may dominate in patients who have neurogenic atrophy related to LDH.

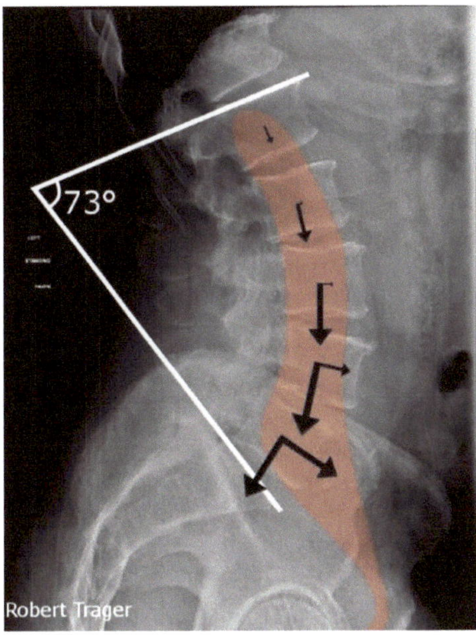

Figure 97: Psoas muscles (red) and forces (arrows) on the lumbar spine; drawn over plain-film standing radiographs. This 60 year-old-man has left L5 & S1 radicular pain related to DS (L4) and LSS (MRI not shown). He also has a bilateral hip flexion contracture seen during gait and Thomas' testing, which contributes to his 73° hyperlordosis. Force vectors created using data from Bogduk[501] are proportionate to the amount of newtons of compression (arrows pointing inferiorly) and shear (arrows facing anteriorly). Image shared with permission of patient by Robert Trager, DC.

The psoas is more resistant to atrophy than the multifidus and erector spinae in those with low back disorders.[506,507] This may be due to its action as a spinal stabilizer,[507] or levels of innervation (L1, L2, L3) being above the most commonly damaged low-lumbar disc levels. The persistence of the psoas could lead to it overpowering the weaker, atrophied posterior lumbar muscles (erectors and multifidus), resulting in a degenerative anterolisthesis.

Hip flexion contractures are often bilateral but are usually worse on the side opposite from sciatica. Discogenic pain stimulates contraction of the **contralateral psoas** through a spinal reflex.[508,509] This causes the psoas to pull the lumbar spine into a concavity on the side away from pain. This may also explain why the contralateral psoas is comparatively larger than psoas on the side of sciatic pain.[303,510]

Functional magnetic resonance imaging studies have found that the psoas muscles may appear asymmetrical in those with low back pain.[511] Higher **metabolic activity** is represented by a brighter signal on T2 weighted imaging. Heightened, asymmetrical signal of the psoas may represent the hip flexor contracture often seen in low back pain and sciatica.

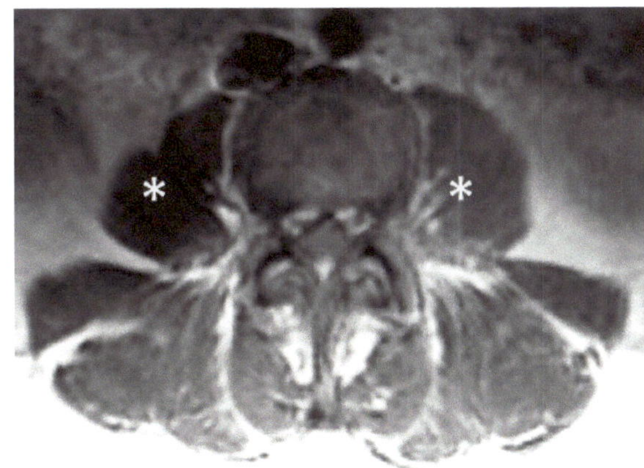

Figure 98: Asymmetrical muscle signal of the psoas on axial MRI indicating asymmetrical muscle activity, in a patient with low back pain. Image CC-BY-2.0 from Clark[511]

Researchers have suggested that hip flexion contractures cause hyperlordosis, which in turn causes **foraminal encroachment**.[483] This is supported by evidence that lumbar extension reduces the size of the intervertebral foramina.[512] Also, limited hip extension causes increased **facet joint loading**.[491] Increased facet joint load may, over time, contribute to joint degeneration, instability, and bony hypertrophy. Hip-flexor-related hyperlordosis may also increase the symptoms of LSS, which typically has a directional preference of lumbar flexion.

Some authors have suggested that hip flexion contractures increase the risk of **spondylolisthesis**[497,513] or worsen already-existing cases.[514] Hip flexion contractures increase lumbar lordosis,[515] which increases loading on the posterior spinal elements (e.g., the facet joints). A psoas-induced spondylolisthesis could theoretically occur with a dominant anterior shear force at the lower lumbar levels combined with other risk factors such as repetitive hyperextension and degenerative changes of the facet joints.

Ischiofemoral impingement

Ischiofemoral impingement is a condition that results from a narrowing of the **ischiofemoral space**, the space between the greater trochanter of the femur and the ischial tuberosity. Anatomic variation, injury, inflammation, instability, or masses may narrow this space.[516] Narrowing of this space may entrap the sciatic nerve either directly or indirectly by crowding it against an abnormal or inflamed quadratus femoris muscle.[516] Ischiofemoral impingement typically causes buttocks pain and rarely sciatic pain that radiates further into the thigh.[517]

Acetabular cysts

Cystic masses of the hip joint can compress the sciatic nerve in its route from the pelvis to the thigh. This is thought to be a rare cause of sciatica, and up to 2016 as few as ten cases had been published.[518–524] These masses include synovial and ganglial cysts from the hip joint or enlarged hip bursa. Sciatica related to hip cysts has been linked to trauma,[523] labrum tears,[519] hip replacement,[521] and hip joint arthritis.

Varicose sciatica

Dysfunction of the venous system may occur in sciatica secondary to spinal pathology, and rarely be a primary cause of symptoms. Lumbar disc herniation and stenosis are associated with increased pressure in the **vertebral vein system**, and compression, thrombosis, or dilation of lumbar vertebral veins. Varicosities in the lumbar spine, pelvis, or sciatic nerve less often result from hypercoagulability, abdominal masses, or congenital variations. Some patients suffer from a combination of spinal and venous pathology.[525]

Vein dysfunction is one of the earliest theories of sciatica. Iranian medical texts around the 9th century CE referred to sciatica as *irq-al-nasa* or *ergho-nasaa*. While irq refers to nerves and sinew, *nasaa* refers to a vein that collects fluid from the hip, increases in diameter, and causes symptoms of sciatica.[526] In 1764, the Italian physician Cotugno associated varicose veins with sciatica.[9] He believed that veins related to the sciatic nerve became "blocked up" or "sluggish."[473]

Practitioners of Traditional Chinese Medicine (TCM) believed that sciatica arose from blood vessel dysfunction. The *Mawangdui Manuscripts* from around 200 BCE[527] state that sciatica arises when qi moves opposite to its normal direction in a condition called **reversal**.[527] Sciatica was said to result from reversal of the Great Yang vessel,[10] which may correspond with the small saphenous vein, or the Foot Minor Yang vessel,[11] which may correspond with the fibular vein.[527]

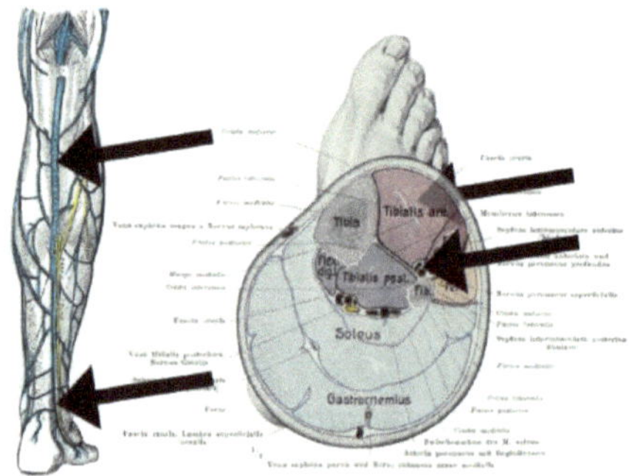

Figure 99: Left: Small saphenous vein (Great Yang vessel), and Right: Anterior tibial vein (Minor Yang vessel). These may be the vessels mentioned in the ancient Chinese Mawangdui and Huangdi Neijing. Sciatica was thought to occur when flow reversed in these vessels. Images from Gray's anatomy (L) and Anatomie des Menschen, public domain.

The terms varicose sciatica or sciatic phlebalgia[528] stem from the Frenchman Quénu's observation in 1890 that sciatica was more prevalent in those with **varicose veins**.[529] Quénu proposed that sciatica began as a chronic phlebitis (vein inflammation).[529] In 1913 the German Reinhardt identified sclerosed sciatic nerve varices in cadavers and proposed these caused sciatic pain.[530]

In 1918 Sicard suggested that mechanical compression of veins in the **intervertebral foramen** contributed to sciatica.[185] Other authors echoed this

---

[9] *If sciatica arises from... an abundance of fluid... cramps are commonly followed by a temporary varicose inflation of the veins... The quantity of fluid that flows into the [sciatic nerve sheath] ... is greater than can be resorbed by the veins... (p. 79-82)*[473]

[10] *Great Yang vessel... attached to the heel, in the outer malleolus... emerges in the [popliteal fossa]. Ascending, it bores the buttock, emerges in the hip joint, and presses laterally on the spine. It emerges at the nape... When this vessel is moved... the ham cannot rotate; the upper side is as if knotted; the calf is as if being ripped... back pain... buttock pain... calf pain; numbness in the little toe... p. 203* [527]

[11] *Minor Yang vessel. It emerges in front of the malleolus. A branch is situated in the bone. The direct path ascends and penetrates the outer... knee. It emerges at the outer... thigh and emerges at the side... The ailments: Ailing from the loss of function in the toe next to the little toe; pain in the outer... shin; coldness in the shin; pain in the outer... knee; pain in the outer... thigh; pain in the outer... ham... numbness in the middle toe... p. 205* [527]

theory, such as Putti, who felt that the superficial venous plexus surrounding the lower lumbar nerve roots was highly susceptible to compression.[531] Also around this time it was discovered that sciatica could result from venous congestion in the pelvis from space-occupying masses.[532]

Venous stasis

Venous stasis of the lumbar spine involves persistent engorgement of the lumbar vertebral veins. It has been described in **lumbar stenosis**,[533] blockages of the inferior vena cava (IVC), and **disc herniation**,[534] and also is thought to occur in radicular pain during pregnancy.[535] Venous stasis may be a common mechanism underlying neurogenic claudication and radicular pain.[536]

Veins within the lumbar spine are valveless and have **bidirectional flow**.[537] They flow freely into one another and may develop stasis even in those without low back disorders, depending on position and thoraco-abdominal pressure.[538] At rest, the vertebral veins normally flow towards the inferior vena cava (IVC). Conditions that increase intra-thoracic or intra-abdominal pressure reduce flow through the IVC and force blood into the vertebral vein system.

The vertebral vein system is normally at a **low pressure** of around 8 mm Hg when lying on the side at rest.[539] This baseline pressure is increased in those with radicular sciatica from about 10 to 20 mm Hg.[540,541] The vertebral venous pressure is maximized in the sitting position, which adds about 10 mm Hg.[540] It is also increased by straining, as in a Valsalva maneuver.

Obstructions to venous flow create a **compartment syndrome** within the lumbosacral nerve roots or dorsal root ganglia.[542,543] The radicular veins are on the surface of nerve roots and therefore more susceptible to compression.[543] When compressed, they no longer drain the nerve roots, leading to increased nerve pressure, swelling, ischemia, and fibrosis.[543] Blockage of the vertebral veins may cause a chain of events resulting in nerve root damage.

Epidural venous stasis increases **ectopic nerve firing**. In animal studies clamping of the vena cava has been shown to increase spontaneous firing of the L5 nerve root.[544] The buildup of venous blood blocks the nerve root microcirculation and oxygen supply.[544] Less extreme versions of venous stasis are suspected of causing ectopic firing in those with LSS and radicular sciatica.[536,545]

Vesper's curse describes the combination of **heart** and/or **lung** pathology with LSS to create nocturnal leg pain and restlessness. This condition is thought to arise when there is resistance to venous return to the heart, which causes a retrograde flow of blood to the vertebral vein system.[546] Engorgement of the vertebral veins worsens the neurological consequences of an already-stenotic spinal canal.

Intraosseous hypertension syndrome is a condition of increased venous pressure within bone. Intraosseous pressure of the lumbar vertebrae is defined as the **hydrostatic pressure** of the venous blood within the cancellous trabecular sinusoids.[541] One study found that patients with spondylotic changes to the lumbar spine had about 3 times greater intraosseous pressure.[539] Increased venous pressure also correlates with a lower pH (increased acidity) of the venous environment.[547]

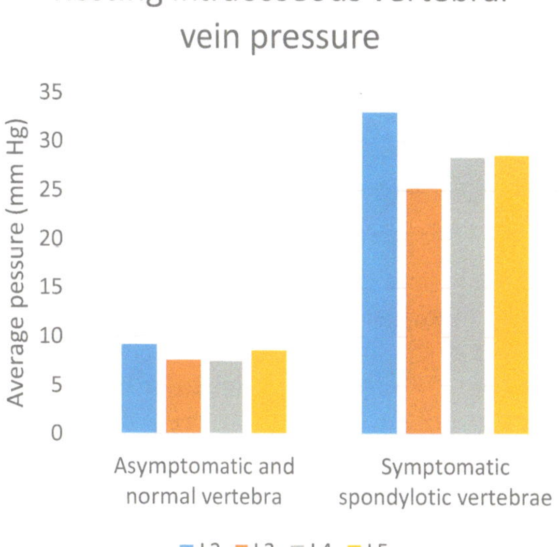

Figure 100: Vertebral vein pressures in patients without symptoms and a normal lumbar radiograph versus those with low back pain or sciatica and degenerative changes seen on radiograph. Data adapted from Arnoldi.[539]

One study found that patients with **spinal trauma** and neurological deficits commonly had diminished venous return through the IVC and increased backflow to the vertebral veins.[548] The mechanism for this was unclear, but the authors suggested it was produced by autonomic dysfunction, diaphragm dysfunction, or chronically raised intra-abdominal pressure.[548]

During **pregnancy** the blood volume increases and the IVC can be partially obstructed by the uterus, causing increased flow to the vertebral veins.[535] This could explain the rise in low-back related sciatica during pregnancy. A fetus, an enlarged or retroverted uterus, or uterine fibroids may create symptoms by compressing neural tissue directly or by obstructing the IVC.

Diagnostic imaging may show vertebral vein abnormalities in sciatic patients. The **basivertebral veins** may be more prominent in those with LSS, possibly due to venous stasis.[533] Those with **type I Modic changes** seen on MRI have intraosseous vertebral venous pressures 73% greater than those without Modic changes.[547] Gadolinium-enhanced MRIs can be used to highlight the venous engorgement in those with LSS.[545]

Chronically elevated **intra-abdominal pressure** may block normal flow through the IVC and lead to increased venous flow to the spine.[548] Elevated vertebral vein pressure in those with low back disorders is thought to be caused by abdominal muscle **guarding**.[541] Patients with LDH have increased resting activity of the abdominal obliques and quadratus lumborum.[549] Increased intra-abdominal pressure, possibly related to guarding, may cause stasis and congestion of the vertebral vein system.

Epidural varicosis

Epidural varicosis can occur in relation to spinal pathology, vascular disease, or developmental anomalies of the inferior vena cava. Narrowed areas of the spine are thought to obstruct epidural veins and cause them to dilate,[550] a process called **venous entrapment**.[545] It is thought that epidural varicosis most often results secondary to spinal pathology such as LDH and LSS.[550]

Epidural varices have been reported in association with **lumbar disc herniations**[550-553] It is thought that disc material compresses foraminal or anterior epidural veins, reduces their outflow, and causes them to dilate.[534,553] **Foraminal veins** are superficially located on nerve roots and dorsal root ganglia and more susceptible to external pressure than deeper vessels.[543]

Epidural varices may arise in those with **lumbar stenosis**. It is thought that occlusion of the spinal canal or intervertebral foramina blocks the outflow of venous blood.[533,545,550,554] This mass effect slows or blocks flow in the vertebral veins, leading to pooling of blood and dilation of veins. Epidural varices have been suggested as a cause of neurogenic claudication, pain, sensory loss, and weakness in those with LSS.[554]

Primary epidural varicosis (without spinal pathology) is an uncommon cause of sciatica.[555] Authors have reported epidural varicosis in those undergoing lumbar spine surgery ranging from 0.3% to 5%.[10,556-558] One surgical series of 100 patients undergoing lumbar spine surgery for sciatica found that in 2% of cases neural compression was from veins and no other cause.[10]

Thrombosis or anomalies of the **inferior vena cava** may cause epidural varicosis and sciatica. Diminished venous return through the vena cava causes reflux of blood into the epidural veins, which act as collaterals around the IVC.[555,559-561] Agenesis or interruption of the IVC as a cause of sciatica is extremely rare, and in one study accounted for only 1 in about 1,000 cases.[555] Patients with **hypercoagulability** such as Factor V Leiden mutation or those taking oral contraceptives may be more likely to develop IVC thrombosis.[555,559,561-563]

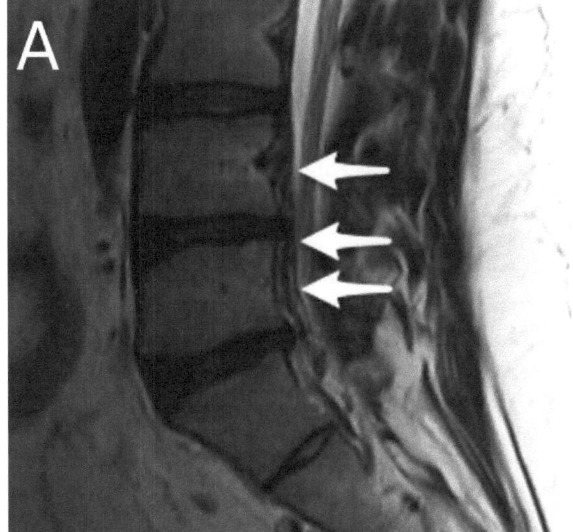

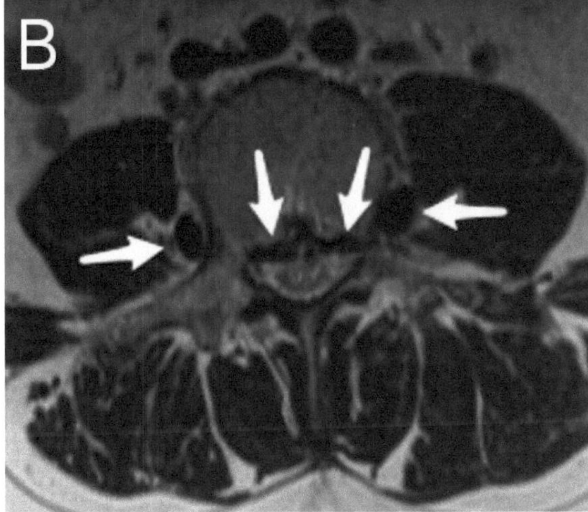

Figure 101: Enlargement of the epidural veins seen on a T2 weighted MRI in a sagittal (A) and axial (B) view, which also shows enlargement of the ascending lumbar veins. This patient had an anomalous inferior vena cava resulting in epidural varicosis and lumbar radiculopathy. Image CC BY 3.0 license from Donmez.[559]

Epidural varicosis may interfere with the **arterial supply** of nutrients and oxygen to nerve roots.[534,543] When venous congestion or pressure elevates to 40 mm Hg, it restricts blood flow through neural **capillaries**.[542,564] Nerve root ischemia is in turn thought to create **fibrosis**, nerve degeneration, and pain.[534] Studies have identified increased fibrin in epidural veins,[550] veins surrounding nerve roots, and within nerve roots adjacent to LDHs.[534,565]

Shrinkage of lumbar veins may explain the **disappearing disc** phenomenon.[552,553,566,567] Epidural varices can mimic or exaggerate the appearance of a herniated disc on MRI. In some instances, surgeons about to operate on an LDH find a smaller herniation than expected on imaging, or varicosities instead of a herniation.[566] Some surgeons also suspect that certain cases of spontaneous regression of LDHs on MRI may relate to regression of epidural varices.[553]

Epidural varicosis may be a side effect of the inflammatory **immune response** to herniated disc material.[550] Displaced nucleus pulposus tissue stimulates the release of macrophages and **pro-inflammatory cytokines**. It is thought that one cytokine, tumor necrosis factor alpha, triggers thrombosis in nerve root capillaries.[568] Other cytokines are abundant in vessels surrounding LDHs and may contribute to vessel damage. These include Willebrand factor, interleukin-1, transforming growth factor-beta, and platelet-derived growth factor.[565]

Space-occupying masses in the pelvis may compress the inferior vena cava (IVC), cause reflux of blood into the lumbar epidural veins, and result in radiculopathy. Examples include the uterus during pregnancy,[561] tumors,[555] and distention of the bladder.[569] Compression of the IVC occurs in later stages of pregnancy when lying in the supine position, but rapidly reverses in the left lateral position.[570]

Some clinics used **epidural venography** in the 1960s and 1970s to assess vertebral venous flow in those with sciatica. This imaging technique used a contrast agent to identify flow obstructions around LDHs.[571] Epidural venography showed indirect signs of LDHs such as the lack of contrast agent in a radicular or anterior internal vertebral vein,[537] or abnormal dilation of epidural veins, which, at the time was called phlebectasia.[537,556,571]

Epidural veins may be a normal finding on MRI depending on the body mass index (BMI) of the patient. Epidural veins are more prominent in those that are **obese**[558] or have greater amounts of epidural fat.[572] Small[12] epidural veins are also seen on those with a normal BMI. One study found that two-thirds of patients with a normal BMI had at least one epidural vein visible that was under 1 millimeter in diameter.[572]

Those with LDH may develop **epidural vein thrombosis**. One study identified those with herniations often had thrombosis of the foraminal veins at the level of LDH on autopsy.[534] Histological research has shown that veins surrounding nerve roots in those

[12] Epidural varicosis is graded on MRI as: Grade 0 (no epidural veins seen), grade 1 (one or more epidural vein seen <1 mm in diameter), grade 2 (epidural vein diameter ≥1 and <3 mm) and grade 3 (≥3 mm).[572]

with LDH have greater levels of **platelets** and **fibrosis**.[565] An inflammatory-immune response to nucleus pulposus is likely to be responsible for thrombus formation.[568]

Pelvic congestion syndrome

Pelvic congestion syndrome is a condition in which veins dilate within the pelvis. These enlarged veins may compress the **lumbosacral plexus** or sciatic nerve within the pelvis.[573] The venous blood is also thought in some cases to **reflux** towards the sciatic nerve, causing varicosities of the sciatic nerve in the thigh or leg.[574] Almost half of patients with sciatic nerve varices have associated varices within the pelvis.[575] Pelvic congestion syndrome causing sciatica has been reported in endometriosis[573] or following pelvic surgery.[576]

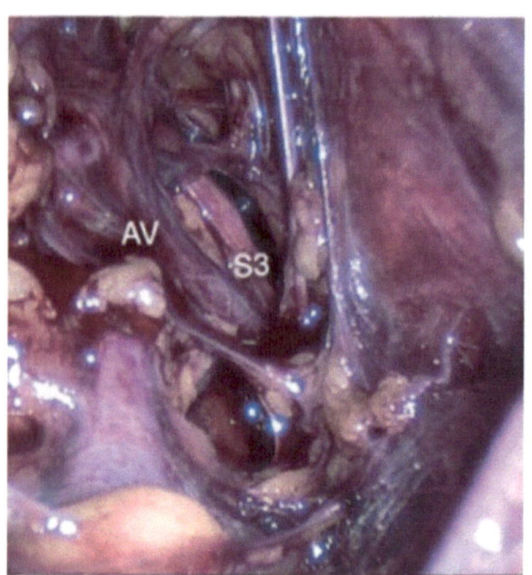

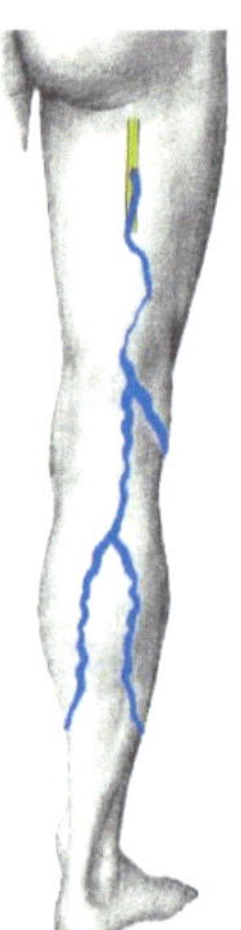

Figure 102: Pelvic congestion syndrome. Varicose veins within the pelvis may directly compress the lumbosacral plexus or cause a reflux or back-up of blood flow into the lower extremity or sciatic nerve vein. Left - abnormal varicose vein (AV) within the pelvis entrapping the S2 (not shown) and S3 nerve roots against the piriformis muscle, image from Lemos and Possover, [577] CC BY 4.0 License. Right - Superficial vein reflux pattern for the sciatic nerve vein, adapted from Labropaulos[578] using Gray's anatomy image by Author.

Vein entrapment

Varicose veins in the gluteal region may compress the sciatic nerve. Varicosities of the inferior gluteal vein, which is adjacent to the sciatic nerve, are the most common to cause sciatica.[579-583] Varicosities of gluteal veins may be caused by compression by the piriformis muscle[583] or trauma.[581] Entrapment occurs typically just distal to the piriformis muscle.[580,582,583] Vein entrapment by the piriformis may also cause sciatic pain with leg swelling and deep venous thrombosis.[584]

Sciatic nerve varicosities

Varicose veins along the course of the sciatic nerve may compress the sciatic nerve or restrict blood flow to it. Sciatic nerve varicosities related to vascular anomalies is rare. However, more mild forms may occur secondary to low back or gluteal disorders, pregnancy, or post-thrombotic disorders. In two studies totaling over 100 patients with varicosities along the sciatic nerve, every patient was found to have pain or other sensory symptoms in the sciatic nerve distribution.[575,585]

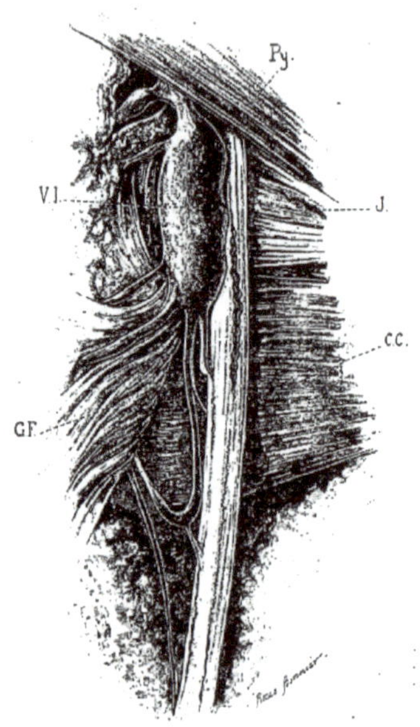

Figure 103: Varicosity of the sciatic vein (VI), seen running along the main trunk of the sciatic nerve. Public domain, from Quénu, 1890(Simon et al., 1890) Py: Piriformis, J: Gemellus muscles, CC: Quadratus femoris, GF: Gluteus maximus.

The sciatic nerve normally has a small vein within its sheath called the sciatic nerve vein.[585] Rarely, there is a persistence of a large embryonic vein of the sciatic nerve called a **persistent sciatic vein**.[585] A persistent sciatic artery may also occur. Those with **Klippel-Trenaunay syndrome** are the most likely to have a persistent sciatic vein and are predisposed to sciatica as well as other systemic problems.[585]

Other risk factors for sciatic varicosities include thrombosis, venous hypertension, hormonal changes during pregnancy, pelvic varicosis or **pelvic congestion syndrome**, and a general predisposition towards varicose veins.[574] Varicose veins of the sciatic nerve are found in 10% of patients with chronic venous disease.[578]

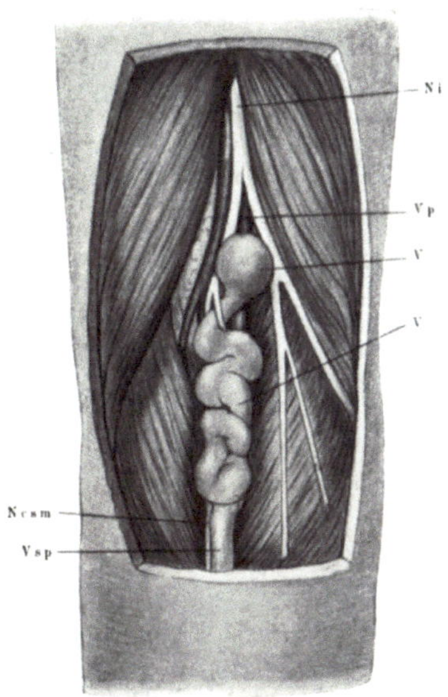

Figure 104: Varicosity of the sciatic nerve at its bifurcation. Ni: Sciatic nerve, Vp: Popliteal vein, Nesm: Medial sural cutaneous nerve. Vsp: Small saphenous vein. V: Varicosity. Public domain from Reinhardt, 1913 (p. 381).

Infection

Bacterial, viral, and fungal infections of the spine, lumbosacral nerves, IVD, and SIJ account for less than 1% of cases of sciatica.[16,340] Evidence is growing that infections may contribute to sciatica when combined with degenerative spinal conditions. Chronic **low-grade infections** of the IVD or nerve cell bodies may be asymptomatic but are common in the general population. Pathogens may invade the **dorsal root ganglia**, the nerve root cell bodies of the lower back, and lumbar discs.

Textbooks from the early 20th century describe infectious causes of sciatica. For example, one text in 1917 stated that sciatica could be caused by any type of general infection or intoxication, including puerperal fever, typhoid, influenza, and gonorrhea.[586]

Herpesviridae

Herpesviridae is a family of viruses of which some have the capability of attacking the cauda equina and causing sciatica. This includes **cytomegalovirus** (CMV),[587,588] **Epstein-Barr virus** (EBV),[589–591] **herpes simplex virus-2** (Elsberg syndrome),[592] and **varicella zoster virus** (VZV).[593] While case reports appeared in the late 1800s linking HSV to sciatica,[594] this topic is still not a major focus of research. One study identified HSV as a possible causative factor in 2.5% of patients with sciatica.[595] Viral cases of sciatica are typically only identified and attributed to these viruses in extreme circumstances of infection, immune suppression, and widespread bodily symptoms such as fever. Despite this, herpesviruses may play a larger role than currently thought and act more as a risk factor in a multifactorial model of sciatica.

Herpesviruses viruses are common and can become latent or dormant in the nerve root ganglia, and when reactivated trigger an attack of sciatica. In general, autopsies show that 40% of **sacral dorsal root ganglia** contain dormant herpes simplex virus-2 (HSV-2).[592] Varicella zoster is another virus known to commonly become latent in these ganglia.[596] All herpesviruses may be capable of becoming latent in the lumbosacral ganglia.[596]

The presence of a herpesvirus in the lumbosacral ganglia does not guarantee the development of sciatica. Varicella zoster and HSV-2 can exist in the spinal nerve ganglia of patients that manifest symptoms of sciatica as well as those that do not. This may be because the viruses need a **trigger** to produce symptoms. Sciatic nerve injury in mice or UV irradiation in guinea pigs can reactivate the herpesvirus from the lumbosacral ganglia.[596] This is evidence that injury along the sciatic nerve pathway could trigger viral-related sciatica.

Sciatica related to herpesvirus infections does not necessarily include the typical symptoms of the virus. Epstein-Barr virus infections of the cauda equina do not typically include symptoms of mononucleosis,[589] herpes simplex virus sciatica does not necessarily involve genital herpes, and Varicella-Zoster infections of the cauda equina do not always cause the typical rash of shingles in the leg. In fact, sciatica may precede the development of the shingles rash by multiple days. The manifestation of nerve root symptoms related to VZV without rash has been called **Zoster sine herpete**.[597] Herpesviruses have also been implicated in degeneration of the lumbar disc. One study found at least one herpesvirus in 81% of lumbar disc samples of patients who underwent discectomy.[598]

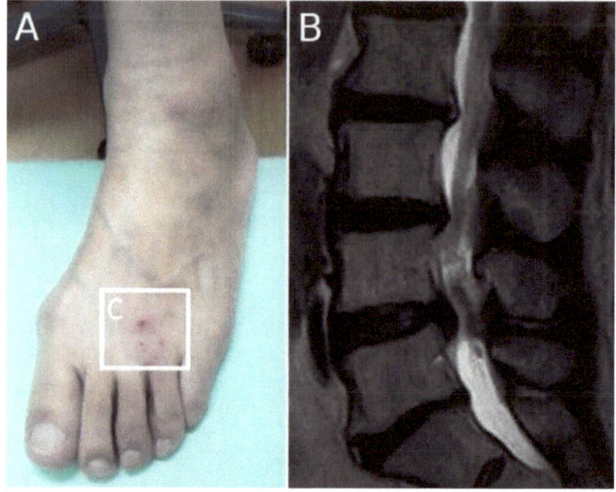

Figure 105: Sciatica caused by herpes zoster. A 74-year-old man presented with a 1-month history of left sided sciatica. X-ray and MRI imaging revealed spinal stenosis (B). The patient's symptoms continued, and the patient and physicians were considering low back surgery, when a vesicular rash (A and C) appeared on the foot. Clinicians diagnosed and treated herpes zoster with famciclovir and NSAIDs and the rash and sciatica went away after 1 week. Image CC BY 4.0 license from Koda et al.[599]

Low-grade disc infection

Low-grade, or **nonpyogenic** infection of the lumbar IVD as a cause of sciatica was first theorized in 2001 by authors of a study that identified ***Propionibacterium acnes*** in 84% of lumbar discectomy samples.[600] Additional studies correlated *P. acnes* with reduced disc space height,[601] annular tears of the disc,[601] and type 1 Modic changes, which is an imaging finding on MRI that shows edema in the endplate near the disc. While *P. acnes* was the most common bacterium identified, there were other less common bacteria cultured from disc samples including coagulase-negative staphylococci.[602]

A systematic review found that positive samples of *P. acnes* were found in a median of 45% of herniated discs.[602] The review concluded that there was moderate evidence for a relationship between the presence of bacteria and both low back pain with LDH and Modic Type 1 change with LDH.[602] The study also found modest evidence for a cause-effect relationship.

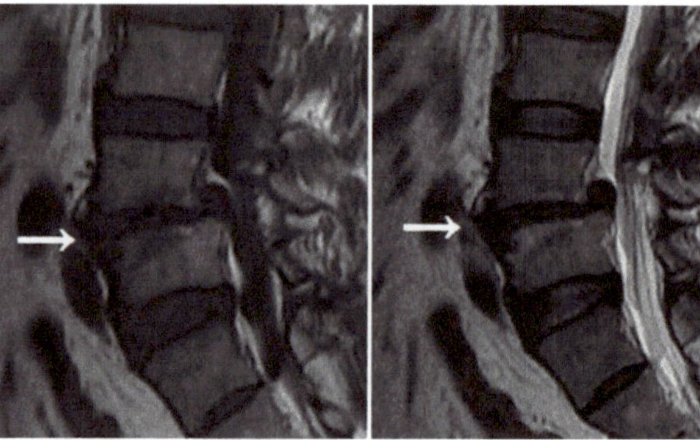

Figure 106: Modic type 1 changes. This gives a hypointense (dark) appearance to the endplate on the T1-weighted MRI (left), and a hyperintense (bright) appearance on T2-weighted MRI (right). These findings represent bone marrow edema and inflammation and have been correlated with low-grade bacterial infection of the IVD. Image from Yu et al,[603] Creative Commons Attribution License.

The theory of a low-grade bacterial infection of the lumbar IVD is based on the notion that the **anaerobic** (low-oxygen) and **avascular** (low-blood supply) environment of the disc can support anaerobic bacteria that thrive under these conditions.[602] It has been suggested that a trauma to the disc enables bacteria to enter from the bloodstream.[600] Once the bacteria are present, they are thought to slowly colonize the disc and contribute to its degeneration.[602]

Low-grade infection of the IVD arises from bacterial and/or viral causes. One study looked at discs that were operated on for herniation and found that most samples (81%) had at least one herpesvirus present.[598] HSV-1 was found in 56%, CMV in 38%, and two patients had both HSV-1 and CMV.[598] Two control samples (without LDH) had no herpesviruses.[598] None of the studied patients had symptoms of acute infection or antibodies in the blood. The study hypothesized that the herpesviruses represented a chronic low-grade infection that contributed to disc degeneration.[598]

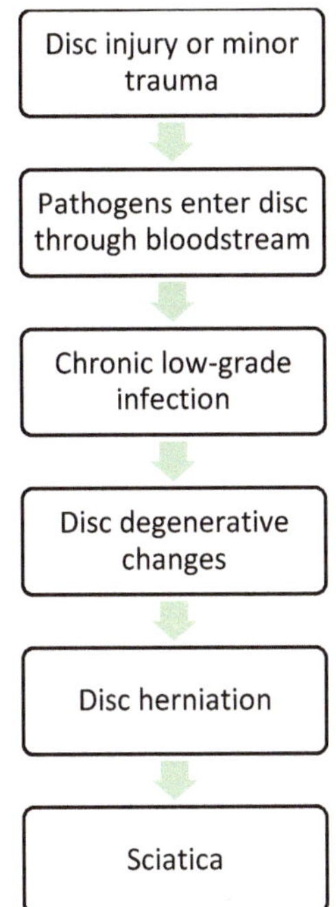

Figure 107: Model of low-grade disc infection. Disc injury may cause a breach in defense, allowing pathogens to enter and establish a chronic-low grade infection, leading to degenerative changes, herniation and sciatica.

Pyogenic infection

Pyogenic (pus-forming) infections are more acute, severe, and clinically recognizable than low-grade bacterial or viral infections. They can rapidly destroy the disc, spine, and spread through the body. Pus, abscess, displaced bone, vascular compromise, and inflammation related to these infections can damage the lumbosacral nerve roots.[604–606] Pyogenic infections are more apparent with constitutional symptoms such as fever.

Pyogenic infections include **discitis** (disc infection), **osteomyelitis** (bone infection), and septic **sacroiliitis** (infection of the SIJ). Abscesses in the buttocks that compress the sciatic nerve are also possible, a condition called gluteal pyomyositis.[607–609] The organisms that cause these infections include bacteria such as *Brucella* and *Mycobacterium tuberculosis*, and fungus such as *Candida*.

Spirochetal illnesses

The two **spirochetes** (coiled bacteria) that can cause sciatica include *Borrelia burgdorferi*, the agent of Lyme disease, and *Treponema pallidum,* the agent of syphilis. **Neuroborreliosis** is Lyme disease involving the nervous system. **Bannwarth's syndrome** is any radicular syndrome from *B. burgdorferi*. Lyme can also damage the IVD and cause sciatica indirectly. While syphilis is fortunately now rare, Lyme disease is common.

Clinicians believed that syphilis was a common cause of sciatica in the late 1800s. In 1914 the French doctor Déjerine felt that the main cause of sciatica was infection and meningitis of the nerve roots, the most common cause being syphilis.[610] It is possible that some of these cases were neuroborreliosis, because Lyme disease was not known until much later.

Lyme disease

Some research suggests that those with Lyme disease are at greater risk of LDH. In one study of patients with sciatica, *B. burgdorferi* antibodies were detected in the **cerebrospinal fluid** of 2.9% of patients.[611] All of the patients with antibodies also had LDH.[611] Another case series identified a correlation between LDH and Lyme disease.[612] An additional study found an association between LDHs and Lyme but described it as a coincidence.[613]

The ability of *Borrelia burgdorferi* to damage **connective tissue** may explain why those with Lyme develop LDHs.[614] Borrelia binds to the proteoglycan **decorin**[614] that is part of the annulus fibrosus, the outer part of the disc. Borrelia also activates enzymes that break down **collagen**,[614] another important part of the annulus.

Patients with Lyme can also develop sciatica from neuroborreliosis. Studies of primates with Lyme disease have shown that *B. burgdorferi* can infect the lumbar **nerve roots** and **dorsal root ganglia**.[615] There is some evidence that the nerve root or roots involved corresponds to the limb of the tick bite (infection site) and erythema migrans rash.[616]

Parasites and helminths

Parasitic and helminth (worm) infection are rare causes of sciatica, with the prevalence depending on geographic distribution and access to clean water and food. The most common parasitic cause of sciatica globally is *Echinococcus granulosus*, the Hydatid worm, which causes Hydatid disease.[617,618] Other parasitic or neurohelminthic (worm infections of the nervous system) diseases that can cause sciatica include *Angiostrongylus cantonensis*, the rat lung worm,[619,620] *Schistosomia*, the blood-fluke (which causes neuro-schistosomiasis),[621,622] and *Spirometra sparganum* (which causes sparganosis).[623]

Hydatid disease spreads through contaminated water and is still endemic in the Mediterranean region. This illness affects the liver, causing obstructive jaundice, and may also cause sciatica by formation of cysts within the pelvis or lumbosacral spine.

Abdominal conditions

Compression of the **lumbosacral plexus** by abdominal or pelvic masses causes a small percentage of sciatica cases. Pelvic tumors, varicose veins, endometriosis, hardened stool, and the fetus in pregnant women rarely compress the lumbosacral plexus.

Hippocrates associated sciatica with constipation. He noted that in sciatica the intestines could only be moved by medicine,[624] and recommended laxatives as a treatment.[454] Many ancient authors, including Pliny, advised purging the bowels and using enemas to treat sciatica.[625] Likewise, the Greek physician Paulus Aegineta (c. 625-690 CE) discussed the removal of "hardened feces."[626]

In the early 1900s, medical authors described that sciatica could be caused by a **mass effect** of feces compressing on lumbosacral nerves in the pelvis.[627] Others described constipation causing a **viscero-somatic reflex** that irritated the sciatic nerve.[628] Prior to the 1930s it was typical for medical literature about constipation to include sciatica as an associated symptom.[629] Regardless of whether constipation is a cause or effect of sciatica or altogether unrelated, it occurs in almost half of patients with sciatica.[630] For comparison, constipation occurs in about 20% of the general population.

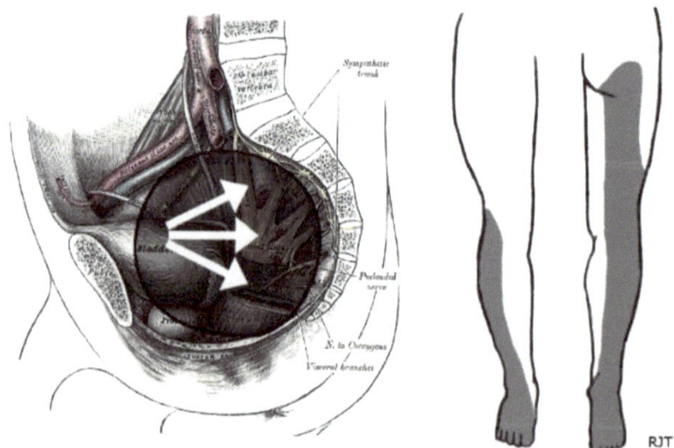

Figure 108: Compression of the lumbosacral plexus by a pelvic mass. Left - image modified from Gray's anatomy, public domain. Right – potential pain distribution in the case of sciatica caused by abdominal or pelvic compression of the lumbosacral plexus, image by Robert Trager, DC.

Endometriosis

Endometriosis is a condition in which tissue similar to the lining of the uterus exists outside of the uterus. The presence of this abnormal endometrial tissue in the pelvic bowl can cause sciatica. This is called **catamenial sciatica**, because the sciatica flares on a **monthly cycle** aligned with bleeding during menses.[631] The sciatica is either caused directly by bleeding that damages the lumbosacral plexus or indirectly through referred pain. About half of the women with endometriosis have cyclical lower extremity pain,[632] which suggests that this syndrome is under-recognized. Endometriosis is the most common of the obstetric or gynecological causes of sciatica in women (52%) followed by pregnancy and labor-related sciatica (31%), and fibroids (3%) and more rare conditions.[631]

Uterine fibroids

Uterine fibroids or **leiomyomas** are the most common solid tumors of the pelvis in women. These tumors do not usually cause symptoms but rarely can cause sciatica due to compressive effects on the lumbosacral plexus.[633-636] A similar but rarer cause of sciatica is a retroverted (backwards-tilted) uterus.[637]

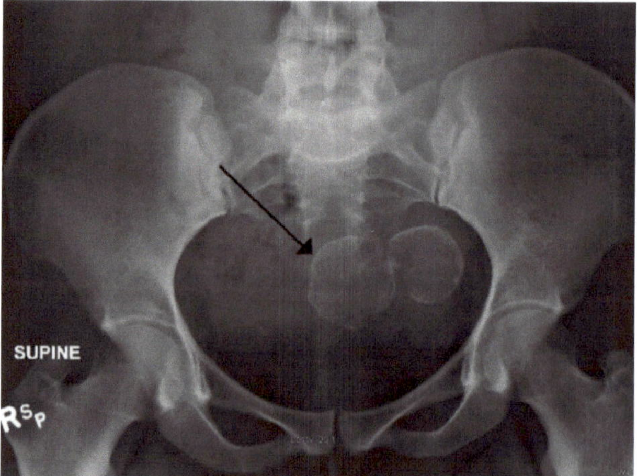

Figure 109: Calcified uterine fibroids can compress the lumbosacral plexus. Image from James Heilman, MD, CC BY 3.0 License.

Pregnancy

Sciatica is uncommon during pregnancy, occurring in about 2.4% of pregnant women.[638] Rarely, enlargement of the uterus by the fetus during pregnancy can compress the lumbosacral plexus, causing a transient sciatica that is alleviated after giving birth.[12] Other theories to explain sciatica during pregnancy include the compression of vascular elements leading to neural ischemia, LDH, excessive vomiting, and sacral stress fractures.[631] Also during labor, extreme positions for long periods of time can over stretch or compress the sciatic nerve. [631]

Retroverted uterus

Only a handful of cases of sciatica caused by a retroverted uterus have been published.[12,15] The uterus may press against **sacral nerves** as they exit the sacral foramina. Symptoms correlate with the **menstrual cycle**,[12,15] being worse just before menses.[15] Further evaluation may also identify endometriosis, ovarian cyst(s) or fluid in Douglas' pouch that could contribute to sciatic symtpoms.[12]

Constipation

Some evidence supports the long-held clinical belief that constipation can compress the **lumbosacral plexus** and cause sciatica. In these cases, the patient can have severe sciatica, with or without neurological deficits, which is relieved by removal of the stool.

In one case, a 12-year-old boy suffered from cauda equina syndrome and abdominal pain, weakness, numbness, and diminished reflexes. The boy was found to have fecal impaction, and his symptoms were relieved after removal of the stool.[639] A similar case of severe constipation in an 11-year-old girl causing megacolon and sciatica was relieved once the bowel was emptied.[640] Patients with congenital megacolon are also predisposed to fecal impactions that cause sciatica.[641]

In another case, a 40-year-old woman with sciatica was found to have an inflamed part of the small intestine near the lumbosacral plexus.[642] The patient's sciatica resolved when this part of the intestine was removed.

Other rare relationships between the gastrointestinal tract and sciatica include diverticulitis, which can cause abscesses that can lead to sciatica,[643] and a sciatic hernia, in which intestines protrude through the greater sciatic notch in the gluteal region and may put pressure on the sciatic nerve.[644]

Referred visceral pain

Referred sciatic pain can arise from pelvic visceral structures when sensory signals from these areas converge with those from the sciatic spinal cord segments. **Viscero-somatic convergence** is the merging of visceral and somatic sensory signals at the spinal cord. Ongoing noxious or nociceptive signals from pelvic viscera can lead to **segmental sensitization**, a form of central sensitization occurring at a specific spinal cord level.

Pain from the **genitourinary organs** can refer into the thigh and leg. Diseases of the **uterus** and **prostate** are the most likely to refer pain into the sciatic distribution. The ureters,[645] colon, ovaries,[12] and bladder[646] only rarely do so. Visceral referral as the sole cause of sciatica is extremely rare. Pelvic visceral pathology more likely combines with somatic pathology such as discogenic pain to create the overall symptom complex.

Clinicians believed visceral pathology to be a more common cause of sciatica in the mid-1800s to early 1900s. In 1887 the English neurologist James Ross suggested that rectal pathology could be referred into the **posterior femoral cutaneous nerve** (PFCN) distribution due to its shared segmental relationship of S3.[647] The English neurologist Henry Head was, in 1893, the first to map urogenital pain referral zones for the prostate, bladder, uterus, and rectum.[648] His research was followed by other reports linking prostatitis to sciatica.[649–651]

Table 14: Segments involved in visceral sciatic pain referral, modified from Head[648]

Segment	Visceral relationship
L5	• Prostate
S1	• Bladder, prostate, uterus
S2	• Rectum, bladder, prostate, uterus
S3	• Rectum, bladder, prostate, uterus

Visceral pathology may contribute to sciatica via **segmental sensitization** of the segments L5-S3. Although the sciatic segments include L4-S3, the fourth lumbar nerve plays a minor role in innervating pelvic viscera. The visceral plexuses of the bladder, prostate, uterus, ovaries, sigmoid colon, and rectum share the sacral segments with the sciatic nerve and PFCN. Sensory information from these pelvic viscera can refer into these nerve distributions due to viscero-somatic convergence at L5-S3.

Another hypothesis for sciatic pain referral is via inflammation of the **pelvic peritoneum**, the fascia that covers the walls of the pelvis. The S2-4 segments innervate the pelvic peritoneum. Of these segments, S2 and S3 also contribute to the sciatic nerve. Peritoneal inflammation likely explains how sciatica arises in some patients with **pelvic endometriosis**.[652] It may also explain referred sciatic pain in other forms of pelvic visceral pathology.

Prostatitis and **chronic pelvic pain syndrome** in men can cause referred sciatic pain and dysfunction of the sacral nerve roots. The prostate can refer pain into the back and occasionally into the posterior thigh and leg,[649–651] including the S2 and S3 segments. Men with chronic pelvic pain syndrome, also called abacterial prostatitis and prostatodynia, have slight neurological deficits of the sacral roots. These men are less able to perform **toe spreading**, which is a function of the S2 and S3 nerve roots. [653] Prostate disease and pain syndromes involve referred pain and neurological deficits of S2 and S3.

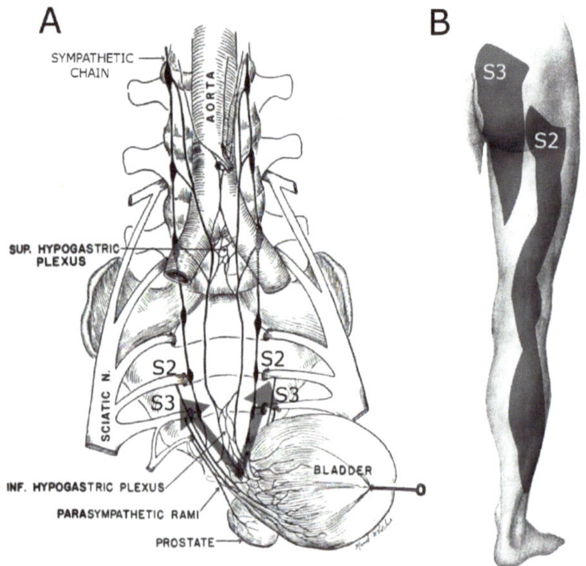

Figure 110: Viscerosomatic convergence causing referred sciatic pain. Sensory information from the pelvic organs and sciatic nerve both share S2 and S3 and these paths converge in the spinal cord. Signals from inflamed pelvic viscera can merge with or refer into the S2 and S3 segments of the sciatic distribution.

Endometriosis can indirectly refer pain to the sciatic nerve. About half of women with endometriosis have some type of sciatic or leg pain.[632] The bleeding and inflammation from ectopic endometrial tissue may inflame the **pelvic peritoneum** and refer pain into the S2-4 segments.[652] Signs that indicate sciatic pain may be caused by endometriosis are tenderness at the sciatic notch, symptoms being worse during menses, and symptoms on the right side.[631]

The cause-effect relationship of spinal or radicular sciatica and visceral pathology[403] is unclear. Visceral pathology may cause referred sciatic pain, and conversely neurological forms of sciatica may cause visceral pathology. One study of MRI-proven discogenic radicular sciatica patients showed that gas discomfort, diarrhea, and constipation were significantly more common than in the general population.[654] Cauda equina syndrome, a rare and severe form of discogenic sciatica, can cause bladder and/or bowel dysfunction. Pelvic visceral pathology can result from intraspinal sciatica as well as contribute to sciatic symptoms independently.

Cerebrospinal fluid pressure

Sciatic symptoms are rarely related to an increase in cerebrospinal fluid (CSF) pressure. An extreme increase in CSF pressure interferes with **blood flow** to the spinal nerve roots and their dorsal ganglia. When pressure in the thecal sac increases above that of the veins on the surface of nerve roots, these veins collapse and arterial flow to the roots is compromised.[655]

The Portuguese physician Lusitanus Zacutus (1575-1642 CE) presented a case of a patient with sciatica that occurred after an attack of tinnitus (ringing in the ears) and migraine. Zacutus claimed this was proof that sciatica originated from the head.[13] Zacutus was the first to report a link between headache, tinnitus, and sciatica, now understood to be an extremely rare condition related to elevated intracranial pressure.

One study found that paresthesias in the extremities of those with **intracranial hypertension** could be resolved with lumbar puncture.[657] Those with idiopathic intracranial hypertension are more likely to suffer from sciatica.[658] A common orthopedic test used to provoke sciatica, Valsalva's test, is thought to work by increasing CSF pressure.[659]

References

1. Kobayashi, S., Yoshizawa, H. & Yamada, S. Pathology of lumbar nerve root compression Part 1: Intraradicular inflammatory changes induced by mechanical compression. *Journal of Orthopaedic Research* **22**, 170–179 (2004).
2. Rogers, M. An analysis of fifty cases of sciatica. *Journal of the American Medical Association* **68**, 425–429 (1917).
3. Fuller, H. W. *On Rheumatism, Rheumatic Gout, and Sciatica: Their Pathology, Symptoms, and Treatment.* (Lindsay & Blakiston, 1864).

[13] One more sign of the illness, he revealed, a sudden preceding attack of tinnitus in the ears with a migraine, which is proof that his condition originates and emanates from the head. (Author's translation, Zacutus, p. 357)[656]

4. Brinjikji, W. *et al.* Systematic Literature Review of Imaging Features of Spinal Degeneration in Asymptomatic Populations. *American Journal of Neuroradiology* **36**, 811–816 (2015).
5. Weishaupt, D., Zanetti, M., Hodler, J. & Boos, N. MR imaging of the lumbar spine: prevalence of intervertebral disk extrusion and sequestration, nerve root compression, end plate abnormalities, and osteoarthritis of the facet joints in asymptomatic volunteers. *Radiology* **209**, 661–666 (1998).
6. Burgstaller, J. M. *et al.* Is There An Association Between Pain and Magnetic Resonance Imaging Parameters in Patients with Lumbar Spinal Stenosis?. *Spine* (2016).
7. Konstantinou, K. *et al.* Characteristics of patients with low back and leg pain seeking treatment in primary care: baseline results from the ATLAS cohort study. *BMC musculoskeletal disorders* **16**, 332 (2015).
8. Koes, B. W., van Tulder, M. W. & Peul, W. C. Diagnosis and treatment of sciatica. *BMJ* **334**, 1313–1317 (2007).
9. Valat, J.-P., Genevay, S., Marty, M., Rozenberg, S. & Koes, B. Sciatica. *Best Practice & Research Clinical Rheumatology* **24**, 241–252 (2010).
10. Kosteljanetz, M., Espersen, J., Halaburt, H. & Miletic, T. Predictive value of clinical and surgical findings in patients with lumbago-sciatica. *Acta neurochirurgica* **73**, 67–76 (1984).
11. Cannon, D. E., Dillingham, T. R., Miao, H., Andary, M. T. & Pezzin, L. E. Musculoskeletal Disorders in Referrals for Suspected Lumbosacral Radiculopathy. *American Journal of Physical Medicine & Rehabilitation* **86**, 957–961 (2007).
12. Yoshimoto, M. *et al.* Diagnostic Features of Sciatica Without Lumbar Nerve Root Compression. *Journal of Spinal Disorders & Techniques* **22**, 328–333 (2009).
13. Saal, J. A., Dillingham, M. F., Gamburd, R. S. & Fanton, G. S. The pseudoradicular syndrome. Lower extremity peripheral nerve entrapment masquerading as lumbar radiculopathy. *Spine* **13**, 926–930 (1988).
14. Laporte, C. *et al.* MRI Investigation of Radiating Pain in the Lower Limbs: Value of an Additional Sequence Dedicated to the Lumbosacral Plexus and Pelvic Girdle. *American Journal of Roentgenology* **203**, 1280–1285 (2014).
15. Gleeson, T. G. *et al.* Coronal oblique turbo STIR imaging of the sacrum and sacroiliac joints at routine MR imaging of the lumbar spine. *Emergency radiology* **12**, 38–43 (2005).
16. Lingawi, S. S. How often is low back pain or sciatica not due to lumbar disc disease? *Neurosciences (Riyadh)* **9**, 94–97 (2004).
17. Guyer, R. *et al.* Extraosseous spinal lesions mimicking disc disease. *Spine* **13**, 328 (1988).
18. Filler, A. G. *et al.* Sciatica of nondisc origin and piriformis syndrome: diagnosis by magnetic resonance neurography and interventional magnetic resonance imaging with outcome study of resulting treatment. *Journal of Neurosurgery: Spine* **2**, 99–115 (2005).
19. Korkiakoski, A. *et al.* Association of Lumbar Arterial Stenosis with Low Back Symptoms: A Cross-Sectional Study Using Two-Dimensional Time-of-Flight Magnetic Resonance Angiography. *Acta Radiologica* **50**, 48–54 (2009).
20. Goddard, M. & Reid, J. Movements induced by straight leg raising in the lumbo-sacral roots, nerves and plexus, and in the intrapelvic section of the sciatic nerve. *Journal of neurology, neurosurgery, and psychiatry* **28**, 12 (1965).
21. Rade, M. *et al.* In Vivo MRI Measurement of Spinal Cord Displacement in the Thoracolumbar Region of Asymptomatic Subjects with Unilateral and Sham Straight Leg Raise Tests. *PloS one* **11**, e0155927 (2016).
22. Rade, M. *et al.* Reduced Spinal Cord Movement with the Straight Leg Raise Test in Patients with Lumbar Intervertebral Disc Herniation. *Spine* (2017).
23. Rade, M. *et al.* Normal multiplanar movement of the spinal cord during unilateral and bilateral straight leg raise: Quantification, mechanisms, and overview. *Journal of Orthopaedic Research* **35**, 1335–1342 (2017).
24. Kobayashi, S., Shizu, N., Suzuki, Y., Asai, T. & Yoshizawa, H. Changes in nerve root motion and intraradicular blood flow during an intraoperative straight-leg-raising test. *Spine* **28**, 1427–1434 (2003).
25. Kobayashi, S. *et al.* Pathomechanisms of sciatica in lumbar disc herniation: effect of periradicular adhesive tissue on electrophysiological values by an intraoperative straight leg raising test. *Spine* **35**, 2004–2014 (2010).
26. Ellis, R. F. Neurodynamic evaluation of the sciatic nerve during neural mobilisation: ultrasound imaging assessment of sciatic nerve movement and the clinical implications for treatment. (Auckland University of Technology, 2011).
27. Akdemir, G. Thoracic and lumbar intraforaminal ligaments: Laboratory investigation. *Journal of Neurosurgery: Spine* **13**, 351–355 (2010).
28. Grimes, P. F., Massie, J. B. & Garfin, S. R. Anatomic and biomechanical analysis of the lower lumbar foraminal ligaments. *Spine* **25**, 2009–2014 (2000).
29. Kallewaard, J. W. *et al.* Epiduroscopy for patients with lumbosacral radicular pain. *Pain Practice* **14**, 365–377 (2014).
30. Min, J.-H., Kang, S.-H., Lee, J.-B., Cho, T.-H. & Suh, J.-G. Anatomic analysis of the transforaminal ligament in the lumbar intervertebral foramen. *Neurosurgery* **57**, 37–41 (2005).
31. Bosscher, H. A. & Heavner, J. E. Incidence and Severity of Epidural Fibrosis after Back Surgery: An Endoscopic Study. *Pain Practice* **10**, 18–24 (2010).
32. Kuilart, K. E., Woollam, M., Barling, E. & Lucas, N. The active knee extension test and Slump test in subjects with perceived hamstring tightness. *International journal of osteopathic medicine* **8**, 89–97 (2005).
33. Turl, S. E. & George, K. P. Adverse neural tension: a factor in repetitive hamstring strain? *Journal of Orthopaedic & Sports Physical Therapy* **27**, 16–21 (1998).
34. Lempainen, L., Sarimo, J., Mattila, K., Vaittinen, S. & Orava, S. Proximal hamstring tendinopathy results of surgical management and histopathologic findings. *The American Journal of Sports Medicine* **37**, 727–734 (2009).
35. Puranen, J. & Orava, S. The hamstring syndrome–a new gluteal sciatica. in *Annales chirurgiae et gynaecologiae* **80**, 212–214 (1990).
36. Lee, G. Y. *et al.* Surgical management of tethered cord syndrome in adults: indications, techniques, and long-term outcomes in 60 patients. *Journal of Neurosurgery: Spine* **4**, 123–131 (2006).
37. Moens, M., De Smedt, A., D'Haese, J., Droogmans, S. & Chaskis, C. Spinal cord stimulation as a treatment for refractory neuropathic pain in tethered cord syndrome: a case report. *Journal of Medical Case Reports* **4**, 74 (2010).
38. Merolli, A., Mingarelli, L. & Rocchi, L. A more detailed mechanism to explain the "bands of Fontana" in peripheral nerves. *Muscle & nerve* **46**, 540–547 (2012).
39. Martin, H. D. *et al.* The effects of hip abduction on sciatic nerve biomechanics during terminal hip flexion. *J Hip Preserv Surg* **4**, 178–186 (2017).
40. Alley, E. A. & Pollock, J. E. Transient Neurologic Syndrome in a Patient Receiving Hypobaric Lidocaine in the Prone Jack-Knife Position: *Anesthesia & Analgesia* **95**, 757–759 (2002).
41. Ha, D. H., Oh, S. K. & Kim, Y. M. Acute Sciatic Nerve Palsy after Sleeping in a Sitting Position -Case Report-. *Journal of Korean Society of Spine Surgery* **18**, 259 (2011).
42. Mulleman, D., Mammou, S., Griffoul, I., Watier, H. & Goupille, P. Pathophysiology of disk-related sciatica. I.—Evidence supporting a chemical component. *Joint Bone Spine* **73**, 151–158 (2006).
43. Ohnmeiss, D. D., Vanharanta, H. & Ekholm, J. Degree of disc disruption and lower extremity pain. *Spine* **22**, 1600–1605 (1997).
44. Younes, M. *et al.* Prevalence and risk factors of disk-related sciatica in an urban population in Tunisia. *Joint Bone Spine* **73**, 538–542 (2006).
45. Kanna, R. M., Shetty, A. P. & Rajasekaran, S. Patterns of lumbar disc degeneration are different in degenerative disc disease and disc prolapse magnetic resonance imaging analysis of 224 patients. *The Spine Journal* **14**, 300–307 (2014).
46. Suthar, P., Patel, R., Mehta, C. & Patel, N. MRI Evaluation of Lumbar Disc Degenerative Disease. *J Clin Diagn Res* **9**, TC04–TC09 (2015).
47. Berg-Johansen, B. Characterization of the Spinal Disc-Vertebra Interface and its Relation to Injury and Back Pain. (UCSF, 2017).
48. Lama, P. *et al.* Do intervertebral discs degenerate before they herniate, or after? *Bone Joint J* **95**, 1127–1133 (2013).
49. Buckwalter, J. A. Aging and Degeneration of the Human Intervertebral Disc. *Spine* **20**, 1307 (1995).
50. Tomaszewski, K., Saganiak, K., G\ladysz, T. & Walocha, J. The biology behind the human intervertebral disc and its endplates. *Folia morphologica* **74**, 157–168 (2015).
51. Yee, A. *et al.* Fibrotic-like changes in degenerate human intervertebral discs revealed by quantitative proteomic analysis. *Osteoarthritis and cartilage* **24**, 503–513 (2016).
52. Sato, K., Kikuchi, S. & Yonezawa, T. In Vivo Intradiscal Pressure Measurement in Healthy Individuals and in Patients With Ongoing Back Problems. *Spine* **24**, 2468 (1999).
53. Antoniou, J. *et al.* The human lumbar intervertebral disc: evidence for changes in the biosynthesis and denaturation of the extracellular matrix with growth, maturation, ageing, and degeneration. *The Journal of clinical investigation* **98**, 996–1003 (1996).
54. Boos, N. *et al.* Classification of Age-Related Changes in Lumbar Intervertebral Discs: 2002 Volvo Award in Basic Science. *Spine* **27**, 2631 (2002).
55. Yang, S.-H. *et al.* Spatial geometric and magnetic resonance signal intensity changes with advancing stages of nucleus pulposus degeneration. *BMC Musculoskeletal Disorders* **18**, 473 (2017).
56. Eyre, D. R. Biochemistry of the Intervertebral Disc. in *International Review of Connective Tissue Research* (eds. Hall, D. A. & Jackson, D. S.) **8**, 227–291 (Elsevier, 1979).
57. Wang, F., Cai, F., Shi, R., Wang, X.-H. & Wu, X.-T. Aging and age related stresses: a senescence mechanism of intervertebral disc degeneration. *Osteoarthritis and Cartilage* **24**, 398–408 (2016).
58. Friedmann, A. *et al.* Microstructure analysis method for evaluating degenerated intervertebral disc tissue. *Micron* **92**, 51–62 (2017).
59. Lama, P., Kulkarni, J. P. & Tamang, B. K. The Role of Cell Clusters in Intervertebral Disc Degeneration and its Relevance behind Repair. *Spine Research* **3**, (2017).
60. Rajasekaran, S. *et al.* Inflammaging determines health and disease in lumbar discs—evidence from differing proteomic signatures of healthy, aging, and degenerating discs. *The Spine Journal* (2019). doi:10.1016/j.spinee.2019.04.023
61. Heraclitus, of E. *et al.* *Hippocrates*. (Heinemann, 1923).
62. Key, A. On paraplegia depending on disease of the ligaments of the spine. *Guy's hospital reports* (1838).

63. Luschka, H. *Die Halbgelenke des menschlichen Körpers: Mit 6 Kupfertafeln*. (Ge. Reimer, 1858).
64. Gray, H. *Anatomy-- descriptive and surgical*. (J.W. Parker and Son, 1858).
65. Vulpian, A. *Maladies du système nerveux: leçons professées a la Faculté de médecine*. (O. Doin, 1879).
66. Kocher, T. *Die Verletzungen der Wirbelsäule zugleich als Beitrag zur Physiologie des menschlichen Rückenmarks*. (G. Fischer, 1896).
67. Krause, F. *Chirurgie des gehirns und rückenmarks nach eigenen erfahrungen*. (Urban & Schwarzenberg, 1911).
68. Middleton, G. S. & Teacher, J. H. Injury of the Spinal Cord Due to Rupture of an Intervertebral Disc During Muscular Effort. *Glasgow Medical Journal* (1911).
69. Goldthwait, J. E. The Lumbo-Sacral Articulation; An Explanation of Many Cases of 'Lumbago,' 'Sciatica' and Paraplegia. *The Boston Medical and Surgical Journal* **164**, 365–372 (1911).
70. Alpers, B. J., Grant, F. C. & Yaskin, J. C. Chondroma of the Intervertebral Disks. *Ann Surg* **97**, 10–18 (1933).
71. Bucy, P. CHondroma of intervertebral disk. *JAMA* **94**, 1552–1554 (1930).
72. Kambin, P. History of surgical management of herniated lumbar discs from cauterization to arthroscopic and endoscopic spinal surgery. in *Arthroscopic and Endoscopic spinal surgery* 1–27 (Springer, 2005).
73. Dandy, W. Loose cartilage from intervertebral disk simulating tumor of the spinal cord. *Arch Surg* **19**, 660–672 (1929).
74. Mixter, W. J. & Barr, J. S. Rupture of the intervertebral disc with involvement of the spinal canal. *N Engl j Med* **211**, 210–5 (1934).
75. Maroudas, A., Stockwell, R., Nachemson, A. & Urban, J. Factors involved in the nutrition of the human lumbar intervertebral disc: cellularity and diffusion of glucose in vitro. *Journal of anatomy* **120**, 113 (1975).
76. Rodriguez, A. G. *et al.* Human Disc Nucleus Properties and Vertebral Endplate Permeability. *Spine (Phila Pa 1976)* **36**, 512–520 (2011).
77. Kepler, C. K., Ponnappan, R. K., Tannoury, C. A., Risbud, M. V. & Anderson, D. G. The molecular basis of intervertebral disc degeneration. *The Spine Journal* **13**, 318–330 (2013).
78. Fields, A. J., Ballatori, A., Liebenberg, E. C. & Lotz, J. C. Contribution of the endplates to disc degeneration. *Current molecular biology reports* **4**, 151–160 (2018).
79. Roberts, S., Menage, J. & Urban, J. P. G. Biochemical and Structural Properties of the Cartilage End-Plate and its Relation to the Intervertebral Disc. *Spine* **14**, 166 (1989).
80. Fields, A. J., Liebenberg, E. C. & Lotz, J. C. Innervation of pathologies in the lumbar vertebral endplate and intervertebral disc. *Spine J* **14**, 513–521 (2014).
81. Newell, N. *et al.* Biomechanics of the human intervertebral disc: A review of testing techniques and results. *Journal of the mechanical behavior of biomedical materials* **69**, 420–434 (2017).
82. Sivan, S.-S. *et al.* Longevity of elastin in human intervertebral disc as probed by the racemization of aspartic acid. *Biochimica et Biophysica Acta (BBA)-General Subjects* **1820**, 1671–1677 (2012).
83. Mwale, F., Roughley, P., Antoniou, J. & others. Distinction between the extracellular matrix of the nucleus pulposus and hyaline cartilage: a requisite for tissue engineering of intervertebral disc. *Eur Cell Mater* **8**, 63–64 (2004).
84. Pattappa, G. *et al.* Diversity of intervertebral disc cells: phenotype and function. *Journal of anatomy* **221**, 480–496 (2012).
85. Liang, L. *et al.* The characteristics of stem cells in human degenerative intervertebral disc. *Medicine (Baltimore)* **96**, (2017).
86. Henriksson, H. B., Svala, E., Skioldebrand, E., Lindahl, A. & Brisby, H. Support of Concept That Migrating Progenitor Cells From Stem Cell Niches Contribute to Normal Regeneration of the Adult Mammal Intervertebral Disc: A Descriptive Study in the New Zealand White Rabbit. *Spine* **37**, 722 (2012).
87. Nerlich, A. G., Schleicher, E. D. & Boos, N. 1997 Volvo Award Winner in Basic Science Studies: Immunohistologic markers for age-related changes of human lumbar intervertebral discs. *Spine* **22**, 2781–2795 (1997).
88. Eyre, D. R. & Muir, H. Quantitative analysis of types I and II collagens in human intervertebral discs at various ages. *Biochimica et Biophysica Acta (BBA) - Protein Structure* **492**, 29–42 (1977).
89. Silagi, E. S., Shapiro, I. M. & Risbud, M. V. Glycosaminoglycan synthesis in the nucleus pulposus: Dysregulation and the pathogenesis of disc degeneration. *Matrix Biology* **71–72**, 368–379 (2018).
90. Wei, Q., Zhang, X., Zhou, C., Ren, Q. & Zhang, Y. Roles of large aggregating proteoglycans in human intervertebral disc degeneration. *Connective Tissue Research* **60**, 209–218 (2019).
91. Wilke, H., Neef, P., Caimi, M., Hoogland, T. & Claes, L. E. New in vivo measurements of pressures in the intervertebral disc in daily life. *Spine* **24**, 755–762 (1999).
92. Hoffman, H. *et al.* Aquaporin-1 expression in herniated human lumbar intervertebral discs. *Global spine journal* **7**, 133–140 (2017).
93. Li, S., Yang, K. & Zhang, Y. Expression of aquaporins 1 and 3 in degenerative tissue of the lumbar intervertebral disc. *Genet Mol Res* **13**, 8225–8233 (2014).
94. Vergroesen, P.-P. A. *et al.* Mechanics and biology in intervertebral disc degeneration: a vicious circle. *Osteoarthritis and Cartilage* **23**, 1057–1070 (2015).
95. Junhui, L. *et al.* Anchorage of annulus fibrosus within the vertebral endplate with reference to disc herniation. *Microscopy research and technique* **78**, 754–760 (2015).
96. Sapiee, N. H., Thambyah, A., Robertson, P. A. & Broom, N. D. New evidence for structural integration across the cartilage-vertebral endplate junction and its relation to herniation. *The Spine Journal* **19**, 532–544 (2019).
97. Tavakoli, J., Elliott, D. M. & Costi, J. J. Structure and mechanical function of the inter-lamellar matrix of the annulus fibrosus in the disc. *Journal of Orthopaedic Research* **34**, 1307–1315 (2016).
98. Sharabi, M., Wade, K. & Haj-Ali, R. Chapter 7 - The Mechanical Role of Collagen Fibers in the Intervertebral Disc. in *Biomechanics of the Spine* (eds. Galbusera, F. & Wilke, H.-J.) 105–123 (Academic Press, 2018). doi:10.1016/B978-0-12-812851-0.00007-0
99. Franklin, L. & Hull, E. W. Lipid content of the intervertebral disc. *Clinical chemistry* **12**, 253–257 (1966).
100. Copius Peereboom, J. W. Some biochemical and histochemical properties of the age pigment in the human intervertebral disc. *Histochemie* **37**, 119–130 (1973).
101. Fields, A. J., Rodriguez, D., Gary, K. N., Liebenberg, E. C. & Lotz, J. C. Influence of biochemical composition on endplate cartilage tensile properties in the human lumbar spine. *Journal of Orthopaedic Research* **32**, 245–252 (2014).
102. Lotz, J., Fields, A. & Liebenberg, E. The role of the vertebral end plate in low back pain. *Global spine journal* **3**, 153–164 (2013).
103. Gullbrand, S. E. *et al.* Low rate loading-induced convection enhances net transport into the intervertebral disc in vivo. *The Spine Journal* **15**, 1028–1033 (2015).
104. Zhang, S.-J. *et al.* Autophagy: A double-edged sword in intervertebral disk degeneration. *Clinica Chimica Acta* **457**, 27–35 (2016).
105. Cisewski, S. E. *et al.* Comparison of Oxygen Consumption Rates of Nondegenerate and Degenerate Human Intervertebral Disc Cells. *Spine* **43**, E60–E67 (2018).
106. Bardonova, L. A. *et al.* ENERGY SUPPLY AND DEMAND IN THE INTERVERTEBRAL DISC. *Coluna/Columna* **17**, 237–239 (2018).
107. Silagi, E. S. Insights into Glycolytic Metabolism and pH Homeostasis in the Hypoxic Intervertebral Disc. (Thomas Jefferson University, 2019).
108. Silagi, E. S., Batista, P., Shapiro, I. M. & Risbud, M. V. Expression of Carbonic Anhydrase III, a Nucleus Pulposus Phenotypic Marker, is Hypoxia-responsive and Confers Protection from Oxidative Stress-induced Cell Death. *Scientific Reports* **8**, 4856 (2018).
109. Liang, C. *et al.* New hypothesis of chronic back pain: low pH promotes nerve ingrowth into damaged intervertebral disks. *Acta Anaesthesiologica Scandinavica* **57**, 271–277 (2013).
110. Nagashima, H. *et al.* High-resolution nuclear magnetic resonance spectroscopic study of metabolites in the cerebrospinal fluid of patients with cervical myelopathy and lumbar radiculopathy. *Eur Spine J* **19**, 1363–1368 (2010).
111. Silagi, E. S. *et al.* Bicarbonate Recycling by HIF-1–Dependent Carbonic Anhydrase Isoforms 9 and 12 Is Critical in Maintaining Intracellular pH and Viability of Nucleus Pulposus Cells. *Journal of Bone and Mineral Research* **33**, 338–355 (2018).
112. Cisewski, S. E. Nutrient Related Mechanisms of Intervertebral Disc Degeneration. (2016).
113. Brock, M., Patt, S. & Mayer, H.-M. The form and structure of the extruded disc. *Spine* **17**, 1457–1461 (1992).
114. Schmid, G. *et al.* Lumbar Disk Herniation: Correlation of Histologic Findings with Marrow Signal Intensity Changes in Vertebral Endplates at MR Imaging. *Radiology* **231**, 352–358 (2004).
115. Willburger, R. E., Ehiosun, U. K., Kuhnen, C., Krämer, J. & Schmid, G. Clinical Symptoms in Lumbar Disc Herniations and Their Correlation to the Histological Composition of the Extruded Disc Material. *Spine* **29**, 1655 (2004).
116. Matveeva, N., Zivadinovik, J., Zdravkovska, M., Jovevska, S. & Bojadzieva, B. Histological composition of lumbar disc herniations related to the type of herniation and to the age. *Bratisl Lek Listy* **113**, 712–717 (2012).
117. Freemont, A. *et al.* Nerve ingrowth into diseased intervertebral disc in chronic back pain. *The Lancet* **350**, 178–181 (1997).
118. Yang, G., Liao, W., Shen, M. & Mei, H. Insight into neural mechanisms underlying discogenic back pain. *Journal of International Medical Research* **46**, 4427–4436 (2018).
119. Das, G., Roy, C. & others. Rami communicans fibers in discogenic low back pain: The controversies. *Indian Journal of Pain* **32**, 60 (2018).
120. Dimitroulias, A. *et al.* An immunohistochemical study of mechanoreceptors in lumbar spine intervertebral discs. *Journal of Clinical Neuroscience* **17**, 742–745 (2010).
121. Roberts, S., Eisenstein, S. M., Menage, J., Evans, E. H. & Ashton, I. K. Mechanoreceptors in intervertebral discs. Morphology, distribution, and neuropeptides. *Spine* **20**, 2645–2651 (1995).
122. Coppes, M. H., Marani, E., Thomeer, R. T. & Groen, G. J. Innervation of" painful" lumbar discs. *Spine* **22**, 2342–2349 (1997).
123. Peng, B., Wu, W., Li, Z., Guo, J. & Wang, X. Chemical radiculitis. *Pain* **127**, 11–16 (2007).
124. Stefanakis, M. *et al.* Annulus fissures are mechanically and chemically conducive to the ingrowth of nerves and blood vessels. *Spine* **37**, 1883–1891 (2012).

125. Binch, A. L. *et al.* Nerves are more abundant than blood vessels in the degenerate human intervertebral disc. *Arthritis research & therapy* **17**, 370 (2015).
126. Lama, P., Maitre, C. L. L., Harding, I. J., Dolan, P. & Adams, M. A. Nerves and blood vessels in degenerated intervertebral discs are confined to physically disrupted tissue. *Journal of Anatomy* **233**, 86–97 (2018).
127. Ohtori, S., Miyagi, M. & Inoue, G. Sensory nerve ingrowth, cytokines, and instability of discogenic low back pain: a review. *Spine Surgery and Related Research* **2**, 11–17 (2018).
128. Mahdi, M. A. E., Latif, F. Y. A. & Janko, M. The Spinal Nerve Root "Innervation", and a New Concept of the Clinicopathological Inter-Relations in Back Pain and Sciatica. *Neurochirurgia* **24**, 137–141 (1981).
129. Milette, P. C., Fontaine, S., Lepanto, L. & Breton, G. Radiating pain to the lower extremities caused by lumbar disk rupture without spinal nerve root involvement. *American journal of neuroradiology* **16**, 1605–1613 (1995).
130. Sivan, S. S. *et al.* Biochemical composition and turnover of the extracellular matrix of the normal and degenerate intervertebral disc. *European Spine Journal* **23**, 344–353 (2014).
131. Segar, A. H., Fairbank, J. C. T. & Urban, J. Leptin and the intervertebral disc: a biochemical link exists between obesity, intervertebral disc degeneration and low back pain—an in vitro study in a bovine model. *Eur Spine J* **28**, 214–223 (2019).
132. Li, Z. *et al.* Melatonin inhibits nucleus pulposus (NP) cell proliferation and extracellular matrix (ECM) remodeling via the melatonin membrane receptors mediated PI3K-Akt pathway. *Journal of Pineal Research* **63**, e12435 (2017).
133. Bertolo, A., Baur, M., Aebli, N., Ferguson, S. J. & Stoyanov, J. Physiological testosterone levels enhance chondrogenic extracellular matrix synthesis by male intervertebral disc cells in vitro, but not by mesenchymal stem cells. *The Spine Journal* **14**, 455–468 (2014).
134. Li, P. *et al.* Estrogen Enhances Matrix Synthesis in Nucleus Pulposus Cell through the Estrogen Receptor β-p38 MAPK Pathway. *CPB* **39**, 2216–2226 (2016).
135. Chou, P.-H. *et al.* Fluid-induced, shear stress-regulated extracellular matrix and matrix metalloproteinase genes expression on human annulus fibrosus cells. *Stem Cell Research & Therapy* **7**, 34 (2016).
136. Handa, T. *et al.* Effects of Hydrostatic Pressure on Matrix Synthesis and Matrix Metalloproteinase Production in the Human Lumbar Intervertebral Disc. *Spine* **22**, 1085 (1997).
137. Wade, K. R., Robertson, P. A., Thambyah, A. & Broom, N. D. "Surprise" Loading in Flexion Increases the Risk of Disc Herniation Due to Annulus-Endplate Junction Failure: A Mechanical and Microstructural Investigation. *Spine* **40**, 891–901 (2015).
138. Hadjipavlou, A. G., Tzermiadianos, M. N., Bogduk, N. & Zindrick, M. R. The pathophysiology of disc degeneration. *Bone & Joint Journal* **90-B**, 1261–1270 (2008).
139. Ameling, W. *et al. Caesarea and the Middle Coast: 1121-2160.* (Walter de Gruyter, 2011).
140. Caelius Aurelianus. *Caelii Aureliani Siccensis, ...De acutis morbis. lib.3. De diuturnis. lib.5. Ad fidem exemplaris manuscripti castigati, & annotationibus illustrati. Cum indice copiosissimo, ac locupletissimo.* (apud Guliel. Rouillium, sub scuto Veneto, 1566).
141. Berger-Roscher, N. *et al.* Influence of Complex Loading Conditions on Intervertebral Disc Failure. *Spine* **42**, E78 (2017).
142. Casaroli, G. *et al.* Numerical prediction of the mechanical failure of the intervertebral disc under complex loading conditions. *Materials* **10**, 31 (2017).
143. Shan, Z. *et al.* A more realistic disc herniation model incorporating compression, flexion and facet-constrained shear: a mechanical and microstructural analysis. Part II: high rate or 'surprise'loading. *European Spine Journal* **26**, 2629–2641 (2017).
144. Harvey-Burgess, M. & Gregory, D. E. The Effect of Axial Torsion on the Mechanical Properties of the Annulus Fibrosus. *Spine* **44**, E195 (2019).
145. Rodrigues, S. A., Thambyah, A. & Broom, N. D. A multiscale structural investigation of the annulus-endplate anchorage system and its mechanisms of failure. *The Spine Journal* **15**, 405–416 (2015).
146. Chooi, W. H. & Chan, B. P. Compression Induced Stress Response of Nucleus Pulposus Cells in 3D Collagen Gel. *Global Spine Journal* **6**, s–0036 (2016).
147. Balkovec, C., Adams, M. A., Dolan, P. & McGill, S. M. Annulus Fibrosus Can Strip Hyaline Cartilage End Plate from Subchondral Bone: A Study of the Intervertebral Disk in Tension. *Global Spine J* **05**, 360–365 (2015).
148. Berg-Johansen, B., Fields, A. J., Liebenberg, E. C., Li, A. & Lotz, J. C. Structure-function relationships at the human spinal disc-vertebra interface. *Journal of Orthopaedic Research®* **36**, 192–201 (2018).
149. Thoreson, O. *et al.* The effect of repetitive flexion and extension fatigue loading on the young porcine lumbar spine, a feasibility study of MRI and histological analyses. *Journal of experimental orthopaedics* **4**, 16 (2017).
150. Rajasekaran, S., Bajaj, N., Tubaki, V., Kanna, R. M. & Shetty, A. P. Anatomy of Failure in Lumbar Disc Herniation. An in Vivo, Multimodal, Prospective Study of 181 Subjects. *Global Spine Journal* **4**, s–0034 (2014).
151. Berg-Johansen, B. *et al.* Tidemark Avulsions are a Predominant Form of Endplate Irregularity. *Spine* **43**, 1095 (2018).
152. Sahoo, M. M., Mahapatra, S. K., Kaur, S., Sarangi, J. & Mohapatra, M. Significance of vertebral endplate failure in symptomatic lumbar disc herniation. *Global spine journal* **7**, 230–238 (2017).
153. Morimoto, M. *et al.* A Rare Case of Progressive Palsy of the Lower Leg Caused by a Huge Lumbar Posterior Endplate Lesion after Recurrent Disc Herniation. *Case Reports in Orthopedics* (2016). doi:10.1155/2016/5963924
154. Kadhim, M. A., Al–Zubaidi, M. E. D. & Yaqub, F. M. MRI Finding of Cartilaginous Endplates Herniation of Lumbar Spine in Patient with Low Back Pain. *Iraqi Postgraduate Medical Journal* **17**, (2018).
155. Wade, K. R., Schollum, M. L., Robertson, P. A., Thambyah, A. & Broom, N. D. A more realistic disc herniation model incorporating compression, flexion and facet-constrained shear: a mechanical and microstructural analysis. Part I: Low rate loading. *Eur Spine J* **26**, 2616–2628 (2017).
156. van Heeswijk, V. M., Thambyah, A., Robertson, P. A. & Broom, N. D. Posterolateral Disc Prolapse in Flexion Initiated by Lateral Inner Annular Failure. *Spine* **42**, 1604–1613 (2017).
157. Tavakoli, J., Amin, D. B., Freeman, B. J. & Costi, J. J. The biomechanics of the inter-lamellar matrix and the lamellae during progression to lumbar disc herniation: which is the weakest structure? *Annals of biomedical engineering* **46**, 1280–1291 (2018).
158. Huang, Y.-C., Urban, J. P. & Luk, K. D. Intervertebral disc regeneration: do nutrients lead the way? *Nature Reviews Rheumatology* **10**, 561–566 (2014).
159. Alpantaki, K., Kampouroglou, A., Koutserimpas, C., Effraimidis, G. & Hadjipavlou, A. Diabetes mellitus as a risk factor for intervertebral disc degeneration: a critical review. *Eur Spine J* (2019). doi:10.1007/s00586-019-06029-7
160. Hormel, S. E. & Eyre, D. R. Collagen in the ageing human intervertebral disc: An increase in covalently bound fluorophores and chromophores. *Biochimica et Biophysica Acta (BBA) - Protein Structure and Molecular Enzymology* **1078**, 243–250 (1991).
161. Staszkiewicz, R. & Bolechala, F. Changes in es sential and trace elements content in degenerat ing human intervertebral discs do not cor respond to patients' clinical status. (2019).
162. Kraemer, J., Kolditz, D. & Gowin, R. Water and electrolyte content of human intervertebral discs under variable load. *Spine* **10**, 69–71 (1985).
163. Wang, C. *et al.* Validation of Sodium MRI of Intervertebral Disc. *Spine (Phila Pa 1976)* **35**, 505–510 (2010).
164. Kubaszewski, \Lukasz *et al.* Atomic absorption spectrometry analysis of trace elements in degenerated intervertebral disc tissue. *Medical science monitor: international medical journal of experimental and clinical research* **20**, 2157 (2014).
165. Karamouzian, S. *et al.* Frequency of Lumbar Intervertebral Disc Calcification and Angiogenesis, and Their Correlation With Clinical, Surgical, and Magnetic Resonance Imaging Findings. *Spine* **35**, 881 (2010).
166. Kubaszewski, \Lukasz *et al.* Chemometric evaluation of concentrations of trace elements in intervertebral disc tissue in patient with degenerative disc disease. *Ann Agric Environ Med* **24**, 610–617 (2017).
167. Nowakowski, A. *et al.* Analysis of trace element in intervertebral disc by atomic absorption spectrometry techniques in degenerative disc disease in the Polish population. *Annals of Agricultural and Environmental Medicine* **22**, (2015).
168. Zioła-Frankowska, A., Kubaszewski, Ł., Dąbrowski, M. & Frankowski, M. Interrelationship between silicon, aluminum, and elements associated with tissue metabolism and degenerative processes in degenerated human intervertebral disc tissue. *Environ Sci Pollut Res* **24**, 19777–19784 (2017).
169. Maltseva, V. Effect of Pb exposure on the cells and matrix of the intervertebral disc of rats. *Regulatory Mechanisms in Biosystems* **2**, (2017).
170. Fardon, D. F. *et al.* Lumbar disc nomenclature: version 2.0: Recommendations of the combined task forces of the North American Spine Society, the American Society of Spine Radiology and the American Society of Neuroradiology. *The Spine Journal* **14**, 2525–2545 (2014).
171. Weiner, B. K. & Patel, R. The accuracy of MRI in the detection of Lumbar Disc Containment. *J Orthop Surg* **3**, 46 (2008).
172. Pneumaticos, S. G., Hipp, J. A. & Esses, S. I. Sensitivity and specificity of dural sac and herniated disc dimensions in patients with low back-related leg pain. *Journal of Magnetic Resonance Imaging* **12**, 439–443 (2000).
173. Beattie, P. F., Meyers, S. P., Stratford, P., Millard, R. W. & Hollenberg, G. M. Associations between patient report of symptoms and anatomic impairment visible on lumbar magnetic resonance imaging. *Spine* **25**, 819–828 (2000).
174. Suri, P., Boyko, E. J., Goldberg, J., Forsberg, C. W. & Jarvik, J. G. Longitudinal associations between incident lumbar spine MRI findings and chronic low back pain or radicular symptoms: retrospective analysis of data from the longitudinal assessment of imaging and disability of the back (LAIDBACK). *BMC musculoskeletal disorders* **15**, 1 (2014).
175. Choi, S.-J. *et al.* The Use of Magnetic Resonance Imaging to Predict the Clinical Outcome of Non-Surgical Treatment for Lumbar Interverterbal Disc Herniation. *Korean Journal of Radiology* **8**, 156 (2007).
176. Kawaguchi, K. *et al.* Effect of cartilaginous endplates on extruded disc resorption in lumbar disc herniation. *PloS one* **13**, e0195946 (2018).
177. Slipman, C. *et al.* Clinical evidence of chemical radiculopathy. *Pain Physician* **5**, 260–265 (2002).

178. Ljunggren, A. E. Discriminant validity of pain modalities and other sensory phenomena in patients with lumbar herniated intervertebral discs versus lumbar spinal stenosis. *Neuro-orthopedics* **11**, 91–99 (1991).
179. Kortelainen, P., Puranen, J., Koivisto, E., Lähde, S. & others. Symptoms and signs of sciatica and their relation to the localization of the lumbar disc herniation. *Spine* **10**, 88 (1985).
180. Mondelli, M. *et al.* Clinical findings and electrodiagnostic testing in 108 consecutive cases of lumbosacral radiculopathy due to herniated disc. *Neurophysiologie Clinique/Clinical Neurophysiology* **43**, 205–215 (2013).
181. Lee, M., McPhee, R. & Stringer, M. An evidence-based approach to human dermatomes. *Clinical Anatomy* **21**, 363–373 (2008).
182. Gardner, A., Gardner, E. & Morley, T. Cauda equina syndrome: a review of the current clinical and medico-legal position. *European Spine Journal* **20**, 690–697 (2011).
183. Maeda, T. *et al.* Factors associated with lumbar spinal stenosis in a large-scale, population-based cohort: The Wakayama Spine Study. *PLOS ONE* **13**, e0200208 (2018).
184. Aurelianus, C., Drabkin, I. E. & Soranus. *On acute diseases and On chronic diseases,*. (Univ. of Chicago Press, 1950).
185. Sicard, J. Névrodocites et funiculites vertébrales. *Presse méd* **26**, 9–11 (1918).
186. Lin, J.-H. *et al.* Diagnostic accuracy of standardised qualitative sensory test in the detection of lumbar lateral stenosis involving the L5 nerve root. *Scientific Reports* **7**, 10598 (2017).
187. Verbiest, H. [Primary stenosis of the lumbar spinal canal in adults, a new syndrome]. *Ned Tijdschr Geneeskd* **94**, 2415–2433 (1950).
188. Kalichman, L. *et al.* Spinal stenosis prevalence and association with symptoms: The Framingham Study. *Spine J* **9**, 545–550 (2009).
189. Ishimoto, Y. *et al.* Prevalence of symptomatic lumbar spinal stenosis and its association with physical performance in a population-based cohort in Japan: the Wakayama Spine Study. *Osteoarthritis and Cartilage* **20**, 1103–1108 (2012).
190. Miyakoshi, N., Hongo, M., Kasukawa, Y., Ishikawa, Y. & Shimada, Y. Prevalence, spinal alignment, and mobility of lumbar spinal stenosis with or without chronic low back pain: a community-dwelling study. *Pain research and treatment* **2011**, (2011).
191. Tomonaga, Y. Relationship Between the Development of the Spinal Canal and the Etiopathogenesis of Lumbar Spinal Stenosis. (Université de Lausanne, Faculté de biologie et médecine, 2012).
192. Watts, R. Lumbar vertebral canal size in adults and children: Observations from a skeletal sample from London, England. *HOMO* **64**, 120–128 (2013).
193. Zhang, H., Sucato, D. J., Nurenberg, P. & McClung, A. Morphometric analysis of neurocentral synchondrosis using magnetic resonance imaging in the normal skeletally immature spine. *Spine* **35**, 76–82 (2010).
194. Tomkins-Lane, C. C., Battié, M. C., Hu, R. & Macedo, L. Pathoanatomical characteristics of clinical lumbar spinal stenosis. *Journal of back and musculoskeletal rehabilitation* **27**, 223–229 (2014).
195. Akuthota, V., Lento, P. & Sowa, G. Pathogenesis of lumbar spinal stenosis pain: why does an asymptomatic stenotic patient flare? *Physical medicine and rehabilitation clinics of North America* **14**, 17–28 (2003).
196. Fogel, G. R. & Esses, S. I. Hip spine syndrome: management of coexisting radiculopathy and arthritis of the lower extremity. *The Spine Journal* **3**, 238–241 (2003).
197. Kong, L., Bai, J., Zhang, B., Shen, Y. & Tian, D. Predictive factors of symptomatic lumbar canal stenosis in patients after surgery for cervical spondylotic myelopathy. *Ther Clin Risk Manag* **14**, 483–488 (2018).
198. Arnoldi, C. *et al.* Lumbar spinal stenosis and nerve root entrapment syndromes. *Clinical Orthopaedics and Related Research®* 4–5 (1976).
199. Schroeder, G. D., Kurd, M. F. & Vaccaro, A. R. Lumbar spinal stenosis: how is it classified? *Journal of the American Academy of Orthopaedic Surgeons* **24**, 843–852 (2016).
200. Fortin, J. D. & Wheeler, M. T. Imaging in lumbar spinal stenosis. *Pain Physician* **7**, 133–139 (2004).
201. Sakai, Y. *et al.* Clinical outcome of lumbar spinal stenosis based on new classification according to hypertrophied ligamentum flavum. *Journal of Orthopaedic Science* **22**, 27–33 (2017).
202. Kim, Y. U. *et al.* Clinical symptoms of lumbar spinal stenosis associated with morphological parameters on magnetic resonance images. *European spine journal* **24**, 2236–2243 (2015).
203. Hong, J. H., Lee, M. Y., Jung, S. W. & Lee, S. Y. Does spinal stenosis correlate with MRI findings and pain, psychologic factor and quality of life? *Korean Journal of Anesthesiology* **68**, 481 (2015).
204. Andrasinova, T. *et al.* Is there a Correlation Between Degree of Radiologic Lumbar Spinal Stenosis and its Clinical Manifestation? (2018). doi:info:doi/10.1097/BSD.0000000000000681
205. Korse, N. S., Kruit, M. C., Peul, W. C. & Vleggeert-Lankamp, C. L. A. Lumbar spinal canal MRI diameter is smaller in herniated disc cauda equina syndrome patients. *PLOS ONE* **12**, e0186148 (2017).
206. Cheung, J. P. Y., Ng, K. K. M., Cheung, P. W. H., Samartzis, D. & Cheung, K. M. C. Radiographic indices for lumbar developmental spinal stenosis. *Scoliosis and Spinal Disorders* **12**, 3 (2017).
207. Hyun, S.-J. *et al.* A Haplotype at the COL9A2 Gene Locus Contributes to the Genetic Risk for Lumbar Spinal Stenosis in the Korean Population. *Spine* **36**, 1273 (2011).
208. Jiang, H., Yang, Q., Jiang, J., Zhan, X. & Xiao, Z. Association between COL11A1 (rs1337185) and ADAMTS5 (rs162509) gene polymorphisms and lumbar spine pathologies in Chinese Han population: an observational study. *BMJ Open* **7**, e015644 (2017).
209. Noponen-Hietala, N. *et al.* Sequence variations in the collagen IX and XI genes are associated with degenerative lumbar spinal stenosis. *Annals of the rheumatic diseases* **62**, 1208–1214 (2003).
210. Hyun, S.-J. *et al.* Progression of lumbar spinal stenosis is influenced by polymorphism of thrombospondin 2 gene in the Korean population. *Eur Spine J* **23**, 57–63 (2014).
211. Cheung, J. P. *et al.* Etiology of developmental spinal stenosis: A genome-wide association study. *Journal of Orthopaedic Research®* **36**, 1262–1268 (2018).
212. Sebastian, A. *et al.* Genetic inactivation of ERK1 and ERK2 in chondrocytes promotes bone growth and enlarges the spinal canal. *Journal of Orthopaedic Research* **29**, 375–379 (2011).
213. Jeong, S.-T. *et al.* MRI study of the lumbar spine in achondroplasia: a morphometric analysis for the evaluation of stenosis of the canal. *The Journal of bone and joint surgery. British volume* **88**, 1192–1196 (2006).
214. Nightingale, S. Developmental spinal canal stenosis and somatotype. *J Neurol Neurosurg Psychiatry* **52**, 887–890 (1989).
215. Griffith, J. F. *et al.* Population reference range for developmental lumbar spinal canal size. *Quantitative imaging in medicine and surgery* **6**, 671 (2016).
216. Callewaert, B., Malfait, F., Loeys, B. & De Paepe, A. Ehlers-Danlos syndromes and Marfan syndrome. *Best practice & research Clinical rheumatology* **22**, 165–189 (2008).
217. Jeffrey, J. E., Campbell, D. M., Golden, M. H. N., Smith, F. W. & Porter, R. W. Antenatal Factors in the Development of the Lumbar Vertebral Canal: A Magnetic Resonance Imaging Study. *Spine* **28**, 1418 (2003).
218. Papp, T., Porter, R. W., Craig, C. E., Aspden, R. M. & Campbell, D. M. Significant antenatal factors in the development of lumbar spinal stenosis. *Spine* **22**, 1805–1810 (1997).
219. Clark, G., Panjabi, M. & Wetzel, F. Can Infant Malnutrition Cause Adult Vertebral Stenosis? *Spine* **10**, 165–170 (1985).
220. Muthuuri, J., Some, E. & Chege, P. Association between early life malnutrition and the size of lumbar spinal canal among adults of coastal region, Kenya. *East African Orthopaedic Journal* **12**, 33–38 (2018).
221. Porter, R. & Pavitt, D. The vertebral canal: I. Nutrition and development, an archaeological study. *Spine* **12**, 901–906 (1987).
222. Porter, R., Drinkall, J., Porter, D. & Thorp, L. The vertebral canal: II. Health and academic status, a clinical study. *Spine* **12**, 907–911 (1987).
223. White, A. Clinical biomechanics of the spine. *Clinical biomechanics of the spine* (1990).
224. Lang, G. *et al.* Preoperative Assessment of Neural Elements in Lumbar Spinal Stenosis by Upright Magnetic Resonance Imaging: An Implication for Routine Practice? *Cureus* **10**,
225. Kanno, H. *et al.* Dynamic change of dural sac cross-sectional area in axial loaded magnetic resonance imaging correlates with the severity of clinical symptoms in patients with lumbar spinal canal stenosis. *Spine* **37**, 207–213 (2012).
226. Lau, Y. Y. O. *et al.* Changes in dural sac caliber with standing MRI improve correlation with symptoms of lumbar spinal stenosis. *Eur Spine J* 1–10 (2017). doi:10.1007/s00586-017-5211-7
227. Finkenstaedt, T. *et al.* Correlation of listhesis on upright radiographs and central lumbar spinal canal stenosis on supine MRI: is it possible to predict lumbar spinal canal stenosis? *Skeletal Radiol* **47**, 1269–1275 (2018).
228. Segebarth, B., Kurd, M. F., Haug, P. H. & Davis, R. Routine Upright Imaging for Evaluating Degenerative Lumbar Stenosis: Incidence of Degenerative Spondylolisthesis Missed on Supine MRI. *Clinical Spine Surgery* **28**, 394 (2015).
229. Kanemura, A. *et al.* The Influence of Sagittal Instability Factors on Clinical Lumbar Spinal Symptoms: *Journal of Spinal Disorders & Techniques* **22**, 479–485 (2009).
230. Pitkanen, M. *et al.* Segmental lumbar spine instability at flexion-extension radiography can be predicted by conventional radiography. *Clinical Radiology* **57**, 632–639 (2002).
231. Chaput, C., Padon, D., Rush, J., Lenehan, E. & Rahm, M. The significance of increased fluid signal on magnetic resonance imaging in lumbar facets in relationship to degenerative spondylolisthesis. *Spine* **32**, 1883–1887 (2007).
232. Bräm, J., Zanetti, M., Min, K. & Hodler, J. MR abnormalities of the intervertebral disks and adjacent bone marrow as predictors of segmental instability of the lumbar spine. *Acta Radiologica* **39**, 18–23 (1998).
233. Yochum, T. R. & Rowe, L. J. *Yochum and Rowe's Essentials of Skeletal Radiology*. (Lippincott Williams & Wilkins A Wolters Kluwer Company, 2005).
234. Frymoyer, J. Degenerative Spondylolisthesis: Diagnosis and Treatment. *The Journal of the American Academy of Orthopaedic Surgeons* **2**, 9 (1994).
235. Wang, Y. X. J., Káplár, Z., Deng, M. & Leung, J. C. S. Lumbar degenerative spondylolisthesis epidemiology: A systematic review with a focus on gender-specific and age-specific prevalence. *Journal of Orthopaedic Translation* **11**, 39–52 (2017).
236. Kim, R., Singla, A. & Samdani, A. F. Classification of Spondylolisthesis. in *Spondylolisthesis: Diagnosis, Non-Surgical Management, and Surgical Techniques* (eds. Wollowick, A. L. & Sarwahi, V.) 95–106 (Springer US, 2015). doi:10.1007/978-1-4899-7575-1_7

237. Marchetti, P. G. *et al.* The surgical treatment of spondylolisthesis. *Chir Organi Mov* **79**, 85–91 (1994).
238. Toyone, T., Tanaka, T., Kato, D., Kaneyama, R. & Otsuka, M. Anatomic Changes in Lateral Spondylolisthesis Associated with Adult Lumbar Scoliosis. *Spine* **30**, E671 (2005).
239. Meyerding, H. Spondylolisthesis. *Surg Gynecol Obstet* **54**, 371–377 (1932).
240. Taillard, W. Le spondylolisthesis chez l'enfant et l'adolescent. *Acta Orthop Scand* **24**, 115–144 (1954).
241. Kepler, C. K. *et al.* Clinical and radiographic degenerative spondylolisthesis (CARDS) classification. *The Spine Journal* **15**, 1804–1811 (2015).
242. Simmonds, A. M. *et al.* Defining the inherent stability of degenerative spondylolisthesis: a systematic review. *Journal of Neurosurgery: Spine* **23**, 178–189 (2015).
243. Labelle, H., Mac-Thiong, J.-M. & Roussouly, P. Spino-pelvic sagittal balance of spondylolisthesis: a review and classification. *Eur Spine J* **20**, 641–646 (2011).
244. Even, J. L., Chen, A. F. & Lee, J. Y. Imaging characteristics of "dynamic" versus "static" spondylolisthesis: analysis using magnetic resonance imaging and flexion/extension films. *The Spine Journal* **14**, 1965–1969 (2014).
245. Wiltse, L. L., Newman, P. H. & Macnab, I. Classification of Spondyloisis and Spondylolisthesis. *Clinical Orthopaedics and Related Research®* **117**, 23 (1976).
246. Kalichman, L. & Hunter, D. J. Diagnosis and conservative management of degenerative lumbar spondylolisthesis. *European Spine Journal* **17**, 327–335 (2007).
247. Ulmer, J. L., Elster, A. D., Mathews, V. P. & King, J. C. Distinction between degenerative and isthmic spondylolisthesis on sagittal MR images: importance of increased anteroposterior diameter of the spinal canal ('wide canal sign'). *American Journal of Roentgenology* **163**, 411–416 (1994).
248. Ver, M. L. P., Dimar, J. R. & Carreon, L. Y. Traumatic Lumbar Spondylolisthesis: A Systematic Review and Case Series. *Global Spine Journal* 2192568218801882 (2018).
249. Jeon, C. *et al.* Degenerative retrolisthesis: Is it a compensatory mechanism for sagittal imbalance? *The bone & joint journal* **95**, 1244–1249 (2013).
250. Denard, P. J. *et al.* Back pain, neurogenic symptoms, and physical function in relation to spondylolisthesis among elderly men. *The Spine Journal* **10**, 865–873 (2010).
251. Kirby, D. J., Dietz, H. C. & Sponseller, P. D. Spondylolisthesis is Common, Early, and Severe in Loeys-Dietz Syndrome. *Journal of Pediatric Orthopaedics* **38**, e455 (2018).
252. Sengupta, D. K. & Herkowitz, H. N. Degenerative spondylolisthesis: review of current trends and controversies. *Spine* **30**, S71–S81 (2005).
253. Matsui, Y. *et al.* The association of lumbar spondylolisthesis with collagen IX tryptophan alleles. *The Journal of bone and joint surgery. British volume* **86**, 1021–1026 (2004).
254. Eroğlu, A., Çarlı, B. A., Pusat, S. & Şimşek, H. The Role of the Features of Facet Joint Angle in the Development of Isthmic Spondylolisthesis in Young Male Patients with L5-S1 Isthmic Spondylolisthesis. *World Neurosurgery* **104**, 709–712 (2017).
255. Liu, Z. *et al.* Variation of facet joint orientation and tropism in lumbar degenerative spondylolisthesis and disc herniation at L4-L5: A systematic review and meta-analysis. *Clinical Neurology and Neurosurgery* **161**, 41–47 (2017).
256. Lin, T.-Y. *et al.* The effects of anterior vacuum disc on surgical outcomes of degenerative versus spondylolytic spondylolisthesis: at a minimum two-year follow-up. *BMC musculoskeletal disorders* **15**, 329 (2014).
257. Huang, K.-Y. *et al.* The roles of IL-19 and IL-20 in the inflammation of degenerative lumbar spondylolisthesis. *Journal of Inflammation* **15**, 19 (2018).
258. Sutovsky, J. *et al.* Cytokine and chemokine profile changes in patients with lower segment lumbar degenerative spondylolisthesis. *International Journal of Surgery* **43**, 163–170 (2017).
259. Elster, A. D. & Jensen, K. M. Computed Tomography of Spondylolisthesis: Patterns of Associated Pathology. *Journal of Computer Assisted Tomography* **9**, 867–874 (1985).
260. Kim, K.-W. *et al.* The Course of the Nerve Root in the Neural Foramen and Its Relationship with Foraminal Entrapment or Impingement in Adult Patients with Lumbar Isthmic Spondylolisthesis and Radicular Pain. *Clinical Spine Surgery* **17**, 220 (2004).
261. Jinkins, J. R., Matthes, J. C., Sener, R. N., Venkatappan, S. & Rauch, R. Spondylolysis, spondylolisthesis, and associated nerve root entrapment in the lumbosacral spine: MR evaluation. *American Journal of Roentgenology* **159**, 799–803 (1992).
262. Lim, J. K. & Kim, S. M. Difference of Sagittal Spinopelvic Alignments between Degenerative Spondylolisthesis and Isthmic Spondylolisthesis. *J Korean Neurosurg Soc* **53**, 96–101 (2013).
263. Roussouly, P. & Pinheiro-Franco, J. L. Biomechanical analysis of the spino-pelvic organization and adaptation in pathology. *Eur Spine J* **20**, 609–618 (2011).
264. Place, H. M. *et al.* Pelvic incidence: a fixed value or can you change it? *The Spine Journal* **17**, 1565–1569 (2017).
265. Lai, Q. *et al.* Correlation between the sagittal spinopelvic alignment and degenerative lumbar spondylolisthesis: a retrospective study. *BMC Musculoskeletal Disorders* **19**, 151 (2018).
266. Oh, J. Y.-L. *et al.* Paradoxical motion in L5-S1 adult spondylolytic spondylolisthesis. *European Spine Journal* **21**, 262–267 (2012).
267. Hanson, D. S., Bridwell, K. H., Rhee, J. M. & Lenke, L. G. Correlation of Pelvic Incidence With Low- and High-Grade Isthmic Spondylolisthesis. *Spine* **27**, 2026 (2002).
268. Jentzsch, T. *et al.* Increased pelvic incidence may lead to arthritis and sagittal orientation of the facet joints at the lower lumbar spine. *BMC Medical Imaging* **13**, 34 (2013).
269. Chokshi, F. H., Quencer, R. & Smoker, W. The "thickened" ligamentum flavum: is it buckling or enlargement? *American Journal of Neuroradiology* **31**, 1813–1816 (2010).
270. Andersen, T. *et al.* Degenerative Spondylolisthesis Is Associated with Low Spinal Bone Density: A Comparative Study between Spinal Stenosis and Degenerative Spondylolisthesis. (2013).
271. Reina, M. A., Lirk, P., Puigdellívol-Sánchez, A., Mavar, M. & Prats-Galino, A. Human Lumbar Ligamentum Flavum Anatomy for Epidural Anesthesia: Reviewing a 3D MR-Based Interactive Model and Postmortem Samples. *Anesthesia & Analgesia* **122**, 903 (2016).
272. Olszewski, A. D., Yaszemski, M. J. & White, A. A. I. The Anatomy of the Human Lumbar Ligamentum Flavum: New Observations and Their Surgical Importance. *Spine* **21**, 2307 (1996).
273. Ramani, P., Perry, R. & Tomlinson, B. Role of ligamentum flavum in the symptomatology of prolapsed lumbar intervertebral discs. *Journal of Neurology, Neurosurgery, and Psychiatry* **38**, 550 (1975).
274. Sairyo, K. *et al.* Pathomechanism of Ligamentum Flavum Hypertrophy: A Multidisciplinary Investigation Based on Clinical, Biomechanical, Histologic, and Biologic Assessments. *Spine* **30**, 2649 (2005).
275. Sairyo, K. *et al.* Lumbar Ligamentum Flavum Hypertrophy Is Due to Accumulation of Inflammation-Related Scar Tissue. *Spine* **32**, E340 (2007).
276. Yoshiiwa, T. *et al.* Analysis of the Relationship between Ligamentum Flavum Thickening and Lumbar Segmental Instability, Disc Degeneration, and Facet Joint Osteoarthritis in Lumbar Spinal Stenosis. *Asian Spine Journal* **10**, 1132–1140 (2016).
277. Abbas, J. *et al.* Ligamentum flavum thickness in normal and stenotic lumbar spines. *Spine* **35**, 1225–1230 (2010).
278. Hur, J. W. *et al.* The mechanism of ligamentum flavum hypertrophy: introducing angiogenesis as a critical link that couples mechanical stress and hypertrophy. *Neurosurgery* **77**, 274–282 (2015).
279. Fukuyama, S., Nakamura, T., Ikeda, T. & Takagi, K. The Effect of Mechanical Stress on Hypertrophy of the Lumbar Ligamentum Flavum. *Clinical Spine Surgery* **8**, 126 (1995).
280. Karavelioglu, E. *et al.* Ligamentum flavum thickening at lumbar spine is associated with facet joint degeneration: an MRI study. *Journal of back and musculoskeletal rehabilitation* **29**, 771–777 (2016).
281. Altinkaya, N., Yildirim, T., Demir, S., Alkan, O. & Sarica, F. B. Factors Associated With the Thickness of the Ligamentum Flavum: Is Ligamentum Flavum Thickening Due to Hypertrophy or Buckling? *Spine* **36**, E1093 (2011).
282. Yabe, Y. *et al.* Decreased elastic fibers and increased proteoglycans in the ligamentum flavum of patients with lumbar spinal canal stenosis. *Journal of Orthopaedic Research* **34**, 1241–1247 (2016).
283. Shemesh, S. *et al.* Diabetes mellitus is associated with increased elastin fiber loss in ligamentum flavum of patients with lumbar spinal canal stenosis: results of a pilot histological study. *European Spine Journal* 1–9 (2018).
284. Luo, J. *et al.* Increased sorbitol levels in the hypertrophic ligamentum flavum of diabetic patients with lumbar spinal canal stenosis. *Journal of Orthopaedic Research* **35**, 1058–1066 (2017).
285. Lotan, R., Oron, A., Anekstein, Y., Shalmon, E. & Mirovsky, Y. Lumbar Stenosis and Systemic Diseases: Is There any Relevance? [Article]. *Journal of Spinal Disorders* **21**, 247–251 (2008).
286. Uesugi, K., Sekiguchi, M., Kikuchi, S. & Konno, S. Relationship between lumbar spinal stenosis and lifestyle-related disorders: a cross-sectional multicenter observational study. *Spine* **38**, E540–E545 (2013).
287. Beckworth, W. J., Holbrook, J. F., Foster, L. G., Ward, L. A. & Welle, J. R. Atherosclerotic Disease and its Relationship to Lumbar Degenerative Disk Disease, Facet Arthritis, and Stenosis With Computed Tomography Angiography. *PM&R* **10**, 331–337 (2018).
288. Kauppila, L. I. Atherosclerosis and Disc Degeneration/Low-Back Pain – A Systematic Review. *European Journal of Vascular and Endovascular Surgery* **37**, 661–670 (2009).
289. LaBan, M. M. & McNeary, L. The Clinical Value of B-Type Natriuretic Peptide (BNP) in Predicting Nocturnal Low Back Pain in Patients with Concurrent Lumbar Spinal Stenosis and Cardiopulmonary Dysfunction (Vesper's Curse): A Clinical Case Series. *American Journal of Physical Medicine & Rehabilitation* **87**, 798 (2008).
290. Asadian, L., Haddadi, K., Aarabi, M. & Zare, A. Diabetes Mellitus, a New Risk Factor for Lumbar Spinal Stenosis: A Case–Control Study. *Clin Med Insights Endocrinol Diabetes* **9**, 1–5 (2016).
291. Cui, G. *et al.* Matrix metalloproteinase 13 in the ligamentum flavum from lumbar spinal canal stenosis patients with and without diabetes mellitus. *Journal of Orthopaedic Science* **16**, 785–790 (2011).
292. Doualla-Bija, M. *et al.* Characteristics and determinants of clinical symptoms in radiographic lumbar spinal stenosis in a tertiary health care centre in sub-Saharan Africa. *BMC Musculoskeletal Disorders* **18**, 494 (2017).
293. Knutsson, B., Sandén, B., Sjödén, G., Järvholm, B. & Michaëlsson, K. Body Mass Index and Risk for Clinical Lumbar Spinal Stenosis: A Cohort Study. *Spine* **40**, 1451 (2015).
294. Inoue, N. & Espinoza Orías, A. A. Biomechanics of Intervertebral Disc Degeneration. *Orthop Clin North Am* **42**, 487–499 (2011).

295. Cotcrini, R., Mancini, F., Bisicchia, S., Maglione, P. & Farsetti, P. The correlation between exaggerated fluid in lumbar facet joints and degenerative spondylolisthesis: prospective study of 52 patients. *J Orthop Traumatol* **12**, 87–91 (2011).
296. Battié, M. C., Niemelainen, R., Gibbons, L. E. & Dhillon, S. Is level- and side-specific multifidus asymmetry a marker for lumbar disc pathology? *The Spine Journal* **12**, 932–939 (2012).
297. Ramos, L. A. V. *et al.* Are lumbar multifidus fatigue and transversus abdominis activation similar in patients with lumbar disc herniation and healthy controls? A case control study. *European Spine Journal* **25**, 1435–1442 (2016).
298. Chen, Y.-Y., Pao, J.-L., Liaw, C.-K., Hsu, W.-L. & Yang, R.-S. Image changes of paraspinal muscles and clinical correlations in patients with unilateral lumbar spinal stenosis. *Eur Spine J* **23**, 999–1006 (2014).
299. Altinkaya, N. & Cekinmez, M. Lumbar multifidus muscle changes in unilateral lumbar disc herniation using magnetic resonance imaging. *Skeletal Radiol* **45**, 73–77 (2016).
300. Hildebrandt, M., Fankhauser, G., Meichtry, A. & Luomajoki, H. Correlation between lumbar dysfunction and fat infiltration in lumbar multifidus muscles in patients with low back pain. *BMC Musculoskeletal Disorders* **18**, 12 (2017).
301. Penning, L. Psoas muscle and lumbar spine stability: a concept uniting existing controversies. *E Spine J* **9**, 577–585 (2000).
302. Barker, K. L., Shamley, D. R. & Jackson, D. Changes in the cross-sectional area of multifidus and psoas in patients with unilateral back pain: the relationship to pain and disability. *Spine* **29**, E515–E519 (2004).
303. Dangaria, T. R. & Naesh, O. Changes in Cross-Sectional Area of Psoas Major Muscle in Unilateral Sciatica Caused by Disc Herniation. *Spine* **23**, 928–931 (1998).
304. Key, J. 'The core': Understanding it, and retraining its dysfunction. *Journal of Bodywork and Movement Therapies* **17**, 541–559 (2013).
305. Daggfeldt, K. & Thorstensson, A. The role of intra-abdominal pressure in spinal unloading. *Journal of Biomechanics* **30**, 1149–1155 (1997).
306. Vostatek, P., Novak, D., Rychnovský, T. & Rychnovská, Š. Diaphragm postural function analysis using magnetic resonance imaging. *PloS one* **8**, e56724 (2013).
307. Postural Function of the Diaphragm in Persons With and Without Chronic Low Back Pain. *J Orthop Sports Phys Ther* **42**, 352–362 (2012).
308. Sihvonen, T. *et al.* Dorsal ramus irritation associated with recurrent low back pain and its relief with local anesthetic or training therapy. *J Spinal Disord* **8**, 8–14 (1995).
309. Kim, S. J. *et al.* Unusual Clinical Presentations of Cervical or Lumbar Dorsal Ramus Syndrome. *Korean Journal of Spine* **11**, 57–61 (2014).
310. Sihvonen, T., Lindgren, K. A., Airaksinen, O. & Manninen, H. Movement disturbances of the lumbar spine and abnormal back muscle electromyographic findings in recurrent low back pain. *Spine* **22**, 289–295 (1997).
311. Sihvonen, T. & Partanen, J. Segmental hypermobility in lumbar spine and entrapment of dorsal rami. *Electromyogr Clin Neurophysiol* **30**, 175–180 (1990).
312. Cornwall, J., John Harris, A. & Mercer, S. R. The lumbar multifidus muscle and patterns of pain. *Manual Therapy* **11**, 40–45 (2006).
313. Kellgren, J. Observations on referred pain arising from muscle. *Clin Sci* **3**, 1937–38 (1938).
314. Kader, D. F., Wardlaw, D. & SMITH, F. W. Correlation Between the MRI Changes in the Lumbar Multifidus Muscles and Leg Pain. *Clinical Radiology* **55**, 145–149 (2000).
315. Hebert, P. R., Barice, E. J. & Hennekens, C. H. Treatment of Low Back Pain: The Potential Clinical and Public Health Benefits of Topical Herbal Remedies. *J Altern Complement Med* **20**, 219–220 (2014).
316. Torstensson, T. *et al.* Referred pain patterns provoked on intra-pelvic structures among women with and without chronic pelvic pain: a descriptive study. *PloS one* **10**, e0119542 (2015).
317. Simons, D. G., Travell, J. G. & Simons, L. S. *Myofascial Pain and Dysfunction 1: The Trigger Point Manual. Upper Half of Body.* (Lippincott Williams & Wilkins, 1999).
318. Adelmanesh, F. *et al.* Is there an association between Lumbosacral radiculopathy and painful Gluteal trigger points?: A cross-sectional study. *American Journal of Physical Medicine & Rehabilitation* **94**, 784–791 (2015).
319. Gunn, C. C. & Milbrandt, W. E. Early and subtle signs in low-back sprain. *Spine* **3**, 267–281 (1978).
320. Takahashi, Y., Hirayama, J., Ohtori, S., Tauchi, T. & Takahashi, K. Anatomical nature of radicular leg pain analyzed by clinical findings. *PAIN RESEARCH* **15**, 87–96 (2000).
321. Maigne, R. & Nieves, W. L. *Diagnosis and Treatment of Pain of Vertebral Origin, Second Edition.* (CRC Press, 2005).
322. Bernard Jr, T. N. & Kirkaldy-Willis, W. H. Recognizing specific characteristics of nonspecific low back pain. *Clinical orthopaedics and related research* **217**, 266–280 (1987).
323. Gunn, C., Milbrandt, W., Little, A. & Mason, K. Dry needling of muscle motor points for chronic low-back pain: a randomized clinical trial with long-term follow-up. *Spine* **5**, 279–291 (1980).
324. Gunn, C. *The Gunn Approach to the Treatment of Chronic Pain: Intramuscular Stimulation for Myofascial Pain of Radiculopathic Origin, 2e.* (Churchill Livingstone, 1996).
325. Gunn, C. C. Neuropathic myofascial pain syndromes. in *Bonica's Management of Pain* 522–529 (Lippincott Williams & Wilkins, Philadelphia, PA, 2001).
326. Skorupska, E., Rychlik, M., Pawelec, W., Bednarek, A. & Samborski, W. Trigger point-related sympathetic nerve activity in chronic sciatic leg pain: a case study. *Acupuncture in Medicine* **32**, 418–422 (2014).
327. Ishihara, K. Spinal imaging abnormality, low back and leg pain, and muscle tension—A five-phase hypothesis considering generative sequence and causal relationship. *Medical hypotheses* **73**, 698–702 (2009).
328. Gunn, C. C. "Prespondylosis" and Some Pain Syndromes Following Denervation Supersensitivity. *Spine* **5**, 185 (1980).
329. Marcus, N. J. Failure to Diagnose Pain of Muscular Origin Leads to Unnecessary Surgery. *Pain Medicine* **3**, 161 (2002).
330. Matsumoto, J. *et al.* Impact of Additional Treatment of Paralumbar Spine and Peripheral Nerve Diseases After Lumbar Spine Surgery. *World Neurosurg* **112**, e778–e782 (2018).
331. King, J. & Lagger, R. Sciatica viewed as a referred pain syndrome. *Surgical neurology* **5**, 46 (1976).
332. Saeidian, S. R., Pipelzadeh, M. R., Rasras, S. & Zeinali, M. Effect of Trigger Point Injection on Lumbosacral Radiculopathy Source. *Anesth Pain Med* **4**, (2014).
333. Tan, L. A. *et al.* High prevalence of greater trochanteric pain syndrome among patients presenting to spine clinic for evaluation of degenerative lumbar pathologies. *Journal of Clinical Neuroscience* (2018).
334. Samuel, A. S., Peter, A. A. & Ramanathan, K. The association of active trigger points with lumbar disc lesions. *Journal of Musculoskelatal Pain* **15**, 11–18 (2007).
335. Were, O. O. The relationship between lumbar radiculopathy and neuropathic heel pain. *Nairobi, Kenya: University of Nairobi* (2013).
336. Orchard, J., Farhart, P., Kountouris, A., James, T. & Portus, M. Pace bowlers in cricket with history of lumbar stress fracture have increased risk of lower limb muscle strains, particularly calf strains. *Open Access J Sports Med* **1**, 177–182 (2010).
337. Orchard, J. W., Farhart, P. & Leopold, C. Lumbar spine region pathology and hamstring and calf injuries in athletes: is there a connection? *Br J Sports Med* **38**, 502–504 (2004).
338. Woodley, S. J. *et al.* Lateral hip pain: findings from magnetic resonance imaging and clinical examination. *journal of orthopaedic & sports physical therapy* **38**, 313–328 (2008).
339. Sayegh, F., Potoupnis, M. & Kapetanos, G. Greater trochanter bursitis pain syndrome in females with chronic low back pain and sciatica. *Acta Orthop Belg* **70**, 423–428 (2004).
340. Tortolani, P. J., Carbone, J. J. & Quartararo, L. G. Greater trochanteric pain syndrome in patients referred to orthopedic spine specialists. *The Spine Journal* **2**, 251–254 (2002).
341. McClinton, S., Weber, C. F. & Heiderscheit, B. Low back pain and disability in individuals with plantar heel pain. *The Foot* **34**, 18–22 (2018).
342. Gunn, C. C. Radiculopathic Pain: Diagnosis and Treatment of Segmental Irritation or Sensitization. *Journal of Musculoskeletal Pain* **5**, 119–134 (1997).
343. Williams, B. S. & Cohen, S. P. Greater trochanteric pain syndrome: a review of anatomy, diagnosis and treatment. *Anesthesia & Analgesia* **108**, 1662–1670 (2009).
344. Hugo, D. & de Jongh, H. R. Greater trochanteric pain syndrome. *SA Orthopaedic Journal* **11**, 28–33 (2012).
345. Africanus, C. *Constantini Africani Post Hippocratem et Galenum.* (Petrus, 1536).
346. Kellgren, J. H. Referred Pains from Muscle. *BMJ* **1**, 325–327 (1938).
347. Kellgren, J. Sciatica. *The Lancet* **237**, 561–564 (1941).
348. Swezey, R. L. Pseudo-radiculopathy in subacute trochanteric bursitis of the subgluteus maximus bursa. *Arch Phys Med Rehabil* **57**, 387–390 (1976).
349. Travell, J. G. & Simons, D. G. *Myofascial Pain and Dysfunction: The Trigger Point Manual; Vol. 2., The Lower Extremities.* (Lippincott Williams & Wilkins, 1992).
350. McRaith. Nerve-Stretching for Cure of Lumbago and Sciatica. *The Medical Times and Gazette* **2**, (1880).
351. Hernando, M. F., Cerezal, L., Pérez-Carro, L., Abascal, F. & Canga, A. Deep gluteal syndrome: anatomy, imaging, and management of sciatic nerve entrapments in the subgluteal space. *Skeletal radiology* **44**, 919–934 (2015).
352. Karmakar, M. *et al.* Three-Dimensional/Four-Dimensional Volumetric Ultrasound Imaging of the Sciatic Nerve: *Regional Anesthesia and Pain Medicine* **37**, 60–66 (2012).
353. Saikku, K., Vasenius, J., Saar, P. & others. Entrapment of the proximal sciatic nerve by the hamstring tendons. *Acta orthopaedica Belgica* **76**, 321 (2010).
354. Jang, J. S., An, S. H. & Lee, S. H. Clinical analysis of extraforaminal entrapment of L5 in the lumbosacral spine. *J Korean Neurosurg Soc* **36**, 383–387 (2004).
355. Arnoldussen, W. & Korten, J. Pressure neuropathy of the posterior femoral cutaneous nerve. *Clinical Neurology and Neurosurgery* **82**, 57–60 (1980).
356. Chhabra, A. *et al.* MR neurography findings of soleal sling entrapment. *American Journal of Roentgenology* **196**, W290–W297 (2011).
357. Williams, E. H., Rosson, G. D., Hagan, R. R., Hashemi, S. S. & Dellon, A. L. Soleal sling syndrome (proximal tibial nerve compression): results of surgical decompression. *Plastic and reconstructive surgery* **129**, 454–462 (2012).
358. Mobbs, R. J., Szkandera, B. & Blum, P. Posterior femoral cutaneous nerve entrapment neuropathy: operative exposure and technique. *British Journal of Neurosurgery* **16**, 309–311 (2002).
359. Aly, T. A., Tanaka, Y., Aizawa, T., Ozawa, H. & Kokubun, S. Medial Superior Cluneal Nerve Entrapment Neuropathy in Teenagers: A Report of Two Cases. *The Tohoku Journal of Experimental Medicine* **197**, 229–231 (2002).

360. Kuniya, H. *et al.* Prospective study of superior cluneal nerve disorder as a potential cause of low back pain and leg symptoms. *Journal of Orthopaedic Surgery and Research* **9**, 139 (2014).
361. Bano, A. *et al.* Persistent sciatica induced by quadratus femoris muscle tear and treated by surgical decompression: a case report. *J Med Case Reports* **4**, 236 (2010).
362. Hopayian, K., Song, F., Riera, R. & Sambandan, S. The clinical features of the piriformis syndrome: a systematic review. *European Spine Journal* **19**, 2095–2109 (2010).
363. Söderberg, L. Prognosis in conservatively treated sciatica. *Acta Orthopaedica* **27**, 3–127 (1956).
364. Beaton, L. E. & Anson, B. J. The relation of the sciatic nerve and of its subdivisions to the piriformis muscle. *Anat. Rec.* **70**, 1–5 (1937).
365. Michel, F. *et al.* Piriformis muscle syndrome: Diagnostic criteria and treatment of a monocentric series of 250 patients. *Annals of Physical and Rehabilitation Medicine* **56**, 371–383 (2013).
366. Lewis, S., Jurak, J., Lee, C., Lewis, R. & Gest, T. Anatomical variations of the sciatic nerve, in relation to the piriformis muscle. *Translational Research in Anatomy* **5**, 15–19 (2016).
367. Varenika, V., Lutz, A. M., Beaulieu, C. F. & Bucknor, M. D. Detection and prevalence of variant sciatic nerve anatomy in relation to the piriformis muscle on MRI. *Skeletal Radiol* 1–7 (2017). doi:10.1007/s00256-017-2597-6
368. Fishman, L. M. *et al.* Piriformis syndrome: diagnosis, treatment, and outcome—a 10-year study. *Archives of physical medicine and rehabilitation* **83**, 295–301 (2002).
369. Jawish, R. M., Assoum, H. A., Khamis, C. F. & others. Anatomical, clinical and electrical observations in piriformis syndrome. *J Orthop Surg Res* **5**, 3 (2010).
370. Battaglia, P. J., Scali, F. & Enix, D. E. Co-presentation of unilateral femoral and bilateral sciatic nerve variants in one cadaver: A case report with clinical implications. *Chiropractic & Manual Therapies* **20**, 34 (2012).
371. Siddiq, M. A. B. *et al.* Piriformis syndrome: a case series of 31 Bangladeshi people with literature review. *European Journal of Orthopaedic Surgery & Traumatology* 1–11 (2016).
372. Sun, C.-H., Lu, S.-C., Wu, Y.-T. & Chang, S.-T. Development of unilateral piriformis syndrome in a female with congenital leg length discrepancy. *Open Journal of Orthopedics* **2**, 135 (2012).
373. Bardeen, C. R. Development and variation of the nerves and the musculature of the inferior extremity and of the neighboring regions of the trunk in man. *Developmental Dynamics* **6**, 259–390 (1906).
374. Chutkow, J. G. Posterior femoral cutaneous neuralgia. *Muscle & nerve* **11**, 1146–1148 (1988).
375. Uluutku, M. & Kurtoğlu, Z. Variations of nerves located in deep gluteal region. *Okajimas folia anatomica Japonica* **76**, 273–276 (1999).
376. Ploteau, S., Salaud, C., Hamel, A. & Robert, R. Entrapment of the posterior femoral cutaneous nerve and its inferior cluneal branches: anatomical basis of surgery for inferior cluneal neuralgia. *Surgical and radiologic anatomy: SRA* (2017).
377. Meng, S. *et al.* High-resolution ultrasound of the posterior femoral cutaneous nerve: visualization and initial experience with patients. *Skeletal radiology* **44**, 1421–1426 (2015).
378. Iyer, V. G. & Shields, C. B. Isolated injection injury to the posterior femoral cutaneous nerve. *Neurosurgery* **25**, 835–838 (1989).
379. Konno, T. *et al.* Anatomical background of 'pseudosciatica' in cluneal neuralgia: GP8. in *Spine Journal Meeting Abstracts* 105–106 (LWW, 2014).
380. Loukas, M. *et al.* Iliolumbar membrane, a newly recognised structure in the back. *Folia morphologica* **65**, 15 (2006).
381. Tubbs, R. S., Levin, M. R., Loukas, M., Potts, E. A. & Cohen-Gadol, A. A. Anatomy and landmarks for the superior and middle cluneal nerves: application to posterior iliac crest harvest and entrapment syndromes: Laboratory investigation. *Journal of Neurosurgery: Spine* **13**, 356–359 (2010).
382. Young, I. J., van Riet, R. P. & Bell, S. N. Surgical release for proximal hamstring syndrome. *The American journal of sports medicine* **36**, 2372–2378 (2008).
383. Bucknor, M. D., Steinbach, L. S., Saloner, D. & Chin, C. T. Magnetic resonance neurography evaluation of chronic extraspinal sciatica after remote proximal hamstring injury: a preliminary retrospective analysis. *J. Neurosurg.* 1–7 (2014). doi:10.3171/2014.4.JNS13940
384. *System of surgery.* (Lea Brothers, 1895).
385. Chapman, V. The Treatment of Sciatica. *Canadian Journal of Medicine and Surgery* **11**, (1902).
386. Martin, H. D., Reddy, M. & Gómez-Hoyos, J. Deep gluteal syndrome. *J Hip Preserv Surg* **2**, 99–107 (2015).
387. Shacklock, M. *Clinical Neurodynamics: A New System of Neuromusculoskeletal Treatment, 1e.* (Butterworth-Heinemann, 2005).
388. Girard PM & Childress HM. Sciatic nerve pressure following rupture and fibrosis of a hamstring muscle. *JAMA* **113**, 2412–2413 (1939).
389. Mastaglia, F. L. Tibial nerve entrapment in the popliteal fossa. *Muscle & nerve* **23**, 1883–1886 (2000).
390. Kang, P. B., Preston, D. C. & Raynor, E. M. Involvement of superficial peroneal sensory nerve in common peroneal neuropathy. *Muscle Nerve* **31**, 725–729 (2005).
391. Trescot, A. M. *Peripheral Nerve Entrapments: Clinical Diagnosis and Management.* (Springer, 2016).
392. Dong, Q. *et al.* Entrapment Neuropathies in the Upper and Lower Limbs: Anatomy and MRI Features. *Radiol Res Pract* **2012**, (2012).
393. Walcott, B. P., Coumans, J.-V. C. & Kahle, K. T. Diagnostic pitfalls in spine surgery: masqueraders of surgical spine disease. *Neurosurgical Focus* **31**, E1 (2011).
394. Reife, M. D. & Coulis, C. M. Peroneal neuropathy misdiagnosed as L5 radiculopathy: a case report. *Chiropractic & Manual Therapies* **21**, 12 (2013).
395. Katirji, B. Peroneal neuropathy. *Neurologic clinics* **17**, 567–591 (1999).
396. Jeon, C.-H., Chung, N.-S., Lee, Y.-S., Son, K.-H. & Kim, J.-H. Assessment of hip abductor power in patients with foot drop: a simple and useful test to differentiate lumbar radiculopathy and peroneal neuropathy. *Spine* **38**, 257–263 (2013).
397. Briggs, C. A. & Chandraraj, S. Variations in the lumbosacral ligament and associated changes in the lumbosacral region resulting in compression of the fifth dorsal root ganglion and spinal nerve. *Clin. Anat.* **8**, 339–346 (1995).
398. Olsewski, J. M., Simmons, E. H., Kallen, F. C. & Mendel, F. C. Evidence from cadavers suggestive of entrapment of fifth lumbar spinal nerves by lumbosacral ligaments. *Spine* **16**, 336–347 (1991).
399. Kanamoto, H. *et al.* The diagnosis of double-crush lesion in the L5 lumbar nerve using diffusion tensor imaging. *The Spine Journal* **16**, 315–321 (2016).
400. Danforth, M. S. & Wilson, P. D. The anatomy of the lumbo-sacral region in relation to sciatic pain. *JBJS* **7**, 109–160 (1925).
401. Larmon, W. A. An Anatomic Study of the Lumbosacral Region in Relation to Low Back Pain and Sciatica. *Ann Surg* **119**, 892–896 (1944).
402. Nathan, H., Weizenbluth, M. & Halperin, N. The lumbosacral ligament (LSL), with special emphasis on the "lumbosacral tunnel" and the entrapment of the 5th lumbar nerve. *International orthopaedics* **6**, 197–202 (1982).
403. Luk, K. D., Ho, H. C. & Leong, J. C. The iliolumbar ligament. A study of its anatomy, development and clinical significance. *Bone & Joint Journal* **68-B**, 197–200 (1986).
404. Zoccali, C. *et al.* The Surgical Anatomy of the Lumbosacroiliac Triangle: A Cadaveric Study. *World neurosurgery* **88**, 36–40 (2016).
405. Protas, M., Loukas, M. & Tubbs, S. The Lumbosacral Tunnel: Cadaveric Study and Review of the Literature. *The Spine Scholar* 3160 (2017).
406. Pitkin, H. & Pheasant, H. Sacrarthrogenetic telalgia 1. A study of referred pain. *Journal of Bone and Joint Surgery* **111**, (1936).
407. Chow, D. H. K., Luk, K. D. K., Leong, J. C. Y. & Woo, C. W. Torsional Stability of the Lumbosacral Junction: Significance of the Iliolumbar Ligament. *Spine* **14**, 611 (1989).
408. Müller, A. & Reulen, H.-J. A Paramedian Tangential Approach to Lumbosacral Extraforaminal Disc Herniations. *Neurosurgery* **43**, 854–861 (1998).
409. Amonoo-Kuofi, H. S., el-Badawi, M. G., Fatani, J. & Butt, M. Ligaments associated with lumbar intervertebral foramina. 2. The fifth lumbar level. *Journal of anatomy* **159**, 1 (1988).
410. Transfeldt, E. E., Robertson, D. & Bradford, D. S. Ligaments of the lumbosacral spine and their role in possible extraforaminal spinal nerve entrapment and tethering. *Journal of spinal disorders* **6**, 507–512 (1993).
411. Sasso, R. C., Kozak, J. A. & Dickson, J. H. The sickle ligament revisited: Release of the lumbosacral ligament via an anterior approach. *Spine* **18**, 2127–2130 (1993).
412. Zhao, Q. *et al.* The morphology and clinical significance of the intraforaminal ligaments at the L5–S1 levels. *The Spine Journal* **16**, 1001–1006 (2016).
413. Wiltse, L., Guyer, R., Spencer, C., Glenn, W. & Porter, I. Alar transverse process impingement of the L5 spinal nerve: the far-out syndrome. *Spine* **9**, 31–41 (1984).
414. Tubbs, R. S. *et al.* Extraforaminal compression of the L5 nerve: an anatomical study with application to failed posterior decompressive procedures. *Journal of Clinical Neuroscience* **41**, 139–143 (2017).
415. Lu, S. *et al.* Clinical anatomy and 3D virtual reconstruction of the lumbar plexus with respect to lumbar surgery. *BMC Musculoskelet Disord* **12**, 76 (2011).
416. Matsumoto, M. *et al.* Posterior decompression surgery for extraforaminal entrapment of the fifth lumbar spinal nerve at the lumbosacral junction: clinical article. *Journal of Neurosurgery: Spine* **12**, 72–81 (2010).
417. Jones, T. L. & Hisey, M. S. L5 radiculopathy caused by L5 nerve root entrapment by an L5-S1 anterior osteophyte. *International Journal of Spine Surgery* **6**, 174–177 (2012).
418. Hashimoto, M., Watanabe, O. & Hirano, H. Extraforaminal stenosis in the lumbosacral spine: efficacy of MR imaging in the coronal plane. *Acta Radiologica* **37**, 610–613 (1996).
419. Ichihara, K. *et al.* The treatment of far-out foraminal stenosis below a lumbosacral transitional vertebra: a report of two cases. *Clinical Spine Surgery* **17**, 154–157 (2004).
420. Kikuchi, K. *et al.* Anterior decompression for far-out syndrome below a transitional vertebra: a report of two cases. *The Spine Journal* doi:10.1016/j.spinee.2013.02.033
421. Weber, J. & Ernestus, R.-I. Transitional lumbosacral segment with unilateral transverse process anomaly (Castellvi type 2A) resulting in extraforaminal impingement of the spinal nerve. *Neurosurgical review* **34**, 143–150 (2011).
422. Bertolotti, M. Contributo alla conoscenze dei vizi di differenzazione regionale del racide con speciale riguardo alla assimilazione sacrale della V. lombare. *Radiologique Medica* **4**, 113–144 (1917).

423. Bertolotti, M. Les syndromes lombo-ischialgiques d'origine vertébrale; leur entitée morphologique, radiographique et clinique. *Rev. neurol* (1922).
424. Castellvi, A. E., Goldstein, L. A. & Chan, D. P. Lumbosacral transitional vertebrae and their relationship with lumbar extradural defects. *Spine* **9**, 493–495 (1984).
425. Nardo, L. *et al.* Lumbosacral Transitional Vertebrae: Association with Low Back Pain. *Radiology* **265**, 497–503 (2012).
426. Tang, M. *et al.* Lumbosacral transitional vertebra in a population-based study of 5860 individuals: prevalence and relationship to low back pain. *European journal of radiology* **83**, 1679–1682 (2014).
427. Porter, N. A. *et al.* Prevalence of extraforaminal nerve root compression below lumbosacral transitional vertebrae. *Skeletal radiology* **43**, 55–60 (2014).
428. Farshad-Amacker, N. A., Herzog, R. J., Hughes, A. P., Aichmair, A. & Farshad, M. Associations between lumbosacral transitional anatomy types and degeneration at the transitional and adjacent segments. *The Spine Journal* **15**, 1210–1216 (2015).
429. Konin, G. & Walz, D. Lumbosacral transitional vertebrae: classification, imaging findings, and clinical relevance. *American Journal of Neuroradiology* **31**, 1778–1786 (2010).
430. de Bruin, F. *et al.* Prevalence and clinical significance of lumbosacral transitional vertebra (LSTV) in a young back pain population with suspected axial spondyloarthritis: results of the SPondyloArthritis Caught Early (SPACE) cohort. *Skeletal radiology* **46**, 633–639 (2017).
431. Hilton, J. *On Rest and Pain: A Course of Lectures on the Influence of Mechanical and Physiological Rest in the Treatment of Accidents and Surgical Diseases, and the Diagnostic Value of Pain.* (Wood, 1879).
432. Gowers, W. R. (William R., Taylor, J. & Schlesinger, E. B. *A manual of diseases of the nervous system.* (Philadelphia : P. Blakiston's Son & Co., 1899).
433. Albee, F. H. A study of the anatomy and the clinical importance of the sacroiliac joint. *Journal of the American Medical Association* **53**, 1273–1276 (1909).
434. Yeoman, W. THE RELATION OF ARTHRITIS OF THE SACRO-ILIAC JOINT TO SCIATICA, WITH AN ANALYSIS OF 100 CASES. *The Lancet* **212**, 1119–1123 (1928).
435. Fortin, J. D., Washington, W. J. & Falco, F. J. E. Three Pathways between the Sacroiliac Joint and Neural Structures. *AJNR Am J Neuroradiol* **20**, 1429–1434 (1999).
436. Slipman, C. W. *et al.* Sacroiliac joint pain referral zones. *Archives of Physical Medicine and Rehabilitation* **81**, 334–338 (2000).
437. Murakami, E., Aizawa, T., Kurosawa, D. & Noguchi, K. Leg symptoms associated with sacroiliac joint disorder and related pain. *Clinical Neurology and Neurosurgery* **157**, 55–58 (2017).
438. Wong, M., Vijayanathan, S. & Kirkham, B. Sacroiliitis presenting as sciatica. *Rheumatology* **44**, 1323–1324 (2005).
439. Margules, K. R. & Gall, E. P. Sciatica-like pain arising in the sacroiliac joint. *JCR: Journal of Clinical Rheumatology* **3**, 9–15 (1997).
440. Kulcu, D. G. & Naderi, S. Differential diagnosis of intraspinal and extraspinal non-discogenic sciatica. *Journal of Clinical Neuroscience* **15**, 1246–1252 (2008).
441. Buijs, E., Visser, L. & Groen, G. Sciatica and the sacroiliac joint: a forgotten concept. *British journal of anaesthesia* **99**, 713–716 (2007).
442. Fortin, J. D. Saoroiliao Joint Innervation and Pain. (1999).
443. Hasankhani, E. G. & Omidi-Kashani, F. Magnetic Resonance Imaging versus Electrophysiologic Tests in Clinical Diagnosis of Lower Extremity Radicular Pain. *ISRN Neuroscience* **2013**, 1–4 (2013).
444. Egli, D. *et al.* Lumbar spinal stenosis: assessment of cauda equina involvement by electrophysiological recordings. *Journal of neurology* **254**, 741 (2007).
445. Micankova Adamova, B. & Vohanka, S. The results and contribution of electrophysiological examination in patients with lumbar spinal stenosis. *Scripta Medica Facultatis Medicae Universitatis Brunensis Masarykianae* **82**, 38–45 (2009).
446. Zheng, C. *et al.* The prevalence of tarsal tunnel syndrome in patients with lumbosacral radiculopathy. *Eur Spine J* **25**, 895–905 (2016).
447. Ang, C.-L. & Foo, L. S. S. Multiple locations of nerve compression: an unusual cause of persistent lower limb paresthesia. *The Journal of Foot and Ankle Surgery* **53**, 763–767 (2014).
448. Kupersmith, M. J., Lieberman, A. N., Spielholz, N., Berczeller, P. & Ransohoff, J. Neuropathy With Susceptibility to Compression Aggravated by Herniated Disk: Early Pathological and Electrodiagnostic Studies. *Arch Neurol* **36**, 645–647 (1979).
449. Yamauchi, T. *et al.* Undiagnosed Peripheral Nerve Disease in Patients with Failed Lumbar Disc Surgery. *Asian Spine J* **12**, 720–725 (2018).
450. Klingman, R. E. The pseudoradicular syndrome: A case report implicating double crush mechanisms in peripheral nerve tissue of the lower extremity. *Journal of Manual & Manipulative Therapy* **7**, 81–91 (1999).
451. Sammarco, G. J., Chalk, D. E. & Feibel, J. H. Tarsal tunnel syndrome and additional nerve lesions in the same limb. *Foot & ankle* **14**, 71–77 (1993).
452. Iwamoto, N. *et al.* Treatment of low back pain elicited by superior cluneal nerve entrapment neuropathy after lumbar fusion surgery. *Spine Surgery and Related Research* **1**, 152–157 (2017).
453. Chodoroff, B. & Ball, R. D. Lumbosacral radiculopathy, reflex sympathetic dystrophy and tarsal tunnel syndrome: An unusual presentation. *Archives of Physical Medicine and Rehabilitation* **66**, 185–187 (1985).
454. Potter, P. *Hippocrates V. Affections, Diseases I & II.* (Harvard University Press, 1988).
455. Sharma, P. V. *Caraka Samhita (Text With English Translation) 4 Volume Set.* (Chaukhambha Orientalia, 2005).
456. De Weerdt, C., Journee, H., Hogenesch, R. & Beks, J. Sympathetic dysfunction in patients with persistent pain after prolapsed disc surgery. A thermographic study. *Acta neurochirurgica* **89**, 34–36 (1987).
457. Hakelius, A., Nilsonne, U., Pernow, B. & Zetterquist, S. The cold sciatic leg. *Acta orthopaedica Scandinavica* **40**, 614 (1969).
458. Gillström, P. Thermography in low back pain and sciatica. *Arch. Orth. Traum. Surg.* **104**, 31–36 (1985).
459. Uematsu, S. *et al.* Quantification of thermal asymmetry. *Journal of Neurosurgery* **69**, 556–561 (1988).
460. Maigne, J.-Y., Treuil, C. & Chatellier, G. Altered lower limb vascular perfusion in patients with sciatica secondary to disc herniation. *Spine* **21**, 1657–1660 (1996).
461. Mizuno, S. *et al.* The effects of the sympathetic nerves on lumbar radicular pain A BEHAVIOURAL AND IMMUNOHISTOCHEMICAL STUDY. *J Bone Joint Surg Br* **89-B**, 1666–1672 (2007).
462. Schmalbruch, H. Fiber composition of the rat sciatic nerve. *The Anatomical Record* **215**, 71–81 (1986).
463. Skorupska, E., Rychlik, M. & Samborski, W. Intensive vasodilatation in the sciatic pain area after dry needling. *BMC Complementary and Alternative Medicine* **15**, 72 (2015).
464. Transfeldt, E. & Macnab, I. *Macnab's Backache.* (Lippincott Williams & Wilkins, 2007).
465. Poskitt, K., Perkin, G. & Greenhalgh, R. A relationship between claudication of the cauda equina and the small aorta syndrome. *Journal of Neurology, Neurosurgery & Psychiatry* **48**, 75–79 (1985).
466. Wilberger Jr, J. E. Lumbosacral radiculopathy secondary to abdominal aortic aneurysms: Report of three cases. *Journal of Neurosurgery* **58**, 965–967 (1983).
467. D'Amour, M. L., Lebrun, L. H., Rabbat, A., Trudel, J. & Daneault, N. Peripheral neurological complications of aortoiliac vascular disease. *Canadian Journal of Neurological Sciences/Journal Canadien des Sciences Neurologiques* **14**, 127–130 (1987).
468. Shields, R., Aaron, J., Postel, G., Gaar, E. & Hourigan, J. A fatal illness presenting as an S1 radiculopathy. Vascular causes of lumbar radicular pain. *The Journal of the Kentucky Medical Association* **95**, 268 (1997).
469. *Hipocrates the Aphorisms of Hippocrates: With a Translation Into Latin and English.* (A. J. Valpy, 1822).
470. (Amidenus), A. *Contractae ex Veteribus medicinae tetrabiblos.* (1549).
471. Shaw, P. *A New Practice of Physic: Wherein the Various Diseases Incident to the Human Body are Describ'd, Their Causes Assign'd, Their Diagnostics and Prognostics Enumerated and the Regimen Proper in Each Deliver'd, with a Competent Number of Medicines for Every Stage and Sympton Thereof ... in Two Volumes.* (T. and T. Longman, 1753).
472. Adams, F. *The extant works of Aretaeus: the Cappadocian.* (Sydenham Society, 1856).
473. Cotugno, D. *A Treatise on the Nervous Sciatica: Or, Nervous Hip Gout ...* (J. Wilkie, 1775).
474. Treves, S. F. *Surgical Applied Anatomy.* (Lea Brothers & Company, 1785).
475. Birnbaum, K., Prescher, A., Hessler, S. & Heller, K. D. The sensory innervation of the hip joint--an anatomical study. *Surg Radiol Anat* **19**, 371–375 (1997).
476. Bruce, W. *Sciatica, a fresh study.* (New York : William Wood, 1913).
477. Bolk, L. Beziehungen zwischen Skelet, Muskulatur und Nerven der Extremitäten, dargelegt am Beckengürtel, an dessen Muskulatur sowie am Plexus lumbo-sacralis. *Morphologisches Jahrbuch* **21**, (1894).
478. Takahashi, Y., Ohtori, S. & Takahashi, K. Human map of the segmental sensory structure ("sensoritomes") in the body trunk and lower extremity. *Pain Res* **23**, 133–141 (2008).
479. Takahashi, Y., Ohtori, S. & Takahashi, K. Sclerotomes in the thoracic and lumbar spine, pelvis, and hindlimb bones of rats. *The Journal of Pain* **11**, 652–662 (2010).
480. Lesher, J. M., Dreyfuss, P., Hager, N., Kaplan, M. & Furman, M. Hip joint pain referral patterns: a descriptive study. *Pain Med* **9**, 22–25 (2008).
481. Hsieh, P.-H. *et al.* Pain distribution and response to total hip arthroplasty: a prospective observational study in 113 patients with end-stage hip disease. *Orthop Sci* **17**, 213–218 (2012).
482. Khan, A., McLoughlin, E., Giannakas, K., Hutchinson, C. & Andrew, J. Hip osteoarthritis: where is the pain? *Annals of the Royal College of Surgeons of England* **86**, 119 (2004).
483. Offierski, C. M. & Macnab, I. Hip-Spine Syndrome. *Spine* **8**, 316 (1983).
484. Saito, J. *et al.* Difficulty of Diagnosing the Origin of Lower Leg Pain in Patients With Both Lumbar Spinal Stenosis and Hip Joint Osteoarthritis. *Spine* **37**, 2089 (2012).
485. Zyl, V. & A, A. Misdiagnosis of hip pain could lead to unnecessary spinal surgery. *SA Orthopaedic Journal* **9**, 54–57 (2010).
486. Hicks, G. E., Sions, J. & Velasco, T. Hip symptoms contribute to low back pain-related disability in older adults with a primary complaint of low back pain: the Delaware spine studies. *Osteoarthritis and Cartilage* **24**, S439 (2016).
487. Prather, H., Cheng, A., Steger-May, K., Maheshwari, V. & Van Dillen, L. Hip and Lumbar Spine Physical Examination Findings in People Presenting With Low Back Pain, With or

Without Lower Extremity Pain. *journal of orthopaedic & sports physical therapy* **47**, 163–172 (2017).

488. Prather, H., Cheng, A., Steger-May, K., Maheshwari, V. & VanDillen, L. Association of Hip Radiograph Findings With Pain and Function in Patients Presenting With Low Back Pain. *PM&R* (2017). doi:10.1016/j.pmrj.2017.06.003
489. Weinberg, D. S., Gebhart, J. J. & Liu, R. W. Hip-spine syndrome: A cadaveric analysis between osteoarthritis of the lumbar spine and hip joints. *Orthopaedics & Traumatology: Surgery & Research* **103**, 651–656 (2017).
490. Gebhart, J. J. *et al.* Hip-spine syndrome: Is there an association between markers for cam deformity and osteoarthritis of the lumbar spine? *Arthroscopy: The Journal of Arthroscopic & Related Surgery* **32**, 2243–2248 (2016).
491. Gómez-Hoyos, J. *et al.* The Hip-Spine Effect: A Biomechanical Study of Ischiofemoral Impingement Effect on Lumbar Facet Joints. *Arthroscopy* **33**, 101–107 (2017).
492. Wang, W., Sun, M., Xu, Z., Qiu, Y. & Weng, W. The low back pain in patients with hip osteoarthritis: current knowledge on the diagnosis, mechanism and treatment outcome. *Annals of Joint* **1**, (2016).
493. Sasagawa, T. & Nakamura, T. Associated Factors for Lumbar Degenerative Spondylolisthesis in Japanese Patients with Osteoarthritis of the Hip: A Radiographic Study. *Asian Spine Journal* **10**, 935–939 (2016).
494. Blizzard, D. J. *et al.* The Impact of Lumbar Spine Disease and Deformity on Total Hip Arthroplasty Outcomes. *ORTHOPEDICS* **40**, e520–e525 (2017).
495. Takeshita, M. *et al.* Sensory innervation and inflammatory cytokines in hypertrophic synovia associated with pain transmission in osteoarthritis of the hip: a case–control study. *Rheumatology (Oxford)* **51**, 1790–1795 (2012).
496. Aurelianus, C. *On acute diseases: And On chronic diseases;* (University of Chicago Press, 1950).
497. Michele, A. A. *Iliopsoas; development of anomalies in man.* (Springfield, Ill., 1962).
498. Mellin, G. Correlations of Hip Mobility with Degree of Back Pain and Lumbar Spinal Mobility in Chronic Low-Back Pain Patients. *Spine* **13**, 668 (1988).
499. Roach, S. M. *et al.* Passive hip range of motion is reduced in active subjects with chronic low back pain compared to controls. *International journal of sports physical therapy* **10**, 13 (2015).
500. Van Dillen, L. R., McDonnell, M. K., Fleming, D. A. & Sahrmann, S. A. Effect of knee and hip position on hip extension range of motion in individuals with and without low back pain. *Journal of Orthopaedic & Sports Physical Therapy* **30**, 307–316 (2000).
501. Bogduk, N., Pearcy, M. & Hadfield, G. Anatomy and biomechanics of psoas major. *Clinical Biomechanics* **7**, 109–119 (1992).
502. Shayesteh Azar, M. *et al.* Association of low back pain with lumbar lordosis and lumbosacral angle. *Journal of Mazandaran University of Medical Sciences* **20**, 9–15 (2010).
503. Yoshimoto, H. *et al.* Spinopelvic Alignment in Patients With Osteoarthrosis of the Hip: A Radiographic Comparison to Patients with Low Back Pain. *Spine* **30**, 1650 (2005).
504. Nachemson, A. The possible importance of the psoas muscle for stabilization of the lumbar spine. *Acta Orthopaedica Scandinavica* **39**, 47–57 (1968).
505. Potvin, J. R., Norman, R. W. & McGill, S. M. Reduction in anterior shear forces on the L4L5 disc by the lumbar musculature. *Clinical Biomechanics* **6**, 88–96 (1991).
506. Chon, J. *et al.* Asymmetric Atrophy of Paraspinal Muscles in Patients With Chronic Unilateral Lumbar Radiculopathy. *Annals of rehabilitation medicine* **41**, 801–807 (2017).
507. Arbanas, J. *et al.* MRI features of the psoas major muscle in patients with low back pain. *European spine journal* **22**, 1965–1971 (2013).
508. Hirayama, J. *et al.* Effects of electrical stimulation of the sciatic nerve on background electromyography and static stretch reflex activity of the trunk muscles in rats: possible implications of neuronal mechanisms in the development of sciatic scoliosis. *Spine* **26**, 602–609 (2001).
509. Suk, K.-S., Lee, H.-M., Moon, S.-H. & Kim, N.-H. Lumbosacral scoliotic list by lumbar disc herniation. *Spine* **26**, 667–671 (2001).
510. Ploumis, A. *et al.* Ipsilateral atrophy of paraspinal and psoas muscle in unilateral back pain patients with monosegmental degenerative disc disease. *The British Journal of Radiology* **84**, 709–713 (2011).
511. Clark, B. C., Walkowski, S., Conatser, R. R., Eland, D. C. & Howell, J. N. Muscle functional magnetic resonance imaging and acute low back pain: a pilot study to characterize lumbar muscle activity asymmetries and examine the effects of osteopathic manipulative treatment. *Osteopathic Medicine and Primary Care* **3**, 7 (2009).
512. Fujiwara, A., An, H. S., Lim, T.-H. & Haughton, V. M. Morphologic changes in the lumbar intervertebral foramen due to flexion-extension, lateral bending, and axial rotation: an in vitro anatomic and biomechanical study. *Spine* **26**, 876–882 (2001).
513. Bachrach, R. M., Micelotta, J. & Winuk, C. The relationship of low back pain to psoas insufficiency. *Journal of Orthopaedic Medicine* **29**, 98–104 (2007).
514. Harms, J. & Stürz. *Severe Spondylolisthesis - Pathology - Diagnosis - Therapy.* (Steinkopff-Verlag Heidelberg, 2002).
515. Jorgensson, A. The iliopsoas muscle and the lumbar spine. *Australian Journal of Physiotherapy* **39**, 125–132 (1993).
516. Hernando, M. F., Cerezal, L., Pérez-Carro, L., Canga, A. & González, R. P. Evaluation and management of ischiofemoral impingement: a pathophysiologic, radiologic, and therapeutic approach to a complex diagnosis. *Skeletal radiology* **45**, 771–787 (2016).
517. Sussman, W. I., Han, E. & Schuenke, M. D. Quantitative assessment of the ischiofemoral space and evidence of degenerative changes in the quadratus femoris muscle. *Surgical and Radiologic Anatomy* **35**, 273–281 (2013).
518. Sherman, P., Matchette, M., Sanders, T. & Parsons, T. Acetabular paralabral cyst: an uncommon cause of sciatica. *Skeletal radiology* **32**, 90–94 (2003).
519. Salunke, A. A. & Panchal, R. A Paralabral Cyst of the Hip Joint Causing Sciatica: Case Report and Review of Literature. *Malays J Med Sci* **21**, 57–60 (2014).
520. Ueo, T. & Hamabuchi, M. Hip pain caused by cystic deformation of the labrum acetabulare. *Arthritis & Rheumatism* **27**, 947–950 (1984).
521. Crawford, J., Van Rensburg, L. & Marx, C. Compression of the sciatic nerve by wear debris following total hip replacement: a report of three cases. *Journal of Bone & Joint Surgery, British Volume* **85**, 1178–1180 (2003).
522. Wu, K.-W., Hu, M.-H., Huang, S.-C., Kuo, K. N. & Yang, S.-H. Giant ganglionic cyst of the hip as a rare cause of sciatica: Case report. *Journal of Neurosurgery: Spine* **14**, 484–487 (2011).
523. Jones, H. G., Sarasin, S. M., Jones, S. A. & Mullaney, P. Acetabular Paralabral Cyst as a Rare Cause of Sciatica. *J Bone Joint Surg Am* **91**, 2696–2699 (2009).
524. Mert, M., Öztürkmen, Y., Ünkar, E. A., Erdoğan, S. & Üzümcügil, O. Sciatic nerve compression by an extrapelvic cyst secondary to wear debris after a cementless total hip arthroplasty: A case report and literature review. *International Journal of Surgery Case Reports* **4**, 805–808 (2013).
525. Tesio, L. The Cause of Back Pain and Sciatica may be a Venous Matter too. *Rheumatology (Oxford)* **30**, 70–71 (1991).
526. Hashemi, M., Halabchi, F. & others. Changing Concept of Sciatica: A Historical Overview. *Iranian Red Crescent Medical Journal* **18**, (2016).
527. Harper. *Early Chinese Medical Literature.* (Routledge, 2013).
528. Kleinschmidt, O. Über Phlebalgia Ischiadica und Ischias. *Klin Wochenschr* **1**, 1730–1732 (1922).
529. Simon, D., Reclus, P., Lejars, F.-M., Berger & Delbet. *Traité de chirurgie. Tome II.* (1890).
530. Reinhardt. Phlebektasien und varizen des nervus ischiadicus. in *Frankfurter Zeitschrift für Pathologie* **13**, (1913).
531. Putti, V. & others. New conceptions in the pathogenesis of sciatic pain. *Lancet* **2**, 30667–0 (1927).
532. Oppenheim, H. *Textbook of nervous diseases ...* (The Darien Press, 1911).
533. Kaiser, M. C. *et al.* Epidural venous stasis in spinal stenosis. *Neuroradiology* **26**, 435–438 (1984).
534. Hoyland, J. A., Freemont, A. & Jayson, M. Intervertebral foramen venous obstruction. A cause of periradicular fibrosis? *Spine* **14**, 558–568 (1989).
535. Fast, A., Weiss, L., Parikh, S. & Hertz, G. Night Backache in Pregnancy: Hypothetical Pathophysiological Mechanisms. *American Journal of Physical Medicine & Rehabilitation* **68**, 227 (1989).
536. Berthelot, J.-M., Le Goff, B. & Maugars, Y. The role for radicular veins in nerve root pain is underestimated: limitations of imaging studies. *Joint, bone, spine: revue du rhumatisme* **78**, 115 (2011).
537. Gargano, F. P., Meyer, J. D. & Sheldon, J. J. Transfemoral ascending lumbar catheterization of the epidural veins in lumbar disk disease: clinical application and results in the diagnosis of herniated intervertebral disks of the lumbar spine. *Radiology* **111**, 329–336 (1974).
538. Anderson, R. Diodrast Studies of the Vertebral and Cranial Venous Systems to Show Their Probable Role in Cerebral Metastases. *Journal of Neurosurgery* **8**, 411–422 (1951).
539. Arnoldi, C. C. Intravertebral pressures in patients with lumbar pain: A preliminary communication. *Acta orthopaedica Scandinavica* **43**, 109–117 (1972).
540. Esses, S. I. & Moro, J. K. Intraosseous vertebral body pressures. *Spine* **17**, S155–9 (1992).
541. Spencer, D. L., Ray, R. D., Spigos, D. G. & Kanakis, C. J. Intraosseous Pressure in the Lumbar Spine. *Spine* **6**, 159 (1981).
542. Kobayashi, S. *et al.* Circulatory dynamics of the cauda equina in lumbar canal stenosis using dynamic contrast-enhanced magnetic resonance imaging. *The Spine Journal* **15**, 2132–2141 (2015).
543. Parke, W. W. & Whalen, J. L. The Vascular Pattern of the Human Dorsal Root Ganglion and Its Probable Bearing on a Compartment Syndrome. *Spine* **27**, 347 (2002).
544. Ikawa, M., Atsuta, Y. & Tsunekawa, H. Ectopic Firing due to Artificial Venous Stasis in Rat Lumbar Spinal Canal Stenosis Model: A Possible Pathogenesis of Neurogenic Intermittent Claudication. *Spine* **30**, 2393 (2005).
545. Jinkins, J. R. Gd-DTPA Enhanced MR of the Lumbar Spinal Canal in Patients with Claudication. *Journal of Computer Assisted Tomography* **17**, 555 (1993).
546. LaBan, M. M., Wilkins, J. C., Wesolowski, D. P., Bergeon, B. & Szappanyos, B. J. Paravertebral venous plexus distention (Batson's): an inciting etiologic agent in lumbar radiculopathy as observed by venous angiography. *American journal of physical medicine & rehabilitation* **80**, 129–133 (2001).

547. Moore, M. R. *et al.* Relationship Between Vertebral Intraosseous Pressure, pH, PO2, pCO2, and Magnetic Resonance Imaging Signal Inhomogeneity in Patients with Back Pain: An in Vivo Study. *Spine* **16**, S239 (1991).
548. Cassar-Pullicino, V. N., Colhoun, E., McLelland, M., McCall, I. W. & el Masry, W. Hemodynamic alterations in the paravertebral venous plexus after spinal injury. *Radiology* **197**, 659–663 (1995).
549. Kuai, S. *et al.* The Effect of Lumbar Disc Herniation on Musculoskeletal Loadings in the Spinal Region During Level Walking and Stair Climbing. *Medical science monitor: international medical journal of experimental and clinical research* **23**, 3869–3877 (2017).
550. Wong, C.-H., Thng, P. L., Thoo, F.-L. & Low, C.-O. Symptomatic spinal epidural varices presenting with nerve impingement: report of two cases and review of the literature. *Spine* **28**, E347–E350 (2003).
551. Acar, F., Kayali, H., Erdogan, E., Kahraman, S. & Timurkaynak, E. Abnormal Dilated Epidural Venous Plexus Mimicking Prolapse of Intervertebral Disc. *Turkish Neurosurgery* **15**, 97–100 (2005).
552. Tofuku, K., Koga, H., Yone, K. & Komiya, S. Spontaneous regression of symptomatic lumbar epidural varix: a case report. *Spine* **32**, E147–E149 (2007).
553. Zimmerman, G. A., Weingarten, K. & Lavyne, M. H. Symptomatic lumbar epidural varices: report of two cases. *Journal of neurosurgery* **80**, 914–918 (1994).
554. Kamogawa, J., Kato, O. & Morizane, T. Three-dimensional visualization of internal vertebral venous plexuses relative to dural sac and spinal nerve root of spinal canal stenosis using MRI. *Japanese journal of radiology* **36**, 351–360 (2018).
555. Paksoy, Y. & Gormus, N. Epidural venous plexus enlargements presenting with radiculopathy and back pain in patients with inferior vena cava obstruction or occlusion. *Spine* **29**, 2419–2424 (2004).
556. Gümbel, U., Pia, H. W. & Vogelsang, H. Lumbosacrale Gefäßanomalien als Ursache von Ischialgien. *Acta neurochir* **20**, 131–151 (1969).
557. Hammer, A., Knight, I. & Agarwal, A. Localized venous plexi in the spine simulating prolapse of an intervertebral disc: a report of six cases. *Spine* **28**, E5–E12 (2003).
558. Slin'ko, E. I. & Al-Qashqish, I. I. Surgical treatment of lumbar epidural varices. *Journal of Neurosurgery: Spine* **5**, 414–423 (2006).
559. Donmez, F. Y. Epidural venous plexus engorgement: what lies beneath? *Case reports in radiology* **2015**, (2015).
560. Dudeck, O. *et al.* Epidural venous enlargements presenting with intractable lower back pain and sciatica in a patient with absence of the infrarenal inferior vena cava and bilateral deep venous thrombosis. *Spine* **32**, E688–E691 (2007).
561. Floman, Y., Smorgick, Y., Rand, N. & Bar-Ziv, J. Inferior Vena Cava Thrombosis Presenting as Lumbar Radiculopathy. *American Journal of Physical Medicine & Rehabilitation* **86**, 952–955 (2007).
562. Kamerath, J. & Morgan, W. Absent Inferior Vena Cava Resulting in Exercise-Induced Epidural Venous Plexus Congestion and Lower Extremity Numbness: A Case Report and Review of the Literature. *Spine August 15, 2010* **35**, (2010).
563. Widge, A. S., Tomycz, N. D. & Kanter, A. S. Sacral preservation in cauda equina syndrome from inferior vena cava thrombosis: Case report. *Journal of Neurosurgery: Spine* **10**, 257–259 (2009).
564. Olmarker, K., Rydevik, B., Holm, S. & Bagge, U. Effects of experimental graded compression on blood flow in spinal nerve roots. A vital microscopic study on the porcine cauda equina. *Journal of Orthopaedic Research* **7**, 817–823 (1989).
565. Cooper, R. *et al.* Herniated intervertebral disc-associated periradicular fibrosis and vascular abnormalities occur without inflammatory cell infiltration. *Spine* **20**, 591–598 (1995).
566. Aoyama, T. *et al.* Radiculopathy Caused by Lumbar Epidural Venous Varix. *Neurologia medico-chirurgica* **48**, 367–371 (2008).
567. Pekindil, G. & Yalniz, E. Symptomatic lumbar foraminal epidural varix. Case report and review of the literature. *British Journal of Neurosurgery* **11**, 159 (1997).
568. Olmarker, K. & Rydevik, B. Selective inhibition of tumor necrosis factor-α prevents nucleus pulposus-induced thrombus formation, intraneural edema, and reduction of nerve conduction velocity: possible implications for future pharmacologic treatment strategies of sciatica. *Spine* **26**, 863–869 (2001).
569. Tuan, A. S., Nabavizadeh, S. A., Pukenas, B., Mohan, S. & Learned, K. O. Reversible dilatation of lumbar epidural venous plexus secondary to pelvic venous compression: mimicker of pathology. *BJR|case reports* **3**, 20150287 (2016).
570. Hirabayashi, Y., Shimizu, R., Fukuda, H., Saitoh, K. & Igarashi, T. Effects of the pregnant uterus on the extradural venous plexus in the supine and lateral positions, as determined by magnetic resonance imaging. *British journal of anaesthesia* **78**, 317–319 (1997).
571. Gershater, R. & St. Louis, E. L. Lumbar epidural venography: Review of 1,200 cases. *Radiology* **131**, 409–421 (1979).
572. Park, S. K. *et al.* Dilatation of the spinal epidural venous plexus in patients with prominent epidural fat. *The British journal of radiology* **89**, 20160064 (2016).
573. Lemos, N. *et al.* Vascular entrapment of the sciatic plexus causing catamenial sciatica and urinary symptoms. *International urogynecology journal* 1–3 (2015).
574. Enrici, E., Mocellin, M. & D'Alotto, C. Varicose veins of external popliteal sciatic nerve. *Phlébologie* 69–76 (2014).
575. Pachêco, K., Magalhaes, F. & Loureiro, A. Les varices du nerf sciatique: pathologie sous-évaluée. *Phlébologie* **65**, 35–44 (2012).
576. Possover, M. & Forman, A. Pelvic Neuralgias by Neuro-Vascular Entrapment: Anatomical Findings in a Series of 97 Consecutive Patients Treated by Laparoscopic Nerve Decompression. *Pain Physician* **18**, E1139-1143 (2015).
577. Lemos, N. & Possover, M. Laparoscopic approach to intrapelvic nerve entrapments. *J Hip Preserv Surg* hnv030 (2015). doi:10.1093/jhps/hnv030
578. Labropoulos, N. *et al.* Nonsaphenous superficial vein reflux. *Journal of Vascular Surgery* **34**, 872–877 (2001).
579. Choudur, H. N., Joshi, R. & Munk, P. L. Inferior Gluteal Vein Varicosities: A Rare Cause of Sciatica. *JCR: Journal of Clinical Rheumatology* **15**, 387 (2009).
580. Hu, M.-H. *et al.* Vascular compression syndrome of sciatic nerve caused by gluteal varicosities. *Annals of vascular surgery* **24**, 1134–e1 (2010).
581. Maniker, A. H., Thurmond, J., Padberg, F. T., Blacksin, M. & Vingan, R. Traumatic Venous Varix Causing Sciatic Neuropathy: Case Report. *Neurosurgery* **55**, 1224 (2004).
582. Pacult, M. A., Henderson, F. C., Wooster, M. D. & Varma, A. K. Sciatica Caused by Venous Varix Compression of the Sciatic Nerve. *World Neurosurgery* **117**, 242–245 (2018).
583. Zhang, Z., Zhang, X., Yang, C. & Wen, X. Refractory sciatica caused by gluteal varicosities. *Orthopäde* **46**, 781–784 (2017).
584. Bustamante, S. & Houlton, P. Swelling of the leg, deep venous thrombosis and the piriformis syndrome. *Pain Res Manag* **6**, 200–203 (2000).
585. Labropoulos, N., Tassiopoulos, A. K., Gasparis, A. P., Phillips, B. & Pappas, P. J. Veins along the course of the sciatic nerve. *Journal of Vascular Surgery* **49**, 690–696 (2009).
586. Forchheimer, F. & Irons, E. E. *Forchheimer's therapeusis of internal disease.* (D. Appleton and Co., 1915).
587. Anders, H.-J. & Goebel, F.-D. Cytomegalovirus polyradiculopathy in patients with AIDS. *Clinical infectious diseases* **27**, 345–352 (1998).
588. Miller, R. *et al.* Acute lumbosacral polyradiculopathy due to cytomegalovirus in advanced HIV disease: CSF findings in 17 patients. *Journal of Neurology, Neurosurgery & Psychiatry* **61**, 456–460 (1996).
589. Sharma, K., Sriram, S., Fries, T., Bevan, H. & Bradley, W. Lumbosacral radiculoplexopathy as a manifestation of Epstein-Barr virus infection. *Neurology* **43**, 2550–2550 (1993).
590. Hottenrott, T., Rauer, S. & Bäuerle, J. Primary Epstein-Barr virus infection with polyradiculitis: a case report. *BMC Neurology* **13**, 96 (2013).
591. Majid, A. *et al.* Epstein–Barr virus myeloradiculitis and encephalomyeloradiculitis. *Brain* **125**, 159–165 (2002).
592. Berger JR & Houff S. Neurological complications of herpes simplex virus type 2 infection. *Arch Neurol* **65**, 596–600 (2008).
593. Wendling, D., Langlois, S., Lohse, A., Toussirot, E. & Michel, F. Herpes zoster sciatica with paresis preceding the skin lesions. Three case-reports. *Joint Bone Spine* **71**, 588–591 (2004).
594. Fagge, C. H. *The Principles and Practice of Medicine.* (J. & A. Churchill, 1888).
595. Jensen, P., Andersen, E., Boesen, F., Dissing, I. & Vestergaard, B. The incidence of herniated disc and varicella zoster virus infection in lumboradicular syndrome. *Acta neurologica Scandinavica* **80**, 142–144 (1989).
596. Gilden, D. H., Mahalingam, R., Cohrs, R. J. & Tyler, K. L. Herpesvirus infections of the nervous system. *Nature Clinical Practice Neurology* **3**, 82–94 (2007).
597. Ter Meulen, B. & Rath, J. Motor radiculopathy caused by varicella zoster virus without skin lesions ('zoster sine herpete'). *Clinical neurology and neurosurgery* **112**, 933 (2010).
598. Alpantaki, K., Katonis, P., Hadjipavlou, A., Spandidos, D. & Sourvinos, G. Herpes virus infection can cause intervertebral disc degeneration A CAUSAL RELATIONSHIP? *Journal of Bone & Joint Surgery, British Volume* **93**, 1253–1258 (2011).
599. Koda, M. *et al.* Herpes zoster sciatica mimicking lumbar canal stenosis: a case report. *BMC research notes* **8**, 320 (2015).
600. Stirling, A., Worthington, T., Rafiq, M., Lambert, P. A. & Elliott, T. S. J. Association between sciatica and Propionibacterium acnes. *Lancet* **357**, 2024 (2001).
601. Zhou, Z. *et al.* Relationship between annular tear and presence of Propionibacterium acnes in lumbar intervertebral disc. *Eur Spine J* **24**, 2496–2502 (2015).
602. Urquhart, D. M. *et al.* Could low grade bacterial infection contribute to low back pain? A systematic review. *BMC Medicine* **13**, 13 (2015).
603. Yu, L.-P., Qian, W.-W., Yin, G.-Y., Ren, Y.-X. & Hu, Z.-Y. MRI Assessment of Lumbar Intervertebral Disc Degeneration with Lumbar Degenerative Disease Using the Pfirrmann Grading Systems. *PLOS ONE* **7**, e48074 (2012).
604. Quinones-Hinojosa, A., Jun, P., Jacobs, R., Rosenberg, W. S. & Weinstein, P. R. General principles in the medical and surgical management of spinal infections: a multidisciplinary approach. *Neurosurg focus* **17**, E1 (2004).
605. Colmenero, J. *et al.* Pyogenic, tuberculous, and brucellar vertebral osteomyelitis: a descriptive and comparative study of 219 cases. *Annals of the rheumatic diseases* **56**, 709–715 (1997).
606. Cottle, L. & Riordan, T. Infectious spondylodiscitis. *Journal of Infection* **56**, 401–412 (2008).

607. Chong, K. W. & Tay, B. K. Piriformis pyomyositis: a rare cause of sciatica. *Singapore Med J* **45**, 229–231 (2004).
608. Hu, M. T., Shaw, C. E., Evans, S. & Britton, T. C. Acute sciatica with an infective cause. *J R Soc Med* **91**, 87–88 (1998).
609. Kamal, T., Hall, M., Moharam, A., Sharr, M. & Walczak, J. Gluteal pyomyositis in a non-tropical region as a rare cause of sciatic nerve compression: a case report. *Journal of medical case reports* **2**, 204 (2008).
610. Dejerine, J. *Sémiologie des affections du système nerveux*. (Masson et Cie., 1914).
611. Schmutzhard, E., Mohsenipour, I. & Stanek, G. Incidence of nervous system Borrelia burgdorferi infection in patients with lumboradicular syndrome. *European neurology* **33**, 149–151 (2008).
612. Dupeyron, A. *et al.* Sciatica, disk herniation, and neuroborreliosis. A report of four cases. *Joint bone spine* **71**, 433–437 (2004).
613. Meier, C., Reulen, H., Huber, P. & Mumenthaler, M. Meningoradiculoneuritis mimicking vertebral disc herniation. A "neurosurgical" complication of lyme-borreliosis. *Acta neurochirurgica* **98**, 42–46 (1989).
614. Müller, K. E. Damage of Collagen and Elastic Fibres by Borrelia Burgdorferi – Known and New Clinical and Histopathological Aspects. *Open Neurol J* **6**, 179–186 (2012).
615. Cadavid, D., O'Neill, T., Schaefer, H. & Pachner, A. R. Localization of Borrelia Burgdorferi in the Nervous System and Other Organs in a Nonhuman Primate Model of Lyme Disease. *Lab Invest* **80**, 1043–1054 (2000).
616. Halperin, J. J. Nervous System Lyme Disease. *Infectious Disease Clinics of North America* **22**, 261–274 (2008).
617. Moro, P. & Schantz, P. M. Echinococcosis: a review. *International Journal of Infectious Diseases* **13**, 125–133 (2009).
618. Turgut, M. Hydatid disease of the spine: a survey study from Turkey. *Infection* **25**, 221–226 (1997).
619. Maretić, T. *et al.* Meningitis and Radiculomyelitis Caused by Angiostrongylus cantonensis. *Emerging Infectious Diseases* **15**, 996–998 (2009).
620. Wood, G., Delamont, S., Whitby, M. & Boyle, R. Spinal sensory radiculopathy due to Angiostrongylus cantonensis infection. *Postgraduate medical journal* **67**, 70–72 (1991).
621. Badr, H. *et al.* Schistosomal myeloradiculopathy due to Schistosoma mansoni: Report on 17 cases from an endemic area. *Annals of Indian Academy of Neurology* **14**, 107–110 (2011).
622. Ferrari, T. C. A. & Moreira, P. R. R. Neuroschistosomiasis: clinical symptoms and pathogenesis. *The Lancet Neurology* **10**, 853–864 (2011).
623. Huang, C.-T. *et al.* Sparganosis of the cauda equina: A rare case report and review of the literature. *Neurology India* **60**, 102 (2012).
624. Hippocrates, Coxe, J. R. & Galen. *The writings of Hippocrates and Galen*. (Philadelphia : Lindsay and Blakiston, 1846).
625. Pliny, the E., Bostock, J. & Riley, H. T. (Henry T. *The natural history of Pliny*. (London, H. G. Bohn, 1856).
626. Aegineta, P. *The Seven Books of Paulus Ægineta*. (Sydenham Society, 1844).
627. Harburn, J. Some Points In The Treatment Of Brachialgia And Sciatica. *British medical journal* **1**, 245 (1905).
628. Kellogg, J. H. *Modern Medicine*. (Modern Medicine Publishing Company, 1902).
629. Earle, S. T. Physiology of Constipation. *California state journal of medicine* **9**, 438 (1911).
630. Ali, M., Shukla, V. D., Dave, A. R. & Bhatt, N. N. A clinical study of Nirgundi Ghana Vati and Matra Basti in the management of Gridhrasi with special reference to sciatica. *Ayu* **31**, 456–460 (2010).
631. Al-Khodairy, A.-W. T., Bovay, P. & Gobelet, C. Sciatica in the female patient: anatomical considerations, aetiology and review of the literature. *European Spine Journal* **16**, 721–731 (2006).
632. Missmer, S. A. & Bove, G. M. A pilot study of the prevalence of leg pain among women with endometriosis. *Journal of bodywork and movement therapies* **15**, 304–308 (2011).
633. Murphy, D. R., Bender, M. I. & Green, G. Uterine Fibroid Mimicking Lumbar Radiculopathy. *Spine* **35**, E1435–E1437 (2010).
634. Heffernan, L., Fraser, R. & Purdy, R. L-5 radiculopathy secondary to a uterine leiomyoma in a primigravid patient. *American journal of obstetrics and gynecology* **138**, 460 (1980).
635. Laman, D., Endtz, L., van Well-Krouwel, H. & Gerretsen, G. A rare cause of lumbosacral plexus neuropathy. *Clinical neurology and neurosurgery* **87**, 47–49 (1985).
636. Acar, B., Kadanali, S. & Acar, U. Rare gynecological condition causing sciatic pain. *International journal of gynaecology and obstetrics: the official organ of the International Federation of Gynaecology and Obstetrics* **42**, 50 (1993).
637. Murata, Y., Takahashi, K., Murakami, M. & Moriya, H. An Unusual Cause of Sciatic Pain. *J Bone Joint Surg Br* **83-B**, 112–113 (2001).
638. Sencan, S., Ozcan-Eksi, E. E., Cuce, I., Guzel, S. & Erdem, B. Pregnancy-related low back pain in women in Turkey: Prevalence and risk factors. *Annals of Physical and Rehabilitation Medicine* **61**, 33–37 (2018).
639. Lawrentschuk, N. & Nguyen, H. Cauda equina syndrome secondary to constipation: an uncommon occurrence. *ANZ journal of surgery* **75**, 498–500 (2005).
640. Frischhut, B., Ogon, M., Trobos, S. & Judmaier, W. Sciatica as a manifestation of idiopathic megacolon: A previously undescribed causal relationship. *The Journal of Pediatrics* **133**, 449 (1998).
641. Hiatt, R. B. The Pathologic Physiology of Congenital Megacolon. *Ann Surg* **133**, 313–320 (1951).
642. Demarquay, J. *et al.* Right-sided sciatalgia complicating Crohn's disease. *The American journal of gastroenterology* **93**, 2296–2298 (1998).
643. Ailianou, A. *et al.* Review of the principal extra spinal pathologies causing sciatica and new MRI approaches. *The British Journal of Radiology* **85**, 672–681 (2012).
644. Chitranjan, Kandpal, H. & Madhusudhan, K. S. Sciatic hernia causing sciatica: MRI and MR neurography showing entrapment of sciatic nerve. *Br J Radiol* **83**, e65-66 (2010).
645. Fetterman, F. S. Referred Pain of Ureteral Origin. *American Journal of Obstetrics and Gynecology* **23**, 259–261 (1932).
646. Warren, J. W. *et al.* Sites of pain from interstitial cystitis/painful bladder syndrome. *The Journal of urology* **180**, 1373–1377 (2008).
647. Ross, J. On the segmental distribution of sensory disorders. *Brain* **10**, 333–361 (1888).
648. Head, H. On disturbances of sensation with especial reference to the pain of visceral disease. *Brain* **16**, 1–133 (1893).
649. Wesson, M. B. Backache Due to Seminal Vesiculitis and Prostatitis. *California and western medicine* **27**, 346 (1927).
650. Player, L. P. The prostate and its influence on low-back pain. *California and western medicine* **23**, 993 (1925).
651. Kutzmann, A. A. Back pain of urologic origin. *California and western medicine* **27**, 208 (1927).
652. Vilos, G. A., Vilos, A. W. & Haebe, J. J. Laparoscopic Findings, Management, Histopathology, and Outcomes in 25 Women with Cyclic Leg Pain. *The Journal of the American Association of Gynecologic Laparoscopists* **9**, 145–151 (2002).
653. Yilmaz, U., Rothman, I., Ciol, M. A., Yang, C. C. & Berger, R. E. Toe spreading ability in men with chronic pelvic pain syndrome. *BMC Urology* **5**, 11 (2005).
654. Grøvle, L. *et al.* Comorbid subjective health complaints in patients with sciatica: a prospective study including comparison with the general population. *Journal of psychosomatic research* **70**, 548–556 (2011).
655. Groves, M. D., McCutcheon, I. E., Ginsberg, L. E. & Kyritsis, A. P. Radicular pain can be a symptom of elevated intracranial pressure. *Neurology* **52**, 1093–1093 (1999).
656. Zacutus, L. *Praxis medica admiranda: in qua, exempla monstrosa, rara, nova, mirabilia, circa abditas morborum causas, signa, eventûs, atque curationes exhibita, diligenttissimè proponuntur*. (apud Joannem-Antonium Huguetan, 1637).
657. Round, R. & Keane, J. R. The minor symptoms of increased intracranial pressure 101 patients with benign intracranial hypertension. *Neurology* **38**, 1461–1461 (1988).
658. Daniels, A. B. *et al.* Profiles of Obesity, Weight Gain, and Quality of Life in Idiopathic Intracranial Hypertension (Pseudotumor Cerebri). *American Journal of Ophthalmology* **143**, 635-641.e1 (2007).
659. Magee, D. J. *Orthopedic Physical Assessment*. (Elsevier Health Sciences, 2014).

Chapter 4 Symptoms of sciatica

Key points

- Symptoms and medical history inform the diagnosis, further testing, prognosis, and treatment of sciatica
- The location and radiation of symptoms and palliative and provocative factors have the highest diagnostic utility

Interpreting symptoms and medical history

Few isolated symptoms and risk factors have a high diagnostic utility in sciatica. These factors have a greater utility when observed in **clusters**.[1,2] Groups of findings may point to a specific condition, and if not, may help classify sciatica as intraspinal or extraspinal.

Likelihood ratios (±LR) help determine if a condition is likely to be present. Likelihood ratios for a positive test (+LR) >10 are large or strong, those > 5 and ≤ 10 are moderate, and those >2 and ≤ 5 small or weak. Likelihood ratios for a negative test (-LR) ≤ 0.1 are large or strong, > 0.1 and ≤ 2 are moderate, > 0.2 and ≤ 0.5 are small or weak. The only symptoms with a large positive likelihood ratio are dermatomal distributions of L4 (+LR 13) and S1 (+LR 11).[3] Only one symptom of sciatica has a large negative likelihood ratio, when standing exacerbates symptoms (-LR 0.04), absence of which helps rule out lumbar spinal stenosis (LSS).[2]

Odds ratios (OR) express the probability of a disease occurring. Odds ratios ≥ 1.68 and <3.47 are considered small, ≥ 3.47 and < 6.71 are medium, and ≥ 6.71 are large.[4] Symptoms with odds greater than 1 indicate a greater probability of the disease while those less than 1 indicate reduced probability of the disease. Examples of symptoms with a large odds ratio include groin pain which implicates the sacroiliac joint (SIJ),[5] and claudication which points to LSS.[6,7] Lifestyle factors such as an occupation involving manual labor with high lumbar loads which provides a large odds ratio for lumbar disc herniation (LDH).[8,9]

Sensitivity (sn) and **specificity** (sp) describe the true positives and true negatives, respectively, given by a test. In general, moderate sensitivity or specificity is ≥ 80% while ≥ 90% is considered high.[10] Tests with over 90% sensitivity may be considered good **screening tests** for low back disorders.[11] Examples of tests with high sensitivity include dermatomal distribution of symptoms for LDH,[12] and provocative factors such as standing and walking for LSS.[2,13] The only highly specific symptom that may be useful for diagnosing extraspinal sciatic symptoms is the alleviation of symptoms while standing, which indicates vascular claudication.[2]

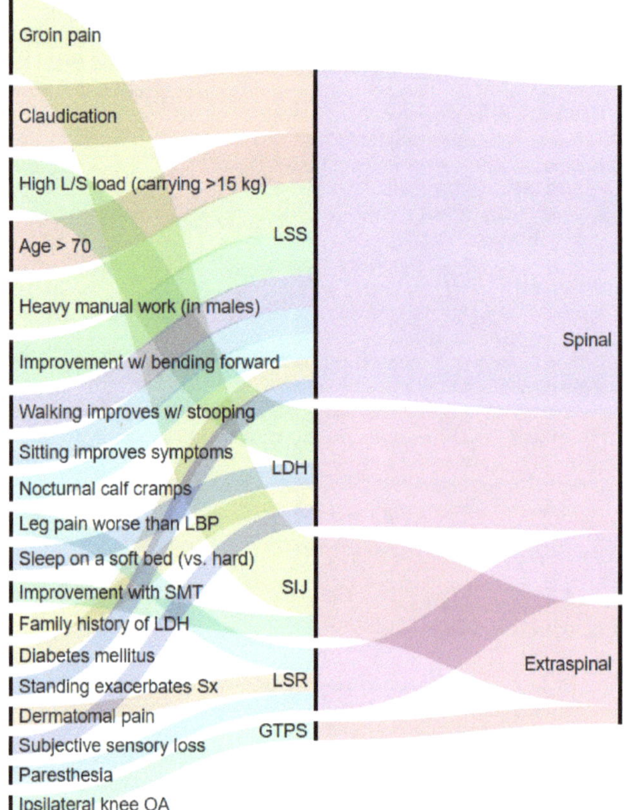

Figure 111: Overview of symptoms and risk factors with the greatest odds ratios for sciatica. Symptoms are categorized by diagnosis and location. Abbreviations include lumbar (L/S), lumbosacral radiculopathy (LSR), LSS (lumbar spinal stenosis), LDH (lumbar disc herniation), GTPS (greater trochanteric pain syndrome), OA (osteoarthritis), spinal manipulative therapy (SMT), sacroiliac joint (SIJ), symptoms (Sx), with (w/). The size of each row correlates with an increasing diagnostic odds ratio (OR), ranging from 3.34 to 14.48. Only studies with ORs were included. Data adapted from multiple authors[2,5–9,13–29]

Demographics

Those **over age 70** have increased odds of having LSS (OR 2.9 to 5.4).[6,13] Those under age 65 are less likely to have LSS (-LR 0.33).[14] Patients **under age**

37 with low back pain are more likely to have lumbar instability (+LR 3.0).[15]

Female gender increases the odds of GTPS by a factor of 3.4.[16] Females also have greater odds of having degenerative spondylolisthesis (OR 2.5).[17] **Males** are only slightly more likely to have lumbar nerve root compression (+LR 1.3) or LDH (+LR 1.2).[18]

Review of systems

Severely abnormal symptoms can be red flags (see above) while mild abnormalities usually point to LSS. **Urinary disturbance** increases the odds of nerve root compression (OR 2.3)[19] and the likelihood of LSS (+LR 6.9).[6] Those with LSS may report **poor balance** (+LR 1.5),[14] **waking up to urinate** at night (+LR 2.3),[13] or having to **walk more slowly** than usual due to their lower extremities (+LR 2.3).[13] Other health problems should be considered as these may affect the prognosis (see chapter 7).

Prior treatments

Those with prior lumbar surgeries are at risk for ongoing low back complications. Those with prior disc surgery have greater odds of **recurrent disc herniation** if they are **diabetic** or **smoke** (OR 1.99).[20] One study using epiduroscopy (minimally invasive video imaging) found that over 90% of those with persistent pain following low back surgery had significant **fibrosis**.[21] A systematic review found that 5.5% of patients undergoing surgical decompression for LSS developed new or **increased lumbar instability.**[22] Those with prior lumbar surgeries may rarely develop infection or hematoma.

Patients that obtain relief from **SIJ manipulation** have 4 times the odds of having suffered from SIJ pain.[23] Patients with pain that **does not centralize** using a directional preference exercise are only slightly more likely to have SIJ pain (+LR 1.1, OR 2.6).[23,24]

Patients that have had **repeated treatments every year** for low-back related symptoms have increased odds of LSS (OR 2.7).[13]

Medical history

Patients with **diabetes mellitus** have greater odds of LSS (OR 3.7).[25] Patients with primary **hip osteoarthritis** have increased odds of degenerative spondylolisthesis (OR 1.9).[17] **Early life malnutrition** may predispose to the development of LSS.[26] Diabetics and smokers with prior disc surgery have a small increase in odds of **recurrent disc herniation.**[20] Those with ipsilateral **knee osteoarthritis** have greater odds of GTPS (OR 3.5).[16]

Social history

Occupation affects the likelihood of disc herniation being present. Patients that perform **heavy physical labor** involving carrying loads over 15 kilograms have greater odds of having a LDH (OR 2.1-9.7).[9,27,28] Likewise, those that regularly perform **heavy lifting** in addition to **extreme forward bending** with over 90 degrees of trunk flexion have increased odds of LDH (OR 3.2). Exposure to **whole-body vibration** is another risk factor for LDH (OR 1.9-2.1).[29]

Those that sleep on a **hard bed** have reduced odds of having a LDH (OR 0.2-0.4) while those that sleep on a soft bed have increased odds (OR 2.8-4.4).[9,28] It is unknown if bed type influences the odds of other types of sciatica such as those related to instability or greater trochanteric pain.

Patients that **exercise** regularly have reduced odds of having LDH (OR 0.4).[28] This is also true for those who have practiced **bodybuilding** for many years or hours (OR 0.5 for ≥ 1,350 hours).[30] Those that do not exercise have increased odds of LDH (OR 2.3).[28] Studies have shown conflicting results regarding the impact of body mass index on the likelihood of LDH.[18,31]

Smokers have a small increase in odds of LDH[32] as well as recurrent disc herniation after surgery.[20] Smoking does not appear to play a significant role in LSS.[8]

Family history

Those with a family history of **lumbar disc herniation** have increased odds of LDH (OR 3.6-5.9).[9,28,31] Family history may also be relevant for LSS. One study found that the size of the central lumbar canal and dural sac are highly heritable traits.[33]

A family history of **connective tissue disorders** such as **Marfan** and **Ehlers-Danlos** syndromes can be relevant, as they are associated with disc herniation and spondylolisthesis.[34] **Neurofibromatosis** is a rare genetic disorder that can cause radicular sciatica by producing nerve root tumors.[34] **Autoimmune disorders** such as ankylosing spondylitis may be relevant considering they can cause sacroiliitis. Those with hereditary multiple osteochondromas may be at risk for compression of the sciatic nerve by bony outgrowths.[35]

Common symptoms

Location and radiation of sciatica

Location and radiation of sciatic pain are among the most useful symptoms in localizing the cause of sciatic pain. Clinicians should ask patients to trace their distribution of symptoms and compare this to a dermatomal (nerve root) pattern. The most specific symptoms of discogenic radicular sciatica include a **single-dermatome pain distribution** (98% specific in the case of S1 radiculopathy[3]), below knee pain (sp 95%),[36] and leg pain worse than back pain (sp 92%).[37] The best symptoms to help rule out discogenic radicular sciatica is the absence of dermatomal pain (-LR 0.42)[38] or absence of below-knee pain (-LR 0.45).[1]

Patients that complain of symptoms **distal to the knee** are more likely to have nerve root involvement. Although patients may report pain in the "leg" it should be determined if they mean the true anatomical leg (the calf and shin below the knee), or rather the thigh. One large study of patients with low back-related lower extremity pain found that 77% of those with radicular pain had pain distal to the knee compared to 41% of those with referred non-radicular pain.[39] The presence of below-knee symptoms increases the odds of radicular sciatica by a factor of at least 2 (ORs from studies range from 2.13 to 3.34).[36,40] Absence of below-knee pain helps rule out radicular sciatica with moderate probability (-LR 0.45).[1]

Leg pain worse than back pain is a sign of radicular sciatica. One large study of patients with low back-related lower extremity pain found that 56% of those with radicular pain had leg pain worse than back pain compared to 41% of those with referred non-radicular pain.[39] Imaging studies have found that those with leg pain worse than back pain have 1.45 to 4.50 times the odds of discogenic radicular sciatica.[1,18,40,41] Absence of this symptom does not help rule out lumbar pathology.[1,18,40,41]

A **dermatomal pain distribution** increases the probability of discogenic radicular sciatica being present. Symptoms that correspond precisely to a single dermatome (either L4, L5, or S1) are highly specific (92-98%) for disc-related sciatica.[3] Symptoms that include more than one dermatome are more sensitive and less specific. Absence of any dermatomal pain helps rule out nerve root compression with moderate probability (-LR 0.42).[38] Presence of any dermatomal pain increases the odds of nerve root compression by a factor of 2.1-3.5.[12,19,38]

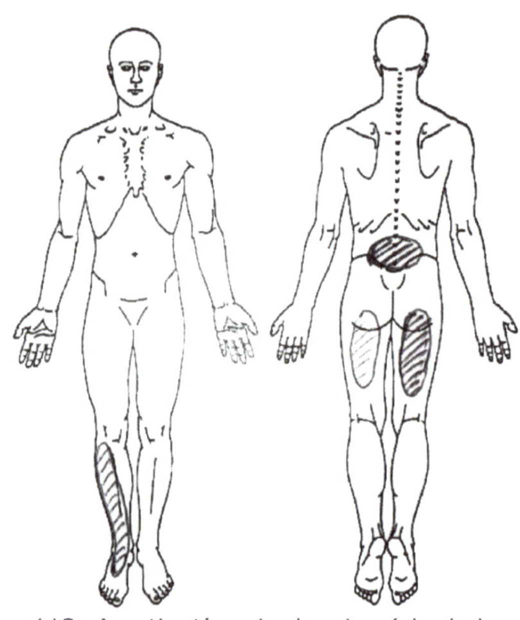

Figure 112: A patient's pain drawing (shaded areas) who suffered from a bilateral L5 radiculopathy, worse on the right side, caused by lumbar stenosis related to a degenerative anterolisthesis of L4. This drawing has typical elements of radiculopathy (L5 dermatome in anterolateral leg) and stenosis (bilateral symptoms). Shared with patient's permission by Robert Trager, DC.

Bilateral symptoms are highly specific for LSS.[6,11,42] These include any bilateral symptoms (sp 98%),[11] bilateral buttock or leg pain (92%),[42] and bilateral plantar numbness.[6] Bilateral symptoms are found more frequently in LSS than LDH or extraspinal causes of sciatica.

Non-dermatomal pain is occasionally specific for diagnoses of sciatica. **Groin pain** increases the odds of hip osteoarthritis by a factor of 3.4[43] and SIJ pain by a factor of 14.5.[5] Pain at the **posterior superior iliac spine** increases the odds of **SIJ pain** by a factor of 2.75.[23] Numbness of the perineal region is highly specific (99%) for LSS.[6,7] In general, gluteal pain and thigh pain[42] lack diagnostic utility.

Non-radicular conditions may create pain patterns that mimic dermatomal symptoms. Some confusion stems from the similarity of peripheral nerve distributions with dermatomes, for example the common peroneal nerve distribution and the L5 dermatome in the leg.[57,58] Certain conditions, such as superior cluneal nerve entrapment or hip arthritis, may create a pain referral pattern that mimics a dermatome. Pain patterns should always be correlated with other physical examination findings.

Table 15: Pain patterns that mimic lumbosacral dermatomal patterns

Condition	**Mimics dermatome(s)**
Superior cluneal nerve entrapment	L3-S3[44]
Hip arthritis	L4[45]
Greater trochanteric pain syndrome	L4, 5[46,47]
Lumbosacral extraforaminal entrapment	L5[48]
Pelvic mass compression of lumbosacral plexus	L4-S3[49,50]
Endometriosis of the lumbosacral plexus or sciatic nerve	L4-S3[51,52]
Sacroiliitis / SIJ pain	L5, S1, S2[53–55]
Sciatic nerve entrapment in piriformis or deep gluteal syndrome	L5, S1, S2[56]
Common peroneal nerve entrapment	L5[57,58]
Sciatic nerve entrapment in hamstring syndrome	S1, S2[59]
Posterior femoral cutaneous nerve entrapment	S1, S2[60,61]
Tibial nerve entrapment / soleal sling syndrome	S1[62,63]

Palliative and provocative symptoms

The combination of sciatic symptoms being **worse standing and better sitting** is moderately predictive of LSS.(+LR 6.1, -LR 0.23, sn 80%, sp 87%).[2] **Coughing, sneezing, and bearing down** provides a specific sign when these actions increase only leg pain (sp 77-79%).[64] These actions are less specific if they increase only low back pain (sp 31-80%).[1,18] When coughing, sneezing, and bearing down increases only leg pain, the odds of disc herniation increase by a factor of 2.5 and odds of nerve root compression increase by 2.3.[64]

Response to sitting helps differentiate discogenic sciatica from LSS. Those with **worse pain while sitting** have greater odds (OR 1.90) of discogenic radicular sciatica.[19] Those with symptom **improvement while sitting** have greater odds of LSS (OR 4.88).[65] Those with **no pain while sitting** have even greater likelihood of LSS (+LR 6.6).[14] Absence of relief while seated helps rule out LSS to a moderate degree (-LR 0.3).[65] Pain with sitting is also associated with sciatic nerve entrapment in the gluteal region.[66]

Patients that **sit down for most of the day** due to lower extremity symptoms have two times the odds of having LSS.[13] **Pain immediately upon sitting down** is highly specific for radiographic instability.[67]

Standing helps distinguish LSS from vascular claudication symptoms. Those with exacerbation of symptoms while standing have 3 to 3.5 times the odds of having LSS[7] while those with alleviation of symptoms (+LR 2.8) are more likely to have vascular claudication.[2] The best symptom to rule out LSS is the absence of symptom exacerbation while standing (-LR 0.04).[2]

Those that obtain relief of lower extremity symptoms when **walking** with a flexed, stooped posture are more likely to have LSS.[68] Patients may also report having to lean on a shopping cart while walking to alleviate pain, a sign called the **shopping cart sign**. Absence of the shopping cart sign helps rule out LSS (-LR 0.38).[2] Those with vascular claudication may require less time (1-2 minutes) to recover from symptoms exacerbated by walking compared to those with LSS (>10 minutes).[2]

Pain while **lying down** is not specific for any diagnosis. Pain exacerbated by lying on the affected side is seen in 75% of those with GTPS,[69] 52% of those with SIJ pain, and 37% of those with LDH or LSS.[5]

Quality

Most individual pain descriptors including burning pain, sharp pain, shooting pain, tingling, and toothache-type pain have poor diagnostic accuracy.[1,70]

The only descriptor that by itself is accurate is **subjective sensory loss**, which increases the odds of LDH by a factor of 3.5 and nerve root compression by a factor of 2.3.[18]

Pain descriptors may have increased diagnostic utility when occurring with **self-reported numbness**. The combination of self-reported numbness and **pins-and-needles** sensation increases the odds of LDH by a small amount (OR 1.7).[1]

Onset

Progressively worsening pain increases the odds having a LDH with an annular tear.[71] Likewise, **non-sudden onset** (gradual-onset) sciatic pain increases the odds of LDH (OR 2.1) and nerve root compression (OR 2.3) by a small amount.[18] Those with sudden-onset sciatic pain are less likely to have LDH and nerve root compression.[18]

Severity

Severity of pain is a non-specific finding in diagnosing LSS or LDH.[1,14] Those with **severe sciatic pain** 7 or more out of 10 on a numeric rating scale are slightly more likely (+LR 1.7) to have a LDH[1] and LSS (+LR 2.0).[14] Those without at least **moderate pain** 4 out of 10 are slightly less likely to have a disc herniation (-LR 0.52).[1]

Timing of sciatica

The frequency of sciatic pain (e.g. constant, intermittent, occasional) has a low diagnostic utility in diagnosing sciatica.[1] Likewise, paroxysmal pain (sudden intensifications) does not increase or decrease the likelihood of disc herniation or nerve root compression.[18]

Pain at night is commonly reported by those with low back pain and sciatica, and by itself does not distinguish LSS from LDH.[72] Night pain correlates with a reduction in the straight-leg raising degree[73] as well as with younger age.[74] Sleeping on a soft bed may increase the odds of developing sciatica compared to a firm bed (OR 2.75).[28]

One study found that those that **wake up at night in pain while not moving** were more likely to have a discogenic radiculopathy and also be flexion intolerant.[75] Those waking up with pain while rolling in bed were more likely to have facet-joint mediated pain. Another study found that **sciatic pain worst in the morning** was predictive of a LDH with an annular tear.[71] Patients with radicular sciatica may also wake up at night with calf spams or cramps (see below).

Cramps and spasms

Calf cramping occurs in a range of types of sciatica. It is common in LSS and vascular claudication and in general does not differentiate the two conditions.[2] Those with LSS often have **nocturnal calf cramps**, with 71% of patients reporting this symptom.[76] Nocturnal calf cramps increase the odds of LSS by a factor of 4.6.[76]

Frequent calf cramping day or night can be caused by LDH or LSS causing **S1 radiculopathy**.[77,78] Patients with frequent calf cramps may have hypertrophy (enlargement) of the cramping calf as opposed to atrophy. Those with deep gluteal syndrome may have **cramping in the buttocks** or thigh.[66]

Subjective or localized weakness

Subjective weakness in general does not provide strong evidence to rule in or out any diagnosis of sciatica.[18,19,70] Subjective sensory loss has a stronger diagnostic utility for LDH and nerve root compression.

Foot drop is a helpful localizing sign in sciatica. In order to have foot drop the ankle dorsiflexion or tibialis anterior strength must be less than grade 3 of 5 on the Medical Research Council Scale.[79] The most common causes of foot drop are **degenerative spinal conditions** (LDH and LSS) affecting the L4-5 level, and **common peroneal neuropathy**.[79] Foot drop occurs in 3-11% of those with discogenic radiculopathy.[80–82]

The complaint of **legs giving out while walking** is most often associated with LSS.[83] Rarely, subjective weakness such as foot drop, dragging of the leg while walking, or the feeling that the legs "misbehave" and do not do what the patient wants can be red flags of serious pathology.[84] Subjective weakness should be correlated with other symptoms and examination findings.

Red flag symptoms

Certain symptoms that occur with sciatica are **red flags**, which suggest the possibility of serious underlying disease such as infection, cancer, fracture, and cauda equina syndrome (CES). **Combinations of red flags** increase the likelihood of serious pathology, whereas individual red flags are prone to being falsely positive or negative.[85] The presence of red flags may require an urgent or emergent medical referral or consultation with a spinal surgeon. Sciatica with symptoms of serious pathology is sometimes called **atypical sciatica**.[53]

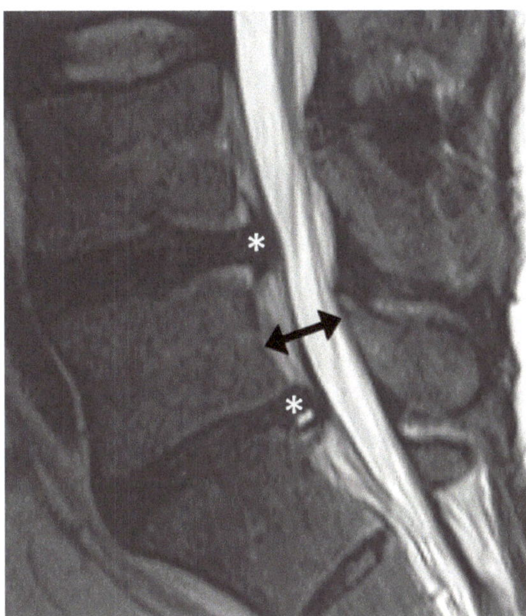

Figure 113: Two disc herniations (*) and a congenitally narrow spinal canal of 14 mm (arrows). This 36-year-old man presented with a 1-week history of constant severe LBP with radiation to the left groin and testicle, and reported not urinating as often as normal. Examination showed severe weakness (≤3/5 strength) of the bilateral gluteal muscles, hamstrings, psoas, and quadriceps, and weakness of the left tibialis anterior and extensor hallucis longus both 4/5. SLR was limited at 10° (L) and 30° (R). The patient was referred to a local hospital for suspected cauda equina syndrome and an emergent MRI. He opted to avoid surgery but made a nearly full recovery regardless. Case shared with permission of patient by Robert Trager, DC.

Medical history

The medical history may reveal red flags in the sciatic patient. The most predictive factor for malignancy in patients with low back pain is a **history of cancer**/malignancy.[86] About half of patients diagnosed with spinal metastasis have a history of malignancy.[87] Those with **osteoporosis** have greater odds of having a spinal fracture (OR 2.5).[88]

Medications

Certain medications may increase the odds of having serious pathology. One study found that patients with a history of taking **anticoagulants** had 15.6 times the odds of having a serious cause of low back pain such as retroperitoneal or aortic bleeding.[89] Those with **prolonged corticosteroid use** have a greater likelihood of having a spinal fracture.[86,88] Medication history is relevant to manual therapists who should avoid certain manipulative techniques if there is suspicion of fracture or bleeding.

Age

One study identified that **older age** of at least 75 years (OR 3.5) and trauma (OR 7.8) individually increased the risk of **vertebral fracture**.[88] Another study found that the combination of trauma and older age was more specific for fracture. They found that trauma and age over 50 was 94% specific for fracture in those with low back pain, whereas trauma and age over 70 was 99% specific.[85]

Sciatica in a **child** is uncommon. Lumbar disc herniation is uncommon in children, and its prevalence in the first two decades of life is 0.8-3.8%.[90] Presence of this symptom requires greater attention and sooner diagnostic testing than for an adult.[91] Cauda equina tumors,[92] spinal tumors including osteoblastomas and osteoid osteomas,[93,94] infections, and vascular malformations rarely cause sciatica in children.

Nocturnal sciatica

Nocturnal sciatica by itself is not specific for serious pathology but may be important when combined with other red flags. One study found that those with low back pain worse at night had 4.3 times the odds of having serious pathology.[89] Another study found that low-back related night pain or pain that awakens from sleep had a low sensitivity (55%) and specificity (42%) for predicting malignancy.[85]

One-third of those with **discogenic sciatica** report that their pain is worse at night,[41] which may be triggered by rolling over in bed.[95] Those with **lumbar stenosis** can also have night pain,[96] as well as aching calf pain, fasciculations, and restless legs at night, a condition called "Vesper's curse."[97]

Night pain rarely represents spondylodiscitis,[98] septic sacroiliitis,[99] or tumors of the spine,[100] pelvis,[49,101] or cauda equina.[102,103] Night pain in conjunction with **sweating** is more indicative of infection.[85]

Weight loss

Unexplained weight loss and a history of malignancy could be signs of cancer. Recent **unexplained weight loss** is highly specific (95.6%) for malignancy in patients with low back pain, but has a low sensitivity (8.2%) as it is not a common symptom.[85] Alternatively, intentional weight loss may increase the risk of common peroneal neuropathy at the fibular neck.[104]

Recent unexplained weight loss can be a symptom of spinal **malignancies** including leptomeningeal metastasis[105] and malignant vertebral[106] or pelvic tumors.[50,107] Those with spinal lymphoma may present with sciatica, weight loss, and night sweats.[108]

Recent unexplained weight loss with sciatica is rarely a symptom of **infections** including spondylodiscitis[98] and septic sacroiliitis[99,109]. It can also be a sign of a **ruptured abdominal aortic aneurysm**.[110,111]

Fever

The combination of **fever**, **chills** or **sweating**, and a **recent infection** is highly specific (99%) for infection in patients with low back pain.[85] Sweating at night is 86% specific for infection in those with low back pain.[85] Those with a history of drug abuse or immunodeficiency may also be at risk of infection-related sciatica.

A fever or history of febrile episode can represent **spinal infections** such as spondylodiscitis[112] and septic sacroiliitis,[113] or nervous system infection such as viral radiculopathy,[114,115] neuroborreliosis,[116] and neurosyphilis.[117]

Immunodeficiency

Immune deficiency is not typically considered a red flag for low back pain[85,87,88] and one study found no correlation between immune suppressing medications and serious pathology-related low back pain.[89] However, these studies have not considered the presence of sciatica or radiculopathy. Those who are immune deficient or have abused intravenous drugs who present with sciatica rarely have an infection such as spondylodiscitis,[118] septic sacroiliitis,[113] viral radiculopathy,[119,120] or neurosyphilis.[117,121]

Cauda equina symptoms

Bladder incontinence or urinary retention, frequent urination, bowel incontinence, decreased sensation of urination or decreased fecal sensation are by themselves poor predictors of cauda equina syndrome (CES).[122] The combination of recent **loss of bladder and bowel control** is highly specific (97%) for cauda equina syndrome in those with low back pain but lacks sensitivity (8.3%).[85] **Constant non-mechanical pain** is the most common red flag symptom, and is experienced by 80% of those with CES.[87] Any suspicion of CES requires emergent referral for possible surgery or other medical treatment.

Rapidly progressive sensory or motor deficits over hours is another sign of cauda equina syndrome. This can be caused by lumbar disc herniation,[123] but more rarely by spinal epidural hematoma,[124] spondylodiscitis with epidural abscess,[125] other types of spinal infections, malignant spinal tumors and pathological fractures.[126,127] Rarely this is caused by Guillain-Barré syndrome which can mimic radicular sciatica.[128]

Trunk pain

Sciatic pain typically involves the lower back and lower extremities and is less likely to affect the thoracic spine, and even less likely to affect the abdominal region. **Band-like trunk pain** or abdominal pain has been associated with **spinal metastatis**.[84,87,129] This band-like pain may represent a thoracic or upper lumbar dermatomal pattern, which is rare for those with low back pain. Disc herniations above L3 account for less than 3% of low back pain.[130] Those with thoracic back pain in addition to low back pain also have increased odds of spinal fracture (OR 2.1).[88]

Yellow flags

Clinicians should screen for yellow flags, also called **psychosocial risk factors** for chronicity or barriers to recovery. These include patient's beliefs, emotional responses, and pain behaviors.[131] These factors affect prognosis rather than diagnosis. Most international low back pain guidelines recommend screening for yellow flags.[132] A survey found that almost 90% of surgeons desire to screen for yellow flags.[133] Taking note of yellow flags is useful in designing a treatment plan that addresses them, typically with an educational component.

Patients with yellow flags may have a **slower recovery** from sciatica. Pain-related fear has been found to inversely correlate with recovery from sciatic pain.[134] In addition, patients whose radiating pain does not centralize with treatment have higher odds of having yellow flags.[135] These findings suggest psychosocial factors interfere with improvement.

Patients with sciatica may have **incorrect beliefs** about their pain. They may feel that their symptoms are uncontrollable[136] or will worsen over time.[137] They may have a poor expectation for improvement with medical treatments and manual therapies.[138,139] Patients may also think that having a disc herniation means they will be disabled for life.[140]

Emotional responses such as worries, fears, anxiety, and distress that does not meet the criteria for a mental disorder are considered yellow flags in low back pain.[131] Patients with sciatica may feel that their life is "on hold" and future is uncertain.[136] Those with chronic sciatica are more prone to have feelings of guilt or shame regarding their symptoms.[141] Patients may believe that they "should have been more careful."[142]

Pain behaviors and **fear avoidance** are thought to be risk factors for chronic sciatic pain.[143] Examples of pain behaviors include groaning, using a cane, rubbing the painful site, and over-reliance on passive treatments such as ice, heat, or analgeiscs.[131,143] Fear-avoidance is the avoidance of activity or movement due to fear of pain and injury.[144] For example patients may hesitate to perform or avoid everyday activities such as bending down or picking up their children.[142] Low back pain patients tend to avoid activities that caused their symptoms, which is thought to create an ongoing cycle of disuse, atrophy, and further pain.[145]

Questionnaires such as the STarT Back Screening Tool,[146,147] Fear Avoidance Beliefs Questionnaire (FABQ),[135,148,149] and Tampa Scale for Kinesiophobia (TSK) [150–152] have been used to identify yellow flags in sciatic patients. These questionnaires ask patients to agree or disagree to questions such as "It's really not safe for a person with a condition like mine to be physically active.(STarT Back Screening Tool)[146] or "My work might harm my back."(FABQ)[153]

Yellow flags are common in patients with sciatica. One study found that about 40% of those with sciatica scored highly on the TSK questionnaire.[152] Another study found that 39% of those with radicular sciatica as well as 39% with referred lower extremity pain had high scores on the STarT Back Screening Tool.[39]

It may be possible to replace yellow flag questionnaires with individual questions.[154] One study found that substituting a single question for the Tampa Scale for Kinesiophobia -- **"How much 'fear' do you have that these complaints would be increased by physical activity?"** predicted clinical outcome to a similar degree as the entire questionnare.[154]

Clinicians may ask open-ended questions or ask patients to agree with statements to reveal potential yellow flags. A response to "**What do you think is causing your pain**?" or "what do you think is going on during a flare?" with a degenerative or structural answer such as "out" or "slipped" or "loss of disc space" is associated with a poorer perception of prognosis.[155] The question "What are you doing to relieve your pain?" aims to determine if there is over-reliance on rest or passive treatments.[156] The questions "Do you believe your condition is going to get better?" and "Are you confident you can cope with your condition?" seeks to determine self-efficacy, expectations, and beliefs.[147]

References

1. Konstantinou, K., Lewis, M. & Dunn, K. M. Agreement of self-reported items and clinically assessed nerve root involvement (or sciatica) in a primary care setting. *Eur Spine J* **21**, 2306–2315 (2012).
2. Nadeau, M. *et al.* The reliability of differentiating neurogenic claudication from vascular claudication based on symptomatic presentation. *Can J Surg* **56**, 372–377 (2013).
3. Hancock, M. J., Koes, B., Ostelo, R. & Peul, W. Diagnostic accuracy of the clinical examination in identifying the level of herniation in patients with sciatica. *Spine* **36**, E712–E719 (2011).
4. Chen, H., Cohen, P. & Chen, S. How big is a big odds ratio? Interpreting the magnitudes of odds ratios in epidemiological studies. *Communications in Statistics—Simulation and Computation®* **39**, 860–864 (2010).
5. Kurosawa, D. *et al.* A Diagnostic Scoring System for Sacroiliac Joint Pain Originating from the Posterior Ligament. *Pain Med* **18**, 228–238 (2017).
6. Konno, S. *et al.* Development of a clinical diagnosis support tool to identify patients with lumbar spinal stenosis. *European Spine Journal* **16**, 1951–1957 (2007).
7. Suri, P. Does This Older Adult With Lower Extremity Pain Have the Clinical Syndrome of Lumbar Spinal Stenosis? *JAMA: The Journal of the American Medical Association* **304**, 2628 (2010).
8. Abbas, J. *et al.* Socioeconomic and physical characteristics of individuals with degenerative lumbar spinal stenosis. *Spine* **38**, E554–E561 (2013).
9. Davtyan, H. Risk Factors of Developing Lumbar Disc Herniation in Armenia: a case-control study. *College of Health Sciences* (2011).

10. Cardinal, L. Diagnostic testing in the context of high-value care: Incorporating prior probability. *Journal of community hospital internal medicine perspectives* **6**, 33674 (2016).
11. Cook, C. *et al.* Clustered clinical findings for diagnosis of cervical spine myelopathy. *Journal of Manual & Manipulative Therapy* **18**, 175–180 (2010).
12. Vroomen, P., de Krom, M., Wilmink, J., Kester, A. & Knottnerus, J. Diagnostic value of history and physical examination in patients suspected of lumbosacral nerve root compression. *Journal of Neurology, Neurosurgery & Psychiatry* **72**, 630–634 (2002).
13. Sugioka, T., Hayashino, Y., Konno, S., Kikuchi, S. & Fukuhara, S. Predictive value of self-reported patient information for the identification of lumbar spinal stenosis. *Family Practice* **25**, 237–244 (2008).
14. Katz, J. N. *et al.* Degenerative lumbar spinal stenosis diagnostic value of the history and physical examination. *Arthritis & Rheumatism* **38**, 1236–1241 (1995).
15. Fritz, J. M., Piva, S. R. & Childs, J. D. Accuracy of the clinical examination to predict radiographic instability of the lumbar spine. *European Spine Journal* **14**, 743–750 (2005).
16. Segal, N. A. *et al.* Greater Trochanteric Pain Syndrome: Epidemiology and Associated Factors. *Arch Phys Med Rehabil* **88**, 988–992 (2007).
17. Sasagawa, T. & Nakamura, T. Associated Factors for Lumbar Degenerative Spondylolisthesis in Japanese Patients with Osteoarthritis of the Hip: A Radiographic Study. *Asian Spine Journal* **10**, 935–939 (2016).
18. Verwoerd, A. J. *et al.* Diagnostic accuracy of history taking to assess lumbosacral nerve root compression. *The Spine Journal* (2013).
19. Coster, S., de Bruijn, S. F. & Tavy, D. L. Diagnostic value of history, physical examination and needle electromyography in diagnosing lumbosacral radiculopathy. *Journal of neurology* **257**, 332–337 (2010).
20. Huang, W., Han, Z., Liu, J., Yu, L. & Yu, X. Risk Factors for Recurrent Lumbar Disc Herniation. *Medicine (Baltimore)* **95**, (2016).
21. Bosscher, H. A. & Heavner, J. E. Incidence and Severity of Epidural Fibrosis after Back Surgery: An Endoscopic Study. *Pain Practice* **10**, 18–24 (2010).
22. Guha, D., Heary, R. F. & Shamji, M. F. Iatrogenic spondylolisthesis following laminectomy for degenerative lumbar stenosis: systematic review and current concepts. *Neurosurgical focus* **39**, E9 (2015).
23. Dreyfuss, P., Michaelsen, M., Pauza, K., McLarty, J. & Bogduk, N. The Value of Medical History and Physical Examination in Diagnosing Sacroiliac Joint Pain. *Spine* **21**, 2594 (1996).
24. Szadek, K. M., van der Wurff, P., van Tulder, M. W., Zuurmond, W. W. & Perez, R. S. G. M. Diagnostic validity of criteria for sacroiliac joint pain: a systematic review. *Journal of Pain* **10**, 354 (2009).
25. Asadian, L., Haddadi, K., Aarabi, M. & Zare, A. Diabetes Mellitus, a New Risk Factor for Lumbar Spinal Stenosis: A Case–Control Study. *Clin Med Insights Endocrinol Diabetes* **9**, 1–5 (2016).
26. Muthuuri, J., Some, E. & Chege, P. Association between early life malnutrition and the size of lumbar spinal canal among adults of coastal region, Kenya. *East African Orthopaedic Journal* **12**, 33–38 (2018).
27. Sun, Z. M. *et al.* [Case-control study of the risk factors of lumbar intervertebral disc herniation in 5 northern provinces of China]. *Nan Fang Yi Ke Da Xue Bao* **30**, 2488–2491 (2010).
28. Zhang, Y., Sun, Z., Zhang, Z., Liu, J. & Guo, X. Risk Factors for Lumbar Intervertebral Disc Herniation in Chinese Population: A Case-Control Study. *Spine* **34**, E918–E922 (2009).
29. Seidler, A. *et al.* Occupational risk factors for symptomatic lumbar disc herniation; a case-control study. *Occup Environ Med* **60**, 821–830 (2003).
30. Schumann, B. *et al.* Lifestyle factors and lumbar disc disease: results of a German multi-center case-control study (EPILIFT). *Arthritis Research & Therapy* **12**, R193 (2010).
31. Saftić, R., Grgić, M., Ebling, B. & Splavski, B. Case-control study of risk factors for lumbar intervertebral disc herniation in Croatian island populations. *Croatian medical journal* **47**, 593–600 (2006).
32. Huang, W., Qian, Y., Zheng, K., Yu, L. & Yu, X. Is smoking a risk factor for lumbar disc herniation? *Eur Spine J* **25**, 168–176 (2016).
33. Battié, M. C. *et al.* Brief Report: Lumbar Spinal Stenosis Is a Highly Genetic Condition Partly Mediated by Disc Degeneration. *Arthritis & Rheumatology* **66**, 3505–3510 (2014).
34. Corey, J. Genetic disorders producing compressive radiculopathy. in *Seminars in neurology* **26**, 515 (2006).
35. Yu, K., Meehan, J. P., Fritz, A. & Jamali, A. A. Osteochondroma of the Femoral Neck: A Rare Cause of Sciatic Nerve Compression. *Orthopedics* (2010). doi:10.3928/01477447-20100625-26
36. Beattie, P. F., Meyers, S. P., Stratford, P., Millard, R. W. & Hollenberg, G. M. Associations between patient report of symptoms and anatomic impairment visible on lumbar magnetic resonance imaging. *Spine* **25**, 819–828 (2000).
37. Cook, C. *et al.* The clinical value of a cluster of patient history and observational findings as a diagnostic support tool for lumbar spine stenosis. *Physiotherapy Research International* **16**, 170–178 (2011).
38. Thapa, S. S., Lakhey, R. B., Sharma, P. & Pokhrel, R. K. Correlation between Clinical Features and Magnetic Resonance Imaging Findings in Lumbar Disc Prolapse. *J Nepal Health Res Counc* **14**, 85–88 (2016).
39. Konstantinou, K. *et al.* Characteristics of patients with low back and leg pain seeking treatment in primary care: baseline results from the ATLAS cohort study. *BMC musculoskeletal disorders* **16**, 332 (2015).
40. Stynes, S., Konstantinou, K., Ogollah, R., Hay, E. M. & Dunn, K. M. Clinical diagnostic model for sciatica developed in primary care patients with low back-related leg pain. *PloS one* **13**, e0191852 (2018).
41. Vroomen, P. C. A. J., Krom, M. C. T. F. M. de & Knottnerus, J. A. Predicting the outcome of sciatica at short-term follow-up. *British Journal of General Practice* **52**, 119–123 (2002).
42. Ljunggren, A. E. Discriminant validity of pain modalities and other sensory phenomena in patients with lumbar herniated intervertebral discs versus lumbar spinal stenosis. *Neuro-orthopedics* **11**, 91–99 (1991).
43. Brown, M. D., Gomez-Marin, O., Brookfield, K. F. W. & Li, P. S. Differential Diagnosis of Hip Disease Versus Spine Disease. *Clinical Orthopaedics and Related Research* **419**, 280–284 (2004).
44. Kuniya, H. *et al.* Prospective study of superior cluneal nerve disorder as a potential cause of low back pain and leg symptoms. *Journal of Orthopaedic Surgery and Research* **9**, 139 (2014).
45. Offierski, C. M. & Macnab, I. Hip-Spine Syndrome. *Spine* **8**, 316 (1983).
46. Swezey, R. L. Pseudo-radiculopathy in subacute trochanteric bursitis of the subgluteus maximus bursa. *Arch Phys Med Rehabil* **57**, 387–390 (1976).
47. Tortolani, P. J., Carbone, J. J. & Quartararo, L. G. Greater trochanteric pain syndrome in patients referred to orthopedic spine specialists. *The Spine Journal* **2**, 251–254 (2002).
48. Matsumoto, M. *et al.* Posterior decompression surgery for extraforaminal entrapment of the fifth lumbar spinal nerve at the lumbosacral junction: clinical article. *Journal of Neurosurgery: Spine* **12**, 72–81 (2010).
49. Thompson, R. & Berg, T. L. Primary bone tumors of the pelvis presenting as spinal disease. *Orthopedics* **19**, 1011–1016 (1996).
50. Wilkes, L., Cannon, C. & Ham, O. Malignant tumors of the pelvic girdle mimicking the herniated disk syndrome. *Clinical orthopaedics and related research* **138**, 217–221 (1979).
51. Floyd, J. R., Keeler, E. R., Euscher, E. D. & McCutcheon, I. E. Cyclic sciatica from extrapelvic endometriosis affecting the sciatic nerve: Case report. *Journal of Neurosurgery: Spine* **14**, 281–289 (2011).
52. Ceccaroni, M. *et al.* Cyclic sciatica in a patient with deep monolateral endometriosis infiltrating the right sciatic nerve. *Journal of Spinal Disorders & Techniques* **24**, 474–478 (2011).
53. Kulcu, D. G. & Naderi, S. Differential diagnosis of intraspinal and extraspinal non-discogenic sciatica. *Journal of Clinical Neuroscience* **15**, 1246–1252 (2008).
54. Buijs, E., Visser, L. & Groen, G. Sciatica and the sacroiliac joint: a forgotten concept. *British journal of anaesthesia* **99**, 713–716 (2007).
55. Margules, K. R. & Gall, E. P. Sciatica-like pain arising in the sacroiliac joint. *JCR: Journal of Clinical Rheumatology* **3**, 9–15 (1997).
56. Lewis AM, L. R. Magnetic resonance neurography in extraspinal sciatica. *Arch Neurol* **63**, 1469–1472 (2006).
57. Walcott, B. P., Coumans, J.-V. C. & Kahle, K. T. Diagnostic pitfalls in spine surgery: masqueraders of surgical spine disease. *Neurosurgical Focus* **31**, E1 (2011).
58. Reife, M. D. & Coulis, C. M. Peroneal neuropathy misdiagnosed as L5 radiculopathy: a case report. *Chiropractic & Manual Therapies* **21**, 12 (2013).
59. Saikku, K., Vasenius, J., Saar, P. & others. Entrapment of the proximal sciatic nerve by the hamstring tendons. *Acta orthopaedica Belgica* **76**, 321 (2010).
60. Arnoldussen, W. & Korten, J. Pressure neuropathy of the posterior femoral cutaneous nerve. *Clinical Neurology and Neurosurgery* **82**, 57–60 (1980).
61. Chutkow, J. G. Posterior femoral cutaneous neuralgia. *Muscle & nerve* **11**, 1146–1148 (1988).
62. Drees, C., Wilbourn, A. J. & Stevens, G. H. Main trunk tibial neuropathies. *Neurology* **59**, 1082–1084 (2002).
63. Mastaglia, F. L. Tibial nerve entrapment in the popliteal fossa. *Muscle & nerve* **23**, 1883–1886 (2000).
64. Verwoerd, A. J. *et al.* A diagnostic study in patients with sciatica establishing the importance of localization of worsening of pain during coughing, sneezing and straining to assess nerve root compression on MRI. *European Spine Journal* 1–4 (2016).
65. Fritz, J. M., Erhard, R. E., Delitto, A., Welch, W. C. & Nowakowski, P. E. Preliminary results of the use of a two-stage treadmill test as a clinical diagnostic tool in the differential diagnosis of lumbar spinal stenosis. *Journal of spinal disorders* **10**, 410–416 (1997).
66. Martin, H. D., Reddy, M. & Gómez-Hoyos, J. Deep gluteal syndrome. *J Hip Preserv Surg* **2**, 99–107 (2015).
67. Maigne, J.-Y., Lapeyre, E., Morvan, G. & Chatellier, G. Pain immediately upon sitting down and relieved by standing up is often associated with radiologic lumbar instability or marked anterior loss of disc space. *Spine* **28**, 1327–1334 (2003).
68. Dong, G. & Porter, R. Walking and cycling tests in neurogenic and intermittent claudication. *Spine* **14**, 965–969 (1989).

69. Woodley, S. J. *et al.* Lateral hip pain: findings from magnetic resonance imaging and clinical examination. *journal of orthopaedic & sports physical therapy* **38**, 313–328 (2008).
70. Lauder, T. D. *et al.* Effect of history and exam in predicting electrodiagnostic outcome among patients with suspected lumbosacral radiculopathy. *American journal of physical medicine & rehabilitation* **79**, 60 (2000).
71. Vucetic, N., Bri, E. de & Svensson, O. Clinical history in lumbar disc herniation: A prospective study in 160 patients. *Acta Orthopaedica Scandinavica* **68**, 116–120 (1997).
72. Jonsson, B. & Stromqvist, B. Symptoms and signs in degeneration of the lumbar spine. A prospective, consecutive study of 300 operated patients. *Journal of Bone & Joint Surgery, British Volume* **75**, 381–385 (1993).
73. Jönsson, B. & Strömqvist, B. The straight leg raising test and the severity of symptoms in lumbar disc herniation. A preoperative evaluation. *Spine (Phila Pa 1976)* **20**, 27–30 (1995).
74. Jönsson, B. & Strömqvist, B. Influence of age on symptoms and signs in lumbar disc herniation. *Eur Spine J* **4**, 202–205 (1995).
75. Sweetman, B. J. & Sweetman, S. J. Various types of sleep disturbance due to different sorts of low back pain: 5: A clinical database analysis. *International Musculoskeletal Medicine* **37**, 153–163 (2015).
76. Matsumoto, M. *et al.* Nocturnal leg cramps: a common complaint in patients with lumbar spinal canal stenosis. *Spine* **34**, E189–E194 (2009).
77. Gross, R. *et al.* Focal myositis of the calf following S1 radiculopathy. in *Seminars in arthritis and rheumatism* **38**, 20–27 (Elsevier, 2008).
78. Ong, V., Jones, J. & Steuer, A. An unusual cause of calf hypertrophy: Severe lumbar canal stenosis with S1 nerve root radiculopathy. *APLAR Journal of Rheumatology* **10**, 316–319 (2007).
79. Wang, Y. & Nataraj, A. Foot drop resulting from degenerative lumbar spinal diseases: clinical characteristics and prognosis. *Clinical neurology and neurosurgery* **117**, 33–39 (2014).
80. Bakhsh, A. Role of conventional lumbar myelography in the management of sciatica: An experience from Pakistan. *Asian Journal of Neurosurgery* **7**, 25 (2012).
81. Rehman, L. *et al.* Correlation between clinical features and magnetic resonance imaging findings in patients with lumbar disc herniation. *Journal of Postgraduate Medical Institute (Peshawar-Pakistan)* **21**, (2011).
82. Schistad, E. i. *et al.* Association between baseline IL-6 and 1-year recovery in lumbar radicular pain. *EJP* **18**, 1394–1401 (2014).
83. Hall, H. Effective spine triage: patterns of pain. *The Ochsner Journal* **14**, 88–95 (2014).
84. Greenhalgh, S. & Selfe, J. A qualitative investigation of Red Flags for serious spinal pathology. *Physiotherapy* **95**, 223–226 (2009).
85. Premkumar, A., Godfrey, W., Gottschalk, M. B. & Boden, S. D. Red Flags for Low Back Pain Are Not Always Really Red: A Prospective Evaluation of the Clinical Utility of Commonly Used Screening Questions for Low Back Pain. *JBJS* **100**, 368 (2018).
86. Downie, A. *et al.* Red flags to screen for malignancy and fracture in patients with low back pain. *Br J Sports Med* **48**, 1518–1518 (2014).
87. Keillar, E. Are we missing any patients with serious spinal pathology? *International Journal of Therapy and Rehabilitation* **20**, 487–494 (2013).
88. Enthoven, W. T. M. *et al.* Prevalence and "Red Flags" Regarding Specified Causes of Back Pain in Older Adults Presenting in General Practice. *Phys Ther* **96**, 305–312 (2016).
89. Thiruganasambandamoorthy, V. *et al.* Risk factors for serious underlying pathology in adult emergency department nontraumatic low back pain patients. *Journal of Emergency Medicine* **47**, 1–11 (2014).
90. Ferrante, L., Mastronardi, L., Lunardi, P., Puzzilli, F. & Fortuna, A. Lumbar disc herniation in teenagers. *Eur Spine J* **1**, 25–28 (1992).
91. Kordi, R. & Rostami, M. Low Back Pain in Children and Adolescents: an Algorithmic Clinical Approach. *Iran J Pediatr* **21**, 259–270 (2011).
92. Mathew, P. & Todd, N. V. Intradural conus and cauda equina tumours: a retrospective review of presentation, diagnosis and early outcome. *Journal of Neurology, Neurosurgery & Psychiatry* **56**, 69–74 (1993).
93. Raskas, D. S., Graziano, G. P., Herzenberg, J. E., Heidelberger, K. P. & Hensinger, R. N. Osteoid osteoma and osteoblastoma of the spine. *Journal of Spinal Disorders & Techniques* **5**, 204–211 (1992).
94. Avadhanam, P. K., Vuyyur, S. & Panigrahi, M. K. A rare occurrence of osteoblastoma in a child. *J Pediatr Neurosci* **5**, 153–156 (2010).
95. Transfeldt, E. & Macnab, I. Differential Diagnosis of Low Back Pain. in *Macnab's Backache* 339–355 (Lippincott Williams & Wilkins, 2007).
96. Frymoyer, J. Degenerative Spondylolisthesis: Diagnosis and Treatment. *The Journal of the American Academy of Orthopaedic Surgeons* **2**, 9 (1994).
97. Laban, M., Sl, V., Af, F. & Rs, T. Restless legs syndrome associated with diminished cardiopulmonary compliance and lumbar spinal stenosis--a motor concomitant of 'Vesper's curse'. *Arch Phys Med Rehabil* **71**, 384–388 (1990).
98. Cottle, L. & Riordan, T. Infectious spondylodiscitis. *Journal of Infection* **56**, 401–412 (2008).
99. Pouchot, J. *et al.* Tuberculosis, of the sacroiliac joint: clinical features, outcome, and evaluation of closed needle biopsy in 11 consecutive cases. *The American journal of medicine* **84**, 622–628 (1988).
100. Sim, F., Dahlin, D., Stauffer, R. & Edward, L. Primary bone tumors simulating lumbar disc syndrome. *Spine* **2**, 65–74 (1977).
101. Kakutani, K., Doita, M., Nishida, K., Miyamoto, H. & Kurosaka, M. Radiculopathy due to malignant melanoma in the sacrum with unknown primary site. *European Spine Journal* **17**, 271–274 (2007).
102. Shimada, Y. *et al.* Clinical features of cauda equina tumors requiring surgical treatment. *The Tohoku journal of experimental medicine* **209**, 1–6 (2006).
103. Fearnside, M. R. & Adams, C. B. Tumours of the cauda equina. *J. Neurol. Neurosurg. Psychiatr.* **41**, 24–31 (1978).
104. Katirji, B. Peroneal neuropathy. *Neurologic clinics* **17**, 567–591 (1999).
105. Schiff, D., O'Neill, B. & Suman, V. J. Spinal epidural metastasis as the initial manifestation of malignancy: clinical features and diagnostic approach. *Neurology* **49**, 452–456 (1997).
106. Esser, S. M. & Baima, J. Ewing Sarcoma Causing Back and Leg Pain in 2 Patients. *PM&R* **4**, 317–321 (2012).
107. Paulson, E. Neoplasms of the bony pelvis producing the sciatica syndrome. *Minnesota medicine* **34**, 1069 (1951).
108. Vanneuville, B. *et al.* Non-Hodgkin's lymphoma presenting with spinal involvement. *Annals of the rheumatic diseases* **59**, 12–14 (2000).
109. Ariza, J. *et al.* Brucellar Sacroiliitis: Findings in 63 Episodes and Current Relevance. *Clin Infect Dis.* **16**, 761–765 (1993).
110. Lodder, J., Cheriex, E., Oostenbroek, R., Soeters, P. & Vreeling, F. Ruptured abdominal aortic aneurysms presenting as radicular compression syndromes. *Journal of neurology* **227**, 121–124 (1982).
111. Keller, A. Chronic contained aortic rupture presenting as anterior thigh pain. *BMJ case reports* **2012**, (2012).
112. Colmenero, J. *et al.* Pyogenic, tuberculous, and brucellar vertebral osteomyelitis: a descriptive and comparative study of 219 cases. *Annals of the rheumatic diseases* **56**, 709–715 (1997).
113. Hermet, M. *et al.* Infectious sacroiliitis: a retrospective, multicentre study of 39 adults. *BMC Infectious Diseases* **12**, 305 (2012).
114. Bathoorn, E. *et al.* Primary Epstein-Barr virus infection with neurological complications. *Scandinavian journal of infectious diseases* **43**, 136–144 (2011).
115. Dworkin, R. H. *et al.* Diagnosis and assessment of pain associated with herpes zoster and postherpetic neuralgia. *The Journal of Pain* **9**, 37–44 (2008).
116. Halperin, J. J. Lyme disease and the peripheral nervous system. *Muscle & nerve* **28**, 133–143 (2003).
117. Winston, A., Marriott, D. & Brew, B. Early syphilis presenting as a painful polyradiculopathy in an HIV positive individual. *Sexually transmitted infections* **81**, 133–134 (2005).
118. Cunningham, M. E., Girardi, F., Papadopoulos, E. C. & Cammisa, F. P. Spinal infections in patients with compromised immune systems. *Clinical orthopaedics and related research* **444**, 73–82 (2006).
119. Gilden, D. H., Kleinschmidt-DeMasters, B., LaGuardia, J. J., Mahalingam, R. & Cohrs, R. J. Neurologic complications of the reactivation of varicella–zoster virus. *New England Journal of Medicine* **342**, 635–645 (2000).
120. Centner, C., Bateman, K. & Heckmann, J. Manifestations of HIV infection in the peripheral nervous system. *Lancet neurology* **12**, 295–309 (2013).
121. Raji, V., Dhanasegaran, S., Subramanian, K. & Sivaprakash, S. Syphilitic myeloradiculopathy and pupillary light near disassociation: an overlap syndrome in a HIV positive individual. *Indian journal of medical sciences* **60**, 421 (2006).
122. Fairbank, J., Hashimoto, R., Dailey, A., Patel, A. A. & Dettori, J. R. Does patient history and physical examination predict MRI proven cauda equina syndrome? *Evidence-based spine-care journal* **2**, 27 (2011).
123. Gardner, A., Gardner, E. & Morley, T. Cauda equina syndrome: a review of the current clinical and medico-legal position. *European Spine Journal* **20**, 690–697 (2011).
124. Hejazi, N., Thaper, P.-Y. & Hassler, W. Nine Cases of Nontraumatic Spinal Epidural Hematoma. *Neurologia medico-chirurgica* **38**, 718–724 (1998).
125. Phillips, G. & Jefferson, A. Acute spinal epidural abscess. Observations from fourteen cases. *Postgraduate medical journal* **55**, 712–715 (1979).
126. Weinstein, J. N. & McLain, R. F. Primary tumors of the spine. *Spine* **12**, 843–851 (1987).
127. Lee, C.-S. & Jung, C.-H. Metastatic Spinal Tumor. *Asian Spine J* **6**, 71–87 (2012).
128. van Doorn, P. A., Ruts, L. & Jacobs, B. C. Clinical features, pathogenesis, and treatment of Guillain-Barré syndrome. *The Lancet Neurology* **7**, 939–950 (2008).
129. Finucane, L. Metastatic disease masquerading as mechanical low back pain; atypical symptoms which may raise suspicion. *Manual Therapy* **18**, 624–627 (2013).
130. Albert, T. J. *et al.* Upper lumbar disc herniations. *Journal of Spinal Disorders & Techniques* **6**, 351–359 (1993).
131. Nicholas, M. K., Linton, S. J., Watson, P. J., Main, C. J. & Group, "Decade of the Flags" Working. Early identification and management of psychological risk factors ("yellow flags") in patients with low back pain: a reappraisal. *Physical therapy* **91**, 737–753 (2011).

132. Koes, B. W., van Tulder, M. W., Ostelo, R., Kim Burton, A. & Waddell, G. Clinical Guidelines for the Management of Low Back Pain in Primary Care. *Spine* **26**, 2504–2513 (2001).
133. Busse, J. W. *et al.* Surgeon attitudes toward nonphysician screening of low back or low back–related leg pain patients referred for surgical assessment: a survey of Canadian spine surgeons. *Spine* **38**, E402–E408 (2013).
134. Haugen, A., Grøvle, L., Brox, J., Natvig, B. & Grotle, M. Pain-related fear and functional recovery in sciatica: results from a 2-year observational study. *J Pain Res* **9**, 925–931 (2016).
135. Werneke, M. W. & Hart, D. L. Centralization: association between repeated end-range pain responses and behavioral signs in patients with acute non-specific low back pain. *Journal of rehabilitation medicine* **37**, 286–290 (2005).
136. Ryan, C. & Roberts, L. 'life on hold': the lived experience of sciatica. *Orthopaedic Proceedings* **100-B**, 22–22 (2018).
137. Holte, J. & Vuoskoski, P. The lived-through experience of spinally referred leg pain: a descriptive phenomenological study. in (36th International Human Science Research Conference, Between Necessity and Choice: Existential Dilemmas in the Human Life-World, Jelenia Gora, Poland, July 11-14, 2017, 2017).
138. Hopayian, K. & Notley, C. A systematic review of low back pain and sciatica patients' expectations and experiences of health care. *The Spine Journal* **14**, 1769–1780 (2014).
139. Ong, B. N., Konstantinou, K., Corbett, M. & Hay, E. Patients' Own Accounts of Sciatica: A Qualitative Study. *Spine* **36**, 1251 (2011).
140. Frederiksen, P. *et al.* Can group-based reassuring information alter low back pain behavior? A cluster-randomized controlled trial. *PLOS ONE* **12**, e0172003 (2017).
141. Turner-Cobb, J. M., Michalaki, M. & Osborn, M. Self-conscious emotions in patients suffering from chronic musculoskeletal pain: A brief report. *Psychology & health* **30**, 495–501 (2015).
142. Darlow, B. *et al.* Easy to harm, hard to heal: patient views about the back. *Spine* **40**, 842–850 (2015).
143. Hasenbring, M., Ulrich, H. W., Hartmann, M. & Soyka, D. The Efficacy of a Risk Factor-Based Cognitive Behavioral Intervention and Electromyographic Biofeedback in Patients with Acute Sciatic Pain: An Attempt to Prevent Chronicity. *Spine* **24**, 2525 (1999).
144. Darlow, B. Beliefs about back pain: the confluence of client, clinician and community. *International Journal of Osteopathic Medicine* **20**, 53–61 (2016).
145. Risch, S. V. *et al.* Lumbar strengthening in chronic low back pain patients. Physiologic and psychological benefits. *Spine* **18**, 232–238 (1993).
146. Hill, J. C. *et al.* A primary care back pain screening tool: Identifying patient subgroups for initial treatment. *Arthritis Care & Research* **59**, 632–641
147. Wertli, M. M., Held, U., Lis, A., Campello, M. & Weiser, S. Both positive and negative beliefs are important in patients with spine pain: findings from the Occupational and Industrial Orthopaedic Center registry. *The Spine Journal* (2017). doi:10.1016/j.spinee.2017.07.166
148. Claus, D. *et al.* An evidence-based information booklet helps reduce fear-avoidance beliefs after first-time discectomy for disc prolapse. *Annals of Physical and Rehabilitation Medicine* **60**, 68–73 (2017).
149. Louw, A., Diener, I. & Puentedura, E. J. The short term effects of preoperative neuroscience education for lumbar radiculopathy: A case series. *International journal of spine surgery* **9**, (2015).
150. Grøvle, L., Haugen, A. J., Natvig, B., Brox, J. I. & Grotle, M. The prognosis of self-reported paresthesia and weakness in disc-related sciatica. *European Spine Journal* **22**, 2488–2495 (2013).
151. Rufa, A., Beissner, K. & Dolphin, M. The use of pain neuroscience education in older adults with chronic back and/or lower extremity pain. *Physiotherapy theory and practice* 1–11 (2018).
152. Verwoerd, A. J. H., Luijsterburg, P. A. J., Koes, B. W., el Barzouhi, A. & Verhagen, A. P. Does Kinesiophobia Modify the Effects of Physical Therapy on Outcomes in Patients With Sciatica in Primary Care? Subgroup Analysis From a Randomized Controlled Trial. *Phys Ther* **95**, 1217–1223 (2015).
153. Waddell, G., Newton, M., Henderson, I., Somerville, D. & Main, C. J. A Fear-Avoidance Beliefs Questionnaire (FABQ) and the role of fear-avoidance beliefs in chronic low back pain and disability. *Pain* **52**, 157–168 (1993).
154. Verwoerd, A. J. H., Luijsterburg, P. A. J., Timman, R., Koes, B. W. & Verhagen, A. P. A single question was as predictive of outcome as the Tampa Scale for Kinesiophobia in people with sciatica: an observational study. *Journal of Physiotherapy* **58**, 249–254 (2012).
155. Sloan, T. J. & Walsh, D. A. Explanatory and Diagnostic Labels and Perceived Prognosis in Chronic Low Back Pain. *Spine* **35**, E1120 (2010).
156. Diener, I., Kargela, M. & Louw, A. Listening is therapy: Patient interviewing from a pain science perspective. *Physiotherapy theory and practice* **32**, 356–367 (2016).

Chapter 5 The clinical examination

Key points

- Combinations of tests help rule the spine and nerve root involvement in or out
- Deficits are more pronounced in those with radicular sciatica compared to extraspinal or myofascial sciatica
- Red flag signs may prompt urgent or emergent referral

Examination flow

The examination helps localize the source or sources of sciatic pain. This influences the treatment plan and decision to obtain further testing. The history and symptoms of sciatica guide the examination. The overarching principle of the sciatica examination is to rule in or out the lumbar spine, the most common source of sciatica. The examination uses a combination of palpation, range of motion (ROM), neurological, and orthopedic tests. Nevertheless, the exact source of symptoms may not be clear.

A **cluster** of positive tests has a greater diagnostic utility than individual tests. Studies have shown that **multiple segmental findings** for S1 radiculopathy including dermatomal pain, plantar flexion weakness, and reduced Achilles reflex, and positive SLR has a high specificity for L5-S1 lumbar disc herniation (LDH) (sp 94-99%).[1,2] Studies have also found that signs of L5 radiculopathy including dermatomal pain, extensor hallucis longus weakness, a positive straight leg raise (SLR), and normal Achilles reflex are highly specific for L4-5 herniation (sp 83-95.5).[1,2] The combination of at least 3 provocative tests for the (SIJ) is more predictive than any individual test for diagnosing SIJ pain.[3] Combinations of tests are more accurate than individual findings.

Figure 114: Examination findings to rule in or out nerve root and spinal involvement in sciatica: Abbreviations: Directional preference (DP), neurological tests (neuro), negative likelihood ratio (-LR), orthopedic and neurodynamic tests (ortho) positive likelihood ratio (+LR), SLR (straight leg raise), trigger point (TrP)

	Rule in nerve root / spine	Rule out nerve root / spine
Palpation	• Gluteal TrPs (+LR 8.6)[4]	• Absence of gluteal TrPs (-LR 0.3)[4]
ROM & DP	• Centralization with DP (+LR infinite)[5]	• Absence of centralization with DP (-LR 0.18 to 0.5)[6,7]
Neuro	• Combination of reflex, motor, and sensory deficit (+LR infinite)[8]	• Absence of any neurological deficit (-LR 0.4-0.5)[9,10]
Ortho	• SLR positive (+LR 2.2-4.7)[11,12] • Slump test causes pain distal to knee (+LR 11.9)[13] • Slump test (+LR 4.9-8.6)[11,12]	• SLR negative (-LR 0.05)[12,14] • Slump test negative (-LR 0.1 to 0.18)[11,13] • Bragard's test negative (-LR 0.5)[15]

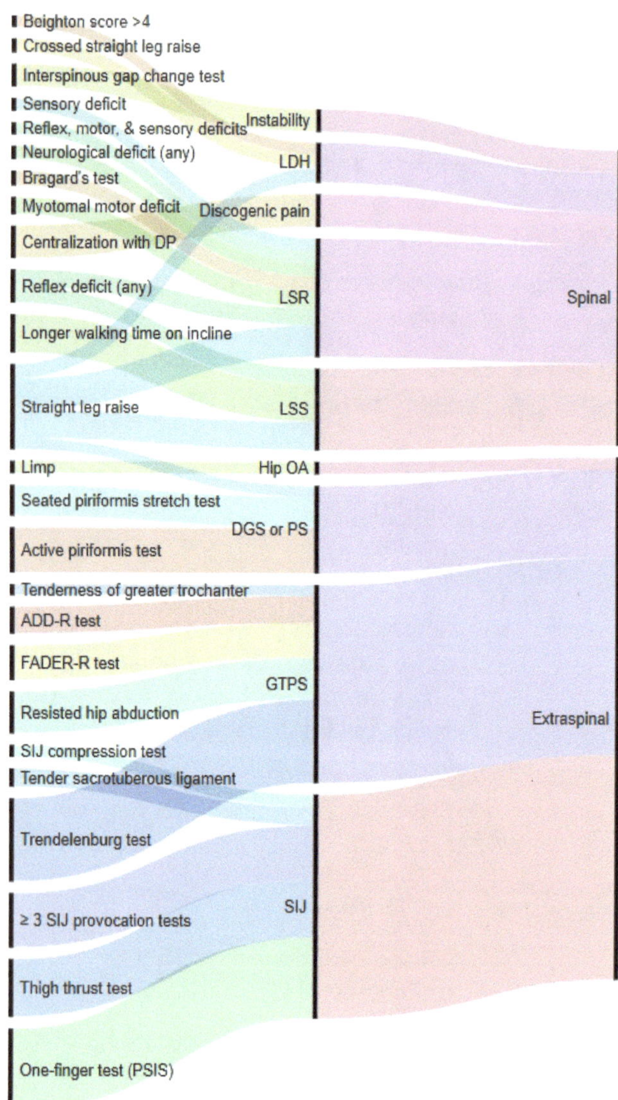

Figure 115: Overview of examination factors with the greatest odds ratios for sciatica, categorized by diagnosis and location. Diagnoses are distinct according to the gold standard test used in the referenced study. Abbreviations include LSR (lumbosacral radiculopathy), LSS (lumbar spinal stenosis), LDH (lumbar disc herniation), GTPS (greater trochanteric pain syndrome), OA (osteoarthritis), NR (nerve root), DGS (deep gluteal syndrome), PS (piriformis syndrome), and SIJ (sacroiliac joint pain). The size of each row correlates with an increasing diagnostic odds ratio (OR), ranging from 3.50 to 26.46. Data adapted from multiple authors.[4,5,7,12,15,16,16-25]

Inspection

Skin

Skin findings may help identify the cause of sciatica or its comorbidities or sequelae. Findings include varicose veins, rashes, birthmarks, and signs of cardiovascular disease. Clinicians should consider these findings within a differential diagnosis although they may be incidental or unrelated to the cause of sciatica.

Patients with sciatica may have signs of vascular or venous disease. One study of 21 patients with LDH found that 62% of patients had **telangiectasias** (small groups of dilated blood vessels) or **reticular veins** (small dilated veins), 10% had varicose veins, and 4% had venous edema. One case reported improvement of leg telangiectasias, reticular veins, and cyanosis following manual therapies to the lumbar spine, which was suggestive that lumbar spine therapies indirectly alleviated these findings.[16]

Rarely varicosities along the course of the sciatic nerve cause sciatica. One study found that sciatic patients with varicose veins in the lower extremity were more likely to have a **sciatic nerve varicosity**.[17] Another study found that in these cases, sciatic nerve pain could be provoked by compression of the end point of a varix in the popliteal fossa.[18] Superficial low-back varicose veins may be seen in those with **epidural varicosis**.[19]

Lower **extremity edema** in sciatica may be a sign of pain-related immobility,[16] injury, or rarely a red flag. Lymphedema may occur in patients with sciatica related to metastasis or tumors of the spine or pelvis, or those who have undergone radiation therapy.[20] Leg edema is also seen in those with sciatic nerve compression palsy, typically after a long period of compression while intoxicated.[21,22] Rarely, piriformis syndrome may cause leg edema related to deep vein thrombosis.[23]

Lower extremity edema in sciatica may be caused by dysfunction of the autonomic nervous system.[16] One animal study found that stimulation of the lumbosacral nerve roots caused **plasma extravasation** in the extremities.[24] This effect was thought to be caused by an antidromic or efferent action of autonomic neurons.[24]

A rash may point to an infectious etiology of sciatica. A **vesicular rash** in a lumbosacral dermatome that correlates with segmental deficits may indicate herpes zoster radiculopathy.[25] Sciatica with **erythema migrans**, also called a bull's-eye rash, points to neuroborreliosis (Lyme disease).[26] **Acrodermatitis chronica atrophicans** (ACA) is a rash with initial skin swelling and erythema followed by thinning, hair loss, telangiectasias, altered pigmentation, and varicose veins. Borrelia burgdorferi, the agent of Lyme disease, may cause this rash and disc herniations by damaging collagen fibers.[27]

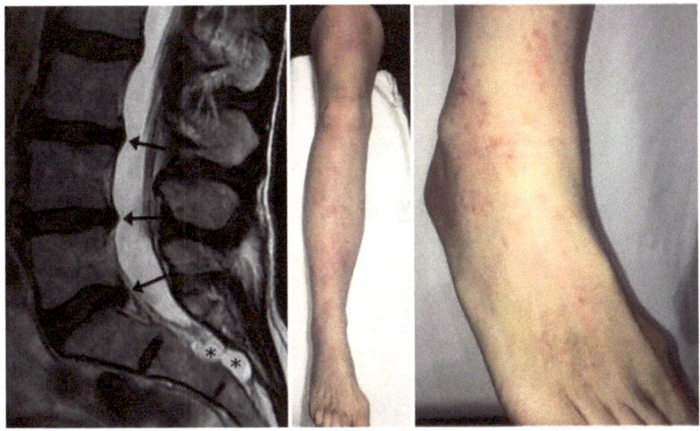

Figure 116: Lyme and disc lesions. This 49-year-old woman presented with chronic aching pain in the low back, and R gluteal region, and thigh. Presence of systemic symptoms such as rash, night sweats, headaches, and brain fog prompted a western blot which showed three positive bands for Borrelia burgdorferi. MRI revealed disc bulges at L3-4, L4-5, and a disc herniation at L5-S1 (arrows) as well as two Tarlov cysts. Her rash is red with bluish spots, with sclerotic areas and swelling, called acrodermatitis chronica atrophicans, and is characteristic of chronic Lyme disease.

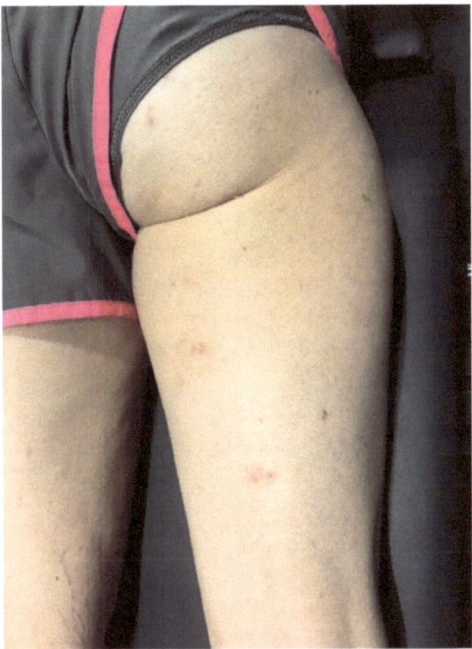

Figure 117: A middle-aged woman presented with a 3-day history of radiating pain and paresthesia in the R S1 dermatome. Further inspection revealed a vesicular dermatomal rash. She was referred to her primary care physician for suspected zoster radiculopathy and rapidly improved with antiviral therapy. Case shared with patient's permission by Robert Trager, DC.

Congenital skin markings rarely point to an underlying anomaly or tumor. Those with multiple **café-au-lait macules** related to neurofibromatosis may have a schwannoma causing sciatica. A **cutaneous hemangioma** over 4 cm in diameter that crosses the midline may relate to underlying spinal anomalies such as a spinal hemangioma, vascular malformation, or tethered spinal cord.[28]

Skin discoloration occasionally points to systemic or metabolic etiologies. Dark bluish discoloration of skin in the ear, hands, or grayish discoloration of the sclera occurs in **ochronosis**, also called alkaptonuria. Ochronosis can cause early degenerative changes in the lumbar spine.[29] **Dependent rubor** (redness) of the legs is seen in those with aortoiliac occlusive disease. Redness and warmth in the extremities may suggest a systemic attack of gout involving the spine or SIJ.

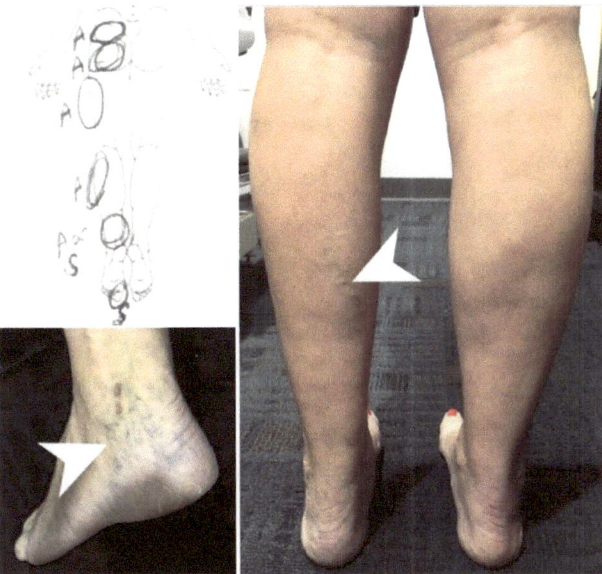

Figure 118: Varicose veins in sciatica. This 49-year old woman presented with a 6-year history of left sided sciatica (aching "A" and stabbing pain "S") and muscle atrophy. She had reduced sensation of the left lateral leg, medial hamstring and Achilles hyporeflexia, and L5-S2 myotomal weakness resulting from a LDH at L5-S1. Varicose veins (arrowheads) in this case were incidental or secondary to the atrophy, disuse, or neurological consequences of the disc lesion. Case from Robert Trager, DC, with patient's permission.

Blanching is the pale skin response to finger pressure. It may relate to the poor blood flow, fascial changes, and subcutaneous edema in those with sciatica. Clinicians can use finger pressure into the lumbar soft tissue to temporarily restrict blood flow and blanch the skin surface. When the skin does not rapidly return to its normal color this is thought to indicate poor blood flow.[30] This sign is called **blood stasis** or **sha stasis** in the gua sha literature, and is thought to indicate that gua sha will help the patient.[31]

Blanching may result from autonomic effects of muscle trigger points.[32] Patients with trigger point-related sciatica often have **vasoconstriction** and reduced temperature in the region of sciatic pain.[33] When trigger points are treated, for example with dry needling, vasodilation occurs and temperature increases in the pain distribution.[33] These effects may relate to the increased sympathetic nervous system activity in those with myofascial pain.

Lumbar **trophedema**, a localized subcutaneous edema, is occasionally reported in those with low back pain and radicular sciatica.[34,35] One study reported an incidence of lumbar trophedema in 50% of cases of sciatica.[34] **Lumbar subcutaneous edema** seen on MRI may relate to the clinical finding of trophedema and is found in over half of low back pain, radiculopathy, and sciatica patients.[36]

Lumbar subcutaneous edema accumulates between the deep thoracolumbar fascia and the subcutaneous fat. It may be caused by inflammation, poor microcirculation, poor lymphatic flow, fat deposition,[37] and instability of the spine.[36] It is more frequently seen in those that are obese.[38] The inflammation and pain may form a cycle of lack of movement[39] followed by weight gain and more edema.

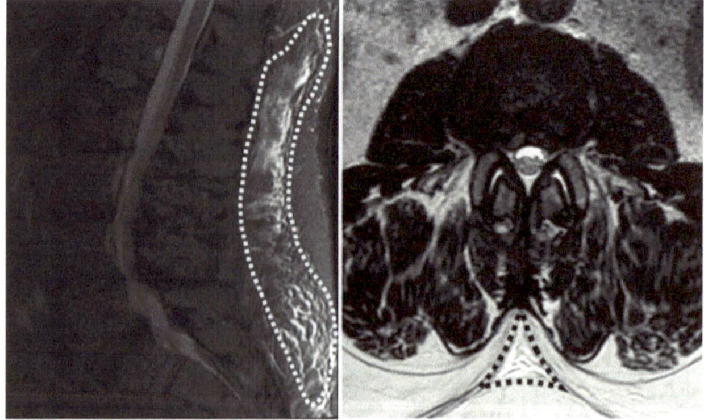

Figure 119: Lumbar subcutaneous edema. This 61-year old male presented with L sided sciatic pain radiating to his L calf. The left image is a sagittal STIR showing subcutaneous edema (dashed line). The right image shows the typical triangle shape of edema just posterior to the spinous processes (dashed line). Case from Robert Trager, DC, with patient's permission.

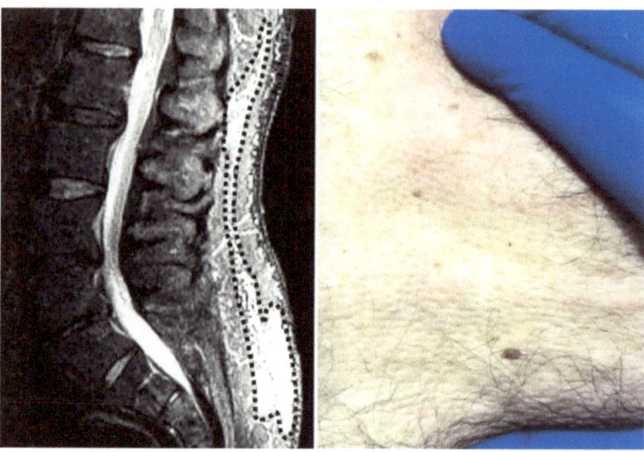

Figure 120: Peau d'orange of lumbar subcutaneous edema. A 52-year-old man presented with chronic radiating pain and numbness from the low back into the R gluteal region and lateral thigh. He had both discogenic radicular signs and myofascial pain. Left: STIR sagittal MRI showing subcutaneous edema (dotted line). Right – dimpling around hair follicles of thickened skin (peau d'orange) is identified by gently squeezing the skin. Symptoms improved most with a combination of instrument-assifsted soft tissue manipulation and lumbar traction. Case shared with patient's permission by Robert Trager, DC.

Trophedema gives a **peau d'orange** (orange peel) appearance of the skin when it is squeezed together, instead of normal wrinkling.[34] Peau d'orange is a **dimpled appearance** created by the hair follicles being surrounded by raised thickened edematous skin. A clinician may also press a blunt object into the skin to reveal subcutaneous edema. The matchstick test is performed by pressing the end of a matchstick into the lower back or thigh.[34] Indentations that remain for minutes indicate subcutaneous edema. Another method is to press the thumb into the lumbar or sacral fascia for 20 seconds and assess for **pitting**.[40] Some clinicians also use a pinch-roll palpation technique to identify lumbar trophedema.[35]

Changes of the toenails may point to comorbidities of sciatica. A blackish discoloration of the nail plate, called **melanochynia**, may indicate vitamin B12 deficiency. **Whitening** or thickening of the nails or absent lunulae are signs of cardiovascular disease and may indicate aortoiliac occlusive disease.

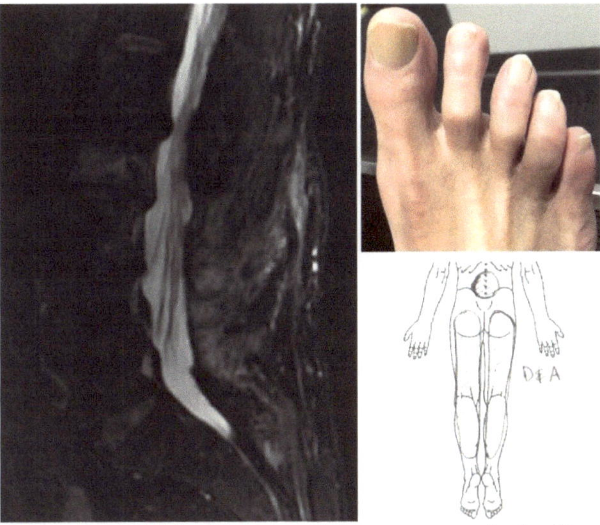

Figure 121: This 68-year-old man presented with a 10-year history of severe lower back pain and bilateral sciatica. A laminectomy for LSS (Left) did not alleviate his symptoms, after which a cardiologist diagnosed him with aortoiliac occlusive disease via angiography. Common iliac artery stents helped alleviate his residual pain. He had increased pain with SLR, diminished dorsal pedal pulses, whitening of the nails and absent lunulae (signs of cardiovascular disease) and did not demonstrate a directional preference. A combination of LSS and vascular pathology caused his symptoms. Case from Robert Trager, DC, images shared with patient's permission.

Posture

Lateral shift

Sciatic scoliosis, also called a lateral shift, lateral trunk shift, trunk list, lateral list, lumbosacral list, or antalgia, is an acute-onset abnormal posture with the torso shifted to one side relative to the pelvis. A lateral shift is a **non-structural scoliosis** related to muscle spasm. It has also been defined as over a 5-degree Cobb angle between L1 and L5 on a standing radiograph.[41] Most cases (about 80%) of sciatic scoliosis involve an **ipsilateral lumbar convexity** on the side of pain with a **contralateral lateral shift** towards the non-painful side.[42–45] This common pattern does not depend of the type or position of disc herniation (e.g. medial or lateral to the nerve root),[44] nor does its severity correlate with degree of disability.[45]

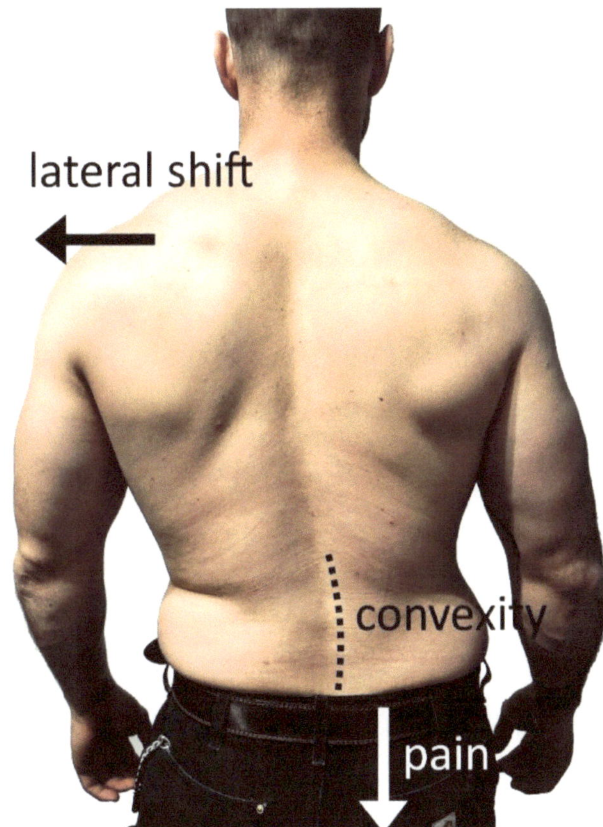

Figure 122: The most common pattern of lateral shift away from the side of sciatica. Image shared with permission of patient by Robert Trager, DC.

The naming of a lateral shift describes the side that the upper torso shifts to, relative to the pelvis. A **plumb line** from C7 or T12 relative to S1 helps measure a lateral shift. If the upper torso moves the plumb line to the left of S1, this is a left lateral shift. If the torso moves right, it is a right lateral shift. The naming (right or left) of scoliosis corresponds to its convex side.

A lateral shift may be differentiated from an idiopathic scoliosis according to the response during Adam's **forward bending test**.[46] If no rib hump is present, this supports a diagnosis of lateral shift opposed to scoliosis.

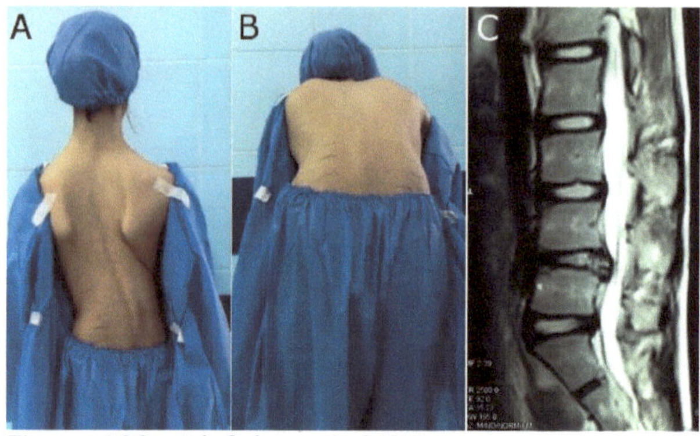

Figure 123: A left lateral shift in response to a right sided LDH at L4-5. The left shift (A) presents with no rib hump during Adam's forward bend (B). MRI (C) reveals the most common disc level of L4-5 for a lateral shift. Images from Omidi-Kashani using CC-BY-3.0 license.[46]

Sciatic scoliosis is a protective neurological reflex that limits or reduces nerve compression. This adaptive response to relieve pressure from spinal pathology has been called **autonomic decompression**.[43] The same-side convexity reduces pressure on the disc and/or nerve lesion by opening the **intervertebral foramen**.[44] The shift also moves **weight-bearing** to the healthy side.[42] Sciatic scoliosis is thought to be caused by a spinal cord reflex that stimulates the contralateral **psoas** and **quadratus lumborm**,[47] and possibly the erector spinae.

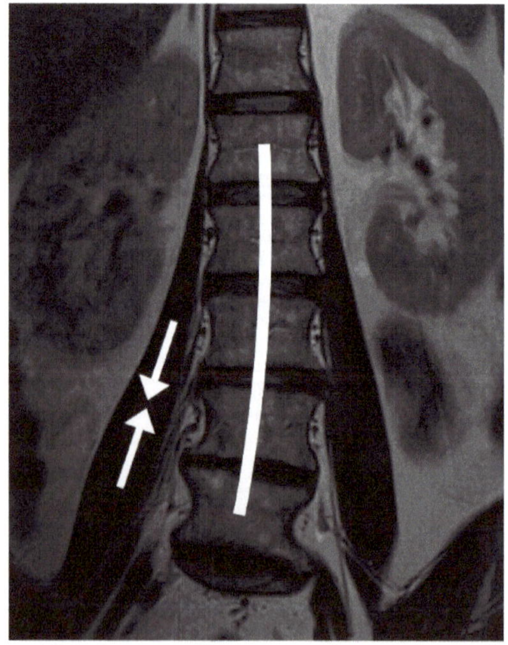

Figure 124: Spasm of the psoas (arrows) may induce a sciatic scoliosis (curve) -schematic.

The most common cause of a lateral shift is a **lumbar disc herniation** (LDH). Lateral shifts occur in 18% of cases of discogenic sciatica.[48,49] Despite the classic appearance, a lateral shift has a low diagnostic utility for radicular sciatica with a sensitivity of 15% and specificity of 53%.[9] The presence of a lateral shift has the strongest association with **L4-5** herniations (odds ratio, OR 5.6),[49] probably because L4-5 has greater coronal plane movement compared to L5-S1.[50] Females are more likely to develop a lateral shift than males (OR 4.3).[49]

A lateral shift occurs in conditions other than LDH. Cases of **annular fissure** or discogenic pain without herniation,[51] muscle spasms,[52] SIJ disorders,[52] and less often in piriformis syndrome,[53] cases of spinal tumors, such as osteoid osteoma and osteoblastoma,[54] and infections of the spine can produce a lateral shift. A lumbar scoliosis related to degenerative LSS typically develops gradually over months or years as opposed to an acute lateral shift.

Lordosis

Hyperlordosis, an increased lumbar lordosis (anterior convex curve) or hypolordosis (reduced lordosis) is not specific for any diagnosis relating to sciatica. Reduction in the lumbar lordosis may be a **pain-avoidance** mechanism as this position causes slackening of the nerve roots.[55] An increase in lordosis may correlate with zygapophyseal joint pain and also been associated with piriformis and deep gluteal syndrome.[56]

The **low midline sill sign** is a wrinkling or thickening of the skin at a point in the lower back that forms a sill or "I" shape, in addition to an anterior change in position of a spinous process compared to the spinous below. The sign is thought to be caused by the anterior position of the spinous process of the vertebra with a spondylolisthesis compared to the inferior vertebra.[57] This sign has a high sensitivity (81%) specificity (89%), positive (79%) and negative (91%) predictive values for lumbar spondylolisthesis.[57]

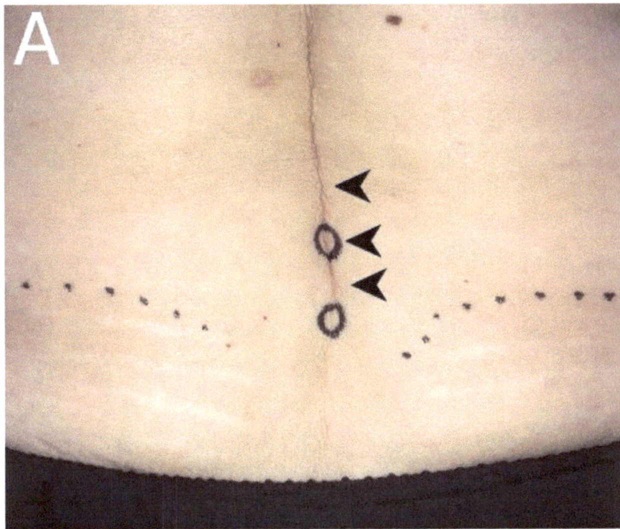

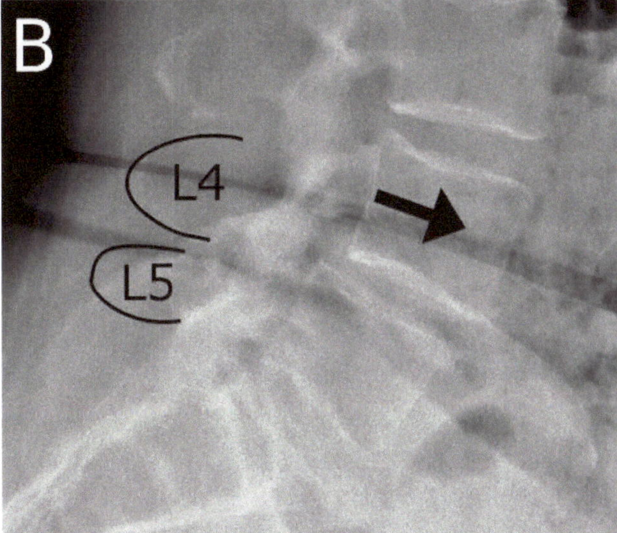

Figure 125: Low midline sill sign. This 63-year-old woman presented with chronic LBP radiating into both thighs and legs, with BL L5/S1 deficits. Examination (A) identified a sill in the skin of the lower back (arrowheads) and anterior position of the L4 spinous in relation to L5 (circled in A, outlined in B). Radiographs (B) demonstrated a degenerative spondylolisthesis of L4 on L5. Case shared with permission of patient by Robert Trager, DC.

Sitting posture

Habitual sitting with the **legs crossed** can compress the common peroneal nerve.[58] Alternatively, sitting with crossed legs could be a pain-avoidance mechanism, as flexion and external rotation of the hip and flexion of the knee reduces sciatic nerve tension. Sitting with a lean with weight on the non-painful buttocks and avoiding weight on the side of sciatica can be a sign of deep gluteal syndrome.[59]

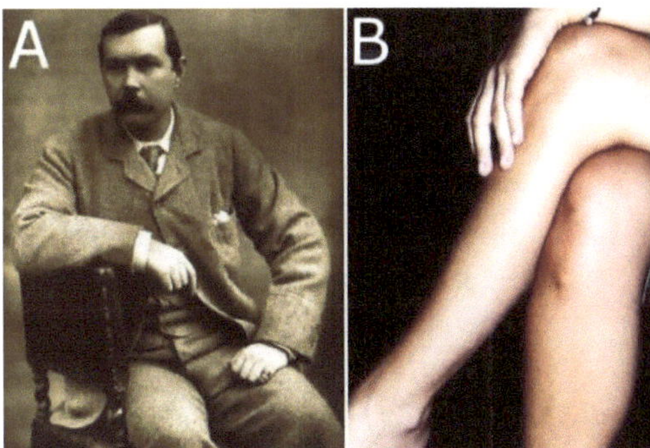

Figure 126:(A) Sitting and leaning away from pain may indicate a deep gluteal syndrome. (B) Habitual leg crossing may indicate common peroneal nerve injury or neural tension. Image (A) of Arthur Conan Doyle public domain. Image (B) CC BY 2.0 by Stefano Mortellaro.

Leg-length discrepancy

Leg-length discrepancy in patients with radiating pain is most often associated with LDH. One study of patients with LDH and radiating pain found that leg length deficiency correlated with the side pain in women but not in men.[60] The study found that pain radiated into the **shorter leg** in about 70% of women with a leg length discrepancy of 1 mm or more.[60] A recent large study found no significant association of leg length with greater trochanteric pain syndrome (GTPS).[61]

Gait

Patients with sciatica may have one or more adaptive gait patterns including changes in walking posture, stride length, speed, or base of support. Gait analysis helps determine if symptoms stem from LSS, LDH, or a deep gluteal syndrome.

Neurogenic claudication

Neurogenic claudication refers to leg pain or numbness that occurs with walking or standing and reduces with sitting or resting with the spine flexed. Dynamic changes of the spine that occur with walking including epidural pressure, lumbar instability, disc bulging, and ligament buckling may account for these symptoms. Neurogenic claudication has a high diagnostic utility for **lumbar spinal stenosis (LSS)**, with a sensitivity of 82%, specificity of 78%, +LR 3.7, -LR 0.2, and odds ratio of 11.4.[62,63]

Caelius Aurelianus may have been the first to describe neurogenic claudication around 450 CE. He discovered that as patients walked they began to feel sciatic pain and thus were either forced to stop or flex forward.[64]

> *...even in the case of one who is able to walk, the first steps are difficult and there is a*

> *burning sensation... all of a sudden the patient has to sit down again... others have their bodies drawn and bent forward (Drabkin p. 909)*

Dynamic changes of the disc and spinal ligaments may explain neurogenic claudication. Walking upright may cause bulging of **discs**[65] and buckling of the **ligamentum flavum**,[66,67] which narrows the spinal canal. Walking upright may also increase **lumbar instability** related to spondylolisthesis,[68] which will further reduce the size of the lumbar canal. Conversely, lumbar flexion increases the size of the **spinal canal** and **intervertebral foramina**, which may reduce pressure on compromised nerve roots in those with LSS.[66] The stooped gait of neurogenic claudication may be an adaptive mechanism that helps avoid radicular pain.

Increases in lumbar **epidural pressure** may explain neurogenic claudication. Walking with a flexed spine reduces the lumbar epidural pressure compared to walking upright.[67] Those with LSS have a more pronounced reduction in epidural pressure with flexion,[67] which may explain why these patients walked stooped. Epidural pressure could also result from the reduction in spinal canal size with an upright or extended posture compared to flexed.

Alternatively, the stooped gait of neurogenic claudication may occur due to **hip flexion** rather than spine flexion.[68] Hip flexion can be a pain-avoidance mechanism to reduce tension in the psoas and anterior shear force on the lumbar spine. Increased hip flexion during walking could reduce symptoms related to instability during walking.

In the **stoop test** the patient walks at least 50 meters while standing straight to determine if sciatic symptoms increase. If symptoms are subsequently abolished by walking stooped (with a flexed spine) or sitting, the test is positive and indicates LSS.[66] Walking tests have a low sensitivity (58%) but high specificity (82%) for LSS.[68] If claudication symptoms reduce by walking with a flexed spine, the odds of LSS being present increase by a factor of 6.2.[68]

The **two-stage treadmill test** involves having the patient walk at a self-determined pace on a level treadmill until claudication symptoms increase, for a maximum of 10 minutes or until they feel the need to stop. The patient then sits until symptoms subside, then repeats the test on a 15° incline. If the patient's symptoms begin sooner and they need a longer recovery period when **walking level** compared to an incline, the test is positive. A positive test has a sensitivity of 76.9%, specificity of 94.7%, and increases the likelihood of LSS by a factor of 14.5.[69]

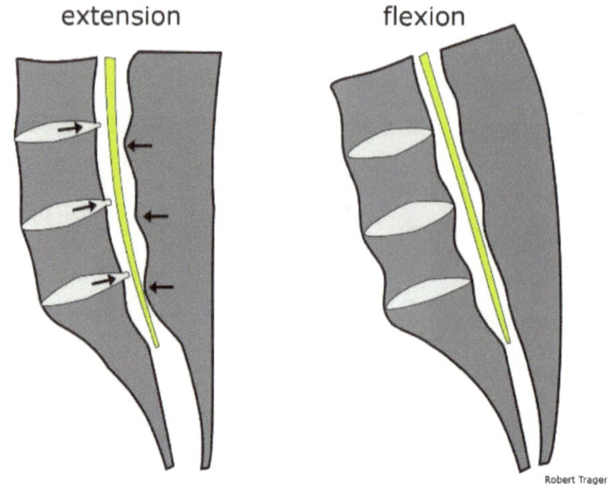

Figure 127: In older patients with LSS, the lumbar canal reduces in diameter during upright walking or extension due to bulging of discs and buckling of spinal ligaments (arrows). The canal diameter increases with flexion and alleviates compression of the lumbosacral nerve roots.

Patients with neurogenic claudication caused by LSS may have less symptoms when walking with a cane, shopping cart, walker, or even a lawnmower. The **shopping cart sign** describes any reduction of symptoms in a supported flexed position. Using a shopping cart increases spinal flexion by 3.4° and unloads the spine by almost 7% of body weight.[70] Unloading the spine may reduce dynamic disc bulging or instability, whereas spinal flexion may widen the spinal canal and IVFs.

Stride length

Hip mobility, neural tension, and pelvic rotation affect stride length. Pain at separate phases of gait may help distinguish between different causes of sciatica. Neural tension and hip immobility may reduce stride length in the same manner that they may restrict a straight leg raise test.

The most common conditions to produce a **shorter stride** in sciatica are LDH, LSS, and hip-spine syndrome. In those with LSS, shorter stride length correlates with a greater level of overall disability.[71] Those with acute or severe LDH may also have reduced stride length. One study of hospitalized patients with discogenic sciatica showed a reduction in stride length by 40%.[72] Patients with **hip-spine syndrome** (hip pathology along with sciatica) may shorten the stride by limiting hip extension to avoid symptoms. These patients tend to lift the foot on the side of sciatic pain before it the hip extends maximally.

A hip flexion contracture causes flexion, adduction, and internal rotation of the involved hip or hips. It also causes a compensatory increase in pelvic and trunk movement to aid in hip movement. When these findings are bilateral it is called a **tight-rope-walker's gait**, and when unilateral this is called a **psoatic limp**.[73] The reduced hip extension limits stride length in patients with hip flexion contracture.

Patients with sciatica from **hamstring tendinopathy** have pain with longer strides, especially when the heel contacts the ground. The **long-stride heel strike test** assesses for pain proximal and lateral to the ischium at heel strike or hip flexion phase of a long-stride gait. A positive test increases the odds of sciatic nerve entrapment by a hamstring tear.[74]

Most patients with chronic LDH have a normal stride length.[75] It is thought that an increase in **pelvic rotation** helps maintain stride length in these patients.[75] Improved neural mobility with improvement of the disc pathology over time may also facilitate longer strides.

Velocity

A reduced gait velocity can be found in both LSS[71] and severe LDH.[72] In those with LSS the gait velocity is inversely related to the level of disability,[71] meaning the worse the disability, the slower the gait.

Hip and pelvis movement

The gait of LDH is **slow and deliberate**.[76] At slower speeds the gait may appear normal but when patients attempt to walk faster they increase **pelvic rotation**.[75,77] This causes rotation of the thorax and lumbar spine with the pelvis,[75] and causes the arms to swing more with the legs (opposite of normal). These movements are less energy-efficient but allow for short-term guarding against pain.

Trendelenburg's sign is when the unaffected pelvis drops lower while walking, or if the patient compensates by leaning toward the affected hip. During the stance phase of gait on the side affected by sciatica, the opposite side hip can dip down due to inability of the hip abductors to stabilize the pelvis. This indicates hip abductor and **gluteus medius** weakness and is most often seen in cases of sciatica caused by GTPS[78] and L5 radiculopathy.

Those with hip-related sciatica often have one of many alterations of gait to reduce pain or adapt for a loss in hip movement. The loss of hip ROM associated with hip disorders may cause a compensatory increase in lumbar and pelvic movement. Low back and sciatic patients with a **limp** have odds of hip-related symptoms increased by a factor of 3.9.[79]

Patients with hip osteoarthritis may be identified by having limited hip extension.[80] These patients may also have a **pelvic wink**, an increased lumbopelvic rotation that compensates for reduced hip extension. Hip-spine syndrome is a cause of pelvic wink in sciatica.

Patients with piriformis syndrome have greater amounts of hip flexion and internal rotation, and less hip extension during gait.[75] These movements could exacerbate symptoms because they tension the sciatic nerve. The gait of piriformis syndrome involves a hip position that may contribute to ongoing symptoms.

Base of support

A **wide-based gait** in a patient with sciatica is a sign of significantly impaired lower extremity sensation and balance. One study of 93 patients with low back pain found that a wide-based gait is highly specific (97%) for LSS and significantly increases its likelihood (+LR 14.3).[81] The width of the base of support is directly related to the level of disability in those with LSS.[71]

Specific weakness

Patients with L4 radiculopathy have increased **knee flexion** after heel strike, possibly due to **quadriceps weakness**.[80] Increased knee flexion with heel strike can help distinguish radiculopathy and LSS from hip symptoms, which do not necessarily cause quadriceps weakness.

Foot drop, a dragging or dropping of the foot during walking, indicates weakness of the dorsiflexors of the ankle. One large study of patients with foot drop found that, excluding central nervous system causes, the majority were caused by **common peroneal nerve** lesions (30.6%), followed by L5 radiculopathies (19.7%), and polyneuropathies (18.3%).[82]

Those with S1 radiculopathy have reduced ability to **push-off** during gait. One study found that patients with L5-S1 disc herniation had a 17% reduction in push-off. The study also found this finding was specific to L5-S1 disc pathology and not seen in lesions at L4-5.[83]

Guarding

Those with LDH have an adaptive gait pattern that involves increased paraspinal and core muscle tone. The erector spinae, multifidus, quadratus lumborum, and abdominal obliques have increased activity which reduces anterior-posterior **shear forces** on L4 and L5.[84] In the short-term, guarding protects against instability and discogenic pain; however long-term guarding during gait may be detrimental because it adds compression to the lumbar intervertebral discs (IVDs).[84] Additional spinal compression could then increase the long-term risk of additional disc herniation.[84]

Muscle inspection

Severe or longstanding cases of sciatica may cause atrophy, a decrease in the size of muscles. Calf atrophy is uncommon and has a low sensitivity in LDH.[85] Atrophy of smaller muscles in the feet may be more common and easier to recognize. Pseudohypertrophy (also called fatty replacement, denervation hypertrophy, and neurogenic hypertrophy) causing enlargement of the calf is also possible in nerve lesions causing sciatica and has most often been reported in LDH.[86,87]

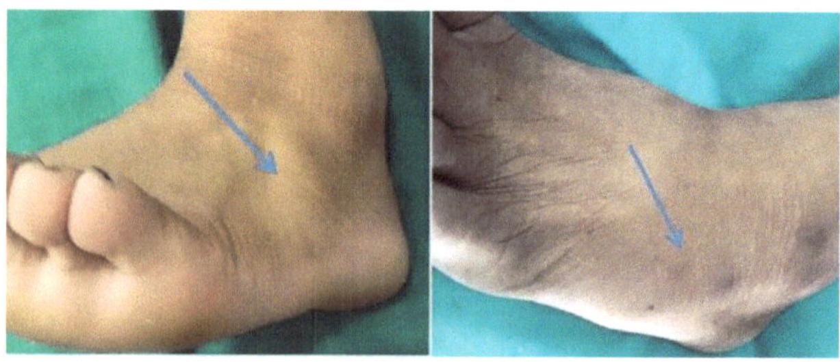

Figure 128: Atrophy of the extensor digitorum brevis (EDB). A normal foot (left) has a bulge caused by the EDB on the lateral foot while an atrophied foot (right) does not. The EDB is the most commonly atrophied muscle in patients with LDH or LSS.[88] Image CC BY 4.0 license from Munakomi.[88]

The Roman physician Caelius Aurelianus gave the first description of muscle atrophy and pseudohypertrophy (enlargement) in sciatica circa 450 CE:

> *When the disease slows [the person] down, nourishment ceases, and the whole leg becomes thin, which the Greeks call atrophian (Author's translation, Aurelianus, p.496)*[89]

Fasciculation (muscle twitching), also called **focal neuromyotonia** can occur in sciatica. This causes a continuous rippling, cramping, or twitching of the muscles in the distribution affected by a nerve lesion. This has been reported in LDH with radiculopathy.[90] Leg muscle fasciculation or cramping can be a sign of partial denervation and hypersensitivity of the motor neurons.[34] Twitching can progress into cramping during the night-time, in particular in those with LSS who inadvertently extend the spine while sleeping. Fasciculation can be both a sign of impending denervation but also recovery from denervation to partial denervation.

Range of motion

Lumbar & trunk

Lumbar and trunk ROM tests help find factors contributing to sciatic pain. Abnormally high or low ROM can be a sign of dysfunction or pathology. The movement pattern, velocity, symptoms during movement, and contribution of the hips and pelvis to trunk motion can also give clues to the source of symptoms. Limited trunk range increases the odds of radiating low back pain. Those unable to touch their **fingertips to the floor** have 3.4 times the odds of having radiating low back pain.[91]

Most **lumbar pathology** will reduce lumbar ROM in all directions,[92] except for those with isthmic spondylolisthesis.[93] Reduced spinal extension while standing is the most common loss of ROM in those with low back pain (LBP) radiating distal to the gluteal fold.[94] Those with **lumbar disc herniation** have the greatest reduction in lumbar flexion in standing compared to other movements and those without disc pathology.[95] Those with LDH have more of a restriction of lumbar extension when there is nerve root compression (as seen on MRI).[96] The greatest limitation of those with LSS,[92] including those with foraminal stenosis,[97] is lumbar extension.

Those with **extraspinal sciatica** may have significant limitations in lumbar ROM. One study found that almost half of patients with a lower extremity **nerve entrapment syndrome** had a limited lumbar ROM.[98] The authors suggested that the entrapped nerves were irritated by movements of the sciatic nerve that corresponded to lumbar motion.[98] Those with superior **cluneal nerve entrapment** commonly have limitations of flexion, rotation, and/or lateral flexion.[99] This condition involves entrapment of one or multiple cluneal nerves at the thoracolumbar and upper gluteal fascia. Limitations in lumbar ROM may occur in extraspinal conditions due to restricted neural or myofascial mobility.

Clinicians most often evaluate lumbar ROM using **standing active ROM** and occasionally using passive ROM or ROM in the sitting or lying positions. The **double inclinometer** method is commonly used by placing inclinometers at T12 and S2 or L1 and S1.[100]

Screening tests include the modified **Schober test**, which involves measuring changes in length from marks 5 cm below and 10 cm above the lumbosacral junction from standing to flexion.[95]

The **finger-floor distance**, also called the fingertip-floor distance, is a screening test for **forward bending**. This motion combines hip, lumbar, and thoracic mobility, hamstring flexibility and neural tension. Clinicians may measure the finger-to-floor distance by having the patient reach for the floor with full knee extension. The distance between middle fingers and the floor is the finger-floor distance. Those with a finger-floor distance of **>25 cm** have 2.8 times greater odds of having **lumbosacral nerve root compression**.[12] A faster method of testing the finger-floor distance is assessing the patient's ability to flex to the point where their hands reach **past the knees**.[101] Inability to reach beyond the knees is a sensitive but nonspecific sign of LDH.[101]

Table 16: Normal values for lumbar ROM. Data for lumbar from Troke et al[100] and trunk flexion from Laird[102]

Movement	Normal range
Trunk flexion	90°-121°
Lumbar flexion	40-72°
Lumbar extension	6-29°
Lumbar lateral flexion	15-29°
Lumbar axial rotation	7°

Trunk flexion is the combination of pelvic, hip, and lumbar flexion. The relative contribution of the pelvic-hip complex versus the lumbar region is referred to as **lumbopelvic rhythm**.[102] This value can be expressed as a percentage calculated by lumbar degrees divided by pelvic & hip degrees. The lumbar contribution to trunk flexion in asymptomatic people ranges from 42-61%,[102] meaning the lumbar spine contributes to about half of the total trunk flexion. A sciatic patient most commonly has reduced lumbar range with increased pelvic-hip range. The pattern can be opposite with increased lumbar contribution, for example in a **pars fracture**.

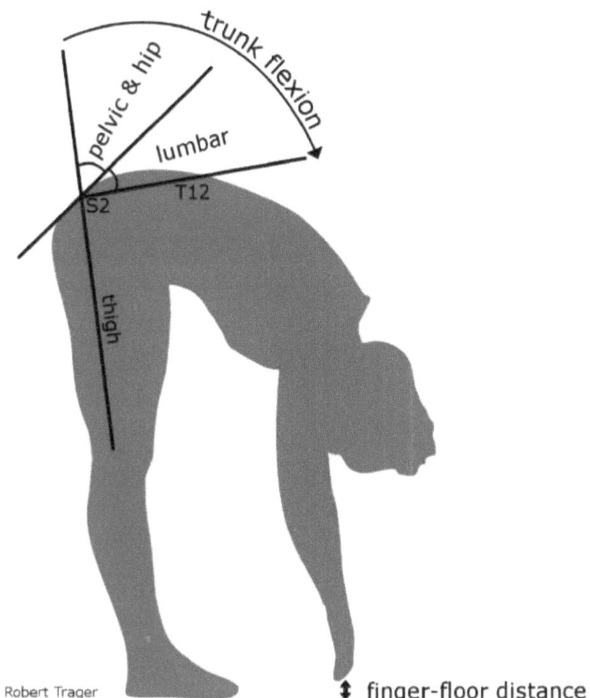

Figure 129: Lumbar flexion, combined with pelvic and hip flexion, make up the total trunk flexion in the sagittal plane

Relative stiffness and **relative flexibility** refer to one body region being more stiff or flexible than another and the potential adverse impact on movement this may have. In the model of **regional interdependence**, movements of the low back depend on neural mobility, hamstring flexibility, hip and pelvis mobility, and many other factors. Lumbar movement patterns may follow the **path of least resistance**, meaning movement happens first in the more flexible regions. Range of motion assessments can help identify relative stiffness or flexibility as it relates to sciatic pain.

Those with LBP and sciatica often have **early lumbar flexion** during forward bending. One study found that LBP sufferers flex the lumbar spine more in the **first 30 degrees** of trunk flexion compared to those without back pain.[103] These patients also have limitations of hamstring flexibility and neural mobility as measured by active knee extension and the straight leg raise.[103]

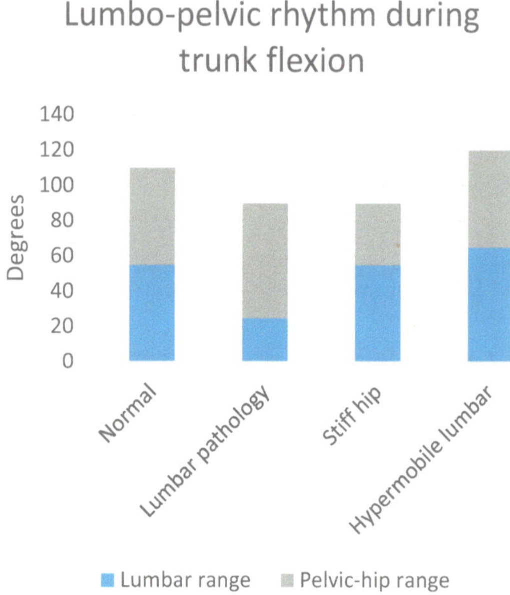

Figure 130: Relative contributions of lumbar and pelvic-hip motion to total trunk flexion. These are typical examples which illustrate the effects of lumbo-pelvic rhythm.

A subset of LBP patients have a greater loss of hip motion compared to low back motion.[104] Those with LBP also begin forward bending with a greater degree of lumbar flexion when picking up objects.[105] Abnormal **early lumbar flexion** is common in LBP and may be due to relative stiffness of the hip,[106] hamstring tightness,[103] or limited neural mobility.[103]

Movement velocity during ROM testing is a more sensitive measure of LBP than ROM itself.[107] Those with degenerative disc disease, disc herniation, spondylolisthesis, and LSS have reduced movement velocity during ROM testing for flexion and extension.[92] People without back pain take 4.4 seconds to go through a cycle of forward and backward bending, whereas those with LBP and a positive SLR take 9.3 seconds, more than double the normal time.[108] Those with LBP with or without a positive SLR also take longer to pick up an object from the floor.[109] Slower movements in those with LBP may relate to increased muscle activity or neural tension.[109]

The **withdrawal test** is a screening test for adverse neural tension and disc pathology. During a forward bend, the pelvis normally moves posteriorly to balance the center of gravity. In those with sciatic neural tension the pelvis does not move posteriorly and lumbar flexion is limited to 45 degrees at most.[110]

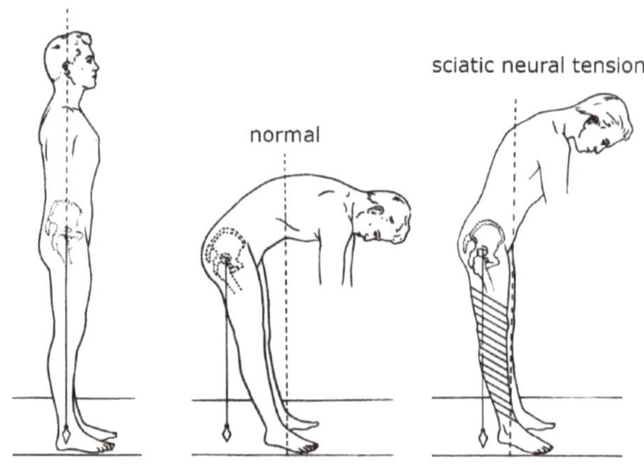

Figure 131: The withdrawal test for sciatic neural tension. Absence of posterior shift of the hips and pelvis and limitation in lumbar flexion during forward bending indicates sciatic nerve tension. Image modified from Michele,[73] public domain.

Persistent **guarding** or activation of the **lumbar paraspinal muscles** may restrict lumbar ROM in those with low back-related leg pain. Those with LDH have greater activity of the erector spinae, lumbar multifidus, semispinalis, and thoracic multifidus during trunk flexion.[111] Patients with low-back related leg pain have been found to lose the **flexion-relaxation response**, in which case the lumbar paraspinal muscles remain abnormally active during flexion.[112] Normally these muscles relax which allows us to reach full flexion. The body may increase paraspinal muscle activity to protect or stabilize injured spinal structures such as the IVD.[113] A reduced lumbar ROM may be a sign of muscle guarding in response to underlying spinal pathology.

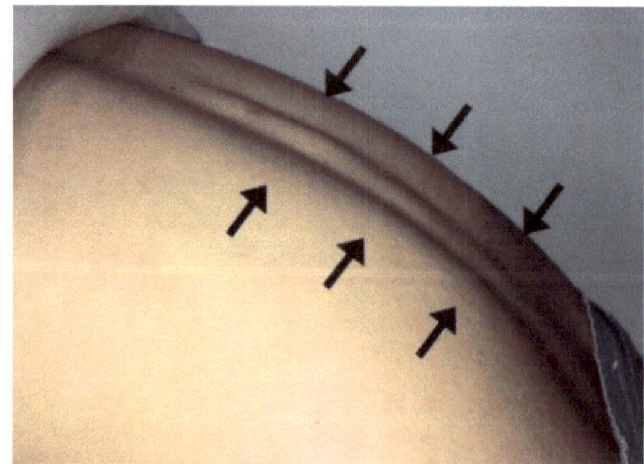

Figure 132: Absent flexion-relaxation response (abnormally increased thoracolumbar erector muscle activity during flexion) in a patient with chronic LBP and 70° of trunk flexion. Shared with permission of patient by Robert Trager DC

Abnormally increased lumbar and trunk ROM can be a sign of underlying **lumbar instability**. One study found that those with greater than 56 degrees of lumbar flexion and greater than 26 degrees of lumbar extension were more likely to have **lumbar instability**.[114] The study also found that those with instability on dynamic radiographs had a significantly higher amount of **total flexion** than those without instability.[114] Those with above-normal lumbar flexion are more likely to have **spondylolysis** (pars fracture).[93] Sciatic patients with ROM above normal range may have lumbar instability and/or pars fracture.

There is a positive correlation between **joint hypermobility** and LDH.[115,116] Joint hypermobility or laxity is measured by the nine-point Beighton scale: Passive dorsiflexion of the 5th finger beyond 90° (1 point each = 2), passive apposition of thumb to flexor part of forearm (1 point each = 2), hyperextension of elbow and knee beyond 10° (1 point each = 4), and **palms-to-floor** during trunk flexion with knees extended (1 point). Those with generalized joint laxity as measured by a **Beighton score > 4** have 3.5 times the odds of having a LDH.[116] Hypermobility may be genetic or acquired, for example during pregnancy.

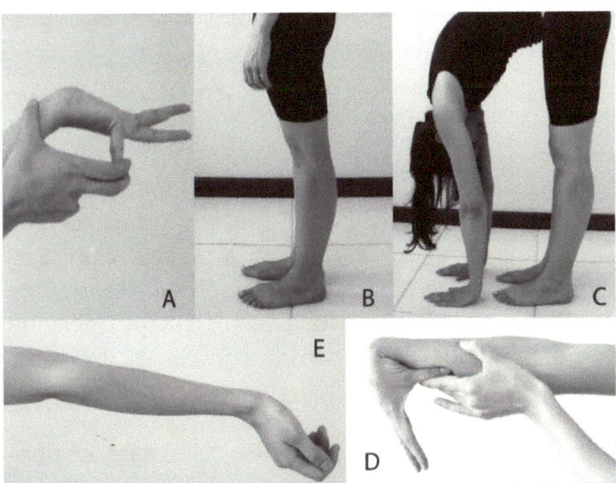

Figure 133: Beighton score for generalized joint hypermobility / ligament laxity. Image from Pasinato et al, 2011, CC BY 4.0 license.

Aberrant movement patterns are abnormal or painful movements that occur during sagittal plane movements. When a patient with back pain has an aberrant movement pattern they are 3.8 times more likely to have lumbar instability.[117] The **instability catch sign** is a sudden pain or inability to move that occurs when extending from a flexed position. This is sometimes referred to as a **painful arc** on return from flexion.[118] A painful arc can also occur during flexion. A **reversed lumbopelvic rhythm** involves moving the pelvis forward while bending the knee to extend from a flexed position.[118] **Gower's sign** is when one must put a hand on their thigh to flex or extend the trunk.[118] Aberrant movements during ROM testing can help identify lumbar instability as a cause of sciatica.

Lumbar ROM testing may be used to monitor **clinical improvement** in sciatica. Improvements in finger-floor distance **>4.5 cm** correlate with improvements in disability related to radicular pain.[119] Improvements in lumbar extension ROM have been found to correlate with **centralization** of sciatica.[120] Other studies have correlated reduction in low back and/or sciatic pain with improvements in ROM following cupping,[121] cryotherapy,[122] and oscillatory manual therapy.[123]

Hip

Hip ROM is often below-average in those with sciatica. Hip extension,[124–126] passive hip flexion, and passive internal rotation are significantly lower in those with LBP.[127] Patients with lower extremity pain with reduced hip **internal ROM** have odds of hip involvement increased by a factor of 7.7.[79] These patients are much less likely to have an isolated pathology of the lumbar spine.[79]

Palpation

Clinicians use palpation to find sites of **hyperalgesia** or **abnormal tissue** along the distribution of the sciatic nerve. Every examination of sciatica should include palpation of the lower back, sciatic nerve, SIJ, gluteal region and hip, thigh, and calf. Palpation helps identify the distribution and severity of symptoms and rarely points to a specific diagnosis.

Clinicians palpate to find areas of increased tenderness as well as structural changes in muscle and fascia. Muscle tenderness is more accurately called **mechanical hyperalgesia of deep somatic structures**.[128] A **trigger point** is a hypersensitive band of muscle that refers pain when stimulated, whereas a tender point does not radiate or refer pain. A muscle spasm is a sudden, involuntary contraction of a muscle. Palpation may also find **allodynia**, pain due to a stimulus that does not normally cause pain. Allodynia can be tactile/mechanical or thermal.

A larger territory of allodynia in the sciatic nerve distribution may reflect a greater degree of **central sensitization**.[129] Symptoms of central sensitization in sciatica include tactile and thermal allodynia[129] as well as pressure sensitivity of muscle (somatic) tissue.[130] Over half (60%) of those with radicular sciatica have allodynia of the lower extremity, whereas those with localized LBP only rarely have this symptom.[129]

Those with **widespread tenderness** are less likely to have discogenic sciatica. One study found that patients with sciatica and more than 8 **tender points** were less likely to have nerve root compression in the lumbar spine (OR 0.15)[131] and more likely to have normal lumbar MRI (OR 1.39).[131] Patients with widespread tenderness may have non-discogenic sciatica and/or an alternative diagnosis such as fibromyalgia.

A **sensitized spinal segment** produces hypertonicity and tenderness within a myotomal or sclerotomal distribution.[133] Some research suggests that **segmental deep mechanical sensitivity** is useful in diagnosing radicular pain.[128,134] Most patients with lumbosacral radicular pain perceive their pain as deep as opposed to on the skin.[134] In addition, muscle tenderness is usually distributed through the proximal and distal extremity.[128] Myotomal pain or tenderness is a palpatory sign of radicular sciatica.

Palpation is not specific to any diagnosis. Areas of tenderness may reflect areas of **secondary hyperalgesia**, an increase in tenderness remote from the area of pathology. In radicular sciatica areas of the gluteal region, thigh, or leg may be tender as a result of central[129] or peripheral sensitization.[135] The sciatic nerve and its branches may be tender in radicular and non-radicular sciatica.[136] Sacral sulcus tenderness is only 9% specific for SIJ pain,[137] while greater trochanter tenderness is only 47% specific for GTPS.[138] Areas of increased tenderness do not necessarily reflect the source of symptoms.

Pinch-roll

The **pinch-and-roll** test is performed by pinching a fold of skin between the thumbs and index fingers, then rolling the skin in one direction and then the other. The trunk is examined from superior to inferior then the lower extremities are examined transversely.[139] In severe cases of pathology, the skin is thickened and difficult to grasp in a fold.[139] In sciatica one may perform pinch-rolling of the trunk, gluteal regions, and any painful regions of the lower extremities.

This test may find **cellulalgia**, also called fibrositis, which is an area of swelling, thickening, hardening, and hypersensitivity. Cellulalgia may be mediated by an **axon reflex** between a spinal segment and its muscles.[139] In this process, injury to a spinal nerve root is thought to stimulate retrograde (backwards) release of inflammatory substances at the sensory nerve endings within the soft tissue. Cellulalgia is a valuable clinical sign if it follows a segmental pattern and may help localize a specific nerve root.

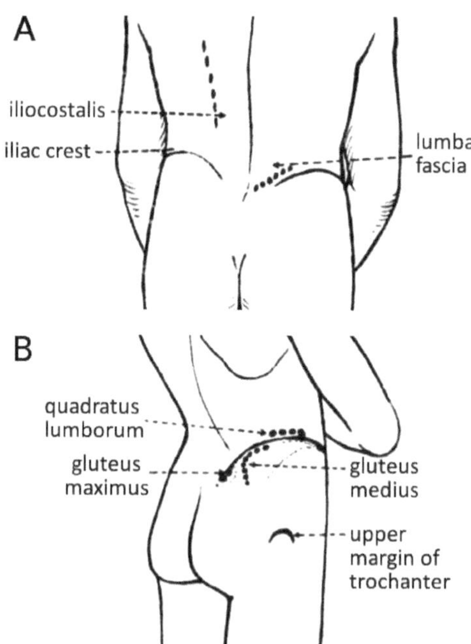

Figure 134: Common locations of cellulalgia (dots) in LBP (A) and sciatica (B), modified from Lewellyn, 1915,[132] public domain.

Pinch-roll technique is an assessment and treatment. Improvement with pinch-roll often coincides with symptomatic improvement of sciatica. One study showed significant improvement of skin tenderness to pinch-roll after four sessions of spinal manipulation for lower back pain compared to sham manipulation.[140]

The distribution of trigger points, cellulalgia, or fibrositis may help determine the origin of sciatica. A segmental pattern of cellulalgia suggests a radicular or spinal origin of pain. Soft tissue changes may also correspond with a peripheral nerve, for example the lateral femoral cutaneous nerve at the lateral thigh in the case of meralgia paresthetica.[139]

Paraspinal points of cellulalgia are thought to relate to sensitization of **the dorsal primary rami** in cases of lumbar radiculopathy.[41,139] Patients with LDH have a lowered pain pressure threshold in paraspinal muscles of the affected side of radiculopathy.[41] This could be due to increased sensitivity or tenderness of the multifidus[41] or other deep paraspinal soft tissue.

Cellulalgia is commonly found at the **crestal point**, an area at the iliac crest 7-8 cm lateral to midline.[139] This point is non-specific and may be tender in cases of radiculopathy, cluneal nerve entrapment, or thoracolumbar fascial thickening. Some authors refer to the relationship between back pain and a tender crestal point as **Maigne's syndrome**.[141] Cellulalgia over the greater trochanter can indicate GTPS (trochanteric bursitis) and L5 radiculopathy.

Trigger points and motor points

A **motor point** is an area of skin that corresponds roughly to the **motor entry point**, an area in which a motor branch of a nerve enters a muscle.[142] This point occurs within the zone of innervation of the muscle, the area with the greatest concentration of neuromuscular junctions.[143] Motor points are also defined as the area where an innervated muscle may be caused to twitch using the least electrical current.[142,143] Motor points vary individually but are identified with the help of landmarks.[142]

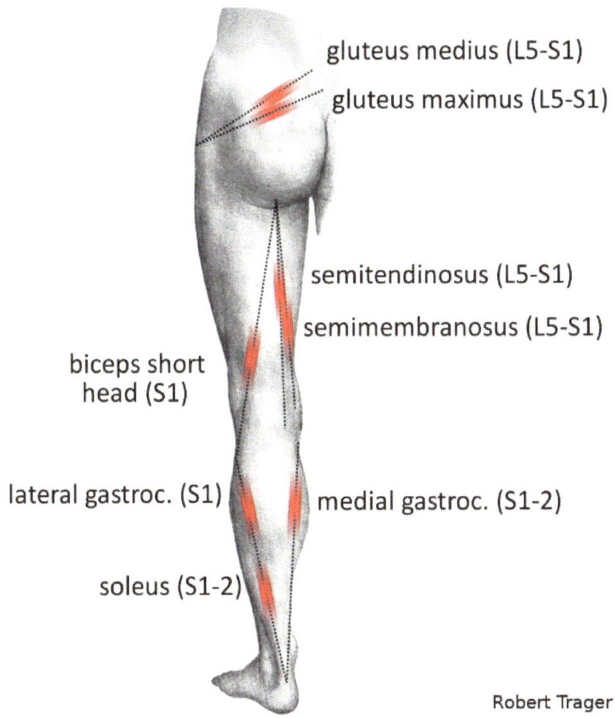

Figure 135: Relative location of motor points of the posterior lower extremity. Data adapted from Gunn,[144] Botter,[142] Botte,[145] and Barbero.[146] A shaded band indicates the zone in which the motor point is typically found. Dotted lines connect bony landmarks and are used to estimate the motor points. Gastroc. = gastrocnemius

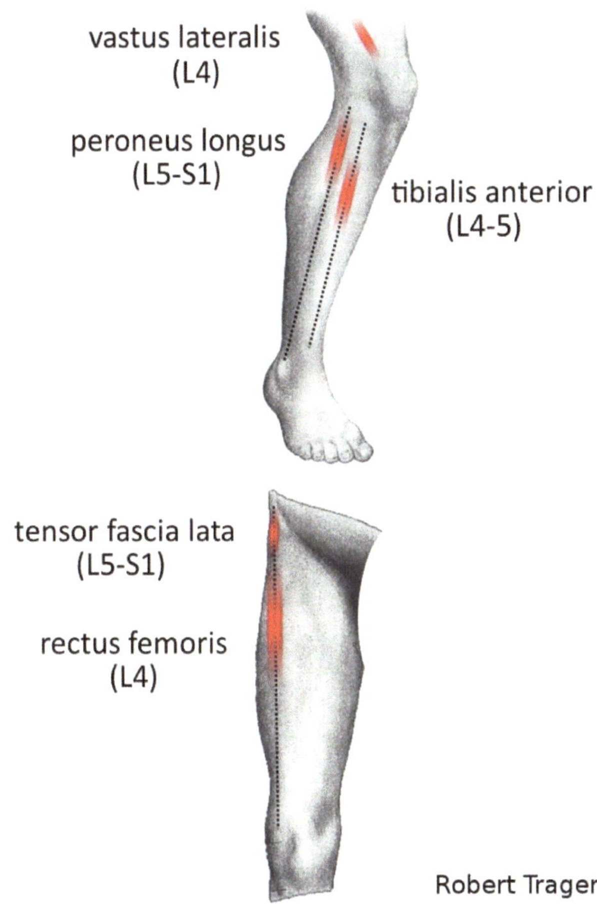

Figure 136: Relative location of motor points of the anterior lower extremity. Data adapted from Gunn,[144] Botter,[142] and Barbero.[146]

Myofascial trigger points or motor points are more common in the **myotome** (group of muscles innervated by a spinal nerve) affected in a radicular sciatica.[34,128,144,147] The pattern of trigger point or motor point tenderness can help localize a nerve lesion. For example, the most common trigger points relating to a L5-S1 disc herniation or S1 radiculopathy include the gluteus maximus and gastrocnemius with at least 90% of patients experiencing these points.[147]

Table 17: Segmental innervation in sciatica

Muscle	L4	L5	S1	S2
Iliopsoas	Medium			
Vastus lateralis	Dark			
Rectus femoris	Dark	Faint		
Tibialis anterior	Dark	Faint	Faint	
Tensor fascia lata		Dark	Dark	
Ext. hallucis longus		Dark	Dark	
Peroneus longus		Dark	Dark	
Gluteus medius		Dark	Dark	
Gluteus maximus		Dark	Dark	
Semimembranosus		Dark	Dark	Medium
Semitendinosus		Dark	Dark	Medium
Biceps femoris		Medium	Dark	Medium
Lateral gastroc.		Faint	Dark	Medium
Medial gastroc.			Dark	Dark
Soleus			Dark	Dark

*L3 and above not shown, to focus on the main roots of the sciatic nerve L4, L5, S1, and S2. Data adapted from Gunn,[143] Barr,[148] and Zhu[149]. Gastroc: Gastrocnemius. Ext: Extensor

Dark = predominant (>25%)

Medium = partial (10-25%)

Faint = slight (<10%)

Trigger point palpation

Sciatica-related trigger points are identified by tenderness to palpation, identification of a taut band of muscle, presence of pain referral into the sciatic distribution, snapping palpation, and a jump sign.[32] **Snapping palpation** is a method of pressing and rolling the finger over a taut muscle band to locate a trigger point to elicit a quick movement of the muscle. One must roll the finger transversely across the direction of the muscle fibers to elicit the snapping response.[32]

The presence of referred sciatic pain from a trigger point (TrP) does not confirm that the sciatica originates from the TrP. It is more likely that the TrP is an effect of a radicular sciatica rather than a cause of it.[150] Palpation-induced pain referral within the sciatic nerve distribution with palpation may represent segmental sensitization. Sciatic distribution TrPs are thought to represent sensitized motor points that relate to an associated spinal nerve level.[147]

One study found that patients with **gluteal muscle trigger points** had a large increase in odds of having discogenic radicular pain verified by MRI (OR 30.4).[4] Absence of gluteal trigger points helped rule out discogenic radicular pain to a moderate degree (-LR 0.28).[4] Despite the association identified in this study, these trigger points may also be seen in piriformis syndrome and GTPS.

The **iliacus** and **psoas** muscles are best palpated starting at the anterior superior iliac spine with the patient lying supine with one or both knees flexed. Initial pressure should be superficial before moving deeper and more medially. One author reported psoas tenderness in more than 90% of sciatic patients.[151] Tenderness of the **iliacus** muscle slightly increases the odds of SIJ pain being present (OR 1.3).[152] Hypertonicity of these muscles may also relate to the hip flexion contractures seen in hip-spine syndrome.

Tender points

Tender points help map out the **distribution of sciatica** rather than its cause. Palpation findings have a high sensitivity and low specificity and are meant to *rule in* rather than *rule out* any given diagnosis. For example, tenderness at the sacral sulcus (at the SIJ medial to the PSIS) has a high sensitivity of 95% but a low specificity of 9% for SIJ pain.[3]

Clinicians may ask the patient to point out the **area of maximal pain**. When a patient with sciatica points to the **SIJ**, infero-medial to the posterior superior iliac spine (PSIS), a sign called the Fortin finger test, it suggests that the pain originates from the SIJ.[153] This has a high sensitivity (76%) but a low specificity (47%).[3] Alternatively, if the patient points to the **PSIS** (the one-finger test), this increases the odds of SIJ pain (OR 25.9).[152] If the patient points to the **greater trochanter**, this is called the **C-sign**, which is a classic finding in GTPS.[154]

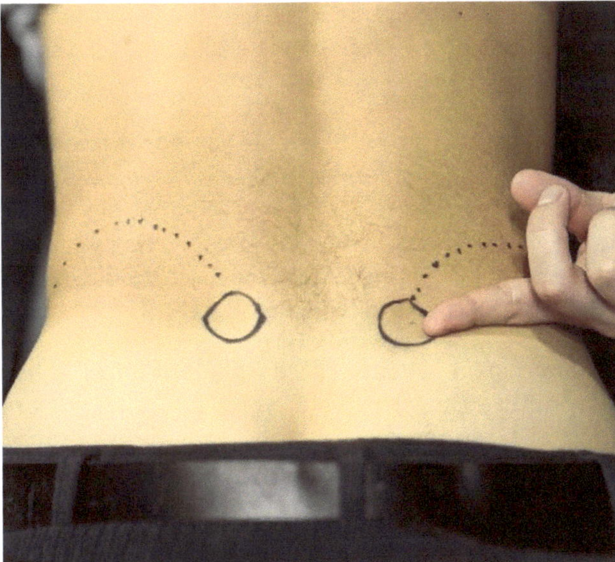

Figure 137: Pointing to the PSIS as the site of maximal pain (the one-finger test), is a sign of SIJ pain. Iliac crests marked with a dotted line.

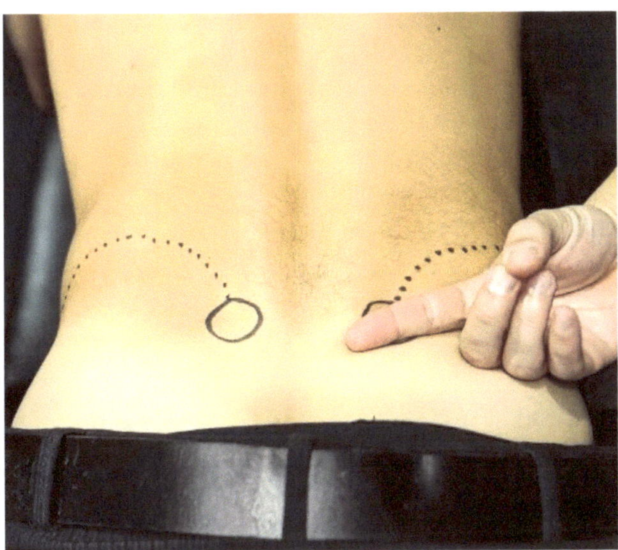

Figure 138: Pointing to the sacroiliac joint as the site of maximal pain (the Fortin finger test), just medial and inferior to the PSIS (circled), is a sign of SIJ pain. Iliac crests are marked with a dotted line.

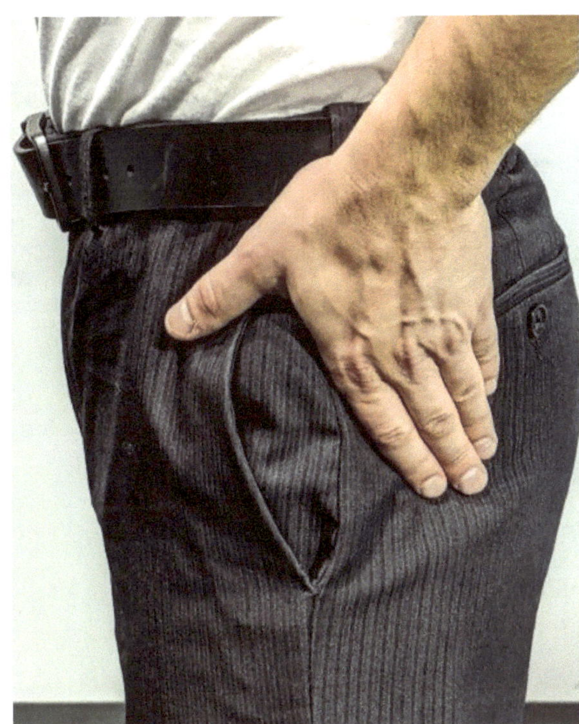

Figure 139: The C-sign of greater trochanteric pain syndrome

Pain and tenderness at the **greater trochanter** is a nonspecific finding that can occur in L5 radicular sciatica[139] and GTPS. Tenderness of the greater trochanter increases the odds of GTPS by a factor of 3.5 and has a sensitivity of 80% and specificity of 47%.[138] This sign is present when there is tenderness around the bony prominence of the trochanter. Trochanteric tenderness may reflect inflammation related to bursitis or tendinitis or alternatively sensitization related to radiculopathy.

Tenderness around the **SIJ** increases the odds of SIJ pain being present. This includes the sacral sulcus (OR 1.9),[3,137] long posterior sacroiliac ligament (1.7), PSIS (OR 2.2), and **sacrotuberous ligament** (OR 5.76).[152]

The **bowstring** or **cram test** is positive when there is tenderness of the tibial nerve at the popliteal fossa with the patient in a straight leg raise position. The **tibial nerve compression** test is another variation, and is positive in 93% of those with neurogenic claudication related to LSS.[156]

Table 18: Musculoskeletal palpation for sciatica

Structure	Differential diagnosis for tenderness
Gastrocnemius, soleus, and plantaris	• Tibial nerve entrapment / soleal sling syndrome • MPS / hypertonicity • Denervation supersensitivity of S1
Gluteal muscles	• DGS / sciatic nerve entrapment • MPS / hypertonicity
Greater trochanter	• GTPS / trochanteric bursitis / gluteal muscle tendon injury / TrPs
Ischial tuberosity / hamstrings	• Hamstring syndrome / hamstring tendinosis / hamstring tear or scar tissue/ sciatic nerve entrapment
Lumbar erector spinae	• MPS / hypertonicity
Peroneal muscles	• MPS / hypertonicity • Denervation supersensitivity of L5-S1
Piriformis muscle & sciatic notch	• PS / DGS / sciatic nerve entrapment • PS secondary to spinal pathology[155]
Psoas and iliacus	• Intraspinal sciatica[151] • SIJ pain[152] • Hip flexor contracture
Sacroiliac joint	• SIJ pain / sacroiliitis
Deep gluteal syndrome (DGS), myofascial pain syndrome (MPS), greater trochanteric pain syndrome (GTPS), piriformis syndrome (PS), trigger points (TrPs)	

Motion palpation

Motion palpation involves pressing on the lumbopelvic and thoracic articulations to determine if there is too much or too little mobility, or by using a combination of static palpation and patient movement. Motion palpation has implications for treatment because a lack of mobility may justify joint manipulation while hypermobility may indicate stabilization exercises.

Clinicians perform the **interspinous gap change** test by palpating the lumbar spinous processes while the patient stands and again when they perform a forward bend. Any abnormality in position from one spinous to the other that is different from the other spaces may represent lumbar instability. This is a sensitive test for instability (sn 82%) but lacks specificity (61%).[57]

Clinicians perform postero-anterior **spring testing** using manual posterior-to-anterior pressure on the lumbar spine. The resulting movement of the articulations is either "hypomobile," "normal," or "hypermobile." Spring testing may also produce pain, which is a non-specific finding.

Low back pain patients with **normal mobility** or **hypomobility** (no hypermobility) to spring testing are most likely to respond favorably to a lumbar stabilization exercise program.[157] Hypomobility of lumbar segments as detected by spring testing increases the likelihood of a positive response to spinal manipulation by a small amount (+LR 1.3).[158]

Hypermobility of the lumbar spine during spring testing of a LBP patient is relatively specific for radiographic instability (sp 81%).[114] Lack of hypomobility is also highly specific (sp 95%).[114] The identification of hypermobility on exam suggests the patient may respond best to treatment involving stabilization-based exercises.[159]

Nerve tenderness

Tenderness of the sciatic nerve or its branches is a common clinical finding in diverse types of sciatica. One study found that 56% those with low-back related leg pain had nerve tenderness in at least two locations,[160] while another study found that 100% of patients had tenderness in at least one location.[161] Sciatic nerve tenderness often result from radiculopathies but can also be caused by peripheral nerve entrapments.

The French pediatrician François Valleix may have been the first to document the tender points associated with sciatica in 1841, which his colleagues called Valleix points. He recognized that predictable points along the course of the sciatic nerve and its branches were often tender. The most common points he identified (in 36 patients) were the SIJ near the PSIS in 97% of cases, around the greater trochanter in 72%, sciatic notch in 44%, and middle of the iliac crest in 22%.[162] The tenderness of these points may relate to peripheral sensitization of the nervi nervorum and/or central sensitization.

> *All these tender points did not exist in every case, but we usually found quite a few [in each case], and the patient designates them accurately when questioned... we first remark the*

multiplicity of these tender points, sown, so to speak, in the course of the [sciatic] nerve and its main branches. (Valleix, p. 515, Author's translation)

Tinel's test is a method of testing for nerve injury by percussing (lightly tapping) on the nerve to elicit paresthesia in the nerve distribution. Sciatic pain reproduced by a Tinel's test is suggestive of peripheral nerve compression but does not rule out a radicular lesion.

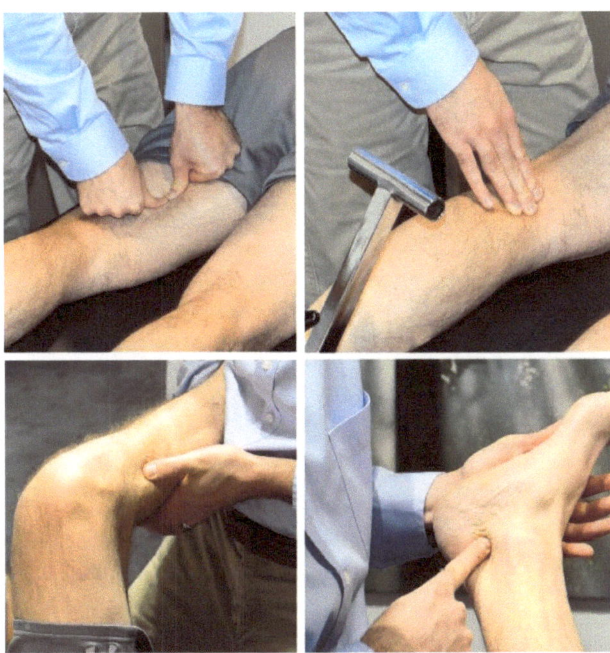

Figure 140: Nerve palpation. Sciatic (top left), tibial at the popliteal fossa (top right), common peroneal (bottom left), and tibial at the tarsal tunnel (bottom right)

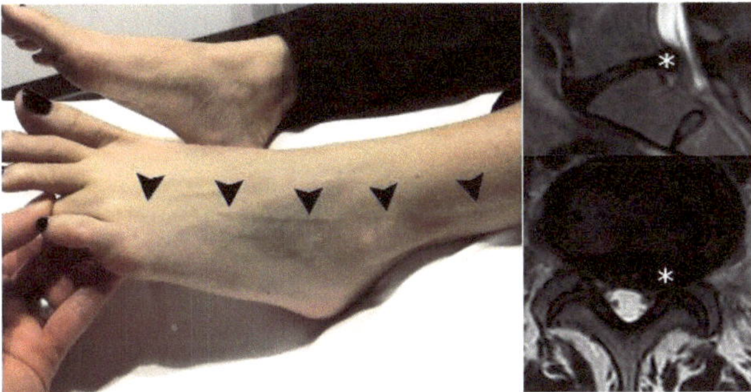

Figure 141: The superficial peroneal nerve 4th toe flexion sign. This 48-year-old woman presented with subacute LBP and sciatica w/ radiation to left leg, lateral ankle, and foot dorsum. MRI revealed L5-S1 disc extrusion compressing the left L5 nerve root (*). Her pain coincided with a tender superficial peroneal nerve in the distribution of symptoms. The nerve was more visible and sensitive (arrowheads) during this test. Case shared with patient's permission by Robert Trager, DC.

A peripheral nerve entrapment may mimic or occur with an intraspinal form of sciatica. Examples of purely extraspinal forms of sciatic pain that may be identified using Tinel's test include common peroneal entrapment,[163] sciatic nerve entrapment,[164] and soleal sling syndrome.[165]

Peripheral nerve tenderness or Tinel signs may correspond to radiculopathy of a spinal nerve(s) from which it derives. One study correlated deep peroneal nerve tenderness with L5 radiculopathy and sural nerve tenderness with S1 radiculopathy.[161] Another study reported that patients with L4-5 LDH (typically causing an L5 radiculopathy) frequently had Tinel signs at the common peroneal nerve.[163] Likewise, Tinel signs have also been reported at superficial peroneal entrapments in those with LSS or disc pathology at L4-5.[166] Peripheral nerve palpation may identify a local entrapment, point to a radiculopathy, or both in the case of a double-crush lesion.

Table 19: Nerve palpation for sciatica

Nerve	Palpation or Tinel's test	Differential diagnosis
Sciatic	Mid-thigh along the sciatic trunk[164]	Low-back related leg pain,[160] injury or entrapment
Common peroneal	Fibular neck[167]	L5 radic[163]
Deep peroneal	Anterior ankle[168] or sinus tarsi for lateral terminal branches [161]	L5 radic,[161] anterior tarsal tunnel syndrome[168]
Superficial peroneal	Lateral midfoot while passively flexing the 4th toe	L5 radic, injury or entrapment
Superior cluneal	Iliac crest (variable)[169]	LSR, injury or entrapment
Sural	Lateral calcaneus	S1 radic,[161] injury or entrapment
Tibial at knee	Popliteal space,[98] or soleal sling[165]	Low-back related leg pain,[160] injury or entrapment
Tibial at ankle	Tarsal tunnel[170]	Posterior tarsal tunnel syndrome[168]
Radiculopathy (radic), lumbosacral radiculopathy (LSR)		

Muscle testing

Motor deficits in sciatic pain usually represent nerve root injury but can also result from extraspinal, myofascial, or referred types of sciatic pain. A motor deficit identified in a sciatic patient increases the odds of nerve root compression or radiculopathy by a factor of 4 to 5.[12,171,172] The highest odds of radiculopathy occur when weakness corresponds to a myotome (OR 5.4).[172]

Myotomal weakness, also called segmental weakness, is the finding of multiple weak muscles that correspond to a spinal nerve root level (e.g. L4, L5, or S1). The hallmark of myotomal weakness is weakness of segmentally related but anatomically distant muscles. Examples include weakness of the rectus femoris (thigh) and tibialis anterior (leg) for L4, weakness of the gluteus medius (hip) and extensor hallucis longus (foot) for L5, or weakness of the gluteus maximus (hip) and calf muscles (leg) for S1.

Non-radicular or myofascial sciatica may cause **localized weakness** rather than segmental weakness. Weakness may occur around pain and pathology instead of in a myotomal pattern. In GTPS, which can mimic L5 radiculopathy, the gluteal muscles are weak in over 70% of patients.[78] In contrast, those with L5 radiculopathy may have gluteal weakness and great toe extensor weakness.[173] Similarly, hamstring syndrome involves hamstring weakness in up to 95% of patients[174] but hip extension is normal, which helps distinguish from S1 radiculopathy.[175]

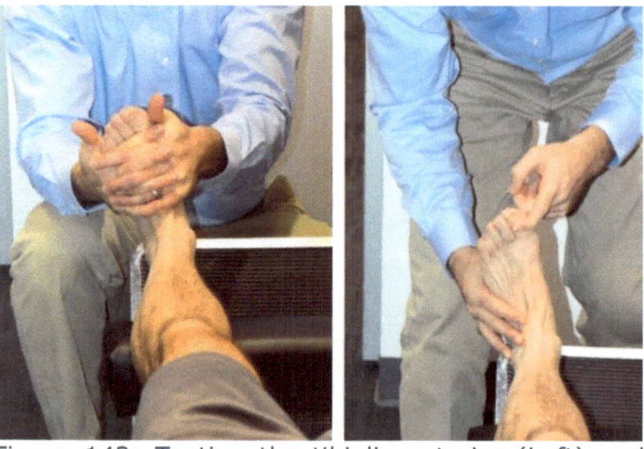

Figure 142: Testing the tibialis anterior (Left) and extensor hallucis longus (Right)

Muscle testing in the foot is more specific than other regions. **Great toe extension** is one of the most accurate muscle tests for radicular sciatica. It assesses the extensor hallucis longus, which extends the great toe. It is most specific for L5 radiculopathy (sn 61%, sp 86%).[173] The **toe abduction test** assesses the dorsal interossei. Difficulty actively separating the toes is a sign of interossei weakness and can indicate a lesion of S1 or S2 or the tibial nerve. **Great toe flexion** likewise assesses the S1 root, with high specificity (82%).[176]

Cramping during muscle testing is a sign of discogenic radiculopathy. Cramping during hamstring muscle testing is a highly specific sign of discogenic radiculopathy (sp 100%),[177] but is less useful in those with LSS.[178] To test for hamstring cramping, knee flexion is resisted with the knee at 90 degrees and the patient prone.[177]

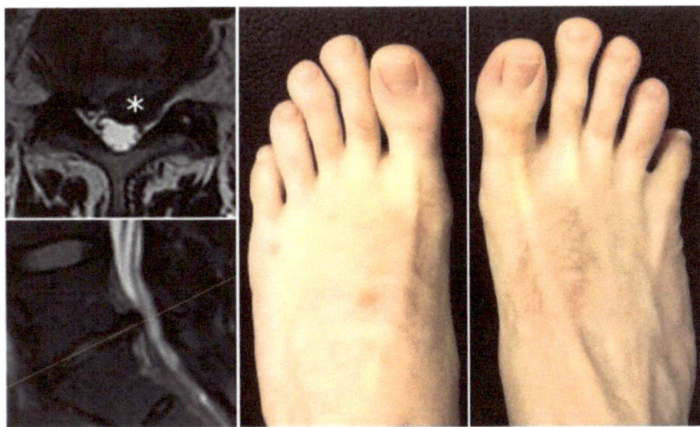

Figure 143: Toe abductor weakness. This 28-year-old man has a disc herniation (*) at L5-S1 compressing the left S1 nerve root, which causes toe abduction weakness of the left foot. Image shared with patient's permission by Robert Trager, DC.

Functional tests or **screening tests** for sciatica are a way to test for weakness by observing the patient complete functional movements or exercises. The **single leg sit-to-stand test** is performed by having the patient rise on one leg from a seated position while allowing them to hold your hand to balance.[173] This test assesses quadriceps strength and weakness in this test is most specific (81%) for the L4 nerve root.[173]

The patient performs the **heel raise test** by completing 10 successive heel raises on one foot, while lightly using a wall to balance. Inability to complete this test has poor sensitivity but high specificity for **L5** or **S1** nerve root impingement (sn 14%, sp 96%).[173] Other signs of weakness are leaning forward or bending the knee.[179] Inability to fully raise the heel against gravity while on one foot is graded a 2/5 muscle strength.[180] The **heel walk** tests the ankle dorsiflexors but has a low likelihood of predicting nerve root impingement (sn 16%, sp 80% +LR 0.69).[173]

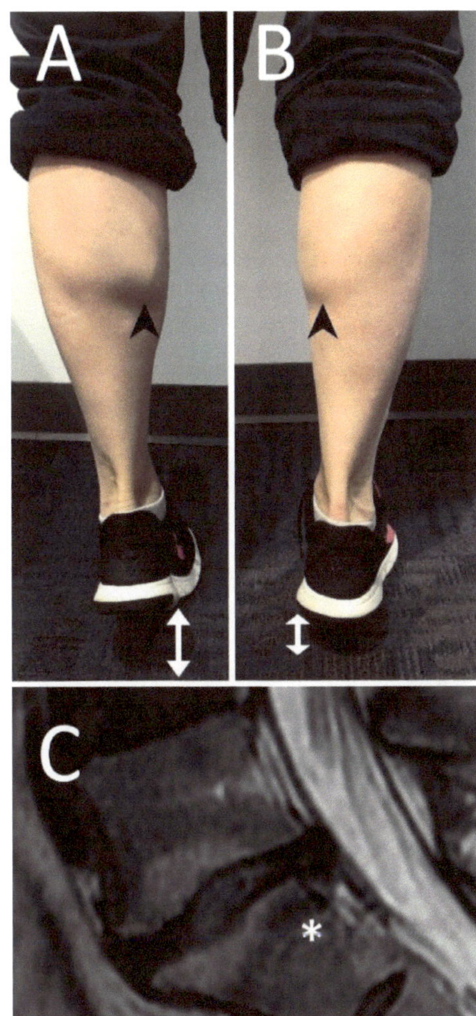

Figure 144: R calf weakness. This 33-year-old woman presented with 3+ year LBP w/ radiation to R calf and S1 myotomal weakness. Left calf (A) shows 5/5 strength, while right calf (B) is 2/5 due to an inability to fully raise (shorter double arrow). Atrophy is evident in B (arrowhead) compared to A. She was diagnosed with discogenic R S1 radiculopathy. Case shared with patient's permission by Robert Trager, DC.

During the **Trendelenburg test** the patient stands on the affected side while the clinician looks for either a drop of the pelvis on the opposite side or a lean to the same side (a compensatory mechanism). The test indicates weakness of the hip abductors (e.g. gluteus medius, maximus, and minimus, tensor fascia lata, piriformis, and obturator internus). The Trendelenburg test may indicate an **L5 radiculopathy** and is the most sensitive and specific test for **greater trochanteric pain syndrome**.[78]

Table 20: Muscle testing for sciatica

Action	Primary nerve root(s) [149]	Non-radicular sciatica weakness
Knee extension (quadriceps)	L4	Hip pathology
Ankle dorsiflexion (tibialis anterior, heel walk)	L4, L5	Common peroneal nerve injury
Great toe extension (extensor hallucis longus)	L5, S1	Common peroneal nerve injury
Hip abduction (gluteal muscles, Trendelenburg)	L5, S1	Greater trochanteric pain syndrome[154]
Ankle eversion	L5, S1	Common or superficial peroneal nerve injury
Hip extension (gluteus maximus)[180]	L5, S1	Hip pathology
Knee flexion (hamstrings)	S1, S2	Hamstring syndrome,[174,175] deep gluteal syndrome[182]
Ankle plantarflexion (calf muscles, heel raise)	S1, S2	Deep gluteal syndrome[183]
Intrinsic foot muscles (abductor hallucis, flexor digitorum brevis)	S2, S3	Soleal sling syndrome[165]

In the **active squatting test**, the patient squats with both knees close together. This assesses hip mobility and strength simultaneously. If the patient cannot complete the squat and begins to fall backwards this can indicate gluteal muscle contracture or deep gluteal syndrome.[184]

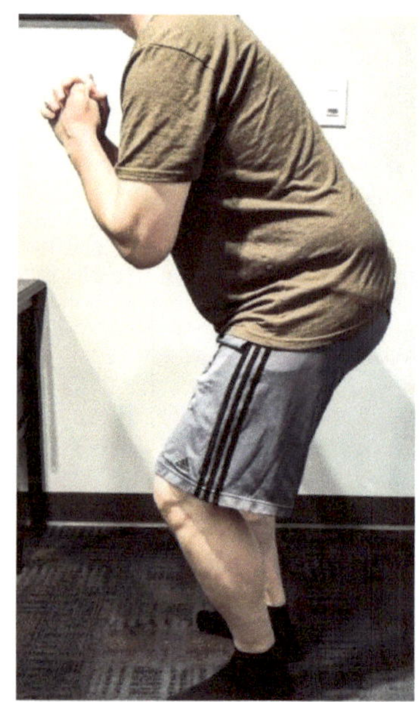

Figure 145: Active squatting test. This 42-year-old man presented with chronic burning gluteal pain that radiated into the posterior-lateral thighs and occasionally the calves. He was unable to squat as shown. Soft tissue manipulation / IASTM and dry needling to the gluteal region significantly reduced his symptoms, suggesting a deep gluteal syndrome. Case shared with patient's permission by Robert Trager, DC.

Orthopedic tests that assess for weakness and pain can be useful in finding the cause of sciatica. The **Pace sign** uses resisted abduction and external rotation of the thigh from the seated position. This test may be positive in GTPS.[154] The **active hamstring test** involves testing the hamstrings from a slightly lengthened position at 30 degrees and can reproduce pain in deep gluteal syndrome[182] and hamstring syndrome.[174] This test is particularly useful in distinguishing hamstring syndrome: While only 30% of patients have hamstring weakness at 90°, 95% will demonstrate weakness at 30°.[174]

Sensory testing and dermatomes

A **dermatomal pattern** (nerve root pattern) of sensory disturbance is suggestive but not diagnostic of a nerve root lesion. Reduced or loss of sensation is found in 50% of those with radicular sciatica and 17% of those with non-radicular sciatica.[185]

The use of dermatomes has evolved since the early 1900s to aid in diagnosing radicular sciatica. In 1904 the French physicians Lortat-Jacob and Sabareanu related sciatica to nerve root inflammation by identifying dermatomal sensory loss.[186] Although dermatome maps were popularly adopted as a means to diagnose discogenic radicular sciatica, it became clear that dermatomes varied or had areas of overlap. Maps of dermatomes have evolved over the years, and newer maps illustrate the most reliable parts of the dermatomes.

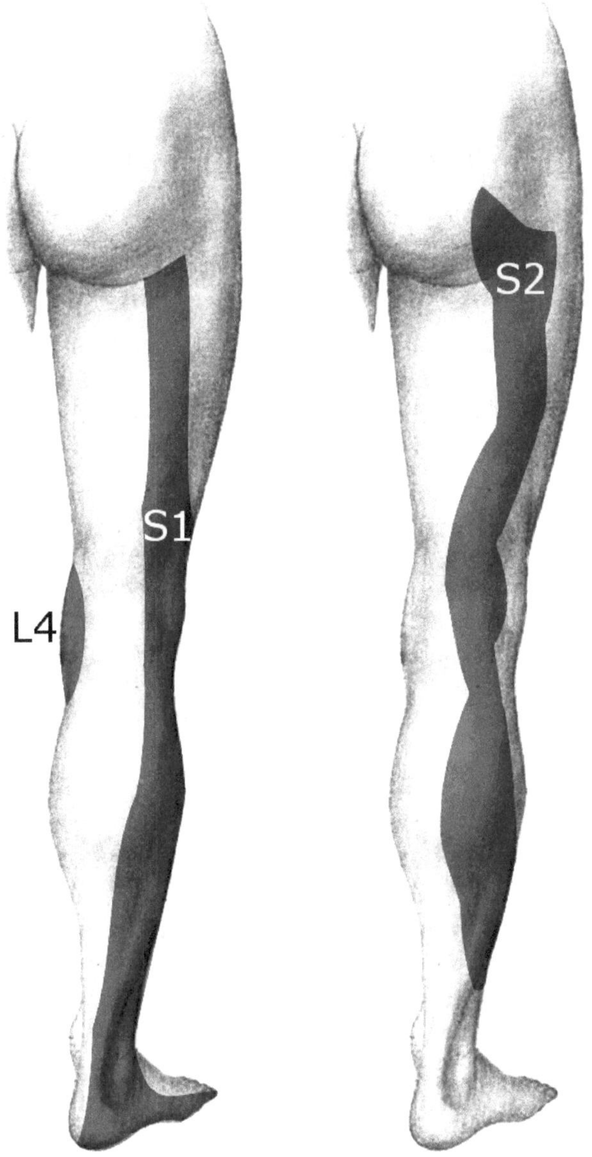

Figure 146: Dermatomes of the posterior lower extremity. Blank regions indicate areas of major variability and overlap. Image by Robert Trager, DC by modification of public domain Gray's anatomy images, using data from Lee's 2008 evidence-based dermatome map.[190] image of leg by Andrea Allen (CC by 2.0), and image of foot by Pixel AddIct (CC BY 2.0).

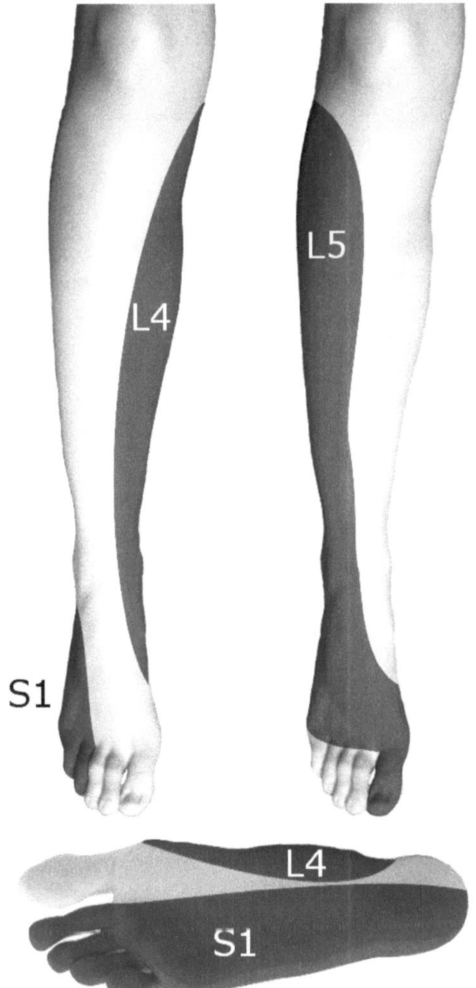

Figure 147: Dermatomes of the anterior leg and foot. Blank regions indicate areas of major variability and overlap. Image by Robert Trager, DC by modification of image of leg by Andrea Allen (CC by 2.0), and image of foot by Pixel AddIct (CC BY 2.0), based on Lee's 2008 evidence-based dermatome map.[190]

Dermatomal sensory loss increases the likelihood of radicular sciatica by, at the most, a small degree (LR + 2.33 for S1).[9] Dermatomal sensory loss is most specific when it is confined to a single dermatome (sp 92-98%) and less specific when it includes areas beyond a single dermatome (sp 30-74%).[1] Absence of sensory loss does not help rule out radicular sciatica.[1,9,176,181] The **S1 dermatome** is the most specific (sp 60-84%) of the common radicular levels of sciatica (L4, L5, S1).[1,9,176,187]

The region of **self-reported sensory loss** does not always correspond with the region of sensory loss on physical examination. One study found a relatively low 62% correlation between symptoms and sensory loss found on examination in those with discogenic sciatica.[128] Another study found self-reported numbness to be more sensitive but less specific than exam-identified numbness.[188]

Dermatome **landmarks** are helpful alternatives for sensory testing in sciatica. Sensory deficit at the **medial ankle** is highly specific for L4 radiculopathy.[173] Studies using the **lateral foot** as a landmark for S1 found it to be highly specific (sp 83-84%).[9,176] These studies also found moderate specificity of the lateral leg or **foot dorsum** for L5. [9,176]

A **non-dermatomal sensory distribution** is common in sciatica. One study examined patients prior to disc surgery and of those with sensory loss, 26% had a **widespread pattern**; the remainder had involvement of one or two dermatomes.[189] Another study found a high prevalence (46%) of non-dermatomal sensory loss in those with chronic LBP over six months.[190] Lumbar stenosis may frequently present as non-dermatomal bilateral buttocks and thigh pain.[191]

Mildly reduced sensation may occur in **neighboring dermatomes** other than those expected via imaging. One study using quantitative sensory testing found sensory disturbances in neighboring ipsilateral and contralateral nerve roots from those affected by a disc herniation.[192] Neighboring dermatomes may be involved due to leakage of inflammatory mediators to nearby nerve roots,[192] neural communications[191] and/or the sensory overlap of adjacent dermatomes.[191]

A bilateral **stocking distribution**, a symmetrical below-knee sensory loss, is most often associated with peripheral neuropathy. It is improbable that radicular sciatica would create a stocking pattern, as there would need to be bilateral involvement of partial L4, L5, and S1 dermatomes. However, patients with radicular sciatica may have a coexisting peripheral neuropathy that complicates their radiculopathy.[193] These patients may have a stocking distribution with one region (e.g. the great toe) more severely affected due to a coexisting nerve root lesion.

Sensory loss due to a **peripheral nerve** injury may mimic a dermatomal pattern. Although peripheral nerve injuries create smaller regions of sensory loss distributions than dermatomes, they may mimic part of a dermatome. For example, common peroneal nerve entrapment and L5 radiculopathy could both cause sensory loss of the lateral leg and foot dorsum. Likewise, sensory loss of the posterior thigh could be from the posterior femoral cutaneous nerve, or S1 or S2 radiculopathy.

Table 21: Sensory deficit landmarks and their differential diagnosis

Landmark	Nerve root	Peripheral nerve(s)
Medial ankle	L4	Saphenous
Lateral leg	L5	Lateral cutaneous of calf, medial sural cutaneous, superficial peroneal, sural
Foot dorsum	L5	Superficial peroneal
Lateral foot	S1	Sural

Rapidly progressive widespread sensory loss is a red flag and can suggest a more severe intraspinal etiology of sciatica. Those with multiple segments involved or an entire-leg distribution could have a space-occupying lesion of the lumbar canal, such as a discogenic cauda equina syndrome, or an infection or inflammatory condition like Guillain-Barre syndrome. Those with insidious-onset sensory loss in multiple dermatomes are most likely to have LSS.

In radicular sciatica **partial-dermatome sensory loss** is the norm while entire-dermatome loss is the exception. One study of patients with disc herniation identified that of those with sensory loss, the majority (72%) of patients had sensory deficits of 25% or less of a dermatome.[194] The study found that only 6% of patients had sensory deficits spanning an entire dermatome.[194]

Dermatomal **cutaneous hyperesthesia** (increased sensitivity to stimuli) is occasionally identified in those with discogenic sciatica[195,196] but also can relate to infections such as **varicella** zoster virus.[197] Patients may have patches of hyperesthesia and hypoalgesia at different parts of the same dermatome.[195] One study reported cutaneous **hyperalgesia** (increased sensitivity to pain) as an early sign of LDH.[198]

Clinicians test for **hypoalgesia** to sharp sensations with a pinprick, safety pin, or sharp toothpick, and test **light touch sensation** with the soft stroke of a finger or a wisp of cotton wool. They may use a metal instrument to test for sensation to cold. Sensation should be tested from **distal to proximal** and along the limb axis.[199] If there is an area of self-reported numbness, it should be tested from the **center outward**.[199] Light touch testing may reveal a larger area of deficit than by pin-prick.[199]

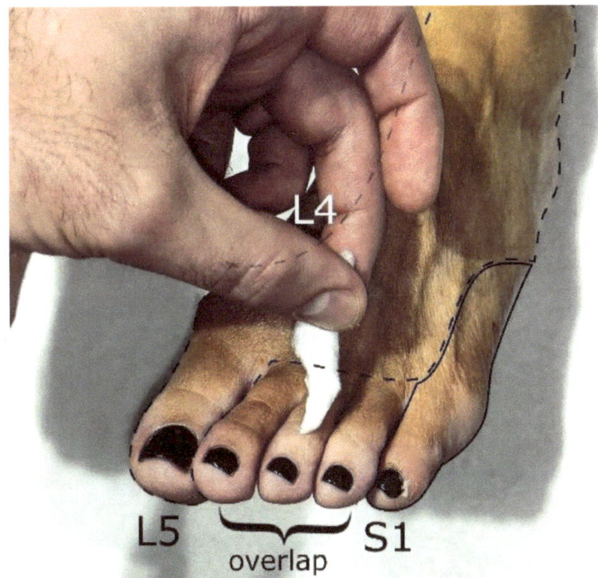

Figure 148: Light touch sensory testing of the dermatomes of the foot and toes. Toes 2-4 are a blend of L5 and S1 whereas the 1st toe and foot dorsum corresponds with the L5 dermatome (bounded by dotted line) and 5th toe corresponds with S1 (bounded by solid line).[191] This patient had both L5 and S1 discogenic radiculopathy with predominant S1 motor and sensory loss, but also had sensory loss in the overlapping zone of L5 and S1 (shown). Image shared with permission of patient by Robert Trager, DC.

Reflex testing

A deep tendon reflex (DTR) examination tests the function of the lumbosacral nerve roots. Radicular, intraspinal, or other nerve-lesion forms of sciatica are more likely to reduce the DTRs compared to myofascial and referred pain. If a DTR is reduced or absent in sciatica the odds of lumbosacral radiculopathy increase by a factor of about 3 to 5.[8,171]

The absence of the **Achilles' tendon reflex** was first identified as a sign of sciatica by Babinski in 1896.[200] He described that patients with sciatica should have a reduced Achilles reflex, and if not they had "hysteria".[200] While this practice continued through the early 1900s, it is now known that patients with sciatica often have a normal Achilles tendon reflex, and it is no longer a requirement for a diagnosis of sciatica.[185]

Deep tendon reflexes have a low sensitivity but high specificity for radicular sciatica.[201,202] Reduction, loss, or asymmetry of a DTR is a specific sign of radicular sciatica. In sciatica, reflexes are only abnormal about 25% of the time.[185] However, reflex abnormalities are highly specific (sp 75%) for radiculopathy.[201]

Normal reflexes are common in sciatica and do not rule out nerve root involvement.

Deep tendon reflexes can also help localize symptoms to a **specific nerve root** level. The patellar reflex is most specific for L4, medial hamstring for L5, and Achilles for S1. Some clinicians also test reflexes for the extensor digitorum brevis reflex, biceps femoris, and adductor muscles.

Table 22: Deep tendon reflexes and their interpretation in sciatica. Hyporeflexia corresponds to an increase in odds or odds ratio (OR) or likelihood ratio (LR) of specific nerve root involvement.

Reflex	Nerve root levels	Nerve injury DDx
Patellar	• L3 or L4 (OR 14.3)[8] • **L4** (+LR 7.7, sp 95%)[173] • L5 (sn 19%, sp 82%)[1]	Femoral[212]
Medial hamstring	• **L5** (+LR 18, sp 85%)[213]	Sciatic (tibial division)[214]
Extensor digitorum brevis	• L5 or S1 (sp 91%)[215]	Common or deep peroneal
Lateral hamstring	• S1, S2	Sciatic (peroneal division)[214]
Achilles	• L5 or S1 (+ LR 7.1, sp 96%)[173] • **S1** (OR 8.44, +LR 3.9, sp 91%)[8,173]	Sciatic
Medial hamstring: Semimembranosus, semitendinosus. Lateral hamstring: Biceps femoris. Differential diagnosis (DDx)		

Larger **peripheral nerve lesions** may reduce or abolish deep tendon reflexes while smaller or cutaneous nerves typically do not. Lesions of the sciatic nerve may affect the Achilles reflex while those of the femoral nerve may affect the patellar. Even though it is possible, hyporeflexia is rarely seen in piriformis syndrome.[203] Lesions of the posterior[204,205] and lateral femoral cutaneous[206] nerves leave the DTRs intact.

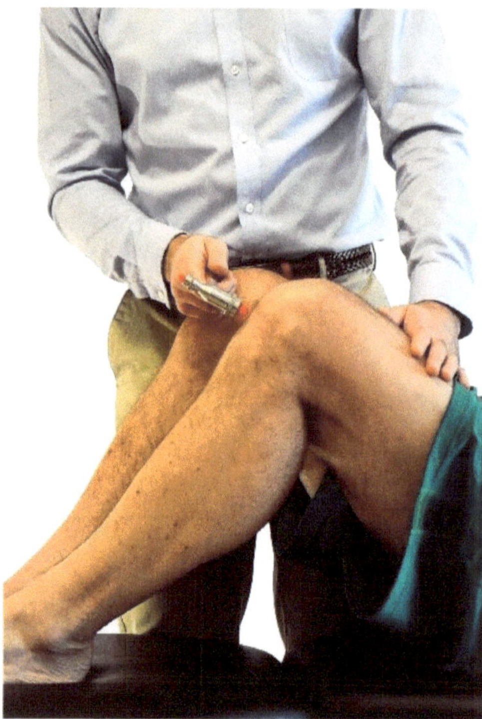

Figure 149: The patellar reflex, tested supine. The non-striking hand may be used to palpate the quadriceps for muscle contraction.

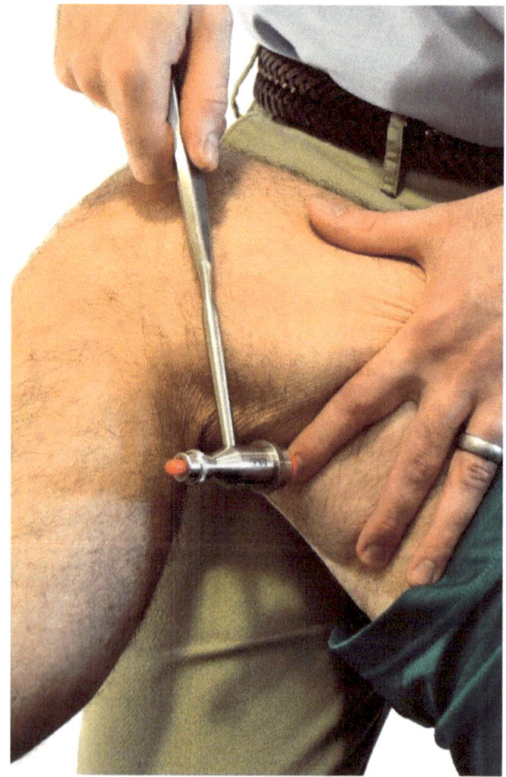

Figure 150: The medial hamstring reflex, tested supine. The non-striking index finger demonstrates the semimembranosus and semitendinosus tendons, and does not need to be in this position to elicit the reflex.

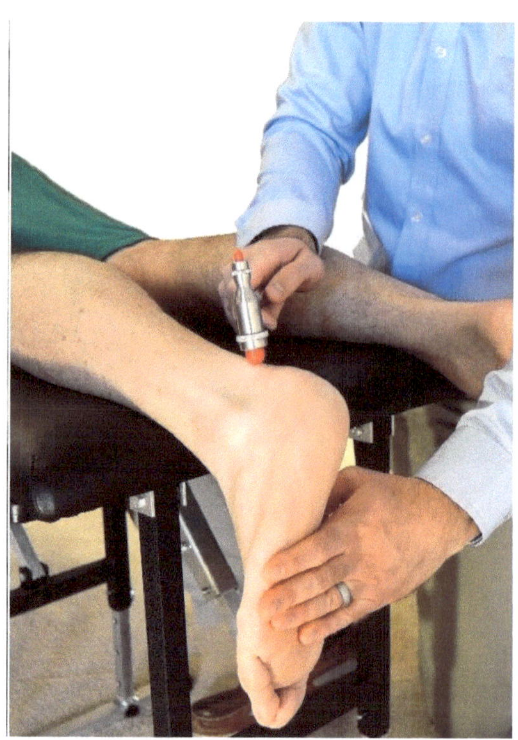

Figure 151: The Achilles reflex, tested prone. The non-striking hand can stabilize the foot in slight dorsiflexion during the test, which enhances the ability to detect the reflex.

Myofascial pain syndromes occasionally reduce DTRs. One study with over 600 patients found hyporeflexia in 5% of non-radicular sciatic patients.[207] Other studies have also reported patients with non-radicular sciatica verified imaging and/or EMG who had reflex deficits.[136,208] One author suggested that trigger points in these patients pain could reduce DTRs.[209] One series found that 14% of patients with **sacroiliac-joint** related sciatica had a diminished patellar reflex while 29% had a diminished Achilles reflex.[210]

Hyperreflexia in the sciatic patient calls for further attention. Radicular sciatica typically reduces or abolishes reflexes rather than increasing them. Tandem stenosis, or stenosis of the cervical and lumbar spine may cause hyperreflexia in sciatica. Rarely **cordonal sciatica** results from cervical or thoracic disc herniations, multiple sclerosis,[211] or amyotrophic lateral sclerosis. Lower extremity reflexes are subject to any systemic illness or comorbidity the patient may have, and should be compared with those of the upper extremity.

Neurodynamic testing

Neurodynamic tests for sciatica assess for **neural tension** and **mechanosensitivity** within the sciatic nerve trunk, branches, or roots. Although LDH is the most common cause of an abnormal neurodynamic test in sciatica, pathology anywhere along the sciatic course can limit neural sliding and elicit pain.

Increased sciatic neural tension is most predictive of spine-related, discogenic radicular sciatica.[171,216] The next most common conditions to limit neural mobility in sciatica are deep gluteal syndrome[217] and piriformis syndrome[218] which restrict movement of the sciatic nerve directly. Peripheral nerve entrapments of the common peroneal and tibial nerves also restrict sciatic nerve mobility.[98]

Pathology of regions far from the sciatic nerve can influence its ability to tolerate stretch. Forward head posture is suspected of increasing low back radicular pain,[219] possibly due to increased spinal cord tension. Cervical and thoracic pathology or disc herniations rarely increase sciatic nerve tension.[220,221]

Table 23: Actions that increase or decrease tension of the sciatic nerve. Data adapted from Butler[222]

Body part	Increases tension	Decreases tension
Neck	Flexion	Extension
Low back	Flexion	Extension
Hip	Flexion Internal rotation Adduction	Extension External rotation Abduction
Knee	Extension	Flexion
Ankle & great toe	Dorsiflexion	Plantarflexion

Straight leg raise

The straight leg raise (SLR), also called the passive straight leg raise (PSLR), is a sciatic neurodynamic test that tenses the sciatic nerve using hip flexion and knee extension. It is the most often used neurodynamic test for sciatica. The SLR is a **screening test**, meaning it has a high sensitivity (91%) but a low specificity (30%).[216] Pain with a SLR increases the odds of radicular sciatica by a factor of 3.7 to 8.9.[171,216] A straight leg raise that does not provoke symptoms helps rule out a radicular lesion (-LR 0.3).[85,216]

The first mention of a test similar to the SLR is in the ancient Egyptian medical text, the Edwin Smith Papyrus (c. 1500 BCE), which described lower back pain caused by extension of the legs in a patient with a back injury.[223] The modern SLR was first formally described by the Serbian physician Lazar Lazarević in 1880 who described an increase in sciatic pain with hip flexion, knee extension, and ankle dorsiflexion.[224] The SLR reached widespread popularity after being published by a student of the French professor Charles Lasègue in 1881.[225]

The SLR causes the sciatic nerve and its roots to undergo movement and stretch. Normally the SLR causes the sciatic nerve to be pulled **distally** towards the knee about 10 mm at 30° of hip flexion and 12 mm at 60° of hip flexion.[226] The sciatic nerve also moves **superficially** (towards the skin surface), **laterally** (towards the outer thigh),[226] and **elongates** a maximum of 8%.[227]

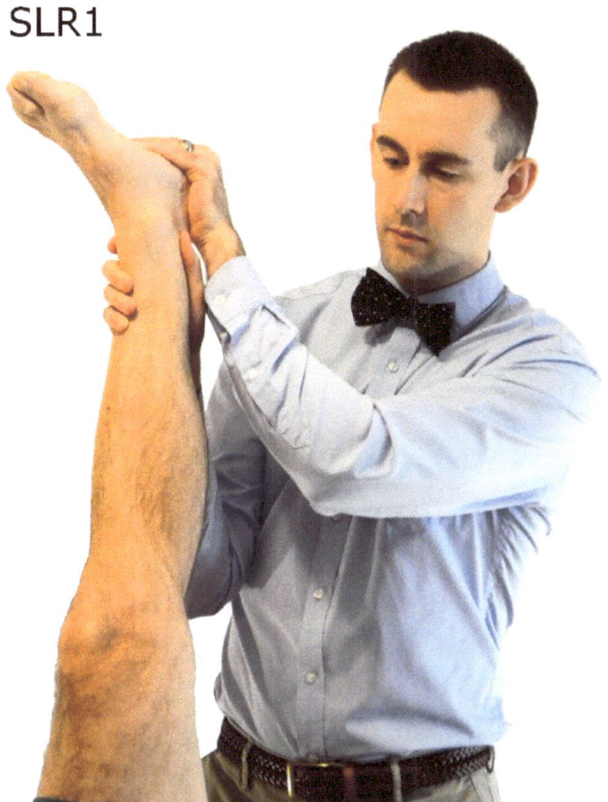

Figure 152: The straight leg raise, also called the SLR or SLR1

The SLR targets the **L5 and S1 nerve roots**. In a 70° SLR these roots slide about 1 to 3 millimeters, in comparison to the L1-4 roots which move on average less than 1 millimeter.[228] Neural tension at S1 and L5 is also significantly greater than the higher nerve roots.[228] Both tension and sliding are most prominent at S1, followed by L5, L4, L3, L2, and L1.[228] The lowest lumbosacral nerve roots undergo more sliding and tension during the SLR than the upper lumbar roots.

The SLR is most sensitive and specific for **L5 and S1 nerve root impingement** (sn 69%, sp 84%, LR+ 4.3).[173] It is not useful for detecting mid-lumbar root impingement (L2, L3, or L4).[173]

Each phase of the straight leg raise affects distinct parts of the sciatic nerve pathway. The initial 30° of hip flexion causes mostly **sciatic nerve sliding** and taking up of slack, while there is typically less than 1 millimeter of nerve root sliding.[228] Most of the **nerve root sliding** occurs between 30-70° of the SLR.[228] After 70° the sciatic nerve is thought to **elongate**.

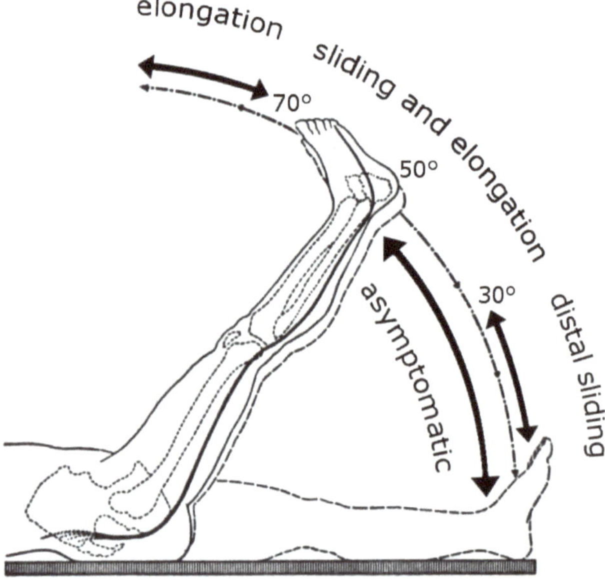

Figure 153: Straight leg raise. Primarily distal sliding of sciatic roots and nerve trunk occurs up to 30 degrees, and primarily elongation or tension beyond 70 degrees. The first 50 degrees should be pain-free. Image modified by author from public domain (Ver Brugghen's Neurosurgery in general practice, 1952).

The SLR should be considered positive when it **reproduces symptoms** in the lower extremity and differs from the asymptomatic side or normal angle or response.[229,230] The most reliable criteria for a positive SLR is the provocation of **radicular pain at any angle**.[231] Although clinicians often consider 45 degrees as the cutoff point for detecting radicular sciatica,[232] the SLR is less reliable below 45 degrees.[231]

The degree of straight leg raising in those without sciatica ranges from 40 to 85 degrees.[229] On average, healthy people should reach nearly 50° before feeling any sensory symptoms (pain, pulling, stretching, etc.).[229] The degree of SLR is reduced with in those with higher body weight.[229] It is increased in women and those that have a high activity level.[229] Because the SLR is influenced by numerous variables, the degree of the test is less important than reproduction of symptoms.

Increased age reduces the likelihood of a positive SLR. Those under age 60 have greater odds of having a positive SLR than those over 60 (OR 5.4).[233] **Height reduction** with aging is thought to decrease the amount of sciatic neural tension.[233] Atrophy of the hamstrings could also play a role in this phenomenon.[233]

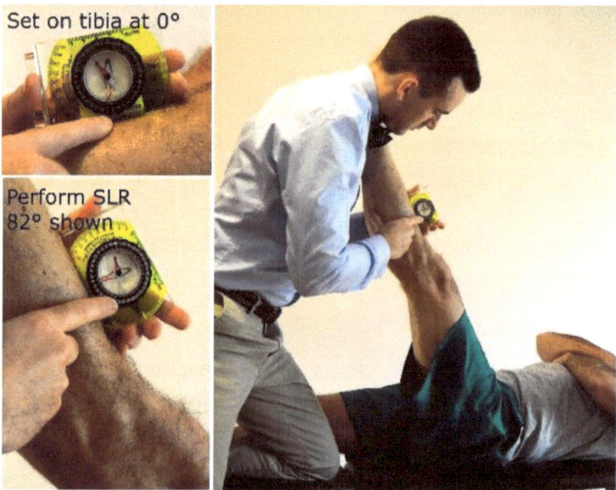

Figure 154: Straight leg raise. The SLR is measured using a petrometer. The petrometer is set to zero on the mid-tibial shaft, then when the leg is raised the dial reflects the SLR angle.

The straight leg raise may provoke pain in extraspinal conditions. A positive SLR is identified in 16% of patients with **SIJ**-related sciatica,[210] and 15% of those with **deep gluteal syndrome**.[217] Tibial or common peroneal nerve entrapments may also cause a positive SLR.[98] Posterior femoral cutaneous nerve entrapments are aggravated by stretching movements and could be exacerbated by the SLR.[234]

Less than a quarter of patients with LSS will have a positive SLR (10-22%).[235,236] If the SLR is positive, the odds of LSS are reduced (OR 0.33).[62] If the SLR is negative, the odds of LSS are increased (OR 2.46).[237] The SLR may reduce the lumbar lordosis,[238] which could explain this phenomenon, as LSS patients often get relief with lumbar flexion. Patients with **foraminal stenosis** are more likely to have a positive SLR than those with central canal stenosis.[239]

The SLR degree is reduced by hamstring tightness.[240] **Tight hamstring syndrome** refers to limitations in hamstring extensibility due to radicular or disc pathology.[241,242] This condition is occasionally the first presenting symptom or sign of disc herniation.[242] Hamstring tightness related to disc herniations may be identified in adolescents by the **board sign**, when SLR causes the buttocks to lift from the table.[241] Hamstring tightness often coincides with sciatic neural tension in the SLR.

There is some evidence that limitations in SLR degree are due to **stretch tolerance**. This has been described as a defense response[238] and voluntary reaction to pain.[238,261,262] Two studies using EMG identified increased activity of the **hamstrings, erector spinae, and gluteus maximus** during the SLR in those with disc herniations and/or LBP.[238,262] One study found that this increased activity went away during general anesthesia, suggesting it was related to the voluntary resistance of the patient.[262]

The central nervous system and spinal cord also influence the SLR degree. In this sense, overactivity of the hamstrings and other **posterior chain** muscles have been described as protective reflex,[261] **reflex spasm**,[241] or involuntary reaction to pain.[238] One study identified this response in rats, even when the spinal cord was cut.[261] This suggests that some limitation of the SLR is related to **central sensitization** leading to increased muscle stretch reflexes.[261]

Table 24: Conditions that cause a positive SLR, provocative of sciatica

Common causes (>80%)

- Lumbar disc bulge, herniation, or annular tear

Moderately common causes (<20%)

- Lumbar stenosis (in 17%)[62]
- Deep gluteal[217] or piriformis syndrome[218]
- Sacroiliitis[210,243]
- Common peroneal,[98] saphenous, [98] or tibial nerve entrapment or lesion[98]

Rare causes (<1%)

- Cordonal sciatica (cervical or thoracic spine)[220,221]
- Diabetic lumbosacral radiculoplexus neuropathy[244]
- Epidural varices[245,246]
- Guillain-Barré Syndrome[247]
- Pelvic disease (e.g. ectopic endometriosis)[248]
- Posterior vertebral apophysis fracture[249]
- Ruptured abdominal aortic aneurysm[250,251]
- Spinal vascular malformation[252]
- Tumors of the cauda equina, conus, and filum terminale[253–255]
- Tumors of the lumbar spine and sacrum[256]
- Vertebral osteomyelitis[257] or septic sacroiliitis[258,259]
- Tethered cord syndrome[260]

The degree of central reflexes limiting the SLR may depend on the severity of the sciatica. One study found that anesthesia with intravenous lidocaine rapidly increased the SLR of patients with discogenic sciatica who were unlikely to require surgery.[263] However, two studies found no difference in the SLR with general or epidural anesthesia in patients about to have disc surgery.[264,265] Patients with severe discogenic sciatica warranting surgery may have SLR limitations maintained by an involuntary central reflex.

Tension of the **superficial back line** of myofascia may limit the SLR. This is a continuous chain of fascia and muscles including the **plantar fascia**, Achilles tendon, gastrocnemius, hamstrings, sacrotuberous ligament, sacral and thoracolumbar fascia, **erector spinae**, semispinalis, and splenius capitis.[266] One study using cadavers found the SLR placed strain on the plantar fascia, which was maximized during ankle dorsiflexion.[267] Other studies found that myofascial release of the suboccipital area, hamstrings, or plantar fascia increased the degree of SLR, possibly because of these myofascial connections.[268,269]

The SLR places tension on smaller nerves in addition to the sciatic. A study using cadavers found that the SLR created most strain on the sciatic nerve, followed by the tibial nerve at the knee, tibial nerve at the ankle, **lateral plantar nerve**, and **medial plantar nerve**.[270] Although the study did not measure the common peroneal nerve, there is clinical evidence that that SLR can provoke pain in those with **peroneal nerve pathology**.[98]

The first and most common method of SLR testing called the **passive straight leg raise** involves hip flexion, knee extension, and ankle dorsiflexion.[267] First, the patient is placed supine on a firm level surface with the cervical spine, trunk, and hips in a neutral position. Next, the leg is gently raised by holding the heel, while keeping the ankle in a neutral position.[272]

SLR sensitizing maneuvers

Variations of the SLR, also called **sensitizing** or **finishing maneuvers**, target certain nerve branches by adding neural tension in specific ways. These tests positive when they reproduce lower extremity pain in the sciatic nerve distribution or course.

Bragard's test is performed by lowering a positive SLR enough that it is no longer provocative of symptoms, then dorsiflexing the ankle.[15] This test is only performed when the SLR is positive. Bragard's test may have a slightly greater specificity than the SLR, and is more accurate in those with **acute symptoms** of less than 3 weeks.[15] This test has been shown to help distinguish discogenic from sacroiliac-joint related sciatica, in which Bragard's test is rarely positive.[210]

A variation called **SLR2** adds ankle eversion and toe extension to the SLR1.[271] This has a bias for **tibial nerve** involvement in sciatica, and may also be positive in those with **tarsal tunnel syndrome**.[270] The **SLR3** adds ankle inversion to the SLR.[271] This test helps identify **sural nerve** pathology.[267]

The **SLR4**, utilizes hip flexion and internal rotation, knee extension, ankle plantarflexion, and foot inversion.[271] This test may help identify patients with **common peroneal nerve** involvement.[271]

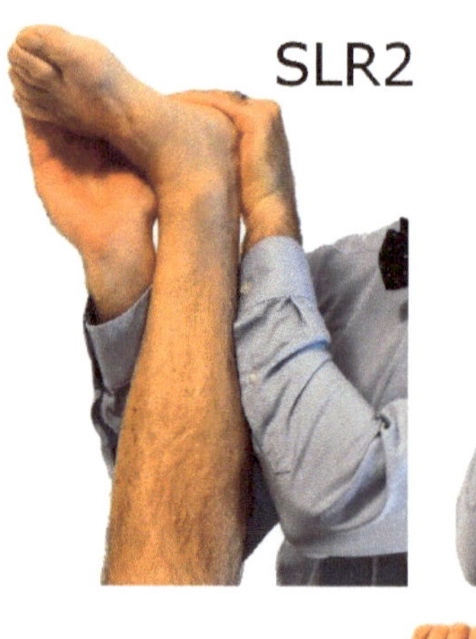

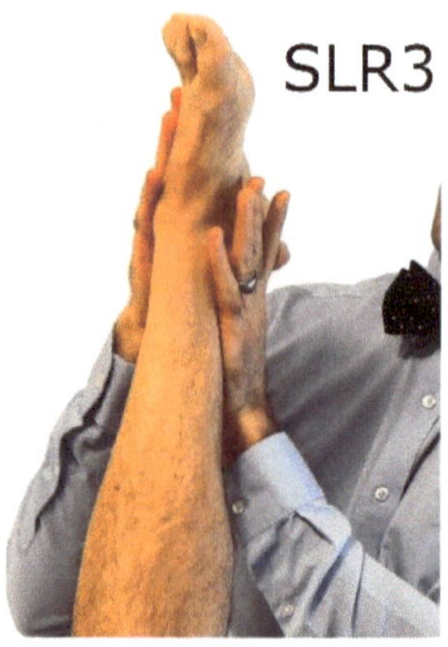

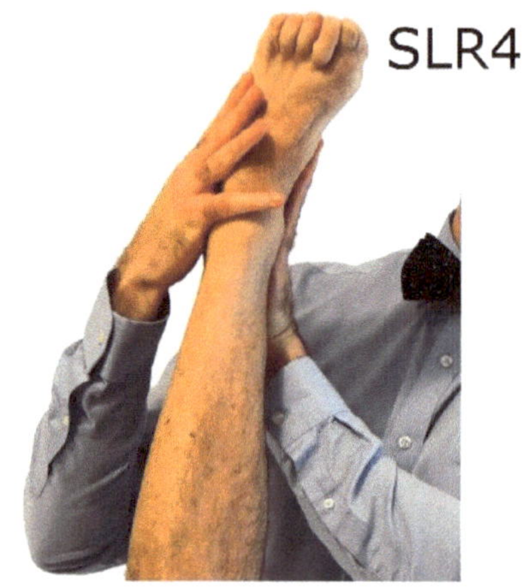

Figure 155: The main SLR variations, SLR2, SLR3, and SLR4

Bonnet's test is performed by adding hip internal rotation and adduction to the SLR.[110] This test has been found to be more useful in those with lumbar intra- or extra-foraminal stenosis. While the SLR is normally negative in those with central canal stenosis, about two-thirds of those with foraminal stenosis have a positive Bonnet's test.[239]

The **SLR5**, is an SLR of the asymptomatic leg.[273] This test is also called the **well-leg raise**, crossed straight leg raise, and crossover sign. This test is seldom positive in cases of sciatica, but when it does, it has a high specificity for L5 or S1 nerve root impingement (sn 7%, sp 96%, LR+ 1.7)[173] and LDH (sn 29%, sp 88%, OR 4.39).[216] It is also more predictive of disc protrusions compared to extrusions (RR 2.56).[274]

There are many other sciatic neural tension tests. **Sicard's test** is similar to a Bragard test except the great toe is dorsiflexed after the SLR instead of the ankle.[275] In **Turyn's test** the great toe is dorsiflexed with the patient supine and legs flat.[276]

Slump testing

The slump test puts tension on the lumbosacral nerve roots and spinal cord with the patient seated. Variations include the seated straight leg raise, sitting root test, and Bechterew's test. The slump test may affect higher lumbar nerve roots than the SLR due to the addition of trunk and neck flexion.[11] When this test causes pain below the knee, the likelihood of radicular sciatica increases greatly (+LR 11.9).[13] When pain is proximal to the knee, the likelihood is only increased by a small degree (+LR 3.0).[13]

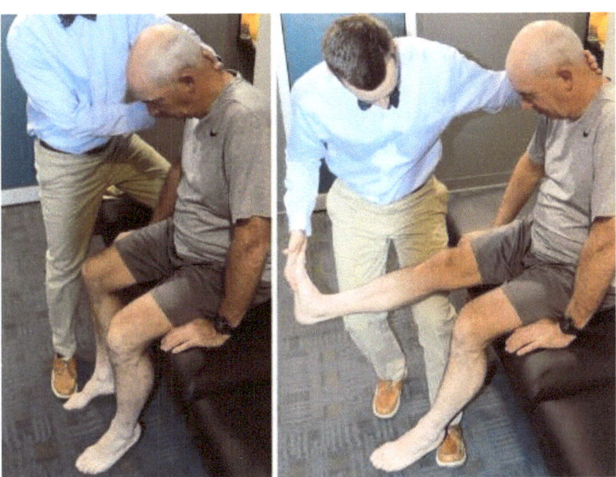

Figure 156: Slump testing, start (left) and finish (right)

The slump test variation 1 (ST1), similar to the sitting root test or Bechterew's test, is performed with a by flexing the patient's spine and hip, then extending one knee and dorsiflexing that ankle.[271] In the slump test variation 4 (ST4) both hips and knees are extended and one ankle is dorsiflexed.[271] The slump test is more sensitive than the straight leg raise and better able to identify patients with LDHs (sn 84%, sp 83%).[11]

Femoral nerve testing

The femoral nerve stretch test (FNST), also called the **prone knee bending test** or Nachlas test, places the femoral nerve and upper lumbar nerve roots under tension. The clinician flexes the knee of the prone patient to perform this test. The FNST is most useful for sciatica that involves the **L4 nerve root**, the only one shared between the sciatic and femoral nerves. This test has a low sensitivity and very high specificity for L2, 3, or 4 nerve root impingement (sn 50%, sp 100%).[173] The crossed variation of this test (crossed FNST) is performed on the asymptomatic side and also has a high specificity for upper lumbar nerve root involvement.[173]

Orthopedic testing

Gluteal-specific tests

Orthopedic tests for the deep gluteal region aim to stretch or contract tendons, muscles, and other fibrous structures to reproduce symptoms of sciatic nerve entrapment.[217] Many of the classic lumbar tests like the straight leg raise and Valsalva's test may be normal in these patients. Tests that increase tension and compression on the sciatic nerve in the gluteal region can reproduce symptoms of deep gluteal syndrome (DGS). **Passive stretching** maneuvers involving hip adduction and/or internal rotation, or **active contraction** using hip abduction and external rotation can elicit symptoms.

Hip **adduction** and **internal rotation** are often painful in any type of deep gluteal syndrome.[217] The **<u>F</u>lexion <u>A</u>dduction <u>I</u>nternal <u>R</u>otation test** or **FAIR** or **FADDIR**, also called the **FADIR** test is the most sensitive and specific test for piriformis syndrome. Clinicians perform the FAIR test by passively flexing the hip to 90 degrees while adducting and internally rotating it. This test is painful in about 90% of those with piriformis syndrome.[277,278] It is moderately specific (sp 83%) and increases the odds of piriformis syndrome by a factor of 2.8.[277] The FAIR test may be painful with other types of DGS.

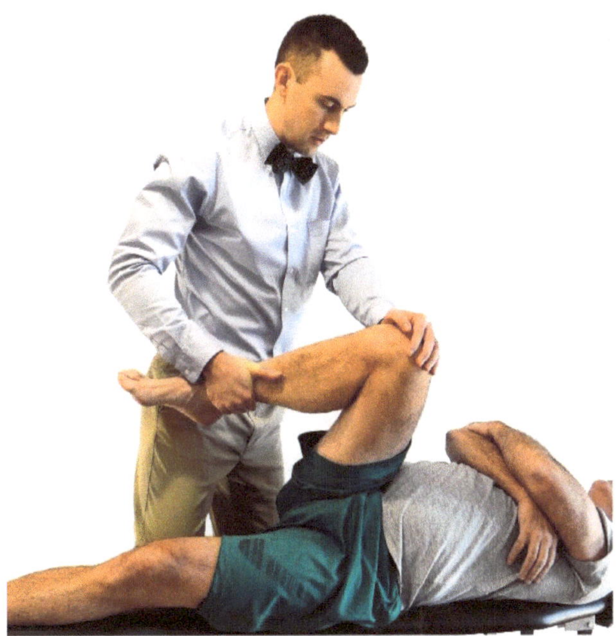

Figure 157: The FADIR test

The **active piriformis test** is performed when the patient actively **abducts** and **externally rotates** the hip against the examiner in the lateral position.[217]

Some authors perform this supine in which case it is easy to perform immediately after the FAIR test. This test is thought to cause the piriformis and other deep rotators including the gemelli and obturator internus to contract and compress the sciatic nerve.[217] This test has a sensitivity of 78%, specificity of 80%, and an odds ratio of 14.4 for the diagnosis of DGS.[217]

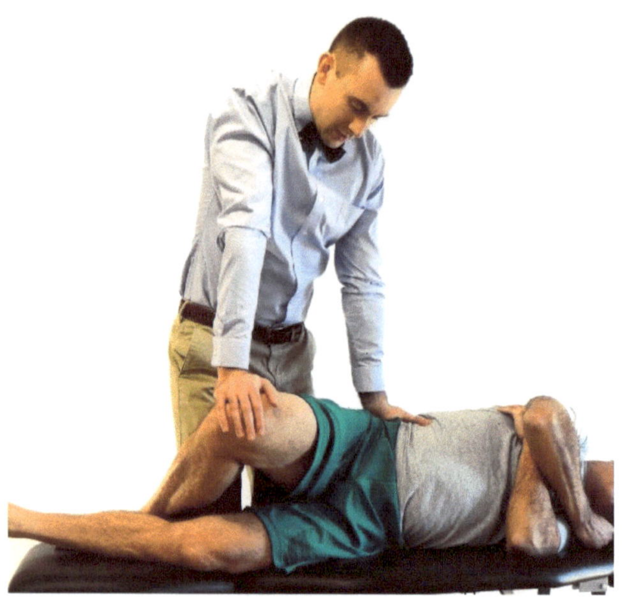

Figure 158: The active piriformis test

The **seated piriformis stretch test** is performed by passively internally rotating the hip with the knee straight while the patient is seated.[217] This test lengthens the piriformis muscle while creating sciatic nerve tension.[217] The common peroneal stretch variation of the SLR may elicit symptoms in a similar manner. Other manual muscle tests such as the Pace sign, Beatty sign, and tonic external rotation of the hip reproduce symptoms with resisted hip abduction.

Physical examination findings may mimic those of discogenic sciatica. The **straight leg raise** is limited and painful in about half of cases of piriformis syndrome.[218] Neurological deficits of reflexes, sensation, and strength each occur in about a third of cases.[218] Patients may have **tonic external rotation of the hip**, which is a visible sign of external rotation of the lower extremity at rest while lying supine.

Active hamstring muscle testing performed at thirty degrees, the **A-30 test**, has a greater sensitivity and accuracy for diagnosing sciatic nerve entrapment caused by proximal hamstring tear and tendinosis than testing at ninety degrees.[74] The test is positive if there is weakness and/or pain at the ischial tuberosity. In a patient with sciatica, a positive A-30 test is highly specific (97%) for **proximal hamstring syndrome** (sciatic nerve entrapment by hamstring pathology).[74]

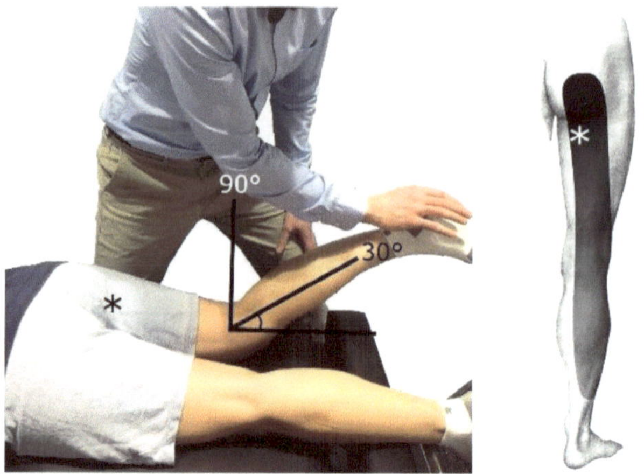

Figure 159: The A-30 test. Pain referral into the lower extremity during the test is strong indicator of proximal hamstring syndrome. This patient had reproduction of her site of maximal pain and tenderness (*), 3/5 strength. and radiating pain (→) with the test. She had slipped on ice a week prior, suffering a grade 2 proximal hamstring strain, and had a radiating sciatic pain referral into the thigh and leg (right image). Case shared with patient's permission.

Sacroiliac-specific tests

Sacroiliac tests can be used to reproduce a patient's SIJ pain and any related sciatica.[210] Many of these tests have a low sensitivity and/or specificity, so combining them is essential to the examination. When **three provocation tests** provoke pain, the odds of symptoms coming from the SIJ increase by a large amount (OR 17.2).[3]

To perform the **thigh thrust test** the clinician directs force posteriorly through the femur of the flexed hip with the patient supine.

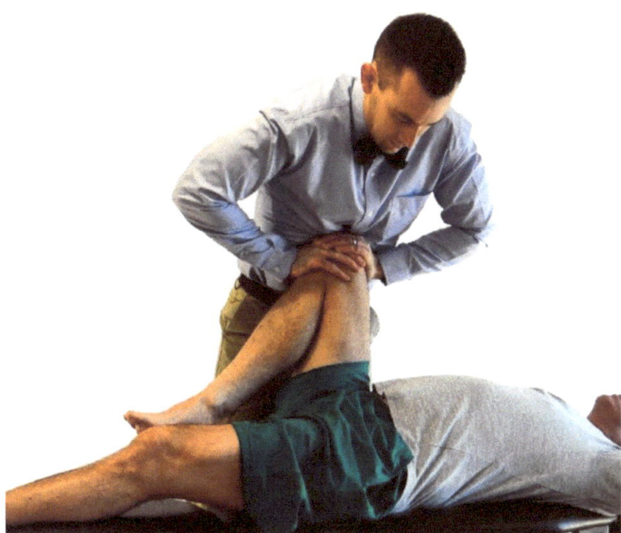

Figure 160: The thigh thrust test

To perform the **SIJ distraction test**, also called the **SIJ gapping test**, the clinician presses posteriorly against the anterior superior iliac spines (ASISs) with the patient supine.[279]

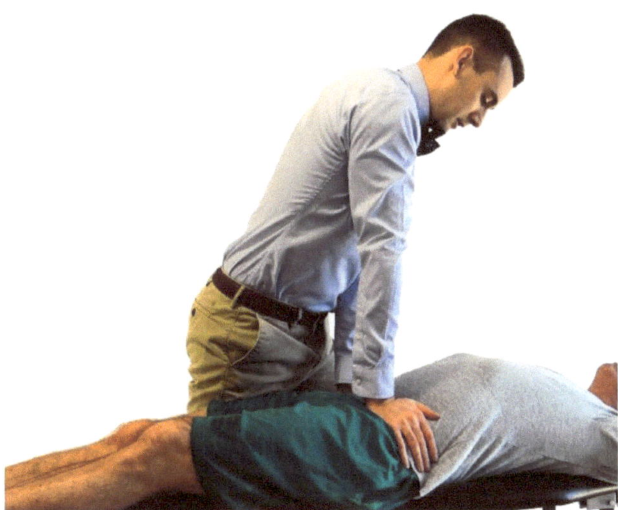

Figure 161: The SIJ distraction test

To perform the **SIJ compression test** the clinician presses medially against the lateral iliac crest while the patient is side-lying.

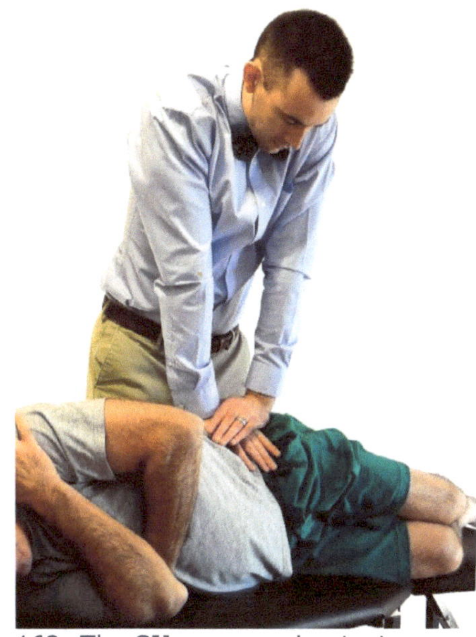

Figure 162: The SIJ compression test

To perform the **sacral thrust** the clinician presses anteriorly on the mid-sacrum with the patient prone.

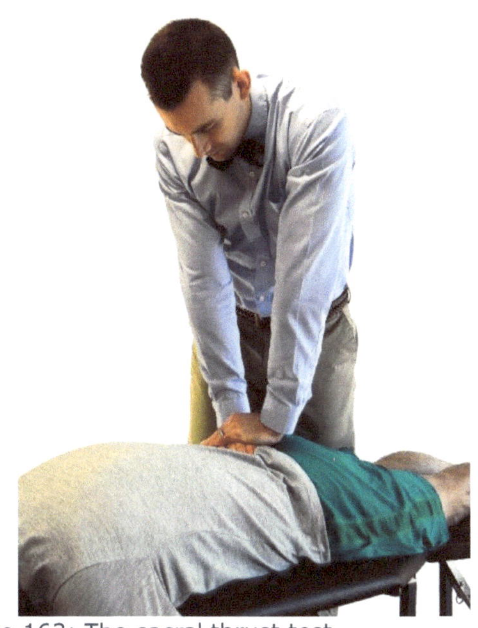

Figure 163: The sacral thrust test

To perform **Gaenslen's test** the clinician flexes one hip while extending the other.

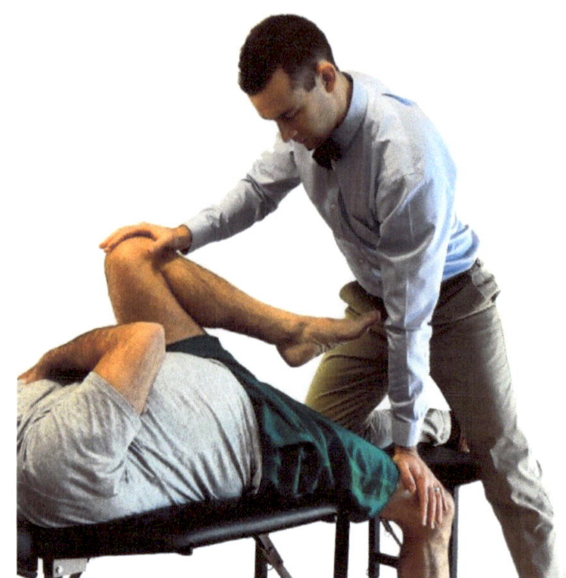
Figure 164: Gaenslen's test

Hip-specific tests

Orthopedic tests targeting the hip joint are often painful in those with LBP. Nearly 80% of LBP sufferers have at least one test provocative of lateral hip, groin, or buttocks pain.[280] Those with LBP and at least one painful hip test have more severe LBP and greater disability levels associated with LBP. [280] These tests may implicate the hip as a source of **pain referral**, or movement restrictions that guide treatment of a concomitant low back disorder.

Clinicians perform the **Flexion ABduction External Rotation Extension test** or **FABERE**, also called the **FABER** test by flexing the patient's knee then passively abducting, externally rotating, and extending the hip so that the ankle rests on the opposite thigh just proximal to the patella.[281] Hip pain indicates a positive test and possible hip pathology. **Groin pain** during FABERE is even more specific for hip pathology and helps distinguish from spinal or radicular sciatica.[260] The FABERE test has a high sensitivity (93%) and specificity (84%) for **hip osteoarthritis**.[282]

This test was first conceived by Dr. Patrick in 1917 to distinguish hip arthritis from spine-related sciatica.[281] The FABERE position minimizes **sciatic nerve tension** so any increase in pain is unlikely to be from sciatic nerve stretching. Only in rare instances such as labral cysts[283] or tumors[284] will the sciatic nerve be compressed by the FABERE position.[260258253] Any increase in lower extremity pain is most likely due to **pain referral** from the hip joint, followed by the **SIJ**, and rarely due to sciatic nerve compression.

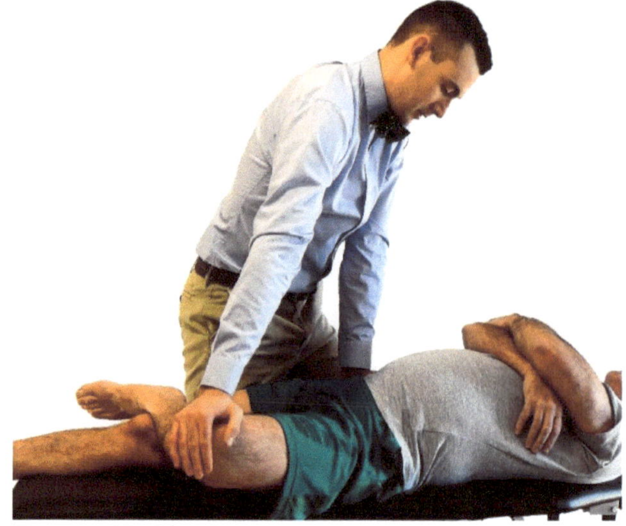
Figure 165: The FABER test

Clinicians perform the hip **Flexion ADuction External Rotation test** or **FADER** test by flexing the hip to 90°, while adducting, and externally rotating it to end range. Pain in the region of the greater trochanter indicates a positive test and possible gluteal tendinopathy. The addition of active patient resistance to this test is called **FADER-R,** which is more sensitive and specific than FADER (sn 44%, sp 93%).[138]

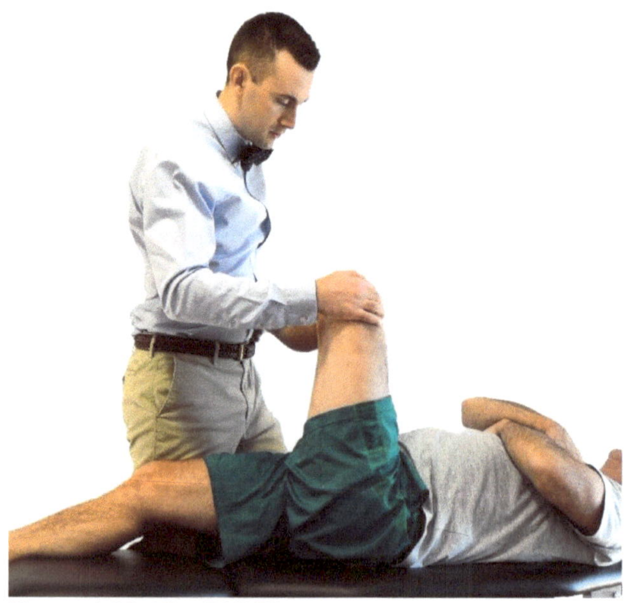
Figure 166: The FADER test

During the **single leg stance,** the patient stands on the side of pain facing the wall, with the other hip flexed to 90°. The patient stands for up to **30 seconds** and can use a finger from the non-painful side hand to help balance. Lateral hp pain within 30 seconds indicates a positive test and possible gluteal tendinopathy. Single-leg-stance is the most specific test for gluteal tendinopathy but has a low sensitivity (sn 38%, sp 100%).[138]

Hip flexor length assessments

The **Thomas test** assesses for hip flexion contracture. To perform this test the clinician places the patient supine and flexes one hip and knee and looks for flexion of the opposite hip. An inability of the thigh to lie flat on the table is a sign of hip flexion contracture. In the second part of the test the clinician presses the thigh against the table. An increase in lumbar lordosis also indicates a hip flexion contracture.

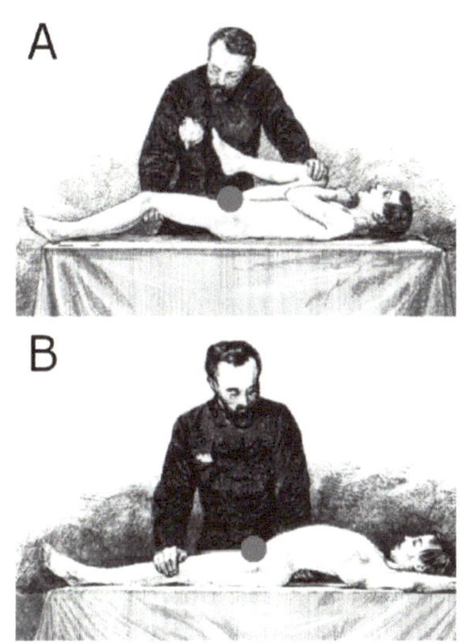

Figure 167: Thomas' test. (A) The knee and hip flex along with the opposite hip. (B) When the clinician extends the patient's hip and knee the lordosis increases. Image from the original description in Hugh Thomas' 1878 book "Diseases of the hip, knee, and ankle joints" (public domain). Modified by Robert James Trager, DC.

The **modified Thomas test** gives a better measure of hip flexor length by allowing the thigh to extend with the help of gravity. The patient lies supine on the edge of the table and holds one hip and knee flexed while allowing the other to extend. The angle of the thigh relative to the table indicates the degree of hip extension. A normal value is three degrees of extension (-3°) while a hip flexor contracture is **five degrees of flexion** (5°) or greater.[285] A rough estimate can be made without using a goniometer by looking for a large gap between the patient's thigh and the table, indicating loss of hip extension.

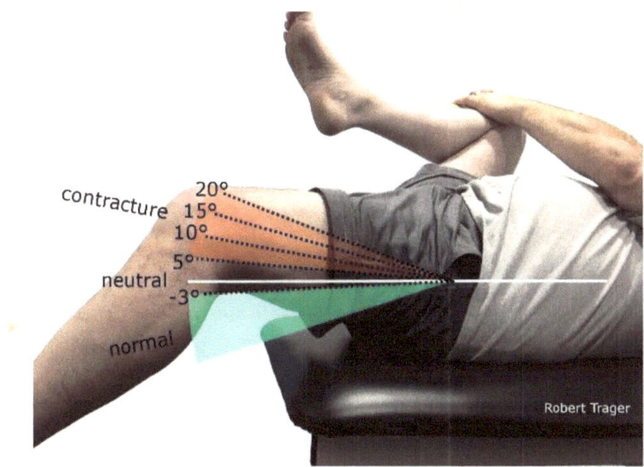

Figure 168: The modified Thomas test. A normal range is at least 3 degrees of hip extension. Hip flexion contracture is five degrees or more of hip flexion. This patient has right sided discogenic sciatic pain with a bilateral hip flexor contracture, more severe 10° contracture on the left side.

Clinicians may use the modified Thomas test to assess the **rectus femoris**. This muscle acts as both a hip flexor and a knee extensor. An inability of the knee to approximate **90° of flexion** during the modified Thomas test indicates rectus femoris contracture. Rectus femoris contracture is thought to contribute to overall hip flexor contracture in those with LBP.[126]

Michele's test is another variation on the Tomas test. Starting in a modified Thomas position, the clinician straightens the tested knee to isolate any effect of the hip contracture to the psoas and exclude the rectus femoris. Typically, extending the knee increases hip extension by reducing stretch on the rectus femoris.[126]

Spinal pressure tests

Spinal fluid pressure tests increase the pressure and/or volume of the vertebral veins and cerebrospinal fluid (CSF) to provoke symptoms of radicular sciatica. These tests include **bearing down** with the vocal cords closed, by **coughing** or **sneezing**, or by compressing the jugular veins. These maneuvers increase vertebral vein and CSF pressure[286] and compress, traction, and irritate sensitized nerve roots.[287] These tests are most sensitive for intraspinal radicular forms of sciatica.

Valsalva's test is the most commonly used pressure test to screen for lumbar pathology. The Italian anatomist Antonio Valsalva (CE 1666 - 1723) initially described this test for examining the ear. The classic traditional Chinese medical text *The Huangdi Neijing*

(100 BC)[i] may have been the first to describe increased LBP related to coughing:[288]

> *When it is the vessel of the flesh structures that lets a person's lower back ache, then the patient cannot cough.¶ When he coughs, the sinews shrink and become tense.¶ (Unschuld p. 621)*

In 1914, the French physician Joseph Déjerine described an increase in sciatic pain with sneezing, coughing, and defacation[289] which has since been called "**Déjerine's triad**." Around 1941 in Germany the **abdominal press** or bauchpresse was identified as a specific sign of LDH.[290]

In 1916 Queckenstedt discovered that jugular vein compression increased CSF pressure, and used this technique to identify tumors of the spinal cord.[291] In 1931, Naffziger performed a similar maneuver to identify nerve root compression.[292]

Anatomy of the vertebral pressure system

Pressure tests work by altering the volume and pressure of the vertebral veins and lumbar cerebrospinal fluid. The **lumbar vertebral vein system** is a communicating network of **valveless**, low-pressure veins with connections anteriorly, superiorly, and inferiorly.[293] This system acts as a **fluid reservoir** that accommodates pressure and volume changes in the thoraco-abdominal cavities. The cerebrospinal fluid pressure and volume changes in response to alterations in the vertebral veins.

The lumbar vertebral vein system includes the **paravertebral** (ascending lumbar), **epidural** (extradural), and **intraosseous** veins. The intraosseous veins originate in the vertebral bodies and connect to the basivertebral vein which in turn connects with the epidural venous plexus. This plexus connects with the paravertebral veins, also called the ascending lumbar veins. The vertebral veins are connected to major vein systems including the caval, pulmonary, and portal veins.[293] They also connect with the adrenals, kidneys, breast, and prostate.[294]

Diagnostic utility

An increase in low back and/or lower extremity pain with coughing, sneezing, or straining is found in just over half of patients with sciatica (52-53%).[295,296] Pain with these maneuvers is most specific for **discogenic** or **intraspinal sciatica**. Those with increased pain upon coughing, sneezing, bearing down have 2 to 2.5 times the odds of having **nerve root compression** on MRI.[295,297,298]

Valsalva maneuvers may not be as useful in patients with LSS, who are typically older. Older patients generate less of an increase in vertebral vein pressure, possibly due to less muscular power with straining.[299] In addition those, with LSS tend to display less mechanosensitivity to neural tension,[233] which is one mechanism of a Valsalva maneuver. Another reason could be the relative absence of an acute inflammatory process compared to an acute LDH.

Those with extraspinal or non-radicular sciatica occasionally have pain with coughing, sneezing, and straining. One study found 42% of patients with **SIJ**-related sciatica had increased pain with these maneuvers.[210] This maneuver may also increase symptoms of an abdominal aortic aneurysm. [302] One study found that pain provocation with coughing, sneezing, or bearing down was a poor predictor of sacroiliitis. None of the patients with this symptom improved with a diagnostic SIJ injection.[137]

Table 25: Conditions that may cause a positive Valsalva's test provocative of sciatica

Common causes
• Lumbar disc pathology
Less common causes
• IVF stenosis[300]
• SIJ pain[210]
Rare causes
• Epidural varices[245,246]
• Leptomeningeal metastasis[301]
• Ruptured abdominal aortic aneurysm[302]
• Spinal epidural hematoma[303]
• Spinal vascular malformation[252]
• Tarlov cyst[304]
• Tumors of the cauda equina, conus, and filum terminale[254,305]
• Tumors of the spine and sacrum[256]

Jugular vein compression tests are less useful in the evaluation of sciatica. This type of test rarely increases discogenic radicular pain.[287] Jugular vein compression only slightly increases CSF pressure in

[i] The term "sinew" could refer to the sciatic nerve as terminology at this time did not distinguish between nerves and connective tissue. The text also describes acupuncture or bloodletting at a location at or near the small saphenous vein near the ankle.

those with LDH, and not at all in those with LSS.[286] Jugular vein compression does not significantly increase the vertebral vein pressure in those with LDH or LSS.[286]

Interpretation

Valsalva's testing may produce **local pain** (LBP) or **lower extremity pain**. Those with only lower extremity pain during this maneuver are more likely to have nerve root compression or LDH. Pain in any location is more sensitive (71%) but less specific (32%) for nerve root compression[298] **Leg pain only** is less sensitive (40%) but more specific (77%) for **nerve root compression.**[298] Leg pain only is likewise more specific (79%) for LDH.[298] Leg pain rather than LBP during a Valsalva is more likely to be caused by radicular sciatica.

Mechanisms of pressure tests

During a Valsalva maneuver the diaphragm and other core muscles become more active.[306] The inferior vena cava (IVC) is flattened, which causes a reflux of venous blood into the spine, displacement of CSF, and narrowing of the thecal sac. Valsalva maneuvers increase thoraco-abdominal, CSF, vertebral vein, and IVC pressure, which compresses and tense the lumbosacral nerves.

A Valsalva maneuver compresses the inferior vena cava (IVC) and increases **IVC pressure**. It is thought that descent of the diaphragm during full inspiration compresses the IVC.[307] One study using CT scans found that a Valsalva flattened the IVC and reduced its diameter.[308] Compression of the IVC rapidly reverses venous flow, forcing it into the vertebral venous system, analogous to a **water-hammer effect.**[309]

Imaging studies show that a Valsalva maneuver diverts venous blood from the IVC towards the lumbar spine. Valsalva's maneuver has been used in lumbar **venography** imaging to cause reflux from the iliac and caval veins into the vertebral veins, making them more visible for diagnostic purposes.[310] A more recent study showed that a Valsalva maneuver increased the prominence of the intradural veins during a single-shot lumbar MRI.[311]

Valsalva maneuvers increase the vertebral **intra-osseous pressures**. This pressure is used as a marker for vertebral venous pressure because intraosseous veins are continuous with epidural veins and have no valves to create a pressure gradient.[312] One study of patients with radicular sciatica found that intraosseous pressure rose on average from 11 to 60 mm Hg during a Valsalva.[312]

A Valsalva maneuver increases **CSF pressure** from a baseline of about 10 mm Hg to 20 mm Hg.[313] The CSF pressure is normally free to move within the spine and increases less than the vertebral veins during a Valsalva. In a healthy patient, cerebrospinal fluid **displaces** cranially into the cervical canal during a Valsalva.[314]

Spinal block pressure is a pathologically increased CSF pressure created by a space-occupying spinal lesion.[315] Studies have shown that there may be focal increases in CSF pressure when the thecal sac is blocked. Any expansile lesion including LDH, LSS, or tumors may create this effect.[315] Spinal block pressure is additionally increased upon straining, voiding, or jugular vein compression.[316]

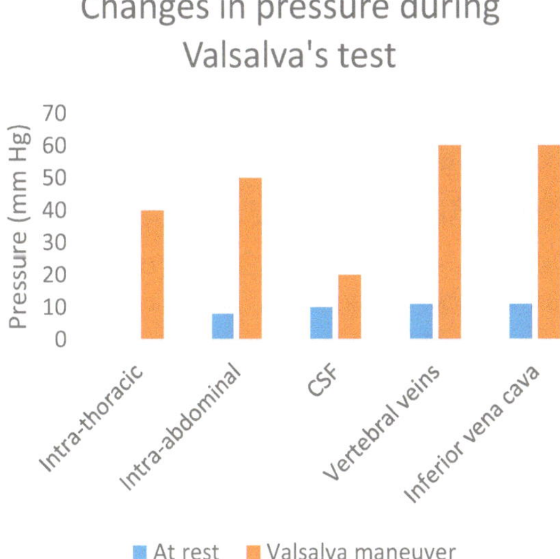

Figure 169: Relative changes in pressure during a Valsalva maneuver. Intrathoracic pressures are from normal subjects and are reported relative to atmospheric pressures. Intra-abdominal pressures are measured from the stomachs of normal subjects. Those of cerebrospinal fluid (CSF) are from patients with neurological pathology. Vertebral vein and inferior vena cava (IVC) pressures are from patients with radicular sciatica. Intra-thoracic and intra-abdominal pressures from Nordenfelt,[320] CSF from Lee,[321] and vertebral vein and IVC from Spencer.[313]

Coughing, sneezing, and bearing down increase the **intra-discal pressure**. One study found that sneezing increased intradiscal pressure by a factor of 3.2, and bearing down (Valsalva) increased pressure by a factor of 1.8.[317] Another study corroborated these findings, and found that a Valsalva increased intradiscal pressure by a factor of about 2.[318]

Valsalva's test increases the lumbar **intra-osseous pressure** by a factor of over 3.[286] Intraosseous pressure is the hydrostatic pressure of the veins within the lumbar vertebrae.[312] The intra-osseous pressure correlates almost exactly with the inferior vena cava pressure.[312] When the IVC pressure is increased during a Valsalva, the intra-osseous pressure simultaneously increases.[312]

Valsalva's test increases the **intra-abdominal pressure** from about 8 to 50 mm Hg and raises **intrathoracic pressure** by about 40 mm Hg.[319] Experiments have shown that **abdominal compression**, which increases intra-abdominal pressure without modifying intra-thoracic pressure, helps shunt venous blood to the vertebral veins.[294] Thoracic and abdominal pressures may be synergistic in compressing the IVC and causing a pressure gradient for venous reflux to the lumbar spine.

A Valsalva maneuver narrows the **dural sac** and reduces the lumbar **CSF volume**.[320] The lumbar CSF reduces by about 30-40 mL (28%) as it displaces towards the cervical region[320] It is thought that the spinal canal volume remains constant, and any loss of CSF is balanced by a roughly equal rise in venous blood.[306] According to this, 30-40 mL (about 2 to 3 tablespoons) of venous blood enters the lumbar spine during a Valsalva maneuver to balance the loss of CSF volume.

The **thecal sac** elongates and narrows as it is compressed by expanded vertebral veins during a Valsalva maneuver.[314] As a result, the lumbar CSF reduces in volume as it shifts towards the upper spine. One study found that abdominal compression (an artificial method of producing a Valsalva effect) reduced lumbar CSF volume by 28%.[320] The reductions in thecal sac and CSF volume reverses rapidly after a Valsalva maneuver.[314]

A Valsalva maneuver places **tension**, **traction**, and **compression** on nerve roots. It is thought that the shrinking of the thecal sac during the Valsalva tractions the lumbar nerve roots proximally and cranially.[287] Because the nerve roots are tethered by connective tissue and unable to move freely, they are also subject to tension.[287] Expansion of the radicular veins may exacerbate a compressive effect of a nerve root against disc material.

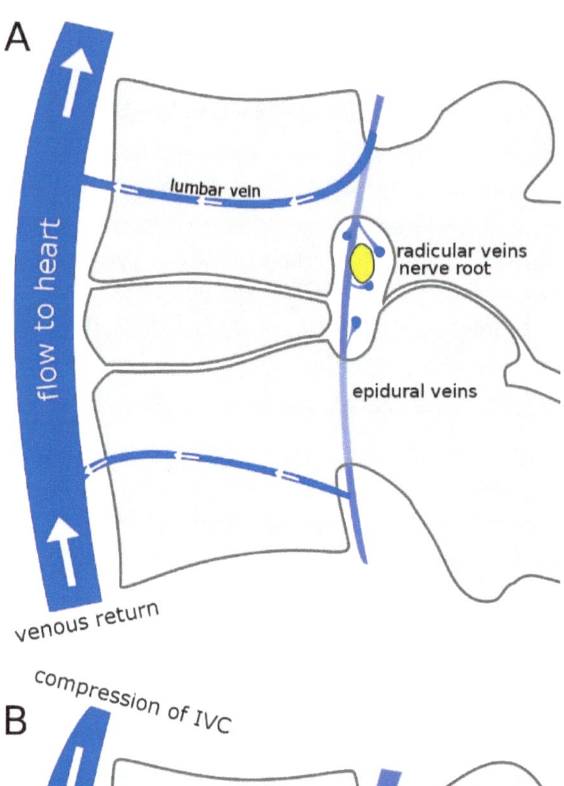

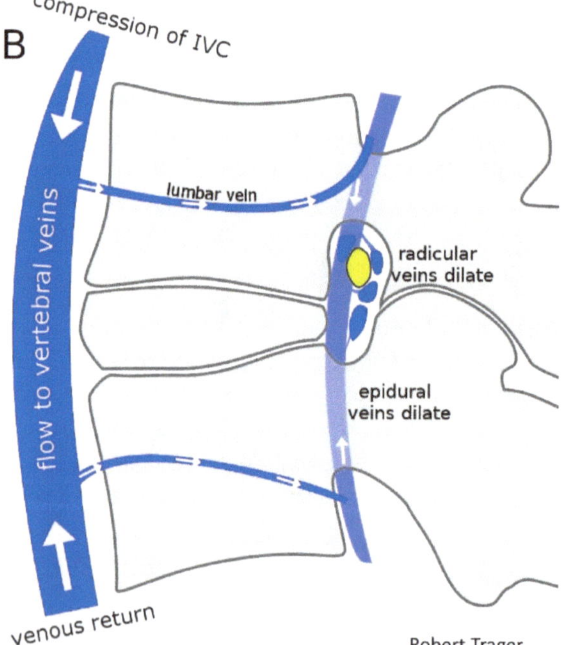

Figure 170: Image A: Normal flow of venous blood in the lumbar spine is towards the inferior vena cava, which flows cranially to the heart. Image B: During a Valsalva maneuver, the IVC is compressed by the diaphragm and intra-abdominal pressure, which reverses the flow of venous blood towards the vertebral veins, causing dilation of these veins and compression of nerve roots.

Increased venous, CSF, and intra-discal pressures may cause pain by activating **nociceptors**. This includes, for example, nociceptors in the annulus fibrosus[321] or dorsal horn of the spinal cord.[129] Elevated venous pressure may also stimulate nociceptors in the lumbar vertebrae.[322] The presence of sensitization may be a requirement to perceive pain during spinal pressure tests.

Elevated vertebral vein or CSF pressures interfere with the **cauda equina microcirculation**. One study used a balloon inserted into the lumbar canal of pigs to simulate increased pressure around nerve roots. The study found that a pressure of 30 mm Hg stopped blood flow through the venules to the nerve roots, while 40 mm Hg stopped flow through the capillaries, and 127 stopped flow through the arterioles.[323] A Valsalva maneuver that increases the CSF pressure to about 20 mm Hg and vertebral vein pressure to about 60 mm Hg would be expected to occlude arterial flow to the lumbosacral nerve roots.

Performing pressure tests

Clinicians may instruct patients to perform the **Valsalva test** by taking a deep breath and bearing down.[273] The clinician may palpate the patient's abdominal muscles to ensure they are contracting.[308] **Straining** has a greater effect on lumbar pressures than coughing, which has more of an effect on elevating thoracic pressure.[324]

An **unsupported**, **seated position** may be the most sensitive method to elicit symptoms during the Valsalva test. In this position, the vertebral veins are at their highest baseline pressure.[325] Sitting while actively straightening the back also increases the intradiscal pressure to a greater degree than lying or standing.[317]

Clinicians may flex or extend the patient's spine prior to the Valsalva maneuver. The "X" sign is the combination of **lumbar flexion** with a Valsalva's test. This test has a high specificity and increases the odds of discogenic sciatica by a large amount (sp 95%, OR 55).[326] Valsalva maneuver during lumbar extension has not been studied but might be useful for those with LSS. Lumbar extension increases the baseline of both CSF and vertebral venous pressures in those with LSS.[286]

Functional and stability testing

Clinicians may evaluate **breathing tests** in multiple positions. They may start by observing the patient in the standing or sitting position. Normally there is proportional expansion of the abdominal wall and chest. Those with sciatica and lower back conditions are more likely to have faulty breathing mechanics and disruption of this normal pattern.

Signs of abnormal breathing include constriction of the abdominal wall towards the umbilicus, called **hour glass syndrome**, activation of accessory muscles of breathing such as the sternocleidomastoid, elevation of the ribcage during inspiration, and **paradoxical breathing**, an inward drawing of the abdomen during inspiration.[327] These movement patterns indicate a reduced ability to stabilize the spine through intra-abdominal pressure and the need to rehabilitate breathing mechanics.

The **diaphragm test** evaluates diaphragm function with the patient seated. The examiner feels for expansion of the anterolateral and posterolateral abdominal wall with inspiration.[327] Faulty breathing mechanics include hollowing of the abdomen or lack of proportional expansion of the abdominal wall during inhalation.[327]

The **supine 90/90 test** evaluates breathing mechanics and the ability to maintain intra-abdominal pressure. The patient lies on their back with hips and knees flexed to 90 degrees. The examiner initially supports the patient's legs then gradually removes support. Signs of failure include an inability to maintain the position, thoracolumbar hyperextension, and lack of lateral and posterior abdominal wall activity with breathing.[327]

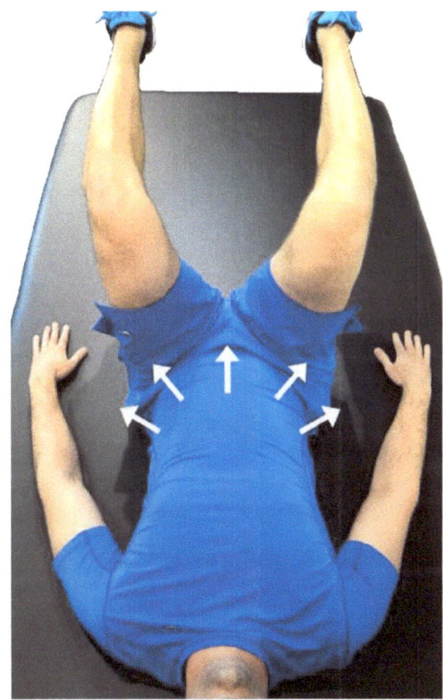

Figure 171: The supine 90/90 test. The patient's abdominal wall should expand diffusely during inspiration.

The **active straight leg raise** (ASLR) tests lumbopelvic stability. It challenges the ability of the deep abdominal muscles to stabilize the lumbar spine and

SIJ during supine hip flexion. The patient is asked to raise the straight leg off the table 20 cm. Signs of failure include **SIJ pain**, **trunk rotation** towards the raised leg, increase in **lumbar lordosis**, and an improved response with active bracing.[327] The clinician may add manual resistance for a **resisted straight leg raise**.[327]

The ASLR can improve with **abdominal bracing**[328] and manual **pelvic compression.**[329] The patient should be allowed to do the exercise without cues, and afterwards may be instructed to stiffen the abdominal muscles, back or stomach. Manual compression can be applied to the ilia bilaterally which may reduce SIJ pain.[329] When verbal cues to brace or manual compression improves the ASLR, these are signs that the patient lacks stability and may benefit from a lumbar spine stabilization exercise program.

An abnormal ASLR can be caused by a problem with the low back, SIJ, or pelvis.[328] The ASLR tests a small ROM while transmitting force through the SIJ. It is frequently abnormal in those with **SIJ pain.**[330] However, those with lumbar spine or pelvic pathology also can have an abnormal ASLR. This could be due poor lumbopelvic stabilization, presence of an irritable disc lesion, or loss of neural mobility.

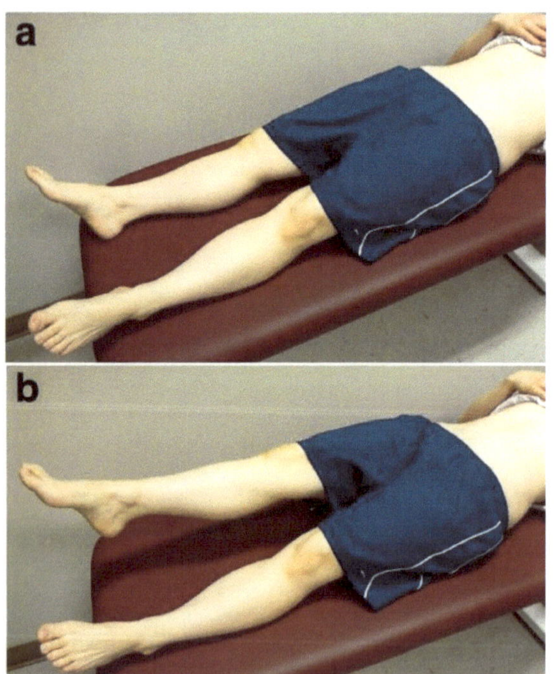

Figure 172: The active straight leg raise, creative commons license from Bruno.[329]

The **prone hip extension test** (PHE) evaluates lumbopelvic stability. To perform this test the examiner places the patient prone and asks them to raise their thigh towards the ceiling to 10-20 degrees of hip extension. Signs of failure include an **anterior pelvic tilt**, increase in **lumbar lordosis**, or **trunk rotation** towards the extended hip during the first 10 degrees.[327] The examiner can add manual resistance at the end of the test.

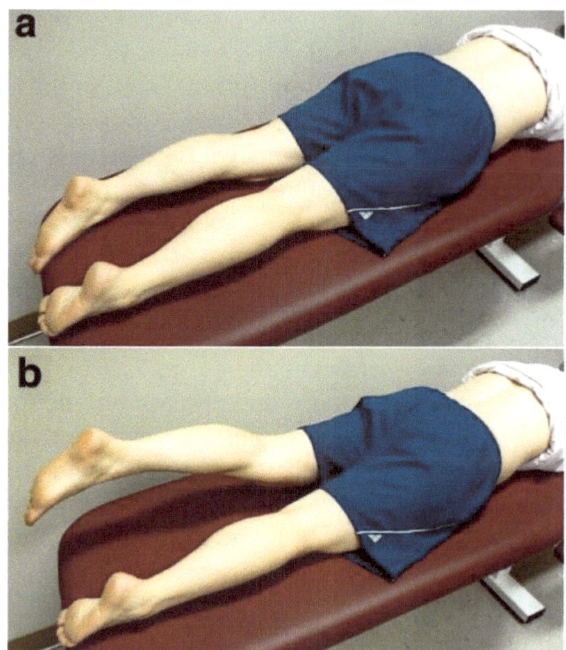

Figure 173: The prone hip extension test, start (a) and finish (b), creative commons license from Bruno.[329]

Those with LBP have much higher activity of the lumbar erector spinae than those without LBP.[331] The abnormal increase in erector activity is thought to be a compensation for lack of stability in the deeper **local stabilizers** such as the **multifidus**. The PHE test can increase LBP symptoms,[332] possibly due to increased tone of the erectors or poor mechanics that lead to irritation of sensitized spinal structures.

The ASLR and PHE tests both have a low sensitivity and high specificity,[333] meaning they best identify those with normal lumbopelvic stability. Patients with sciatica and normal ASLR and PHE tests may be less likely to need a lumbar spine stabilization exercise program. Those with sciatica and abnormal ASLR and/or PHE tests need further testing to find the source of symptoms. These tests are useful to monitor improvement and response to treatment.

Directional preference examination

Patients can be examined using **static** (stationary) or repeated **end-range movements** in positions of flexion, extension, side gliding, and rotation to determine which position(s), if any, alleviate symptoms.[334]

In the case of sciatica, the goal is to determine which position or movement allows for **centralization**, a retreat of radiating pain towards the spine. The **directional preference** (**DP**) is the position or end-range movement that helps centralize pain.

In 1937 Paul Williams, who became known for **Williams flexion exercises**, described how those with discogenic pain obtained relief if they lied or slept supine with the knees and hips flexed.[335] In 1944, doctor Norman Capener described exacerbation or relief of symptoms in flexion and extension. He was one of the first to promote the idea of nucleus pulposus retropulsion, a **posterior migration** of the gelatinous core of the IVD during spinal flexion.[ii] Robin Mckenzie developed Mechanical diagnosis and therapy in 1956 after observing that a patient's radiating LBP improved after lying in lumbar extension.

Lumbar flexion can either relieve or worsen sciatic pain. Lumbar flexion increases the diameter of the spinal canal and intervertebral foramina and often relieves sciatica caused by LSS. Conversely, lumbar flexion under load (e.g. flexed sitting) can encourage posterior migration of the nucleus pulposus and exacerbate discogenic sciatica.[337] Flexion may also increase sciatic pain by increasing neural tension.

Table 26: Effects of flexion and extension on the lumbar spine.

Structure	Flexion	Extension
Meninges and cauda equina	Tensed	Relaxed
Intervertebral foramina	Widened[340]	Narrowed[340]
Spinal canal	Widened[341]	Narrowed[341]
Nucleus pulposus of normal disc	Posterior migration[339]	Anterior migration[339]
Epidural pressure	Decreased[67]	Increased
Posterior longitudinal ligament	Tensed[342,343]	Relaxed
Moderately degenerated disc	No movement[339]	Posterior bulging[339]

Table 27: Clinical utility of the directional preference examination.

Position or movement	Interpretation
30 seconds of extension aggravates sciatica	LSS more likely (OR 5.86) [344]
Bending forward alleviates sciatica	LSS more likely (OR 2.1)[62]
Bending forward aggravates sciatica	LSS less likely (OR 0.36)[62]
Standing aggravates sciatica	LSS more likely (OR 1.3)[62]
Centralization of sciatic pain using DP	Discogenic pain (sn 37%, sp 90%, +LR 4.1),[345] better prognosis for recovery[334,346]

Lumbar flexion can relieve or alleviate symptoms depending on the primary etiology of sciatica. Lumbar stenosis (usually relieved by flexion) and LDH (usually relieved by extension) occur in two different populations. Stenosis patients are generally older (mean age 65) and herniation patients are usually younger (mean age 43).[338] The **hydration** of the IVDs reduces with aging while the typical preference changes from extension to flexion.

[ii] *"In some patients relief from pain is given by hyperextension; in others, by flexion. In [hyperextension], relief may be due to relaxation of the cauda equina and meningeal tension... while in flexion relief may result because there is greater room for the foraminal contents. On the contrary, flexion may increase disc and nuclear retropulsion, while by hyperextension one may aggravate pain by constricting foraminal contents." (Capener)*[336]

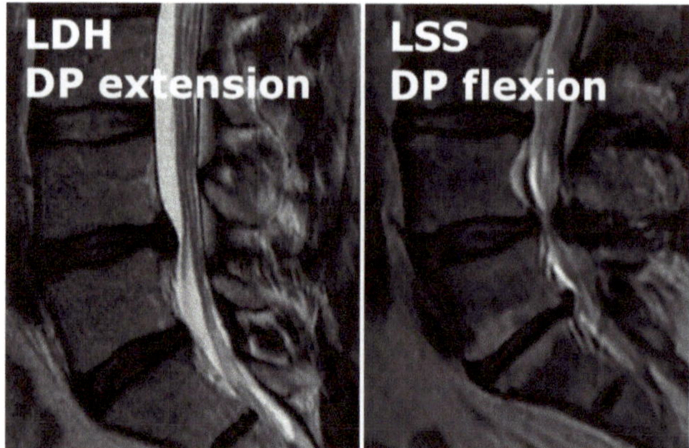

Figure 174: Directional preference (DP) typically changes from extension to flexion with increasing age, disc degeneration, reduction of disc hydration, and narrowing of the spinal canal. Both patients presented with severe bilateral sciatic pain, numbness, and weakness. Left image shows LDH in a 44-year-old man with a DP of extension. Right image shows LSS in a 65-year-old patient with a DP of flexion. Both patients improved with the help of home exercises. Cases shared with permission from patients by Robert Trager, DC.

Discs behave differently with flexion and extension depending on presence of **disc degeneration** which typically occurs with age. Older, degenerated discs bulge in extension, compared to younger non-degenerated discs which move anteriorly in extension.[339] Patients with sciatica should undergo an examination to determine DP in order to guide diagnosis and treatment.

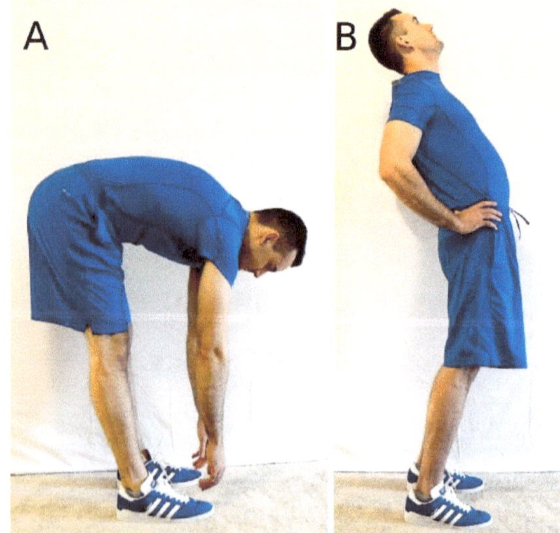

Figure 175: Directional preference examination of flexion in standing (A) and extension in standing (B)

Centralization is when pain moves towards its origin and retreats from a distal to proximal location. Centralization of sciatic pain is when it moves from the foot to the leg, thigh, then buttocks and/or spine. Centralization has been best validated for predicting discogenic pain.[6] One study found that centralization has a sensitivity of 37%, specificity of 90%, and positive likelihood ratio of 4.1 for predicting **discogenic sciatica**.[345]

Centralization with end-range or DP exercises most often occurs with intraspinal sciatica such as disc pathology and LSS. Centralization can occur in other extraspinal conditions such as SIJ pain and myofascial pain. Some patients with sciatica that have normal lumbar discs can still demonstrate centralization.[7]

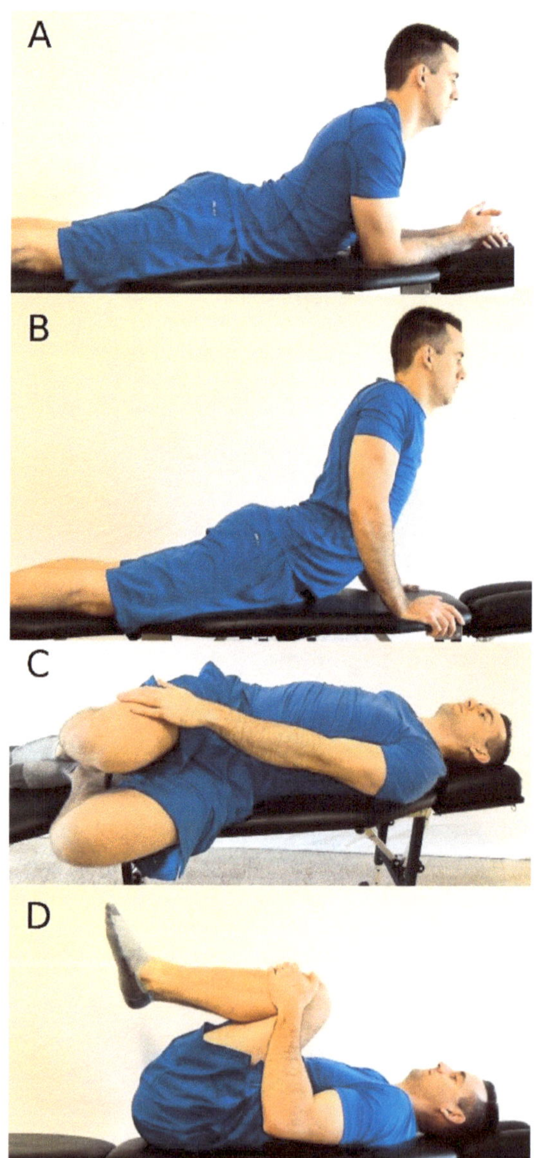

Figure 176: Directional preference examination of partial extension prone (A) maximal extension prone (B) rotation in flexion supine (C) and flexion supine (D)

The ability for a patient's pain to centralize is an indicator they will recover faster and be less likely to undergo surgery. Studies have found that those who centralize have a faster return to work, greater functional improvement, fewer doctor visits, and greater improvements in pain.[334,346] The inability to centralize sciatic pain is associated with an increased odds of higher pain intensity, failure to return to work, interference with daily activities, and need for further health care.[347]

Sensory processing & proprioception tests

Tactile acuity

Those with sciatica may have a lessened ability to distinguish between points touching the skin in the region of pain. One systematic review found that those with LBP had reduced tactile acuity of the low back.[348] Another study found that the extremity affected by sciatica also had diminished tactile acuity.[349] One theory to explain diminished tactile acuity is that nociceptive signals from the lower back directly interfere with tactile acuity, a concept called the "**touch-gate**" phenomenon.[350] Another theory is that pain-related reorganization of the somatosensory cortex of the brain reduces acuity.[351]

The **point-to-point test** is a clinical screening tool for decreased tactile acuity.[352] The clinician should touch a point on the patient's back then instruct the patient to use a pen to touch that point as accurately as they can.[352,353] They should lift the pen rather than slide it. Afterwards, the clinician slides the pen from where the patient placed it to the original point (if they differ), which creates error-lines that measure distance between the two points.

The **two-point discrimination test** is another measure of tactile acuity. The clinician stimulates the skin with two points that are close together and gradually moves them apart until the patient feels two distinct points.[354] Some authors advise comparing the painful side of the lower back to the non-painful side, or comparing the lumbar to the thoracic spine, due to there being a large range of variation between individuals regarding what is considered normal.[354] A difference of 13 millimeters if measured horizontally or 17 millimeters if measured vertically indicates an abnormal result.[354]

Vibration sense

Patients with neuropathic forms of sciatica are more likely to have **hypopallesthesia** (reduced vibration sense) or apallesthesia (loss of vibration sense) than those with referred pain. Clinical testing for vibration is perceived by specialized mechanoreceptors called **Pacinian corpuscles**.[355] Because these corpuscles reside in the periosteum of bone and other layers of fascia,[355] certain authors have interpreted lumbosacral vibration sense using **sclerotomes**.[356,357] The vibration testing zones roughly correspond to dermatomes, which become more distinct in the distal extremity.[358]

Vibrations in the **distal extremity** may be more specific than those more proximal. [358,359] For example, the 5th toe reliably localizes to the S1 nerve root and 2nd and 3rd toes relate to L5.[358] Vibration testing points in the leg may be less reliable for specific nerve root levels as vibration spreads rapidly along the periosteum of bone.[355] For example vibrations spreading along the tibial shaft could encounter periosteum relating to L3, L4, and L5.

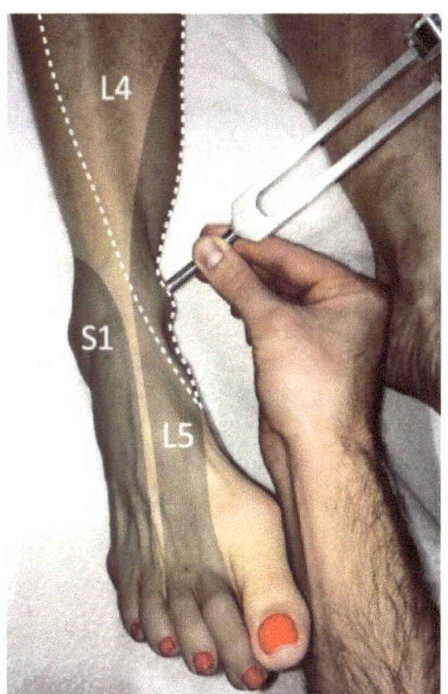

Figure 177: Vibration sense testing of the sclerotome regions most specific for L4 (dashed line), L5 (shaded), and S1 (shaded). The tuning fork is at the medial malleolus, an area that includes both L4 and L5. Image by Robert Trager DC with patient's permission.

Loss of vibration sense can occur in those with **non-radicular sciatica** as well as some healthy patients. One study using a highly sensitive form of testing called quantitative sensory testing (QST) found that 73% those with radicular sciatica had apallesthesia compared to 47% of those with pseudoradicular (referred) sciatica.[208] Another study found diminished sensation to tuning fork vibration in 10% of healthy patients without a history of lumbosacral radicular symptoms.[360] It is also considered normal for those over 70 years of age to have apallesthesia over the great toe.[355]

Lumbosacral vibration sense is typically measured with a **128 Hz tuning fork** over bony prominences of the lower extremities.[355,361] Some authors have reported diminished tuning fork sensation over the lumbar and sacral spinous processes[362,363] and up to 2 cm paraspinally.[362] The tuning fork can be held in place for up to five seconds at each point during which time the patient is asked if they can distinguish between vibrating and not vibrating.[363]

Table 28: Sclerotomal correlation of vibration sense testing

Vibration testing site	Correlation
Patella	L3[364]
Tibial tuberosity	L4[364]
Medial malleolus	L4, L5[358,364]
First metatarsal	L4, L5[358,364]
Dorsal ilium	L5[364]
Second and third metatarsal	L5[358]
Fourth metatarsal	L5 and S1[358]
Lateral malleolus	S1[358,364]
Fifth metatarsal[365]	S1[358,364]

The most commonly documented causes of loss of vibration sense for sciatica relate to **intraspinal** radicular causes including LDH and LSS. One study found that patients with lumbosacral radiculopathy were more likely to have reduced sensation to tuning fork vibration at the great toe or heel.[365] Another study found that diminished vibration sense of 128-Hz tuning fork increased the likelihood of radicular pain compared to other causes of LBP.[366] Loss of vibration sense using a 128 Hz tuning fork at the first metatarsal head has a 53% sensitivity and 81% specificity for diagnosis of LSS.[81] Loss of vibration sense also correlates with increasing neurological severity of LSS.[360]

Deficits of vibration sense correlate with diminished **balance**. One study found that lumbosacral radicular patients with reduced vibration sense were more likely to have impaired balance.[365] Another study found that loss of vibration sense correlated with subjective loss of balance in those with LSS.[367]

Proprioception

Patients with sciatica often have reductions in proprioception, as measured by balance and position sense. Most research showing this phenomenon has focused on those with discogenic radicular sciatica. Deficits of proprioception are thought to relate to denervation of the multifidus,[368] or a reduced capacity to process visual information using **short term memory**.[369]

One study found that patients with discogenic radicular sciatica have a reduced ability to perceive rotation when placed in a slowly rotating seat.[368] Another similar study found that those with LDH had impaired proprioception as measured by **repositioning error**.[370]

Multiple studies have found that patients with discogenic radicular sciatica have impaired balance as measured by postural stability or sway.[368,371] One study of patients with LDH found that the ability to **balance** with the eyes closed was inversely related to the level of self-reported pain.[372] This meant that those with more severe pain had worse balance. Other studies have found that those with discogenic radiculopathy have delayed lower extremity[373] or paraspinal postural muscle activation[369] in response to movement challenges.

Left-right hand judgement

Left-right hand imagery testing, also called **motor imagery testing** involves asking patients to indicate the side of the body or side a figure is turning towards in an image, while assessing for both accuracy and speed. One study found that patients with LBP, in particular those with bilateral back pain, had a greater number of errors when labeling images of a person rotating his trunk either towards the right or left side (using the program Recognise®).[374] A high error rate in motor imagery testing may indicate with **cortical reorganization** in the brain.[374]

References

1. Hancock, M. J., Koes, B., Ostelo, R. & Peul, W. Diagnostic accuracy of the clinical examination in identifying the level of herniation in patients with sciatica. *Spine* **36**, E712–E719 (2011).
2. Reihani-Kermani, H. & Hospitl, B. Correlation of clinical presentation with intraoperative level diagnosis in lower lumbar disc herniation. *Annals of Saudi medicine* **24**, 273–275 (2004).

3. Szadek, K. M., van der Wurff, P., van Tulder, M. W., Zuurmond, W. W. & Perez, R. S. G. M. Diagnostic validity of criteria for sacroiliac joint pain: a systematic review. *Journal of Pain* **10**, 354 (2009).
4. Adelmanesh, F. *et al.* Is there an association between Lumbosacral radiculopathy and painful Gluteal trigger points?: A cross-sectional study. *American Journal of Physical Medicine & Rehabilitation* **94**, 784–791 (2015).
5. Young, S., Aprill, C. & Laslett, M. Correlation of clinical examination characteristics with three sources of chronic low back pain. *The spine journal* **3**, 460–465 (2003).
6. Donelson, R., Aprill, C., Medcalf, R. P. & Grant, W. E. A Prospective Study of Centralization of Lumbar and Referred Pain: A Predictor of Symptomatic Discs and Anular Competence. *Spine May 15, 1997* **22**, 1115–1122 (1997).
7. Kilpikoski, S., Laslett, M., Airaksinen, O. & Kankaanpää, M. Pain centralization and lumbar disc MRI findings in chronic low back pain patients. *International Journal of Mechanical Diagnosis and Therapy* **6**, 3–11 (2011).
8. Lauder, T. D. *et al.* Effect of history and exam in predicting electrodiagnostic outcome among patients with suspected lumbosacral radiculopathy. *American journal of physical medicine & rehabilitation* **79**, 60 (2000).
9. Savage, N. J., Fritz, J. M. & Thackeray, A. The relationship between history and physical examination findings and the outcome of electrodiagnostic testing in patients with sciatica referred to physical therapy. *journal of orthopaedic & sports physical therapy* **44**, 508–517 (2014).
10. Thapa, S. S., Lakhey, R. B., Sharma, P. & Pokhrel, R. K. Correlation between Clinical Features and Magnetic Resonance Imaging Findings in Lumbar Disc Prolapse. *J Nepal Health Res Counc* **14**, 85–88 (2016).
11. Majlesi, J., Togay, H., Ünalan, H. & Toprak, S. The sensitivity and specificity of the slump and the straight leg raising tests in patients with lumbar disc herniation. *JCR: Journal of Clinical Rheumatology* **14**, 87–91 (2008).
12. Vroomen, P., de Krom, M., Wilmink, J., Kester, A. & Knottnerus, J. Diagnostic value of history and physical examination in patients suspected of lumbosacral nerve root compression. *Journal of Neurology, Neurosurgery & Psychiatry* **72**, 630–634 (2002).
13. Urban, L. M. & MacNeil, B. J. Diagnostic accuracy of the slump test for identifying neuropathic pain in the lower limb. *journal of orthopaedic & sports physical therapy* **45**, 596–603 (2015).
14. Cook, C. & Hegedus, E. Diagnostic utility of clinical tests for spinal dysfunction. *Manual therapy* **16**, 21–25 (2011).
15. Homayouni, K., Jafari, S. H. & Yari, H. Sensitivity and Specificity of Modified Bragard Test in Patients With Lumbosacral Radiculopathy Using Electrodiagnosis as a Reference Standard. *Journal of Chiropractic Medicine* **17**, 36–43 (2018).
16. Chu, E. C. & Wong, J. T. Subsiding of Dependent Oedema Following Chiropractic Adjustment for Discogenic Sciatica. *European Journal of Molecular & Clinical Medicine* **5**, (2018).
17. Pachêco, K., Magalhaes, F. & Loureiro, A. Les varices du nerf sciatique: pathologie sous-évaluée. *Phlébologie* **65**, 35–44 (2012).
18. Ricci, S., Georgiev, M., Jawien, A. & Zamboni, P. Sciatic Nerve Varices. *European Journal of Vascular and Endovascular Surgery* **29**, 83–87 (2005).
19. Foti, C. *et al.* Correlazioni cliniche tra reticolo venoso superficiale lombare e congestione venosa profonda del plesso epidurale di Batson nel paziente con lombalgia cronica: analisi di 2 case reports. *G Ital Med Lav Erg* **30**, 377–381 (2008).
20. Jaeckle, K. A. Neurological manifestations of neoplastic and radiation-induced plexopathies. in *Seminars in neurology* **24**, 385–393 (2004).
21. Hynes, J. & Jackson, A. Atraumatic gluteal compartment syndrome. *Postgraduate medical journal* **70**, 210–212 (1994).
22. Tyrrell, P., Feher, M. & Rossor, M. Sciatic nerve damage due to toilet seat entrapment: another Saturday night palsy. *Journal of neurology, neurosurgery, and psychiatry* **52**, 1113 (1989).
23. Bustamante, S. & Houlton, P. Swelling of the leg, deep venous thrombosis and the piriformis syndrome. *Pain Res Manag* **6**, 200–203 (2000).
24. Szolcsanyi, J. Antidromic vasodilatation and neurogenic inflammation. *Agents and actions* **23**, 4–11 (1988).
25. Wendling, D., Langlois, S., Lohse, A., Toussirot, E. & Michel, F. Herpes zoster sciatica with paresis preceding the skin lesions. Three case-reports. *Joint Bone Spine* **71**, 588–591 (2004).
26. Halperin, J. J. Lyme disease and the peripheral nervous system. *Muscle & nerve* **28**, 133–143 (2003).
27. Müller, K. E. Damage of Collagen and Elastic Fibres by Borrelia Burgdorferi – Known and New Clinical and Histopathological Aspects. *Open Neurol J* **6**, 179–186 (2012).
28. Drolet, B. A. Cutaneous signs of neural tube dysraphism. *Pediatric Clinics of North America* **47**, 813–823 (2000).
29. Al-Shudifat, A. & Alkharazi, K. A Prolapsed Intervertbral Disc as the Presenting Feature for Alkaptouria: Case Report. *Journal of Neurological Disorders* **04**, (2016).
30. Nielsen, A., Knoblauch, N. T. M., Dobos, G. J., Michalsen, A. & Kaptchuk, T. J. The effect of Gua Sha treatment on the microcirculation of surface tissue: a pilot study in healthy subjects. *Explore (NY)* **3**, 456–466 (2007).
31. Nielsen, A. *Gua sha: A Traditional Technique for Modern Practice, 2e*. (Churchill Livingstone, 2013).
32. Travell, J. G. & Simons, D. G. *Myofascial Pain and Dysfunction: The Trigger Point Manual; Vol. 2., The Lower Extremities.* (Lippincott Williams & Wilkins, 1992).
33. Skorupska, E., Rychlik, M. & Samborski, W. Intensive vasodilatation in the sciatic pain area after dry needling. *BMC Complementary and Alternative Medicine* **15**, 72 (2015).
34. Gunn, C. C. & Milbrandt, W. E. Early and subtle signs in low-back sprain. *Spine* **3**, 267–281 (1978).
35. Rahbar, M., Shimia, M., Toopchizadeh, V. & Abed, M. Association between knee pain and low back pain. *JPMA* **65**, 626–628 (2015).
36. Quattrocchi, C. C. *et al.* Lumbar subcutaneous edema and degenerative spinal disease in patients with low back pain: a retrospective MRI study. *Musculoskelet Surg* **99**, 159–163 (2015).
37. Genu, A. *et al.* Factors influencing the occurrence of a T2-STIR hypersignal in the lumbosacral adipose tissue. *Diagnostic and Interventional Imaging* **95**, 283–288 (2014).
38. Shi, H., Schweitzer, M. E., Carrino, J. A. & Parker, L. MR Imaging of the Lumbar Spine: Relation of Posterior Soft-Tissue Edema-Like Signal and Body Weight. *American Journal of Roentgenology* **180**, 81–86 (2003).
39. Langevin, H. M. *et al.* Ultrasound evidence of altered lumbar connective tissue structure in human subjects with chronic low back pain. *BMC Musculoskeletal Disorders* **10**, 151 (2009).
40. Cooper, M., Hacking, J. C. & Dixon, A. K. Sacral edema: Computed tomographic and anatomical observations. *Clin. Anat.* **8**, 56–60 (1995).
41. Hirayama, J. *et al.* Relationship between low-back pain, muscle spasm and pressure pain thresholds in patients with lumbar disc herniation. *European Spine Journal* **15**, 41–47 (2006).
42. Zhu, Z. *et al.* Scoliotic posture as the initial symptom in adolescents with lumbar disc herniation: its curve pattern and natural history after lumbar discectomy. *BMC Musculoskeletal Disorders* **12**, 216 (2011).
43. Suk, K.-S., Lee, H.-M., Moon, S.-H. & Kim, N.-H. Lumbosacral scoliotic list by lumbar disc herniation. *Spine* **26**, 667–671 (2001).
44. Matsui, H., Ohmori, K., Kanamori, M., Ishihara, H. & Tsuji, H. Significance of sciatic scoliotic list in operated patients with lumbar disc herniation. *Spine* **23**, 338–342 (1998).
45. Khallaf, M. E. Three dimensional analysis of spino-pelvic alignment in individuals with acutely herniated lumbar intervertebral disc. *Journal of Back and Musculoskeletal Rehabilitation* **30**, 759–765 (2017).
46. Omidi-Kashani, F. Reverse Sagittal Thoracolumbar Alignment Combined with Trunk List in a Young Patient with Lumbar Disc Herniation. *Research* (2014).
47. Hirayama, J. *et al.* Effects of electrical stimulation of the sciatic nerve on background electromyography and static stretch reflex activity of the trunk muscles in rats: possible implications of neuronal mechanisms in the development of sciatic scoliosis. *Spine* **26**, 602–609 (2001).
48. Khuffash, B. & Porter, R. Cross leg pain and trunk list. *Spine* **14**, 602–603 (1989).
49. Kim, R. *et al.* The incidence and risk factors for lumbar or sciatic scoliosis in lumbar disc herniation and the outcomes after percutaneous endoscopic discectomy. *Pain physician* **18**, 555–564 (2015).
50. Lorio, M. P., Bernstein, A. J. & Simmons, E. H. Sciatic spinal deformity-lumbosacral list: an" unusual" presentation with review of the literature. *Clinical Spine Surgery* **8**, 201–205 (1995).
51. Takasaki, H., May, S., Fazey, P. J. & Hall, T. Nucleus pulposus deformation following application of mechanical diagnosis and therapy: a single case report with magnetic resonance imaging. *J Man Manip Ther* **18**, 153–158 (2010).
52. Tenhula, J. A., Rose, S. J. & Delitto, A. Association between direction of lateral lumbar shift, movement tests, and side of symptoms in patients with low back pain syndrome. *Physical therapy* **70**, 480–486 (1990).
53. Park, H. W., Jahng, J. S. & Lee, W. H. Piriformis syndrome: a case report. *Yonsei medical journal* **32**, 64–68 (1991).
54. Ozaki, T. *et al.* Osteoid osteoma and osteoblastoma of the spine: experiences with 22 patients. *Clinical orthopaedics and related research* **397**, 394–402 (2002).
55. Goddard, M. & Reid, J. Movements induced by straight leg raising in the lumbo-sacral roots, nerves and plexus, and in the intrapelvic section of the sciatic nerve. *Journal of neurology, neurosurgery, and psychiatry* **28**, 12 (1965).
56. Trescot, A. M. *Peripheral Nerve Entrapments: Clinical Diagnosis and Management*. (Springer, 2016).
57. Ahn, K. & Jhun, H.-J. New physical examination tests for lumbar spondylolisthesis and instability: low midline sill sign and interspinous gap change during lumbar flexion-extension motion. *BMC musculoskeletal disorders* **16**, 97 (2015).
58. Stewart, J. D. Foot drop: where, why and what to do? *Practical Neurology* **8**, 158–169 (2008).
59. Hernando, M. F., Cerezal, L., Pérez-Carro, L., Abascal, F. & Canga, A. Deep gluteal syndrome: anatomy, imaging, and management of sciatic nerve entrapments in the subgluteal space. *Skeletal radiology* **44**, 919–934 (2015).

60. ten Brinke, A., van der Aa, H. E., van der Palen, J. & Oosterveld, F. Is leg length discrepancy associated with the side of radiating pain in patients with a lumbar herniated disc? *Spine* **24**, 684–686 (1999).
61. Segal, N. A. *et al.* Leg-length inequality is not associated with greater trochanteric pain syndrome. *Arthritis Research and Therapy* **10**, R62 (2008).
62. Konno, S. *et al.* Development of a clinical diagnosis support tool to identify patients with lumbar spinal stenosis. *European Spine Journal* **16**, 1951–1957 (2007).
63. Suri, P. Does This Older Adult With Lower Extremity Pain Have the Clinical Syndrome of Lumbar Spinal Stenosis? *JAMA: The Journal of the American Medical Association* **304**, 2628 (2010).
64. Aurelianus, C., Drabkin, I. E. & Soranus. *On acute diseases and On chronic diseases,.* (Univ. of Chicago Press, 1950).
65. Nguyen, H. S. *et al.* Upright magnetic resonance imaging of the lumbar spine: Back pain and radiculopathy. *J Craniovertebr Junction Spine* **7**, 31–37 (2016).
66. Dyck, P. The stoop-test in lumbar entrapment radiculopathy. *Spine* **4**, 89–92 (1979).
67. Takahashi, K. *et al.* Changes in epidural pressure during walking in patients with lumbar spinal stenosis. *Spine* **20**, 2746–2749 (1995).
68. Dong, G. & Porter, R. Walking and cycling tests in neurogenic and intermittent claudication. *Spine* **14**, 965–969 (1989).
69. Fritz, J. M., Erhard, R. E., Delitto, A., Welch, W. C. & Nowakowski, P. E. Preliminary results of the use of a two-stage treadmill test as a clinical diagnostic tool in the differential diagnosis of lumbar spinal stenosis. *Journal of spinal disorders* **10**, 410–416 (1997).
70. Comer, C. M., White, D., Conaghan, P. G., Bird, H. A. & Redmond, A. C. Effects of Walking With a Shopping Trolley on Spinal Posture and Loading in Subjects With Neurogenic Claudication. *Archives of Physical Medicine and Rehabilitation* **91**, 1602–1607 (2010).
71. Conrad, B. P. *et al.* Associations of self-report measures with gait, range of motion and proprioception in patients with lumbar spinal stenosis. *Gait & posture* **38**, 987–992 (2013).
72. Moldoveanu, S. A., Munteanu, F., Lazar, A. M., Tarasi, C. & Turliuc, D. Establishing a baseline for gait pattern that can be linked to lumbar disk herniation and recurrent lumbar disk herniation. in *E-Health and Bioengineering Conference (EHB), 2015* 1–4 (IEEE, 2015).
73. Michele, A. A. *Iliopsoas; development of anomalies in man.* (Springfield, Ill., 1962).
74. Martin, R. L. *et al.* Accuracy of 3 Clinical Tests to Diagnose Proximal Hamstrings Tears With and Without Sciatic Nerve Involvement in Patients With Posterior Hip Pain. *Arthroscopy: The Journal of Arthroscopic & Related Surgery* **34**, 114–121 (2018).
75. Huang, Y. P. *et al.* Gait adaptations in low back pain patients with lumbar disc herniation: trunk coordination and arm swing. *European Spine Journal* **20**, 491–499 (2011).
76. Andersson, G. B. & Deyo, R. A. History and Physical Examination in Patients With Herniated Lumbar Discs. *Spine* **21**, 10S–18S (1996).
77. Kuai, S. *et al.* Influences of lumbar disc herniation on the kinematics in multi-segmental spine, pelvis, and lower extremities during five activities of daily living. *BMC Musculoskeletal Disorders* **18**, 216 (2017).
78. Bird, P. A., Oakley, S. P., Shnier, R. & Kirkham, B. W. Prospective evaluation of magnetic resonance imaging and physical examination findings in patients with greater trochanteric pain syndrome. *Arthritis & Rheumatism* **44**, 2138–2145 (2001).
79. Brown, M. D., Gomez-Marin, O., Brookfield, K. F. W. & Li, P. S. Differential Diagnosis of Hip Disease Versus Spine Disease. *Clinical Orthopaedics and Related Research* **419**, 280–284 (2004).
80. Yokogawa, N. *et al.* Differences in Gait Characteristics of Patients with Lumbar Spinal Canal Stenosis (L4 Radiculopathy) and Those with Osteoarthritis of the Hip. *PLOS ONE* **10**, e0124745 (2015).
81. Katz, J. N. *et al.* Degenerative lumbar spinal stenosis diagnostic value of the history and physical examination. *Arthritis & Rheumatism* **38**, 1236–1241 (1995).
82. Van Langenhove, M., Pollefliet, A. & Vanderstraeten, G. A retrospective electrodiagnostic evaluation of footdrop in 303 patients. *Electromyography and clinical neurophysiology* **29**, 145 (1989).
83. Morag, E., Hurwitz, D. E., Andriacchi, T. P., Hickey, M. & Andersson, G. B. J. Abnormalities in Muscle Function During Gait in Relation to the Level of Lumbar Disc Herniation. *Spine* **25**, 829 (2000).
84. Kuai, S. *et al.* The Effect of Lumbar Disc Herniation on Musculoskeletal Loadings in the Spinal Region During Level Walking and Stair Climbing. *Medical science monitor: international medical journal of experimental and clinical research* **23**, 3869–3877 (2017).
85. Vroomen, P., de Krom, M. & Knottnerus, J. Diagnostic value of history and physical examination in patients suspected of sciatica due to disc herniation: a systematic review. *Journal of neurology* **246**, 899 (1999).
86. Walcott, B. P. *et al.* Pathological mechanism of lumbar disc herniation resulting in neurogenic muscle hypertrophy. *J Clin Neurosci* **18**, 1682–1684 (2011).
87. Kottlors, M., Mueller, K., Kirschner, J. & Glocker, F. X. Muscle hypertrophy of the lower leg caused by L5 radiculopathy. *Joint Bone Spine* **76**, 562–564 (2009).
88. Munakomi, S. & Kumar, B. M. Extensor digitorum brevis wasting-a decisive preoperative clinical indicator of lumbar canal stenosis. *EC Orthopaedics* **2**, 133–138 (2015).
89. Caelius Aurelianus. *Caelii Aureliani Siccensis, ...De acutis morbis. lib.3. De diuturnis. lib.5. Ad fidem exemplaris manuscripti castigati, & annotationibus illustrati. Cum indice copiosissimo, ac locupletissimo.* (apud Guliel. Rouillium, sub scuto Veneto, 1566).
90. Garg, R., Chaudhari, T., Malhotra, H., Singh, M. & Raut, T. Focal neuromyotonia as a presenting feature of lumbosacral radiculopathy. *Annals of Indian Academy of Neurology* **16**, 693 (2013).
91. Kääriä, S.-M., Mälkiä, E. A., Luukkonen, R. A. & Leino-Arjas, P. I. Pain and clinical findings in the low back: A study of industrial employees with 5-, 10-, and 28-year follow-ups. *European Journal of Pain* **14**, 759–763 (2010).
92. McGregor, A. H., McCarthy, D., Doré, C. J. & Hughes, S. P. Quantitative assessment of the motion of the lumbar spine in the low back pain population and the effect of different spinal pathologies on this motion. *Eur Spine J* **6**, 308–315 (1997).
93. McGregor, A. H., Cattermole, H. R. & Hughes, S. P. F. Global Spinal Motion in Subjects With Lumbar Spondylolysis and Spondylolisthesis: Does the Grade or Type of Slip Affect Global Spinal Motion? *Spine* **26**, 282 (2001).
94. Thomas, E., Silman, A. J., Papageorgiou, A. C., Macfarlane, G. J. & Croft, P. R. Association Between Measures of Spinal Mobility and Low Back Pain: An Analysis of New Attenders in Primary Care. *Spine* **23**, 343 (1998).
95. Stankovic, R., Johnell, O., Maly, P. & Wilmer, S. Use of lumbar extension, slump test, physical and neurological examination inthe evaluation of patients with suspected herniated nucleurs pulposus. A prospective clinical study. *Manual therapy* **4**, 25–32 (1999).
96. Wang, W. T.-J. Comparison of Lumbar Range of Motion in Patients Having Herniated Nucleus Pulposus with and without Nerve Root Compression. 物理治療 **25**, 311–316 (2000).
97. Jenis, L. G., An, H. S. & Gordin, R. Foraminal stenosis of the lumbar spine: a review of 65 surgical cases. *Am J. Orthop.* **30**, 205–211 (2001).
98. Saal, J. A., Dillingham, M. F., Gamburd, R. S. & Fanton, G. S. The pseudoradicular syndrome. Lower extremity peripheral nerve entrapment masquerading as lumbar radiculopathy. *Spine* **13**, 926–930 (1988).
99. Kuniya, H. *et al.* Prospective study of superior cluneal nerve disorder as a potential cause of low back pain and leg symptoms. *Journal of Orthopaedic Surgery and Research* **9**, 139 (2014).
100. Troke, M., Moore, A. P., Maillardet, F. J. & Cheek, E. A normative database of lumbar spine ranges of motion. *Manual therapy* **10**, 198–206 (2005).
101. Albeck, M. A critical assessment of clinical diagnosis of disc herniation in patients with monoradicular sciatica. *Acta neurochirurgica* **138**, 40–44 (1996).
102. Laird, R. A., Kent, P. & Keating, J. L. How consistent are lordosis, range of movement and lumbo-pelvic rhythm in people with and without back pain? *BMC Musculoskeletal Disorders* **17**, 403 (2016).
103. Esola, M. A., McClure, P. W., Fitzgerald, G. K. & Siegler, S. Analysis of lumbar spine and hip motion during forward bending in subjects with and without a history of low back pain. *Spine* **21**, 71–78 (1996).
104. Porter, J. L. & Wilkinson, A. Lumbar-hip flexion motion: a comparative study between asymptomatic and chronic low back pain in 18-to 36-year-old men. *Spine* **22**, 1508–1513 (1997).
105. Marich, A. V., Hwang, C.-T., Salsich, G. B., Lang, C. E. & Van Dillen, L. R. Consistency of a lumbar movement pattern across functional activities in people with low back pain. *Clinical Biomechanics* **44**, 45–51 (2017).
106. Luomajoki, H., Kool, J., de Bruin, E. D. & Airaksinen, O. Movement control tests of the low back; evaluation of the difference between patients with low back pain and healthy controls. *BMC Musculoskeletal Disorders* **9**, 170 (2008).
107. McGregor, A., McCarthy, I. & Hughes, S. Motion Characteristics of Normal Subjects and People with Low Back Pain. *Physiotherapy* **81**, 632–637 (1995).
108. Wong, T. K. & Lee, R. Y. Effects of low back pain on the relationship between the movements of the lumbar spine and hip. *Human movement science* **23**, 21–34 (2004).
109. Shum, G. L. K., Crosbie, J. & Lee, R. Y. W. Movement coordination of the lumbar spine and hip during a picking up activity in low back pain subjects. *Eur Spine J* **16**, 749–758 (2007).
110. Michele, A. A. Determinations of Sciatic Nerve Tension. *Postgraduate medicine* **28**, 488–502 (1960).
111. Kuai, S., Liu, W., Ji, R. & Zhou, W. The Effect of Lumbar Disc Herniation on Spine Loading Characteristics during Trunk Flexion and Two Types of Picking Up Activities. *Journal of Healthcare Engineering* (2017). doi:10.1155/2017/6294503
112. Owens, E. F., Gudavalli, M. R. & Wilder, D. G. Paraspinal Muscle Function Assessed with the Flexion-Relaxation Ratio at Baseline in a Population of Patients with Back-Related Leg Pain. *Journal of Manipulative & Physiological Therapeutics* **34**, 594–601 (2011).
113. Colloca, C. J. & Hinrichs, R. N. The Biomechanical and Clinical Significance of the Lumbar Erector Spinae Flexion-Relaxation Phenomenon: A Review of Literature. *Journal of Manipulative and Physiological Therapeutics* **28**, 623–631 (2005).
114. Fritz, J. M., Piva, S. R. & Childs, J. D. Accuracy of the clinical examination to predict radiographic instability of the lumbar spine. *European Spine Journal* **14**, 743–750 (2005).
115. Aktas, I., Ofluoglu, D. & Akgun, K. Relationship between lumbar disc herniation and benign joint hypermobility syndrome/Lomber disk hernisi ile benign eklem hipermobilite

sendromu arasindaki iliski. *Turkish Journal of Physical Medicine and Rehabilitation* **57**, 85–89 (2011).

116. Han, W. J. *et al.* Generalized Joint Laxity is Associated with Primary Occurrence and Treatment Outcome of Lumbar Disc Herniation. *Korean Journal of Family Medicine* **36**, 141–145 (2015).
117. Ferrari, S., Vanti, C., Piccarreta, R. & Monticone, M. Pain, Disability, and Diagnostic Accuracy of Clinical Instability and Endurance Tests in Subjects With Lumbar Spondylolisthesis. *Journal of Manipulative & Physiological Therapeutics* **37**, 647–659 (2014).
118. Kasai, Y., Akeda, K., Kono, T., Matsumura, Y. & Uchida, A. Symptoms and clinical examinations for assessment of lumbar spinal instability. *Critical Reviews™ in Physical and Rehabilitation Medicine* **20**, (2008).
119. Ekedahl, H., Jönsson, B. & Frobell, R. B. Fingertip-to-Floor Test and Straight Leg Raising Test: Validity, Responsiveness, and Predictive Value in Patients With Acute/Subacute Low Back Pain. *Archives of Physical Medicine and Rehabilitation* **93**, 2210–2215 (2012).
120. Bybee, R. F., Olsen, D. L., Cantu-Boncser, G., Allen, H. C. & Byars, A. Centralization of symptoms and lumbar range of motion in patients with low back pain. *Physiotherapy theory and practice* **25**, 257–267 (2009).
121. Markowski, A. *et al.* A Pilot Study Analyzing the Effects of Chinese Cupping as an Adjunct Treatment for Patients with Subacute Low Back Pain on Relieving Pain, Improving Range of Motion, and Improving Function. *The Journal of Alternative and Complementary Medicine* **20**, 113–117 (2013).
122. Ma, S.-Y. Effect of whole body cryotherapy with spinal decompression on lumbar disc herniation by functional assessment measures. *Journal of the Korean Data and Information Science Society* **21**, 1101–1108 (2010).
123. López-Díaz, J. V., Arias-Buría, J. L., Lopez-Gordo, E., Lopez Gordo, S. & Aros Oyarzún, A. P. Effectiveness of continuous vertebral resonant oscillation using the POLD method in the treatment of lumbar disc hernia". A randomized controlled pilot study. *Manual Therapy* **20**, 481–486 (2015).
124. Mellin, G. Correlations of Hip Mobility with Degree of Back Pain and Lumbar Spinal Mobility in Chronic Low-Back Pain Patients. *Spine* **13**, 668 (1988).
125. Roach, S. M. *et al.* Passive hip range of motion is reduced in active subjects with chronic low back pain compared to controls. *International journal of sports physical therapy* **10**, 13 (2015).
126. Van Dillen, L. R., McDonnell, M. K., Fleming, D. A. & Sahrmann, S. A. Effect of knee and hip position on hip extension range of motion in individuals with and without low back pain. *Journal of Orthopaedic & Sports Physical Therapy* **30**, 307–316 (2000).
127. Prather, H., Cheng, A., Steger-May, K., Maheshwari, V. & VanDillen, L. Association of Hip Radiograph Findings With Pain and Function in Patients Presenting With Low Back Pain. *PM&R* (2017). doi:10.1016/j.pmrj.2017.06.003
128. Takahashi, Y., Hirayama, J., Ohtori, S., Tauchi, T. & Takahashi, K. Anatomical nature of radicular leg pain analyzed by clinical findings. *PAIN RESEARCH* **15**, 87–96 (2000).
129. Defrin, R., Devor, M. & Brill, S. Tactile allodynia in patients with lumbar radicular pain (sciatica). *PAIN®* **155**, 2551–2559 (2014).
130. O'Neill, S., Manniche, C., Graven-Nielsen, T. & Arendt-Nielsen, L. Generalized deep-tissue hyperalgesia in patients with chronic low-back pain. *European journal of pain* **11**, 415–420 (2007).
131. Jensen, O. K., Nielsen, C. V. & Stengaard-Pedersen, K. Low back pain may be caused by disturbed pain regulation: A cross-sectional study in low back pain patients using tender point examination. *European Journal of Pain* **14**, 514–522 (2010).
132. Llewellyn, R. L. J. & Jones, A. B. *Fibrositis (gouty, Infective, Traumatic): So Called Chronic Rheumatism Including Villous Synovitis of Knee and Hip, and Sacro-iliac Relaxation.* (Rebman Company, 1915).
133. Suputtitada, A. Myofascial pain syndrome and sensitization. *Physical Medicine and Rehabilitation Research* **1**, 1–4 (2016).
134. Bove, G. M., Zaheen, A. & Bajwa, Z. H. Subjective Nature of Lower Limb Radicular Pain. *Journal of Manipulative and Physiological Therapeutics* **28**, 12–14 (2005).
135. Lin, J.-H. Lumbar radiculopathy and its neurobiological basis. *World Journal of Anesthesiology* **3**, 162 (2014).
136. Kara, M. *et al.* Sonographic evaluation of sciatic nerves in patients with unilateral sciatica. *Arch Phys Med Rehabil* **93**, 1598–1602 (2012).
137. Dreyfuss, P., Michaelsen, M., Pauza, K., McLarty, J. & Bogduk, N. The Value of Medical History and Physical Examination in Diagnosing Sacroiliac Joint Pain. *Spine* **21**, 2594 (1996).
138. Grimaldi, A. *et al.* Utility of clinical tests to diagnose MRI-confirmed gluteal tendinopathy in patients presenting with lateral hip pain. *Br J Sports Med* **51**, 519–524 (2017).
139. Maigne, R. & Nieves, W. L. *Diagnosis and Treatment of Pain of Vertebral Origin, Second Edition.* (CRC Press, 2005).
140. Elleuch, M.-H. & Ghroubi, S. Vertebral manipulation in chronic low back pain: a prospective randomised study of 85 cases. *International Musculoskeletal Medicine* **31**, 57–62 (2009).
141. Bernard Jr, T. N. & Kirkaldy-Willis, W. H. Recognizing specific characteristics of nonspecific low back pain. *Clinical orthopaedics and related research* **217**, 266–280 (1987).
142. Botter, A. *et al.* Atlas of the muscle motor points for the lower limb: implications for electrical stimulation procedures and electrode positioning. *European journal of applied physiology* **111**, 2461 (2011).
143. Gunn, C., Milbrandt, W., Little, A. & Mason, K. Dry needling of muscle motor points for chronic low-back pain: a randomized clinical trial with long-term follow-up. *Spine* **5**, 279–291 (1980).
144. Gunn, C. C. & Milbrandt, W. E. Tenderness at motor points. A diagnostic and prognostic aid for low-back injury. *J Bone Joint Surg Am* **58**, 815–825 (1976).
145. Botte, M. J., Nakai, R. J., Waters, R. L., McNeal, D. R. & Rubayi, S. Motor point delineation of the gluteus medius muscle for functional electrical stimulation: an in vivo anatomic study. *Archives of physical medicine and rehabilitation* **72**, 112–114 (1991).
146. Barbero, M., Merletti, R. & Rainoldi, A. *Atlas of Muscle Innervation Zones: Understanding Surface Electromyography and Its Applications.* (Springer, 2012).
147. Samuel, A. S., Peter, A. A. & Ramanathan, K. The association of active trigger points with lumbar disc lesions. *Journal of Musculoskelatal Pain* **15**, 11–18 (2007).
148. Barr, K. & others. Electrodiagnosis of Lumbar Radiculopathy. *Physical medicine and rehabilitation clinics of North America* **24**, 79–91 (2013).
149. Zhu, L., Lin, H. & Chen, A. Accurate segmental motor innervation of human lower-extremity skeletal muscles. *Acta neurochirurgica* **157**, 123–128 (2015).
150. Cannon, D. E., Dillingham, T. R., Miao, H., Andary, M. T. & Pezzin, L. E. Musculoskeletal Disorders in Referrals for Suspected Lumbosacral Radiculopathy. *American Journal of Physical Medicine & Rehabilitation* **86**, 957–961 (2007).
151. Cables, H. The use of quinine and urea hydrochloride in sciatica and allied conditions, with a report of a number of cases. *The Lancet Clinic* (1915).
152. Kurosawa, D. *et al.* A Diagnostic Scoring System for Sacroiliac Joint Pain Originating from the Posterior Ligament. *Pain Med* **18**, 228–238 (2017).
153. Fortin, J. D. & Falco, F. J. The Fortin finger test: an indicator of sacroiliac pain. *AMERICAN JOURNAL OF ORTHOPEDICS-BELLE MEAD-* **26**, 477–480 (1997).
154. Meknas, K., Johansen, O. & Kartus, J. Retro-trochanteric sciatica-like pain: current concept. *Knee Surg Sports Traumatol Arthrosc* **19**, 1971–1985 (2011).
155. Kean Chen, C. & Nizar, A. J. Prevalence of piriformis syndrome in chronic low back pain patients. A clinical diagnosis with modified FAIR Test. *Pain Practice* **13**, 276–281 (2013).
156. Adachi, S. *et al.* The tibial nerve compression test for the diagnosis of lumbar spinal canal stenosis—A simple and reliable physical examination for use by primary care physicians. *Acta orthopaedica et traumatologica turcica* (2017).
157. Hicks, G. E., Fritz, J. M., Delitto, A. & McGill, S. M. Preliminary Development of a Clinical Prediction Rule for Determining Which Patients With Low Back Pain Will Respond to a Stabilization Exercise Program. *Archives of Physical Medicine and Rehabilitation* **86**, 1753–1762 (2005).
158. Flynn, T. *et al.* A clinical prediction rule for classifying patients with low back pain who demonstrate short-term improvement with spinal manipulation. *Spine* **27**, 2835–2843 (2002).
159. Fritz, J. M., Cleland, J. A. & Childs, J. D. Subgrouping patients with low back pain: evolution of a classification approach to physical therapy. *journal of orthopaedic & sports physical therapy* **37**, 290–302 (2007).
160. Walsh, J. & Hall, T. Reliability, validity and diagnostic accuracy of palpation of the sciatic, tibial and common peroneal nerves in the examination of low back related leg pain. *Manual Therapy* **14**, 623–629 (2009).
161. Gore, S. & Nadkarni, S. Sciatica: Detection and Confirmation by New Method. *International journal of spine surgery* **8**, 1 (2014).
162. Valleix, F. L. I. *Traité des névralgies, ou, Affections douloureuses des nerfs.* (Baillière, 1841).
163. Yamauchi, T. *et al.* Undiagnosed Peripheral Nerve Disease in Patients with Failed Lumbar Disc Surgery. *Asian Spine J* **12**, 720–725 (2018).
164. Merrild, U. & Søgaard, I. Sciatica caused by perifibrosis of the sciatic nerve. *J Bone Joint Surg Br* **68**, 706 (1986).
165. Chhabra, A. *et al.* MR neurography findings of soleal sling entrapment. *American Journal of Roentgenology* **196**, W290–W297 (2011).
166. Matsumoto, J. *et al.* Clinical features and surgical treatment of superficial peroneal nerve entrapment neuropathy. *Neurologia medico-chirurgica* **58**, 320–325 (2018).
167. Katirji, B. Peroneal neuropathy. *Neurologic clinics* **17**, 567–591 (1999).
168. Zheng, C. *et al.* The prevalence of tarsal tunnel syndrome in patients with lumbosacral radiculopathy. *Eur Spine J* **25**, 895–905 (2016).
169. Morimoto, D. *et al.* Long-term outcome of surgical treatment for superior cluneal nerve entrapment neuropathy. *Spine* **42**, 783–788 (2017).
170. Oh, S. J. & Meyer, R. D. Entrapment neuropathies of the tibial (posterior tibial) nerve. *Neurologic clinics* **17**, 593–615 (1999).
171. Lee, J. & Lee, S. Physical examination, magnetic resonance image, and electrodiagnostic study in patients with lumbosacral disc herniation or spinal stenosis. *Journal of rehabilitation medicine: official journal of the UEMS European Board of Physical and Rehabilitation Medicine* (2012).
172. Mondelli, M. *et al.* Clinical findings and electrodiagnostic testing in 108 consecutive cases of lumbosacral radiculopathy due to herniated disc. *Neurophysiologie Clinique/Clinical Neurophysiology* **43**, 205–215 (2013).

173. Suri, P. *et al.* The Accuracy of the Physical Examination for the Diagnosis of Midlumbar and Low Lumbar Nerve Root Impingement. *Spine* 1 (2010). doi:10.1097/BRS.0b013e3181c953cc
174. Young, I. J., van Riet, R. P. & Bell, S. N. Surgical release for proximal hamstring syndrome. *The American journal of sports medicine* **36**, 2372–2378 (2008).
175. Benazzo, F., Marullo, M., Zanon, G., Indino, C. & Pelillo, F. Surgical management of chronic proximal hamstring tendinopathy in athletes: a 2 to 11 years of follow-up. *Journal of Orthopaedics and Traumatology* 1–7 (2013).
176. Bertilson, B. C., Brosjö, E., Billing, H. & Strender, L.-E. Assessment of nerve involvement in the lumbar spine: agreement between magnetic resonance imaging, physical examination and pain drawing findings. *BMC Musculoskeletal Disorders* **11**, 202 (2010).
177. Demircan, M., Çolak, A., Kutlay, M., Kıbıcı, K. & Topuz, K. Cramp finding: can it be used as a new diagnostic and prognostic factor in lumbar disc surgery? *European Spine Journal* **11**, 47–51 (2002).
178. Nishant, Chhabra, H. S. & Kapoor, K. S. Nocturnal Cramps in Patients with Lumbar Spinal Canal Stenosis Treated Conservatively: A Prospective Study. *Asian Spine J* **8**, 624–631 (2014).
179. Kendall, F. P., McCreary, E. K., Provance, P. G., Rodgers, M. M. & Romani, W. A. *Muscles: Testing and Function, with Posture and Pain.* (LWW, 2005).
180. FAPTA, H. H. P. S. & PT, J. M. M. *Daniels and Worthingham's Muscle Testing: Techniques of Manual Examination, 8e.* (Saunders, 2007).
181. Iversen, T. *et al.* Accuracy of physical examination for chronic lumbar radiculopathy. *BMC musculoskeletal disorders* **14**, 206 (2013).
182. Martin, H. D., Reddy, M. & Gómez-Hoyos, J. Deep gluteal syndrome. *J Hip Preserv Surg* **2**, 99–107 (2015).
183. Lewis AM, L. R. Magnetic resonance neurography in extraspinal sciatica. *Arch Neurol* **63**, 1469–1472 (2006).
184. Chen, C. K. H., Yeh, L., Chang, W.-N., Pan, H.-B. & Yang, C.-F. MRI Diagnosis of Contracture of the Gluteus Maximus Muscle. *American Journal of Roentgenology* **187**, W169–W174 (2006).
185. Konstantinou, K. *et al.* Characteristics of patients with low back and leg pain seeking treatment in primary care: baseline results from the ATLAS cohort study. *BMC musculoskeletal disorders* **16**, 332 (2015).
186. Lortat-Jacob, L. & Sabareanu, G. Les Sciatiques Radiculaires. *Revue de médecine* **25**, 917–938
187. Murphy, D. R., Hurwitz, E. L., Gerrard, J. K. & Clary, R. Pain patterns and descriptions in patients with radicular pain: Does the pain necessarily follow a specific dermatome? *Chiropr Osteopat* **17**, 9 (2009).
188. Lauder, T. D. Musculoskeletal disorders that frequently mimic radiculopathy. *Physical Medicine and Rehabilitation Clinics of North America* **13**, 469–485 (2002).
189. Blower, P. W. Neurologic Patterns in Unilateral Sciatica: A Prospective Study of 100 New Cases. *Spine* **6**, 175 (1981).
190. Rosomoff, H. L., Fishbain, D. A., Goldberg, M., Santana, R. & Rosomoff, R. S. Physical findings in patients with chronic intractable benign pain of the neck and/or back. *Pain* **37**, 279–287 (1989).
191. Lee, M., McPhee, R. & Stringer, M. An evidence-based approach to human dermatomes. *Clinical Anatomy* **21**, 363–373 (2008).
192. Nygaard, Ø. P. & Mellgren, S. I. The function of sensory nerve fibers in lumbar radiculopathy: use of quantitative sensory testing in the exploration of different populations of nerve fibers and dermatomes. *Spine* **23**, 348–352 (1998).
193. Hasankhani, E. G. & Omidi-Kashani, F. Magnetic Resonance Imaging versus Electrophysiologic Tests in Clinical Diagnosis of Lower Extremity Radicular Pain. *ISRN Neuroscience* **2013**, 1–4 (2013).
194. Mittal, A., Chandrasekhar, A., Mohan, R., Rallapalli, R. & Prasad, S. Analysis of the Functional Outcome of Discectomy in Lumbar Disc Prolapse. *IOSR Journal of Dental and Medical Sciences* **14**, 73–80 (2015).
195. Falconer, M. A., Glasgow, G. L. & Cole, D. S. Sensory disturbances occurring in sciatica due to intervertebral disc protrusions: some observations on the fifth lumbar and first sacral dermatomes. *Journal of neurology, neurosurgery, and psychiatry* **10**, 72 (1947).
196. Wojtysiak, M. *et al.* Pre- and Postoperative Evaluation of Patients With Lumbosacral Disc Herniation by Neurophysiological and Clinical Assessment. *Spine* **39**, 1792 (2014).
197. Burkman, K., Gaines Jr, R., Kashani, S. & Smith, R. Herpes zoster: a consideration in the differential diagnosis of radiculopathy. *Archives of physical medicine and rehabilitation* **69**, 132–134 (1988).
198. Morrell, R. M. Herniated Lumbar Intervertebral Disc—Cutaneous Hyperalgesia as an Early Sign. *Mil Med* **124**, 257–269 (1959).
199. Apok, V., Gurusinghe, N. T., Mitchell, J. D. & Emsley, H. C. A. Dermatomes and dogma. *Pract Neurol* **11**, 100–105 (2011).
200. Kakitani, F. T., Collares, D., Kurozawa, A. Y., Lima, P. M. G. de & Teive, H. A. G. How many Babinski's signs are there? *Arquivos de Neuro-Psiquiatria* **68**, 662–665 (2010).
201. Al Nezari, N. H., Schneiders, A. G. & Hendrick, P. A. Neurological examination of the peripheral nervous system to diagnose lumbar spinal disc herniation with suspected radiculopathy: a systematic review and meta-analysis. *The Spine Journal* **13**, 657–674 (2013).
202. Tawa, N., Rhoda, A. & Diener, I. Accuracy of clinical neurological examination in diagnosing lumbo-sacral radiculopathy: a systematic literature review. *BMC Musculoskeletal Disorders* **18**, 93 (2017).
203. Singh, A. & Singh, O. A preliminary clinical evaluation of external snehan and asanas in the patients of sciatica. *International Journal of Yoga* **6**, 71 (2013).
204. Reid, V. & Cros, D. Proximal sensory neuropathies of the leg. *Neurologic clinics* **17**, 655–667 (1999).
205. Chutkow, J. G. Posterior femoral cutaneous neuralgia. *Muscle & nerve* **11**, 1146–1148 (1988).
206. Grossman, M. G., Ducey, S. A., Nadler, S. S. & Levy, A. S. Meralgia paresthetica: diagnosis and treatment. *Journal of the American Academy of Orthopaedic Surgeons* **9**, 336–344 (2001).
207. Konstantinou, K. & Dunn, K. M. Sciatica: Review of Epidemiological Studies and Prevalence Estimates. *Spine* **33**, 2464–2472 (2008).
208. Freynhagen, R. *et al.* Pseudoradicular and radicular low-back pain – A disease continuum rather than different entities? Answers from quantitative sensory testing. *PAIN* **135**, 65–74 (2008).
209. Vulfsons, S., Bar, N. & Eisenberg, E. Back Pain with Leg Pain. *Current pain and headache reports* **21**, 32 (2017).
210. Visser, L., Nijssen, P., Tijssen, C., van Middendorp, J. & Schieving, J. Sciatica-like symptoms and the sacroiliac joint: clinical features and differential diagnosis. *European spine journal: official publication of the European Spine Society, the European Spinal Deformity Society, and the European Section of the Cervical Spine Research Society* (2013).
211. Marchettini, P., Formaglio, F. & Lacerenza, M. Pain as heralding symptom in multiple sclerosis. *Neurological Sciences* **27**, s294–s296 (2006).
212. Busis, N. A. Femoral and obturator neuropathies. *Neurologic clinics* **17**, 633–653 (1999).
213. Esene, I. N. *et al.* Diagnostic performance of the medial hamstring reflex in L5 radiculopathy. *Surgical neurology international* **3**, (2012).
214. Patten, J. P. Nerve Root and Peripheral Nerve Lesions Affecting the Leg. in *Neurological Differential Diagnosis* (ed. Patten, J. P.) 299–314 (Springer Berlin Heidelberg, 1996). doi:10.1007/978-3-642-58981-2_17
215. Dillingham, T. R., Marin, R., Belandres, P. V. & Chang, A. Extensor digitorum brevis reflex in normals and patients with radiculopathies. *Muscle & Nerve: Official Journal of the American Association of Electrodiagnostic Medicine* **18**, 52–59 (1995).
216. Devillé, W. L. J. M., van der Windt, D. A. W. M., Dzaferagic, A., Bezemer, P. & Bouter, L. M. The test of Lasegue: systematic review of the accuracy in diagnosing herniated discs. *Spine* **25**, 1140 (2000).
217. Martin, H. D., Kivlan, B. R., Palmer, I. J. & Martin, R. L. Diagnostic accuracy of clinical tests for sciatic nerve entrapment in the gluteal region. *Knee Surgery, Sports Traumatology, Arthroscopy* **22**, 882–888 (2014).
218. Hopayian, K., Song, F., Riera, R. & Sambandan, S. The clinical features of the piriformis syndrome: a systematic review. *European Spine Journal* **19**, 2095–2109 (2010).
219. Moustafa, I. M. & Diab, A. A. The effect of adding forward head posture corrective exercises in the management of lumbosacral radiculopathy: a randomized controlled study. *Journal of manipulative and physiological therapeutics* **38**, 167–178 (2015).
220. Ito, T., Homma, T. & Uchiyama, S. Sciatica caused by cervical and thoracic spinal cord compression. *Spine* **24**, 1265 (1999).
221. Pal, B. & Johnson, A. Paraplegia due to thoracic disc herniation. *Postgraduate medical journal* **73**, 423–425 (1997).
222. Butler, D. & Gifford, L. The concept of adverse mechanical tension in the nervous system part 1: testing for "dural tension". *Physiotherapy* **75**, 622–629 (1989).
223. Breasted, J. H. *The Edwin Smith Surgical Papyrus: Published in Facsimile and Hieroglyphic Transliteration with Translation and Commentary in 2 Vol.* (University of Chicago Press, 1930).
224. Drača, S. Lazar K. Lazarević, the author who first described the straight leg raising test. *Neurology* **85**, 1074–1077 (2015).
225. Center, H. P. J. K. A. M., Leiden, G. W. B. E. P. of N. U. of & Infirmary, J. M. S. P. E. C. N. H. R. *Neurological Eponyms.* (Oxford University Press, 2000).
226. Ridehalgh, C., Moore, A. & Hough, A. Normative sciatic nerve excursion during a modified straight leg raise test. *Manual therapy* **19**, 59–64 (2014).
227. Boyd, B. S., Topp, K. S. & Coppieters, M. W. Impact of movement sequencing on sciatic and tibial nerve strain and excursion during the straight leg raise test in embalmed cadavers. *journal of orthopaedic & sports physical therapy* **43**, 398–403 (2013).
228. Ko, H.-Y. *et al.* Intrathecal movement and tension of the lumbosacral roots induced by straight-leg raising. *American journal of physical medicine & rehabilitation* **85**, 222–227 (2006).
229. Boyd, B. S. & Villa, P. S. Normal inter-limb differences during the straight leg raise neurodynamic test: a cross sectional study. *BMC musculoskeletal disorders* **13**, 1 (2012).
230. Nee, R. J. & Butler, D. Management of peripheral neuropathic pain: integrating neurobiology, neurodynamics, and clinical evidence. *Physical Therapy in sport* **7**, 36–49 (2006).
231. Vroomen, P. C. A. J., de Krom, M. C. T. F. M. & Knottnerus, J. A. Consistency of History Taking and Physical Examination in Patients With Suspected Lumbar Nerve Root Involvement. *Spine* **25**, 91 (2000).

232. Pande, K. The Use of Passive Straight Leg Raising Test: A Survey of Clinicians. *Malaysian orthopaedic journal* **9**, 44 (2015).
233. Tabesh, H., Tabesh, A., Fakharian, E., Fazel, M. & Abrishamkar, S. The effect of age on result of straight leg raising test in patients suffering lumbar disc herniation and sciatica. *J Res Med Sci* **20**, 150–153 (2015).
234. Kasper, J. M., Wadhwa, V., Scott, K. M. & Chhabra, A. Clunealgia: CT-guided therapeutic posterior femoral cutaneous nerve block. *Clinical imaging* **38**, 540–542 (2014).
235. Hall, S. *et al.* Lumbar spinal stenosis: clinical features, diagnostic procedures, and results of surgical treatment in 68 patients. *Annals of internal medicine* **103**, 271–275 (1985).
236. Konno, S. *et al.* A diagnostic support tool for lumbar spinal stenosis: a self-administered, self-reported history questionnaire. *BMC Musculoskeletal Disorders* **8**, 102 (2007).
237. Genevay, S. *et al.* Clinical classification criteria for neurogenic claudication caused by lumbar spinal stenosis. The N-CLASS criteria. *The Spine Journal* (2017). doi:10.1016/j.spinee.2017.10.003
238. Halbertsma, J. P. K., Göeken, L. N. H., Hof, A. L., Groothoff, J. W. & Eisma, W. H. Extensibility and stiffness of the hamstrings in patients with nonspecific low back pain. *Archives of Physical Medicine and Rehabilitation* **82**, 232–238 (2001).
239. Yamada, H. *et al.* Development of a support tool for the clinical diagnosis of symptomatic lumbar intra-and/or extra-foraminal stenosis. *Journal of Orthopaedic Science* **20**, 811–817 (2015).
240. Miyamoto, N., Hirata, K., Kimura, N. & Miyamoto-Mikami, E. Contributions of hamstring stiffness to straight-leg-raise and sit-and-reach test scores. *International journal of sports medicine* **39**, 110–114 (2018).
241. Atalay, A., Akbay, A., Atalay, B. & Akalan, N. Lumbar disc herniation and tight hamstrings syndrome in adolescence. *Child's Nervous System* **19**, 82–85 (2003).
242. Kia, F. & Schreiber, A. L. Poster 168: Hamstring Shortening and Pain as an Initial Presentation of Lumbosacral Radiculopathy: A Case Report. *PM&R* **2**, S77–S78 (2010).
243. Buijs, E., Visser, L. & Groen, G. Sciatica and the sacroiliac joint: a forgotten concept. *British journal of anaesthesia* **99**, 713–716 (2007).
244. Hirsh, L. F. Diabetic polyradiculopathy simulating lumbar disc disease: report of four cases. *Journal of neurosurgery* **60**, 183–186 (1984).
245. Paksoy, Y. & Gormus, N. Epidural venous plexus enlargements presenting with radiculopathy and back pain in patients with inferior vena cava obstruction or occlusion. *Spine* **29**, 2419–2424 (2004).
246. Hammer, A., Knight, I. & Agarwal, A. Localized venous plexi in the spine simulating prolapse of an intervertebral disc: a report of six cases. *Spine* **28**, E5–E12 (2003).
247. Moulin, D., Hagen, N., Feasby, T., Amireh, R. & Hahn, A. Pain in Guillain-Barré syndrome. *Neurology* **48**, 328–331 (1997).
248. Yoshimoto, M. *et al.* Diagnostic Features of Sciatica Without Lumbar Nerve Root Compression. *Journal of Spinal Disorders & Techniques* **22**, 328–333 (2009).
249. Epstein, N. E. Lumbar surgery for 56 limbus fractures emphasizing noncalcified type III lesions. *Spine* **17**, 1489–1496 (1992).
250. Gutman, H., Zelikovski, A., Gadoth, N., Lahav, M. & Reiss, R. Sciatic pain: a diagnostic pitfall. *The Journal of cardiovascular surgery* **28**, 204 (1987).
251. Wilberger Jr, J. E. Lumbosacral radiculopathy secondary to abdominal aortic aneurysms: Report of three cases. *Journal of Neurosurgery* **58**, 965–967 (1983).
252. Roncaroli, F., Scheithauer, B. W. & Krauss, W. E. Hemangioma of spinal nerve root. *Journal of Neurosurgery: Spine* **91**, 175–180 (1999).
253. Fearnside, M. R. & Adams, C. B. Tumours of the cauda equina. *J. Neurol. Neurosurg. Psychiatr.* **41**, 24–31 (1978).
254. Ker, N. B. & Jones, C. B. Tumours of the cauda equina. The problem of differential diagnosis. *J Bone Joint Surg Br* **67-B**, 358–362 (1985).
255. Shimada, Y. *et al.* Clinical features of cauda equina tumors requiring surgical treatment. *The Tohoku journal of experimental medicine* **209**, 1–6 (2006).
256. Sim, F., Dahlin, D., Stauffer, R. & Edward, L. Primary bone tumors simulating lumbar disc syndrome. *Spine* **2**, 65–74 (1977).
257. Buranapanitkit, B., Lim, A. & Geater, A. Misdiagnosis in vertebral osteomyelitis: problems and factors. *Journal of the Medical Association of Thailand= Chotmaihet thangphaet* **84**, 1743 (2001).
258. Chen, W.-S. Chronic sciatica caused by tuberculous sacroiliitis: a case report. *Spine* **20**, 1194–1196 (1995).
259. Dayan, L., Deyev, S., Palma, L. & Rozen, N. Long-standing, neglected sacroiliitis with remarked sacro-iliac degenerative changes as a result of Brucella spp. infection. *The Spine Journal* **9**, e1–e4 (2009).
260. Kulcu, D. G. & Naderi, S. Differential diagnosis of intraspinal and extraspinal non-discogenic sciatica. *Journal of Clinical Neuroscience* **15**, 1246–1252 (2008).
261. Hirayama, J., Yamagata, M., Takahashi, K. & Moriya, H. Effect of Noxious Electrical Stimulation of the Peroneal Nerve on Stretch Reflex Activity of the Hamstring Muscle in Rats: Possible Implications of Neuronal Mechanisms in the Development of Tight Hamstrings in Lumbar Disc Herniation. *Spine* **30**, 1014 (2005).
262. Yamada, T. & Yoshizawa, H. Electromyographical study of the straight leg raising test in lumbar disc herniation. *Nihon Seikeigeka Gakkai zasshi* **57**, 507–518 (1983).
263. Medrik-Goldberg, T., Lifschitz, D., Pud, D., Adler, R. & Eisenberg, E. Intravenous lidocaine, amantadine, and placebo in the treatment of sciatica: A double-blind, randomized, controlled study. *Regional Anesthesia and Pain Medicine* **24**, 534–540 (1999).
264. Kobayashi, S. Pathophysiology, diagnosis and treatment of intermittent claudication in patients with lumbar canal stenosis. *World Journal of Orthopedics* **5**, 134 (2014).
265. Zhu, Q. *et al.* Adolescent Lumbar Disc Herniation and Hamstring Tightness: Review of 16 Cases. *Spine* **31**, 1810 (2006).
266. Myers, T. W. *Anatomy Trains: Myofascial Meridians for Manual and Movement Therapists.* (Churchill Livingstone, 2009).
267. Coppieters, M. W. *et al.* A modified straight leg raise test to differentiate between sural nerve pathology and Achilles tendinopathy. A cross-sectional cadaver study. *Manual therapy* **20**, 587–591 (2015).
268. Do, K., Kim, J. & Yim, J. Acute effect of self-myofascial release using a foam roller on the plantar fascia on hamstring and lumbar spine superficial back line flexibility. *Phys Ther Rehabil Sci* **7**, 35–40 (2018).
269. Jung, J. *et al.* Immediate effect of self-myofascial release on hamstring flexibility. *Phys Ther Rehabil Sci* **6**, 45–51 (2017).
270. Coppieters, M. W. *et al.* Strain and excursion of the sciatic, tibial, and plantar nerves during a modified straight leg raising test. *Journal of Orthopaedic Research* **24**, 1883–1889 (2006).
271. Butler, D. *Mobilisation of the Nervous System, 1e.* (Churchill Livingstone, 1991).
272. Rebain, R., Baxter, G. D. & Mcdonough, S. A systematic review of the passive straight leg raising test as a diagnostic aid for low back pain (1989 to 2000). *Spine* **27**, E388–E395 (2002).
273. Magee, D. J. *Orthopedic Physical Assessment.* (Elsevier Health Sciences, 2014).
274. Reihani-Kermani, H. Clinical aspects of sciatica and their relation to the type of lumbar disc herniation. (2005).
275. Evans, R. C. *Illustrated Orthopedic Physical Assessment.* (Elsevier Health Sciences, 2008).
276. White, F. A. *Physical Signs in Medicine and Surgery: An Atlas of Rare, Lost and Forgotten Physical Signs.* (Museum Press Books, 2009).
277. Fishman, L. M. *et al.* Piriformis syndrome: diagnosis, treatment, and outcome—a 10-year study. *Archives of physical medicine and rehabilitation* **83**, 295–301 (2002).
278. Singh, U. S. *et al.* Prevalence of piriformis syndrome among the cases of low back/buttock pain with sciatica: A prospective study. *Journal of Medical Society* **27**, 94 (2013).
279. Laslett, M. Evidence-based diagnosis and treatment of the painful sacroiliac joint. *Journal of Manual & Manipulative Therapy* **16**, 142–152 (2008).
280. Prather, H., Cheng, A., Steger-May, K., Maheshwari, V. & Van Dillen, L. Hip and Lumbar Spine Physical Examination Findings in People Presenting With Low Back Pain, With or Without Lower Extremity Pain. *journal of orthopaedic & sports physical therapy* **47**, 163–172 (2017).
281. Patrick, H. T. THE CHICAGO NEUROLOGICAL SOCIETY: A NOTE ON BRACHIAL NEURITIS AND SCIATICA. *The Journal of Nervous and Mental Disease* **45**, 265 (1917).
282. Morimoto, T., Sonohata, M. & Mawatari, M. VALIDITY OF THE PATRICK TEST FOR OSTEOARTHRITIS OF THE HIP AND SCIATICA: GP138. *Spine Journal Meeting Abstracts* (2011).
283. Lakhotia, D., Prashant, K. & Shon, W. Y. Ganglion cyst of the hip mimicking lumbar disk herniation–A case report. *Journal of Clinical Orthopaedics and Trauma* (2017).
284. Gökkuş, K., Aydın, A. T. & Sağtaş, E. Solitary osteochondroma of ischial ramus causing sciatic nerve compression. *Eklem Hastalik Cerrahisi* **24**, 49–52 (2013).
285. Jorgensson, A. The iliopsoas muscle and the lumbar spine. *Australian Journal of Physiotherapy* **39**, 125–132 (1993).
286. Hanai, K. *et al.* Simultaneous measurement of intraosseous and cerebrospinal fluid pressures in lumbar region. *Spine* **10**, 64–68 (1985).
287. Eaton, L. M. Pain caused by disease involving the sensory nerve roots (root pain): its characteristics and the mechanics of its production. *Journal of the American Medical Association* **117**, 1435–1439 (1941).
288. Unschuld, P. U. & Tessenow, H. *Huang Di Nei Jing Su Wen: An Annotated Translation of Huang Di's Inner Classic – Basic Questions, 2 Volumes, Volumes of the Huang Di Nei Jing Su Wen Project. Paul U. Unschuld, General Editor.* (University of California Press, 2011).
289. Dejerine, J. *Sémiologie des affections du système nerveux.* (Masson et Cie., 1914).
290. Busch, E. Luftmyelographie Zur Diagnose Des Lumbalen Discusprolapsus Und Der Ligamentaren Wurzelkompression. *Acta Radiologica* **22**, 556–562 (1941).
291. Pearce, J. M. S. Queckenstedt's manoeuvre. *J Neurol Neurosurg Psychiatry* **77**, 728 (2006).
292. Jones Jr, O. & Naffziger, H. C. Tumors on the Spinal Cord: Their Diagnosis: An Analysis of Fifty-Nine Cases. *California and western medicine* **45**, 17 (1936).
293. Batson, O. V. The function of the vertebral veins and their role in the spread of metastases. *Annals of surgery* **112**, 138 (1940).
294. Anderson, R. Diodrast Studies of the Vertebral and Cranial Venous Systems to Show Their Probable Role in Cerebral Metastases. *Journal of Neurosurgery* **8**, 411–422 (1951).

295. Coster, S., de Bruijn, S. F. & Tavy, D. L. Diagnostic value of history, physical examination and needle electromyography in diagnosing lumbosacral radiculopathy. *Journal of neurology* **257**, 332–337 (2010).
296. Verwoerd, A. J. *et al.* Diagnostic accuracy of history taking to assess lumbosacral nerve root compression. *The Spine Journal* (2013).
297. Stynes, S., Konstantinou, K. & Dunn, K. M. Classification of patients with low back-related leg pain: a systematic review. *BMC Musculoskelet Disord* **17**, 226 (2016).
298. Verwoerd, A. J. *et al.* A diagnostic study in patients with sciatica establishing the importance of localization of worsening of pain during coughing, sneezing and straining to assess nerve root compression on MRI. *European Spine Journal* 1–4 (2016).
299. Hanai, K. Dynamic measurement of intraosseous pressures in lumbar spinal vertebrae with reference to spinal canal stenosis. *Spine* **5**, 568–574 (1980).
300. Reynolds, A. F., Weinstein, P. R. & Wachter, R. D. Lumbar monoradiculopathy due to unilateral facet hypertrophy. *Neurosurgery* **10**, 480–486 (1982).
301. Kienstra, G. E. *et al.* Prediction of spinal epidural metastases. *Archives of neurology* **57**, 690 (2000).
302. Lodder, J., Cheriex, E., Oostenbroek, R., Soeters, P. & Vreeling, F. Ruptured abdominal aortic aneurysms presenting as radicular compression syndromes. *Journal of neurology* **227**, 121–124 (1982).
303. Benny, B. V., Nagpal, A. S., Singh, P. & Smuck, M. Vascular causes of radiculopathy: a literature review. *The Spine Journal* **11**, 73–85 (2011).
304. Mieke, H. *et al.* Electromyography and a review of the literature provide insights into the role of sacral perineural cysts in unexplained chronic pelvic, perineal and leg pain syndromes. *Int J Phys Med Rehab* **5**, (2017).
305. Milnes, J. N. The early diagnosis of tumours of the cauda equina. *Journal of Neurology, Neurosurgery, and Psychiatry* **16**, 158 (1953).
306. Batson, O. V. The Valsalva maneuver and the vertebral vein system. *Angiology* **11**, 443–447 (1960).
307. Kimura, B. J. *et al.* The effect of breathing manner on inferior vena caval diameter. *Eur J Echocardiogr* **12**, 120–123 (2011).
308. Laborda, A. *et al.* Influence of breathing movements and Valsalva maneuver on vena caval dynamics. *World J Radiol* **6**, 833–839 (2014).
309. LaBan, M. M., Wilkins, J. C., Wesolowski, D. P., Bergeon, B. & Szappanyos, B. J. Paravertebral venous plexus distention (Batson's): an inciting etiologic agent in lumbar radiculopathy as observed by venous angiography. *American journal of physical medicine & rehabilitation* **80**, 129–133 (2001).
310. Gershater, R. & St. Louis, E. L. Lumbar epidural venography: Review of 1,200 cases. *Radiology* **131**, 409–421 (1979).
311. Paldor, I. *et al.* Intradural lumbar varix resembling a tumor: case report of a magnetic resonance imaging-based diagnosis. *Spine* **35**, E864–E866 (2010).
312. Spencer, D. L., Ray, R. D., Spigos, D. G. & Kanakis, C. J. Intraosseous Pressure in the Lumbar Spine. *Spine* **6**, 159 (1981).
313. Zhang, Z. *et al.* Valsalva manoeuver, intra-ocular pressure, cerebrospinal fluid pressure, optic disc topography: Beijing intracranial and intra-ocular pressure study. *Acta ophthalmologica* **92**, e475–e480 (2014).
314. Martins, A. N., Wiley, J. K. & Myers, P. W. Dynamics of the cerebrospinal fluid and the spinal dura mater. *Journal of Neurology, Neurosurgery & Psychiatry* **35**, 468–473 (1972).
315. Magnaes, B. Clinical recording of pressure on the spinal cord and cauda equina: Part 1: The spinal block infusion test: method and clinical studies. *Journal of neurosurgery* **57**, 48–56 (1982).
316. Magnaes, B. Clinical recording of pressure on the spinal cord and cauda equina: Part 2: Position changes in pressure on the cauda equina in central lumbar spinal stenosis. *Journal of neurosurgery* **57**, 57–63 (1982).
317. Wilke, H., Neef, P., Caimi, M., Hoogland, T. & Claes, L. E. New in vivo measurements of pressures in the intervertebral disc in daily life. *Spine* **24**, 755–762 (1999).
318. Sato, K., Kikuchi, S. & Yonezawa, T. In Vivo Intradiscal Pressure Measurement in Healthy Individuals and in Patients With Ongoing Back Problems. *Spine* **24**, 2468 (1999).
319. Nordenfelt, O. Studien über Valsalvas Versuch in seiner Anwendung als» Bürgers Pressdruckprobe». *Acta Medica Scandinavica* **82**, 465–491 (1934).
320. Lee, R. R., Abraham, R. A. & Quinn, C. B. Dynamic Physiologic Changes in Lumbar CSF Volume Quantitatively Measured By Three-Dimensional Fast Spin-Echo MRI. *Spine* **26**, 1172 (2001).
321. Stefanakis, M. *et al.* Annulus fissures are mechanically and chemically conducive to the ingrowth of nerves and blood vessels. *Spine* **37**, 1883–1891 (2012).
322. Moore, M. R. *et al.* Relationship Between Vertebral Intraosseous Pressure, pH, PO2, pCO2, and Magnetic Resonance Imaging Signal Inhomogeneity in Patients with Back Pain: An in Vivo Study. *Spine* **16**, S239 (1991).
323. Olmarker, K., Rydevik, B., Holm, S. & Bagge, U. Effects of experimental graded compression on blood flow in spinal nerve roots. A vital microscopic study on the porcine cauda equina. *Journal of Orthopaedic Research* **7**, 817–823 (1989).
324. Usubiaga, J., Moya, F. & Usubiaga, L. Effect of thoracic and abdominal pressure changes on the epidural space pressure. *British journal of anaesthesia* **39**, 612 (1967).
325. Esses, S. I. & Moro, J. K. Intraosseous vertebral body pressures. *Spine* **17**, S155–9 (1992).
326. Cecin, H. A. Cecin's Sign ('X' Sign): improving the diagnosis of radicular compression by herniated lumbar disks. *Revista Brasileira de Reumatologia* **50**, 44–55 (2010).
327. Liebenson, C. *Functional Training Handbook*. (LWW, 2014).
328. Liebenson, C., Karpowicz, A. M., Brown, S. H., Howarth, S. J. & McGill, S. M. The active straight leg raise test and lumbar spine stability. *PM&R* **1**, 530–535 (2009).
329. Beales, D. J., O'Sullivan, P. B. & Briffa, N. K. The effects of manual pelvic compression on trunk motor control during an active straight leg raise in chronic pelvic girdle pain subjects. *Manual Therapy* **15**, 190–199 (2010).
330. Shadmehr, A., Jafarian, Z. & Talebian, S. Changes in recruitment of pelvic stabilizer muscles in people with and without sacroiliac joint pain during the active straight-leg-raise test. *Journal of back and musculoskeletal rehabilitation* **25**, 27–32 (2012).
331. Arab, A. M., Ghamkhar, L., Emami, M. & Nourbakhsh, M. R. Altered muscular activation during prone hip extension in women with and without low back pain. *Chiropractic & Manual Therapies* **19**, 18 (2011).
332. Van Dillen, L. R. *et al.* Effect of active limb movements on symptoms in patients with low back pain. *Journal of Orthopaedic & Sports Physical Therapy* **31**, 402–418 (2001).
333. Bruno, P. A., Millar, D. P. & Goertzen, D. A. Inter-rater agreement, sensitivity, and specificity of the prone hip extension test and active straight leg raise test. *Chiropractic & manual therapies* **22**, 23 (2014).
334. McKenzie, R. A. & May, S. *The Lumbar Spine: Mechanical Diagnosis & Therapy, 2 Vol Set.* (Orthopedic Physical Therapy Products, 2003).
335. Williams, P. C. Lesions of the Lumbosacral Spine. *J Bone Joint Surg Am* **19**, 690–703 (1937).
336. Capener, N. Sciatica An Anatomical and Mechanical Study of the Lumbosacral Region. *Ann Rheum Dis* **4**, 29–36 (1944).
337. Alexander, L. A., Hancock, E., Agouris, I., Smith, F. W. & MacSween, A. The response of the nucleus pulposus of the lumbar intervertebral discs to functionally loaded positions. *Spine* **32**, 1508–1512 (2007).
338. Jonsson, B. & Stromqvist, B. Symptoms and signs in degeneration of the lumbar spine. A prospective, consecutive study of 300 operated patients. *Journal of Bone & Joint Surgery, British Volume* **75**, 381–385 (1993).
339. Zou, J. *et al.* Dynamic bulging of intervertebral discs in the degenerative lumbar spine. *Spine* **34**, 2545–2550 (2009).
340. Fujiwara, A., An, H. S., Lim, T.-H. & Haughton, V. M. Morphologic changes in the lumbar intervertebral foramen due to flexion-extension, lateral bending, and axial rotation: an in vitro anatomic and biomechanical study. *Spine* **26**, 876–882 (2001).
341. Inufusa, A. *et al.* Anatomic Changes of the Spinal Canal and Intervertebral Foramen Associated With Flexion-Extension Movement. *Spine* **21**, 2412–2420 (1996).
342. Henmi, T. *et al.* Natural history of extruded lumbar intervertebral disc herniation. *J. Med. Invest.* **49**, 40–43 (2002).
343. Sarı, H., Akarırmak, Ü., Karacan, I. & Akman, H. Computed tomographic evaluation of lumbar spinal structures during traction. *Physiotherapy Theory and Practice* **21**, 3–11 (2005).
344. Genevay, S. & Atlas, S. J. Lumbar spinal stenosis. *Best Practice & Research Clinical Rheumatology* **24**, 253–265 (2010).
345. Laslett, M., Öberg, B., Aprill, C. N. & McDonald, B. Centralization as a predictor of provocation discography results in chronic low back pain, and the influence of disability and distress on diagnostic power. *The spine journal* **5**, 370–380 (2005).
346. Skytte, L. P., May, S. & Petersen, P. Centralization: Its Prognostic Value in Patients With Referred Symptoms and Sciatica. *Spine June 1, 2005* **30**, (2005).
347. Werneke, M. & Hart, D. L. Centralization phenomenon as a prognostic factor for chronic low back pain and disability. *Spine* **26**, 758–764 (2001).
348. Adamczyk, W., Luedtke, K. & Saulicz, E. Lumbar Tactile Acuity in Patients With Low Back Pain and Healthy Controls. (2018). doi:info:doi/10.1097/AJP.0000000000000499
349. Saeidian, S. R., Moghaddam, H. F., Ahangarpour, A. & Latifi, S. M. Two-Point Discrimination Test in the Treatment of Right-handed Females with Lumbosacral Radiculopathy. *Iran J Med Sci* **36**, 296–299 (2011).
350. Adamczyk, W. M., Saulicz, O., Saulicz, E. & Luedtke, K. Tactile acuity (dys) function in acute nociceptive low back pain: a double-blind experiment. *Pain* **159**, 427–436 (2018).
351. Hotz-Boendermaker, S., Marcar, V. L., Meier, M. L., Boendermaker, B. & Humphreys, B. K. Reorganization in secondary somatosensory cortex in chronic low back pain patients. *Spine* **41**, E667–E673 (2016).
352. Adamczyk, W., S\lugocka, A., Saulicz, O. & Saulicz, E. The point-to-point test: A new diagnostic tool for measuring lumbar tactile acuity? Inter and intra-examiner reliability study of pain-free subjects. *Manual therapy* **22**, 220–226 (2016).
353. Adamczyk, W. M., Luedtke, K., Saulicz, O. & Saulicz, E. Sensory dissociation in chronic low back pain: Two case reports. *Physiotherapy theory and practice* 1–9 (2018).
354. Wand, B. M. *et al.* Lumbar tactile acuity is near identical between sides in healthy pain-free participants. *Manual therapy* **19**, 504–507 (2014).
355. Gilman, S. Joint position sense and vibration sense: anatomical organisation and assessment. *Journal of Neurology, Neurosurgery & Psychiatry* **73**, 473–477 (2002).

356. Gasik, R., Styczyński, T. & Pyskło, B. Examining proprioception in the knee joint area of patients suffering from lumbar spine discopathy. *Reumatologia/Rheumatology* **45**, 186–189 (2007).
357. Ruzikowski, E. [Value of testing vibration sensation in diagnosing spondylogenic pain syndromes]. *Neurol Neurochir Pol* **20**, 553–557 (1986).
358. Wise, B. L. Disturbances of vibratory sense (pallesthesia) associated with nerve root compression due to herniated nucleus pulposus. *AMA Archives of Neurology & Psychiatry* **68**, 377–379 (1952).
359. Zervopoulos, G. Diagnosis and Localization of Herniated Intervertebral Disks. *Neurology* **6**, 754–754 (1956).
360. Adamova, B. M. *et al.* Neurological impairment score in lumbar spinal stenosis. *Eur Spine J* **22**, 1897–1906 (2013).
361. Iversen, M. D. & Katz, J. N. Examination Findings and Self-Reported Walking Capacity in Patients With Lumbar Spinal Stenosis. *Phys Ther* **81**, 1296–1306 (2001).
362. Geletka*, B. J., O'Hearn, M. A. & Courtney, C. A. Quantitative sensory testing changes in the successful management of chronic low back pain. *J Man Manip Ther* **20**, 16–22 (2012).
363. Rabey, M., Slater, H., O'Sullivan, P., Beales, D. & Smith, A. Somatosensory nociceptive characteristics differentiate subgroups in people with chronic low back pain: a cluster analysis. *Pain* **156**, 1874–1884 (2015).
364. Takahashi, Y., Ohtori, S. & Takahashi, K. Human map of the segmental sensory structure ("sensoritomes") in the body trunk and lower extremity. *Pain Res* **23**, 133–141 (2008).
365. Frost, L. R., Bijman, M., Strzalkowski, N. D., Bent, L. R. & Brown, S. H. Deficits in foot skin sensation are related to alterations in balance control in chronic low back patients experiencing clinical signs of lumbar nerve root impingement. *Gait & posture* **41**, 923–928 (2015).
366. Scholz, J. *et al.* A Novel Tool for the Assessment of Pain: Validation in Low Back Pain. *PLoS Med* **6**, e1000047 (2009).
367. Stucki, G. *et al.* Measurement properties of a self-administered outcome measure in lumbar spinal stenosis. *Spine* **21**, 796–803 (1996).
368. Leinonen, V. *et al.* Lumbar paraspinal muscle function, perception of lumbar position, and postural control in disc herniation-related back pain. *SPINE-PHILADELPHIA-HARPER AND ROW PUBLISHERS THEN JB LIPPINCOTT COMPANY THEN LIPPENCOTT WILLIAMS AND WILKINS-* **28**, 842–848 (2003).
369. Leinonen, V. *et al.* Disc Herniation-related Back Pain Impairs Feed-forward Control of Paraspinal Muscles. *Spine* **26**, (2001).
370. Shenouda, M. M. S., Draz, A. H. & Shendy, W. Relationship between Proprioception and Trunk Muscles Strength at Different Trunk Velocities in Patients with Lumbar Disc Prolapse. *Bulletin of Faculty of Physical Therapy* **16**, (2011).
371. Truszczyńska, A., Dobrzyńska, M., Trzaskoma, Z., Drza\l-Grabiec, J. & Tarnowski, A. Assessment of postural stability in patients with lumbar spine chronic disc disease. *Acta of Bioengineering and Biomechanics* **18**, 71–77 (2016).
372. Sipko, T. & Kuczyński, M. Intensity of chronic pain modifies postural control in low back patients. *European Journal of Pain* **17**, 612–620 (2013).
373. Frost, L. R. & Brown, S. H. Muscle activation timing and balance response in chronic lower back pain patients with associated radiculopathy. *Clinical Biomechanics* **32**, 124–130 (2016).
374. Bray, H. & Moseley, G. L. Disrupted working body schema of the trunk in people with back pain. *British Journal of Sports Medicine* **45**, 168–173 (2011).

Chapter 6 Diagnostic testing

Key points

- Imaging is necessary given certain signs or symptoms or a lack of response to treatment
- Imaging findings should correlate with the patient's symptoms; lack of correlation should prompt further investigation for the source of pain
- Laboratory testing may help diagnose the source of sciatica and find barriers to recovery

Diagnostic imaging

Those with sciatica do not always need imaging studies. There is no standard imaging protocol for sciatica, although it most often begins with imaging the lumbar spine, followed by the pelvis, hip, and then other regions. Clinicians should order imaging when symptoms worsen during treatment, do not respond to treatment, or there are **red flag** symptoms or signs present (warning signs of pathology).[1]

Plain film radiography is the most appropriate initial imaging study to evaluate for **vertebral compression fractures** in elderly patients or those with **osteoporosis**, chronic **steroid use**, and/or low-velocity **trauma**.[1] An MRI is the most appropriate imaging study when patients have a history of **cancer** or **immunosuppression**, or have suspected cauda equina syndrome or rapidly progressive neurologic deficit.[1] An MRI with and without contrast should be performed when patients are suspected of having cancer or have had **prior lumbar surgery**.[1]

The presence of widespread neurologic deficits with sciatica suggests **cauda equina syndrome** (CES) and may prompt an urgent MRI. Any new-onset **urinary symptoms**,[2] impairment of the bladder, bowels, or perineal "saddle" numbness are indications for MRI. Clinicians should order imaging if sciatic symptoms are **multifocal** and include deficits in multiple nerve root levels or bilaterally. Acute-onset bilateral sciatica is another sign of CES[3] that should prompt MRI.

Imaging is appropriate when sciatic symptoms persist or progress over **6 weeks** of conservative treatment.[1] An MRI should be obtained for those with severe or progressive neurological deficits. If patients show ongoing signs of improvement such as reduced pain severity or frequency, centralization, improvement in range of motion, straight leg raising, or lessening of neurological deficits, then imaging is unnecessary.

Table 29: Red flags that may prompt imaging (adapted from Patel, 2016)

Cancer or infection	• History of cancer • Unexplained weight loss • Immunosuppression • Urinary infection • Intravenous drug use • Prolonged use of corticosteroids • Back pain not improved with conservative management
Spinal fracture	• History of significant trauma • Minor fall in a potentially osteoporotic or elderly individual • Prolonged use of steroids
Cauda equina syndrome or severe neurologic compromise	• Acute onset urinary retention or overflow incontinence • Loss of anal sphincter tone or fecal incontinence • Saddle anesthesia • Global or progressive motor weakness in the lower limbs

The most commonly imaged region for sciatica is the lumbar spine. In cases without urgency or red flags, the first test is usually **plain film radiography**. Plain film views for sciatica should include anteroposterior (AP) and lateral lumbar view and AP pelvis. The pelvic view assesses the sacroiliac joints (SIJs) and rarely may show intra-pelvic pathology causing lumbosacral plexopathy. Oblique lumbar views are useful for evaluating for fractures of the pars interarticularis. Dynamic views with flexion and extension in the standing position are useful for evaluating lumbar instability.

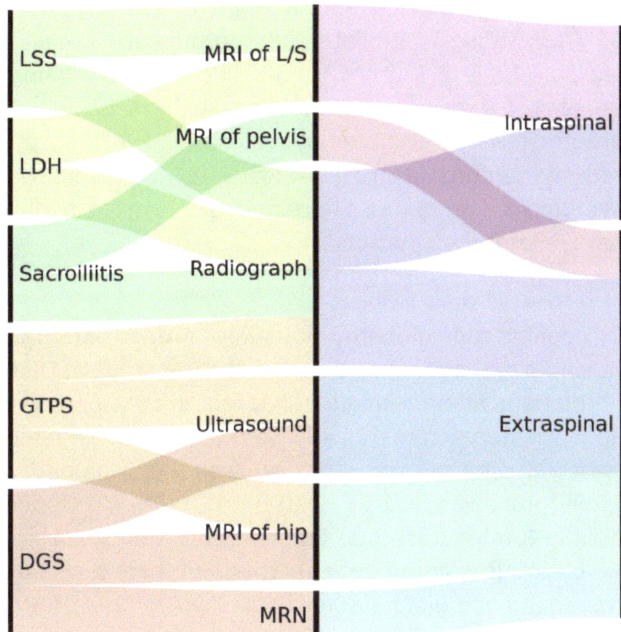

Figure 178: Typical imaging tests performed for select common causes of sciatica. Abbreviations: lumbar spinal stenosis (LSS), lumbar disc herniation (LDH), greater trochanteric pain syndrome (GTPS), deep gluteal syndrome (DGS), magnetic resonance imaging (MRI), lumbar spine (L/S), magnetic resonance neurography or lumbosacral plexus MRI (MRN)

Correlation of imaging with symptoms

Clinicians should determine if sciatic symptoms correspond to imaging findings. Spinal imaging often shows degenerative changes that are **incidental** or **false-positive** findings. Spine-related sciatica imaging findings should correlate with the clinically suspected disc and nerve root level, side, and number of nerve roots involved. Further evaluation may be necessary if signs and symptoms do not correlate with imaging findings. Correlation of imaging with clinical findings reduces misdiagnosis and helps guide treatment towards the responsible pathology.

Misdiagnosis of sciatica

The most common diagnostic errors in sciatica are **overdiagnosis** of **spinal pathology** and **under-diagnosis** of **extraspinal pathology**. Deep gluteal syndrome is the most commonly misdiagnosed disorder.[6] Clinicians may mistakenly ascribe symptoms to the lumbar spine which is the most common cause of sciatica.[4] This problem is compounded by the high prevalence of asymptomatic findings such as degenerative disc changes seen on imaging studies. Imaging for sciatica typically begins with the lumbar spine, which omits extraspinal conditions by default. The lumbar imaging pathway too easily shows incidental findings and disregards conditions outside of the spine.

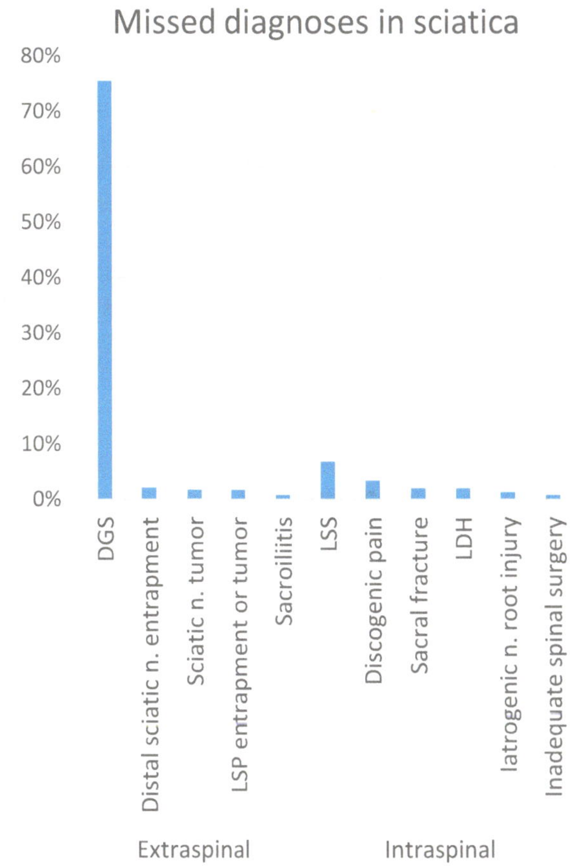

Figure 179: Missed diagnoses in chronic sciatica. Data adapted from Filler's[6] study of 239 patients who did not respond to treatment and had additional magnetic resonance neurography. Abbreviations: deep gluteal syndrome (DGS), nerve (n.), lumbosacral plexus (LSP), lumbar spinal stenosis (LSS), lumbar disc herniation (LDH)

One large study found that although 74% of patients with low back-related leg pain were **clinically diagnosed** with radicular sciatica, MRI was only able to show nerve compression in 61%.[4] The study showed that lumbar radicular sciatica is clinically **over-diagnosed** by 13%.[4] Another study found that clinicians were more likely to identify sensory loss if they had already seen a lumbar MRI showing disc pathology prior to examining the patients.[5]

One large study of patients with chronic, treatment-refractory sciatica used magnetic resonance neurography to search for alternative diagnoses. The study found that extraspinal causes of sciatica were the most frequently missed diagnoses.[6] This study has been corroborated by another, both of which show that the most common missed diagnosis in sciatica is **piriformis syndrome**, a type of deep gluteal syndrome.[6,7]

Disc and nerve level

One study found that clinicians overall impression of diagnosing L4, L5, or S1 radiculopathy was relatively inaccurate.[13] Clinicians had the highest specificity when diagnosing L4 radiculopathy (95%) but were less specific with L5 (75%) and S1 (43%) radiculopathies.[13] Another study found that neurologists clinical diagnosis of the level of lumbar disc herniation (LDH) was moderately accurate.[14] This study found higher accuracy in diagnosing central LDHs compared to lateral LDHs.[14] The more common pattern of discs affecting the traversing nerve root may be easier to diagnose.

Laterality of sciatica

Sciatica can occur unilaterally (on one side) or bilaterally (on both sides). The most common cause of **bilateral sciatica** is lumbar stenosis (LSS), in which 76% of cases are bilateral.[8] The most common cause of **unilateral sciatica** is LDH, in which 91% of cases are unilateral.[15]

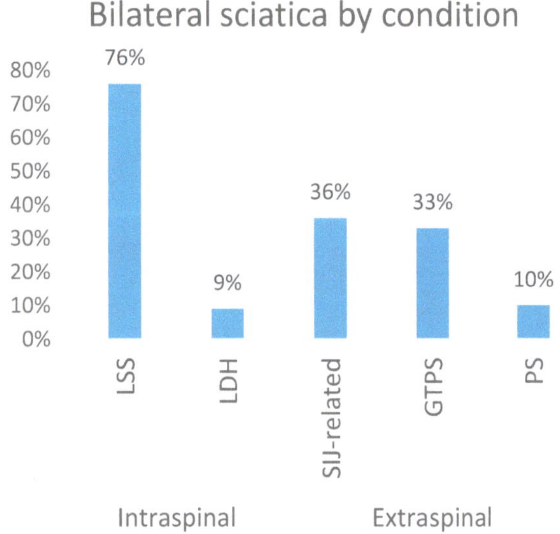

Figure 180: Percentage of bilateral symptoms in the five most common causes of sciatica. Data sources: Lumbar stenosis (LSS),[8] sacroiliac (SIJ),[9] greater trochanteric pain syndrome (GTPS),[10] piriformis syndrome (PS),[11] and lumbar disc herniation (LDH).[12] Data, for example, is interpreted as 9% of symptomatic LDHs cause bilateral symptoms

Bilateral sciatica is a specific sign of LSS (sp. 92-98%).[16] Those with bilateral symptoms of back and leg pain have 2.3 times the likelihood of LSS being present.[17] Extraspinal conditions such as SIJ pain, greater trochanteric pain syndrome (GTPS), and piriformis syndrome are less likely to have bilateral symptoms. Lumbar disc herniations only occasionally have bilateral symptoms.

Number of nerve roots

Discogenic radiculopathy is usually **monoradicular** (a single nerve root) or **biradicular** (two roots). Disc herniations affect a single nerve root in 60% of cases and two nerve roots in 40% of cases.[18] Discogenic radicular sciatica most often causes L5 radiculopathy (54%), followed by S1 (39%) then L4 (7%).[12] Upper or mid-lumbar disc herniations (L1-2, L2-3, L3-4), which are less common, can affect multiple levels of traversing and distal nerve roots. Involvement of the S2 level is rare and is only seen in 4% of cases[iii] of spine-related sciatica.[19,20]

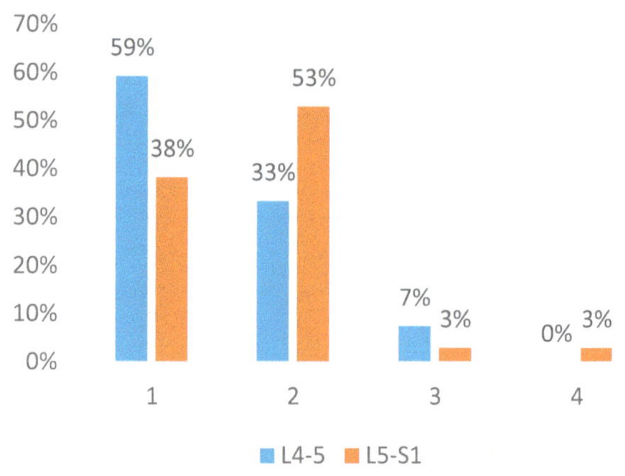

Figure 181: The number of nerve roots affected by L4-5 and L5-S1, shown as a % of 61 cases. Data produced from multiple sources[19-23]

Degenerative LSS is most often **polyradicular**. Stenosis affects at least **three nerve roots** in 71% of cases, two nerve roots in 19% of cases, and a single-level nerve root in only 10% of cases.[24] Stenosis most commonly affects L5 (in 52% of cases), followed by S1 (51%) and L4 (37%).[25] Cases of sciatica that involve more than two nerve roots should be evaluated for spinal stenosis. A young patient with multiple levels of radicular sciatica may be regarded

[iii] The two reference studies only had two cases of S2 in 56 cases of radicular sciatica

as a red flag as this demographic is unlikely to have stenosis.

Intervertebral **foraminal stenosis** affects a single exiting nerve root,[26] except for rare cases with conjoined nerve roots exiting the same foramen.[27] This type of stenosis is common in patients with **degenerative scoliosis**. Stenosis of the lumbar intervertebral foramen compresses the nerve of the cephalad number, for example L4-5 foraminal stenosis affects the L4 nerve root, and L5-S1 foraminal stenosis affects the L5 nerve root.

Conditions affecting the **lumbosacral plexus** may have a broad distribution spanning more than one nerve root level. Unfortunately, these conditions may be difficult to distinguish clinically from intraspinal radiculopathies.[7,28] Additional imaging of the pelvis or lumbosacral plexus may identify the cause of sciatica when lumbar imaging fails to do so, or does not correlate with the patient's symptoms.[7,28,29]

Exiting vs. traversing root

Discogenic sciatica most often affects at least one **traversing nerve root** passing inferior to the disc lesion, and less often one or more **exiting nerve roots** at the level of herniation,[iv] in a ratio of nearly 2:1.[19-23] Disc herniations can also migrate superiorly or inferiorly and affect proximal and distal roots. Higher lumbar disc lesions from L1 to L3 can produce symptoms at any traversing or distal level due to the proximity of the cauda equina.[30]

Lumbar stenosis tends to affect the nerve related to the **lowest spinal segment** of involvement.[v] Lumbar stenosis of L3-L5 most often affects the L5 nerve root. Stenosis of L4-L5 most often affects the L5 nerve root. Stenosis of L4-S1 most often affects the S1 nerve root.[8,19,31-37]

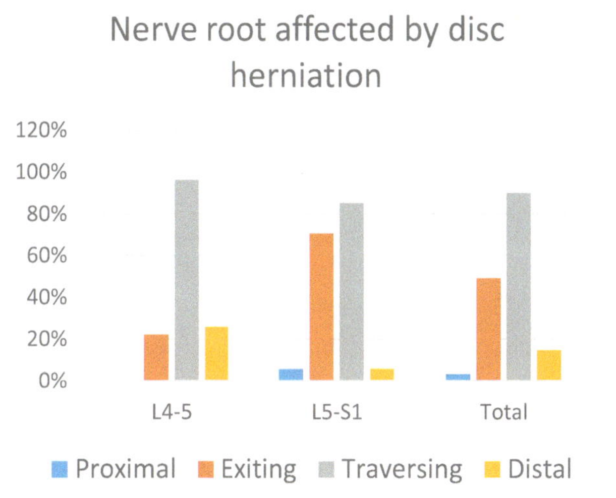

Nerve root affected by disc herniation

120%
100%
80%
60%
40%
20%
0%

L4-5 L5-S1 Total

Proximal Exiting Traversing Distal

Figure 182: Distribution of nerve involvement in LDHs at L4-5 and L5-S1, shown as a % of 61 cases. In degenerative foraminal stenosis related to scoliosis, radicular symptoms relate to the exiting nerve root on the side of concavity 72% of the time and the convexity 29% of the time.[38]. Data produced from a combination of sources[19-23] The most common pattern is involvement of the traversing root, followed by the exiting root.

Descriptive imaging findings

The strongest MRI predictors of radicular leg pain include **disc extrusions**, presence of **nerve root compression**, and **lateral recess stenosis**. Further analysis may help quantify these imaging findings to determine if they are clinically significant.

Quantifiable imaging findings

Only a few quantifiable MRI findings are specific to radicular sciatic leg pain. Findings that are **continuous variables**, rather than a binary "yes" or "no" answer may help determine if a LDH or stenosis is symptomatic. These measurements may help determine if imaging findings are **clinically relevant** or merely incidental.

[iv] The review summarized sixty-one cases of radiculopathy related to single-level disc herniation were from the referenced studies.

[v] The review summarized forty-nine cases of spinal stenosis without disc herniation from the referenced studies: L3-5 stenosis affects at least one side of the root of L3 (11%), L4 (67%), L5 (89%) and S1 (22%). L4-5 stenosis affects L4 (27%), L5 (91%), and S1 (18%). L4-S1 stenosis affects L4 (71%), L5 (93%), and S1 (100%).

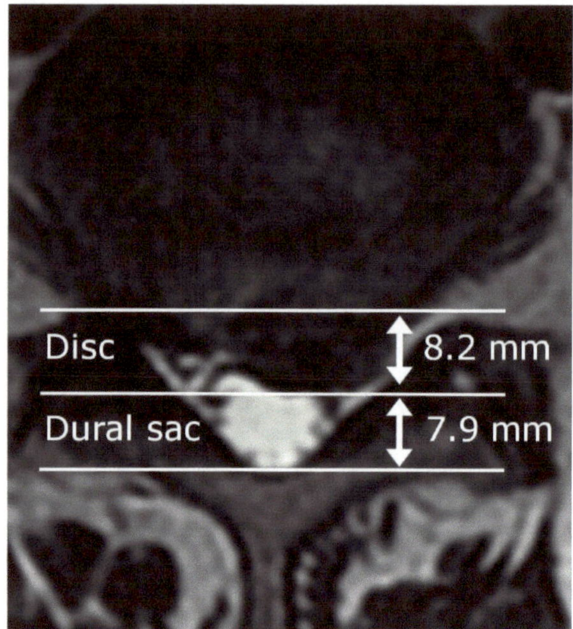

Figure 183: Measurements of AP disc and dural sac in an L5-S1 LDH. In this case both measurements correlate with disc lesion, based on the study by Pneumaticos.[41] AP disc dimension exceeds 6.8 mm while dural sac dimension is less than 10.2 mm. Case shared with permission of patient by Robert Trager, DC.

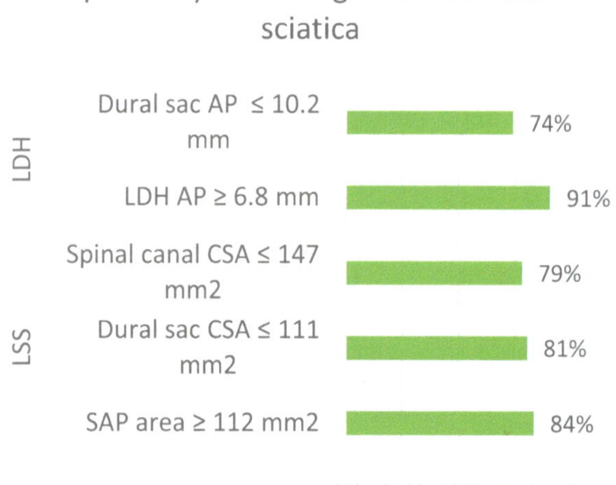

Figure 184: Specific and quantifiable MRI findings that correlate with radicular sciatic leg pain. Data cited in text from multiple authors.[39-41] Abbreviations: anteroposterior measurement (AP), cross-sectional area (CSA), lumbar disc herniation (LDH), lumbar spinal stenosis (LSS), superior articular process (SAP).

Larger disc lesions are more likely to cause sciatica. Disc herniations that are at least **6.8 mm anteroposterior (AP) diameter** have a 91% specificity for sciatica and increase odds of symptoms by a factor of 15.[41] Although disc extrusion-type herniations have the strongest association with sciatica,[42] an extrusion of 2 millimeters or less in AP diameter may not be clinically relevant. Conversely, a disc bulge may be large enough to create symptoms and/or neurological deficit. While it is important to know if a disc herniation is present, it is more important to know if the size is enough to cause symptoms.

The location of disc pathology influences the ability to cause sciatica. Disc herniations that compress a nerve root or cause compression in the **lateral recess** or **intervertebral foramen** are more likely to cause radicular sciatic pain.[43,44] **Central disc herniations** are less likely to cause symptoms.[44]

Lumbar stenosis symptoms correlate with the size of the **dural sac**, **canal cross-sectional area**, and area of the **superior articular process**. The size of the lumbar spinal canal correlates poorly with symptoms. While some studies have found a correlation between a narrow lumbar spinal canal and buttocks and leg pain,[45] other studies have found that moderate stenosis is more symptomatic than severe stenosis,[46] only lateral stenosis correlates with symptoms,[47] or there is no clinical correlation at all.[48]

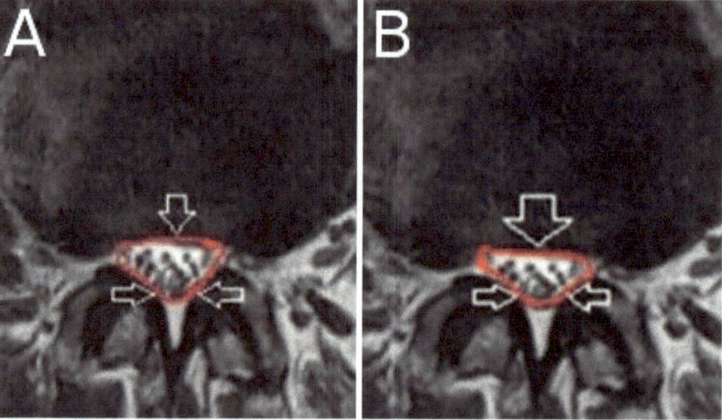

Figure 185: The severity of LSS symptoms correlates with the cross-sectional area of the dural sac (arrows and outline). Image A shows a normal dural sac, image B shows a reduced area in a stenosis patient. Images from Lim,[40] CC-BY-4.0

Signs of instability correlate with sciatica related to LDH and LSS. Listhesis of a vertebra over 3 millimeters during standing **flexion/extension radiographs** correlates with back and/or leg pain.[49]

Extraspinal imaging findings

Diagnosis of extraspinal sciatica often begins with ruling out the lumbar spine and radiculopathy. Sciatica stemming from the deep gluteal space,[6] greater trochanteric region[50] and SIJ[51] is most often identified in patients with prolonged sciatica in whom lumbar imaging is normal and a diagnostic injection alleviates pain. Diagnosis of extraspinal sciatica relies on a clinical diagnosis, finding a lack of correlation of symptoms with lumbar imaging, and/or confirming with advanced imaging for the extraspinal region.

Plain radiography, computed tomography (CT), and magnetic resonance imaging (MRI) may identify **sacroiliitis**. Of these modalities, MRI may best show **SIJ edema** (representing inflammation) which correlates with sciatic pain.[52] Only rarely do bone spurs from the SIJ as seen on plain film impinge upon the lumbosacral plexus.[53] While bony changes can show up on plain radiography and CT, these changes do not necessarily reflect pathology affecting the sciatic nerve.

Magnetic resonance neurography (MRN) is the best imaging study to identify **deep gluteal syndrome**. Imaging signs of piriformis asymmetry and sciatic nerve hypersensitivity at the sciatic notch using MRN has a high specificity (93%) for piriformis syndrome.[6] Sciatic neuropathy caused by hamstring tendon pathology may also be best diagnosed with MRN.[54]

MRI or **diagnostic ultrasound** can identify **greater trochanteric pain syndrome**. Treatment of the gluteal region, for example using diagnostic injection or manual therapy techniques, can corroborate the imaging findings.

Contralateral symptoms

Imaging abnormalities occasionally appear on the side **opposite from symptoms**. In this situation it is difficult to determine if the abnormality is coincidental or a true symptom generator. If every symptom and clinical finding correlates except for the side of symptoms, then further evaluation such as testing with electromyography will help localize the source of symptoms.[55]

Lumbar disc herniations rarely create symptoms on the contralateral side. It is thought that a LDH affects the contralateral root neurodynamics, either by a **traction force** or by **nerve root fibrosis**.[55] Other theories for LDH with contralateral symptoms include venous congestion, migration of epidural fat, and facet hypertrophy.[55]

Mirror image pain describes the co-occurrence of symptoms on the ipsilateral and contralateral side of nerve injury. There are many hypotheses to explain mirror image pain, such as spread of signals across the spinal cord by **commissural interneurons** and release of **pro-inflammatory cytokines** into the cerebrospinal fluid and blood.[56] Studies using animal models of sciatic nerve and root injury have identified immune system responses that may explain mirror image pain.[57] Co-occurrence of symptoms ipsilateral and contralateral to spinal or sciatic nerve injury may be mediated indirectly via the immune and nervous systems.

Upper motor neuron signs

Radiating lower extremity pain rarely stems from the cervical or thoracic spine, in which case it is called **cordonal sciatica** or **funicular leg pain**.[58] Upper motor neuron signs such as hyperreflexia are almost never seen in the common causes of sciatica relating to the lumbar spine, gluteal region, and SIJ. Any cause of radicular sciatica or myofascial sciatica will either decrease or not change reflexes. Upper motor neuron signs call for further evaluation even when lumbar imaging seems to correlate with sciatic symptoms.

Cordonal sciatica can be caused by cervical or thoracic disc herniation or stenosis[59–61] as well as neurological diseases. Lumbosacral radiculopathy is the most common misdiagnosis of patients with Amyotrophic lateral sclerosis.[62] Nearly 4% of those with multiple sclerosis also have a form of radicular pain relating to spinal cord damage.[63]

Upper motor neuron signs that help identify cordonal sciatica include **hyperreflexia**, presence of **pathological reflexes**, **crossed reflexes**, excessive twitching in the lower extremity muscles, and **L'hermitte's symptom**, in which neck flexion causes radiating pain from the back into the lower extremity.[64,65]

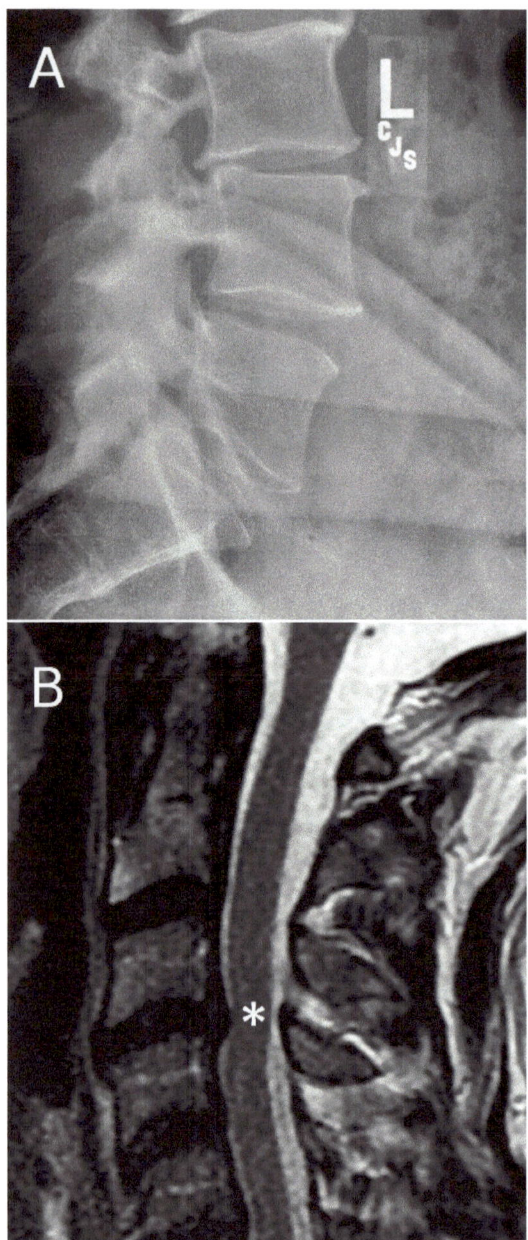

Figure 186: Cervical myelopathy misdiagnosed as LSS. This 63-year-old man presented with chronic LBP radiating to both gluteal regions, hip/thigh weakness, and bilateral cervical-thoracic pain. He was diagnosed with LSS by another clinician, based on symptoms and degenerative changes on radiograph (A) and given L/S exercises which did not help. Examination revealed diffuse hyperreflexia; cervical MRI (B) revealed disc-related cord compression. Case shared with permission of patient by Robert Trager, DC.

Those with **tandem stenosis** have stenosis of two regions of the spine, most often the cervical and lumbar spine. These patients can present with a mix of upper and lower motor neuron signs. These patients need evaluation and treatment of both regions.

Laboratory testing

Laboratory testing may identify the etiology of sciatica, comorbidities, or factors that delay its recovery. Those with persistent sciatica should have tests for inflammatory markers and nutrients involved in nerve healing and musculoskeletal pain. Clinicians should refer those with red-flag signs of acute infections for emergency workup.

Vitamin D deficiency is common and may predispose to sciatica. One study found 85% of those with radicular sciatic pain were either deficient or insufficient in vitamin D.[66] Deficiency of vitamin D causes nerves to become **hypersensitive** to pain.[67,68] Those deficient in vitamin D (<20 ng/ml) have 3.6 times greater odds of having severe leg pain compared to those with normal vitamin D levels (>30 ng/ml).[69]

Magnesium deficiency affects nearly half of the US population.[70] Deficiency in magnesium causes inflammation, **muscle spasms** and cramps, and weakness. The best test for magnesium is the **RBC magnesium** test, which shows a more long-term measure of the mineral in the body compared to serum magnesium. Those with lower magnesium may suffer from greater levels of mast cell activation and subsequent inflammatory histamine release in the lumbar disc and sciatic nerve pathway. Testing for magnesium helps optimize treatment strategies to minimize inflammation and muscle hypertonicity.

Vitamin B12 deficiency can cause bilateral leg paresthesia. This deficiency typically causes a glove and **stocking distribution**, which may mix with dermatomal numbness in radicular sciatica. Testing for B12 helps optimize treatment strategies. Some research has shown that supplementation with B12 improves sciatic pain[71] and improves **walking distance** in those with lumbar spinal stenosis.[72]

Autoimmune markers may help identify an autoimmune or inflammatory arthritide as the cause of sciatica. An elevated erythrocyte sedimentation rate (**ESR**) or C-reactive protein (**CRP**) occurs in a variety of inflammatory arthritides. Antinuclear Antibodies (**ANAs**) occur in ankylosing spondylitis, gout, and sacroiliitis.

Inflammatory markers help determine the severity and progression of discogenic sciatica. C-reactive protein correlates with pain severity in those with **discogenic sciatica**. Those with pain levels over

4.5/10 have 2.5 times the odds of having CRP elevated over 2.9 mg/L.[73] Interleukin-6 and interleukin-8[74,75] also correlate with sciatic pain severity. Those with elevated inflammatory markers may have more severe disc pathology and symptoms.

About 40% of patients with spinal infections lack classic signs such as fever[76] or constitutional symptoms.[77] Laboratory testing for spondylodiscitis or septic sacroiliitis may be based solely on risk factors, for example diabetes mellitus or prior surgeries. In this case a **complete blood count** (CBC), ESR, and CRP should be ordered.[78-80] These may be followed by blood and urine cultures.

Bacterial **antibody tests** may help identify chronic infections causing sciatica. Lyme disease antibodies should be tested when a radicular sciatica coincides with plausible tick exposure, an erythema migrans rash, a flu-like illness, fever, malaise, arthralgias, and/or headache.[81] Testing for Lyme co-infections such as Bartonella and Babesia may also be necessary.

Tests for viruses may identify the cause of sciatica in those with **constitutional symptoms** including fatigue, lymphadenopathy, rash, or **immunocompromise**. Sciatic pain with hyperesthesia can be a warning sign of lumbosacral shingles. Qualitative PCR and antibody testing for the **Herpesviridae** family including **Epstein-Barr** Virus (EBV), **Varicella-Zoster** Virus (VZV), Herpes Simplex Virus (HSV), and cytomegalovirus (CMV) are rarely positive in sciatic patients.

References

1. Patel, N. D. *et al.* ACR appropriateness criteria low back pain. *Journal of the American College of Radiology* **13**, 1069–1078 (2016).
2. Bell, D., Collie, D. & Statham, P. Cauda equina syndrome-What is the correlation between clinical assessment and MRI scanning? *British journal of neurosurgery* **21**, 201–203 (2007).
3. Gardner, A., Gardner, E. & Morley, T. Cauda equina syndrome: a review of the current clinical and medico-legal position. *European Spine Journal* **20**, 690–697 (2011).
4. Konstantinou, K. *et al.* Characteristics of patients with low back and leg pain seeking treatment in primary care: baseline results from the ATLAS cohort study. *BMC musculoskeletal disorders* **16**, 332 (2015).
5. Suri, P., Hunter, D. J., Katz, J. N., Li, L. & Rainville, J. Bias in the physical examination of patients with lumbar radiculopathy. *BMC Musculoskeletal Disorders* **11**, 275 (2010).
6. Filler, A. G. *et al.* Sciatica of nondisc origin and piriformis syndrome: diagnosis by magnetic resonance neurography and interventional magnetic resonance imaging with outcome study of resulting treatment. *Journal of Neurosurgery: Spine* **2**, 99–115 (2005).
7. Yoshimoto, M. *et al.* Diagnostic Features of Sciatica Without Lumbar Nerve Root Compression. *Journal of Spinal Disorders & Techniques* **22**, 328–333 (2009).
8. Zileli, B., Ertekin, C., Zileli, M. & Yünten, N. Diagnostic value of electrical stimulation of lumbosacral roots in lumbar spinal stenosis. *Acta neurologica scandinavica* **105**, 221–227 (2002).
9. Slipman, C. W. *et al.* Sacroiliac joint pain referral zones. *Archives of Physical Medicine and Rehabilitation* **81**, 334–338 (2000).
10. Segal, N. A. *et al.* Greater Trochanteric Pain Syndrome: Epidemiology and Associated Factors. *Arch Phys Med Rehabil* **88**, 988–992 (2007).
11. Fishman, L. M. *et al.* Piriformis syndrome: diagnosis, treatment, and outcome—a 10-year study. *Archives of physical medicine and rehabilitation* **83**, 295–301 (2002).
12. Mondelli, M. *et al.* Clinical findings and electrodiagnostic testing in 108 consecutive cases of lumbosacral radiculopathy due to herniated disc. *Neurophysiologie Clinique/Clinical Neurophysiology* **43**, 205–215 (2013).
13. Iversen, T. *et al.* Accuracy of physical examination for chronic lumbar radiculopathy. *BMC musculoskeletal disorders* **14**, 206 (2013).
14. Hancock, M. J., Koes, B., Ostelo, R. & Peul, W. Diagnostic accuracy of the clinical examination in identifying the level of herniation in patients with sciatica. *Spine* **36**, E712–E719 (2011).
15. Murade, E. C. M., Neto, J. S. H. & Avanzio, O. Estudo da relação e da importância entre a semiologia clínica, tomografia axial computadorizada e eletroneuromiografia nas radiculopatias lombares. *Acta Ortop Bras* **10**, 18–25 (2002).
16. de Schepper, E. I. T. *et al.* Diagnosis of Lumbar Spinal Stenosis: An Updated Systematic Review of the Accuracy of Diagnostic Tests. *Spine April 15, 2013* **38**, (2013).
17. Cook, C. *et al.* The clinical value of a cluster of patient history and observational findings as a diagnostic support tool for lumbar spine stenosis. *Physiotherapy Research International* **16**, 170–178 (2011).
18. Kortelainen, P., Puranen, J., Koivisto, E., Lähde, S. & others. Symptoms and signs of sciatica and their relation to the localization of the lumbar disc herniation. *Spine* **10**, 88 (1985).
19. Khatri, B. O., Baruah, J. & McQuillen, M. P. Correlation of electromyography with computed tomography in evaluation of lower back pain. *Archives of neurology* **41**, 594–597 (1984).
20. Tsonidis, C. *et al.* Comparison of dermatomal SEPs and operative findings in lumbar disc disease. *International journal of psychophysiology* **24**, 267–270 (1996).
21. Ross, M. K. & Swain, D. Dermatomal SEP Testing in the Workup of Lumbosacral Radiculopathy. *American Journal of Electroneurodiagnostic Technology* **37**, 185–195 (1997).
22. Sitzoglou, K. *et al.* Dermatomal SEPs — a complementary study in evaluating patients with lumbosacral disc prolapse. *International Journal of Psychophysiology* **25**, 221–226 (1997).
23. Wojtysiak, M. *et al.* Pre- and Postoperative Evaluation of Patients With Lumbosacral Disc Herniation by Neurophysiological and Clinical Assessment. *Spine* **39**, 1792 (2014).
24. Epstein, N. E., Epstein, J. A., Carras, R. & Lavine, L. S. Degenerative spondylolisthesis with an intact neural arch: a review of 60 cases with an analysis of clinical findings and the development of surgical management. *Neurosurgery* **13**, 555–561 (1983).
25. Micankova Adamova, B. & Vohanka, S. The results and contribution of electrophysiological examination in patients with lumbar spinal stenosis. *Scripta Medica Facultatis Medicae Universitatis Brunensis Masarykianae* **82**, 38–45 (2009).
26. Jenis, L. G. & An, H. S. Spine update: lumbar foraminal stenosis. *Spine* **25**, 389–394 (2000).
27. Taghipour, M., Razmkon, A. & Hosseini, K. Conjoined Lumbosacral Nerve Roots: Analysis of Cases Diagnosed Intraoperatively. *Journal of Spinal Disorders* **22**, 413–416 (2009).
28. Chhabra, A. *et al.* Incremental value of magnetic resonance neurography of Lumbosacral plexus over non-contributory lumbar spine magnetic resonance imaging in radiculopathy: A prospective study. *World journal of radiology* **8**, 109 (2016).
29. Laporte, C. *et al.* MRI Investigation of Radiating Pain in the Lower Limbs: Value of an Additional Sequence Dedicated to the Lumbosacral Plexus and Pelvic Girdle. *American Journal of Roentgenology* **203**, 1280–1285 (2014).
30. Kim, D.-S. *et al.* Clinical Features and Treatments of Upper Lumbar Disc Herniations. *Journal of Korean Neurosurgical Society* **48**, 119 (2010).
31. Colloca, C. J., Keller, T. S. & Gunzburg, R. Neuromechanical characterization of in vivo lumbar spinal manipulation. Part II. Neurophysiological response. *Journal of Manipulative & Physiological Therapeutics* **26**, 579–591 (2003).
32. Colloca, C. J., Keller, T. S. & Gunzburg, R. Biomechanical and neurophysiological responses to spinal manipulation in patients with lumbar radiculopathy. *Journal of Manipulative & Physiological Therapeutics* **27**, 1–15 (2004).
33. Di Lazzaro, V. *et al.* Role of motor evoked potentials in diagnosis of cauda equina and lumbosacral cord lesions. *Neurology* **63**, 2266–2271 (2004).
34. Katifi, H. & Sedgwick, E. Evaluation of the dermatomal somatosensory evoked potential in the diagnosis of lumbo-sacral root compression. *Journal of Neurology, Neurosurgery & Psychiatry* **50**, 1204–1210 (1987).
35. Onofrio, B. M. & Mih, A. D. Synovial Cysts of the Spine. *Neurosurgery* **22**, 642–647 (1988).
36. Shah, R. V. & Lutz, G. E. Lumbar intraspinal synovial cysts: conservative management and review of the world's literature. *Spine J* **3**, 479–488 (2003).
37. Tsitsopoulos, P., Fotiou, F., Papakostopoulos, D., Sitzoglou, C. & Tavridis, G. Comparative study of clinical and surgical findings and cortical somatosensory evoked potentials in patients with lumbar spinal stenosis and disc protrusion. *Acta neurochirurgica* **84**, 54–63 (1987).
38. Ploumis, A. *et al.* Radiculopathy in degenerative lumbar scoliosis: correlation of stenosis with relief from selective nerve root steroid injections. *Pain Medicine* **12**, 45–50 (2011).

39. Lim, T.-H. *et al.* Optimal Cut-Off Value of the Superior Articular Process Area as a Morphological Parameter to Predict Lumbar Foraminal Stenosis. *Pain Research and Management* (2017). doi:10.1155/2017/7914836
40. Lim, Y. S. *et al.* Dural sac area is a more sensitive parameter for evaluating lumbar spinal stenosis than spinal canal area. *Medicine (Baltimore)* **96**, (2017).
41. Pneumaticos, S. G., Hipp, J. A. & Esses, S. I. Sensitivity and specificity of dural sac and herniated disc dimensions in patients with low back-related leg pain. *Journal of Magnetic Resonance Imaging* **12**, 439–443 (2000).
42. Suri, P., Boyko, E. J., Goldberg, J., Forsberg, C. W. & Jarvik, J. G. Longitudinal associations between incident lumbar spine MRI findings and chronic low back pain or radicular symptoms: retrospective analysis of data from the longitudinal assessment of imaging and disability of the back (LAIDBACK). *BMC musculoskeletal disorders* **15**, 1 (2014).
43. Beattie, P. F., Meyers, S. P., Stratford, P., Millard, R. W. & Hollenberg, G. M. Associations between patient report of symptoms and anatomic impairment visible on lumbar magnetic resonance imaging. *Spine* **25**, 819–828 (2000).
44. Janardhana, A. P., Rajagopal, S. R. & Kamath, A. Correlation between clinical features and magnetic resonance imaging findings in lumbar disc prolapse. *Indian journal of orthopaedics* **44**, 263 (2010).
45. Iwahashi, H. *et al.* The Association between the Cross-Sectional Area of the Dural Sac and Low Back Pain in a Large Population: The Wakayama Spine Study. *PLOS ONE* **11**, e0160002 (2016).
46. Kuittinen, P. *et al.* Visually assessed severity of lumbar spinal canal stenosis is paradoxically associated with leg pain and objective walking ability. *BMC Musculoskeletal Disorders* **15**, 348 (2014).
47. Kuittinen, P. *et al.* Correlation of lateral stenosis in MRI with symptoms, walking capacity and EMG findings in patients with surgically confirmed lateral lumbar spinal canal stenosis. *BMC Musculoskeletal Disorders* **15**, 247 (2014).
48. Weber, C. *et al.* Is there an association between radiological severity of lumbar spinal stenosis and disability, pain, or surgical outcome?: A multicenter observational study. *Spine* **41**, E78–E83 (2016).
49. Kanemura, A. *et al.* The Influence of Sagittal Instability Factors on Clinical Lumbar Spinal Symptoms: *Journal of Spinal Disorders & Techniques* **22**, 479–485 (2009).
50. Tortolani, P. J., Carbone, J. J. & Quartararo, L. G. Greater trochanteric pain syndrome in patients referred to orthopedic spine specialists. *The Spine Journal* **2**, 251–254 (2002).
51. Buijs, E., Visser, L. & Groen, G. Sciatica and the sacroiliac joint: a forgotten concept. *British journal of anaesthesia* **99**, 713–716 (2007).
52. Wong, M., Vijayanathan, S. & Kirkham, B. Sacroiliitis presenting as sciatica. *Rheumatology* **44**, 1323–1324 (2005).
53. Bhaskaranand Kumar, K. & George, C. Osteophyte at the sacroiliac joint as a cause of sciatica: a report of four cases. *Journal of Orthopaedic Surgery* **10**, 73–76 (2002).
54. Bucknor, M. D., Steinbach, L. S., Saloner, D. & Chin, C. T. Magnetic resonance neurography evaluation of chronic extraspinal sciatica after remote proximal hamstring injury: a preliminary retrospective analysis. *J. Neurosurg.* 1–7 (2014). doi:10.3171/2014.4.JNS13940
55. Kim, P., Ju, C. I., Kim, H. S. & Kim, S. W. Lumbar Disc Herniation Presented with Contralateral Symptoms. *Journal of Korean Neurosurgical Society* **60**, 220 (2017).
56. Jancalek, R. Signaling mechanisms in mirror image pain pathogenesis. *Annals of neurosciences* **18**, 123 (2011).
57. Hatashita, S., Sekiguchi, M., Kobayashi, H., Konno, S. & Kikuchi, S. Contralateral neuropathic pain and neuropathology in dorsal root ganglion and spinal cord following hemilateral nerve injury in rats. *Spine* **33**, 1344–1351 (2008).
58. Chan, C. K., Lee, H.-Y., Choi, W.-C., Cho, J. Y. & Lee, S.-H. Cervical cord compression presenting with sciatica-like leg pain. *European Spine Journal* **20**, 217–221 (2010).
59. Ito, T., Homma, T. & Uchiyama, S. Sciatica caused by cervical and thoracic spinal cord compression. *Spine* **24**, 1265 (1999).
60. Kobayashi, S. ' Tract pain syndrome' associated with chronic cervical disc herniation. *Hawaii medical journal* **33**, 376 (1974).
61. Langfitt TW, E. F. PAin in the back and legs caused by cervical spinal cord compression. *JAMA* **200**, 382–385 (1967).
62. Belsh, J. M. & Schiffman, P. L. Misdiagnosis in patients with amyotrophic lateral sclerosis. *Archives of internal medicine* **150**, 2301 (1990).
63. Ramirez-Lassepas, M., Tulloch, J. W., Quinones, M. R. & Snyder, B. D. Acute radicular pain as a presenting symptom in multiple sclerosis. *Archives of neurology* **49**, 255 (1992).
64. Noseworthy, J., Heffernan, L. & others. Motor radiculopathy–an unusual presentation of multiple sclerosis. *The Canadian journal of neurological sciences. Le journal canadien des sciences neurologiques* **7**, 207 (1980).
65. Moulin, D. E., Foley, K. M. & Ebers, G. C. Pain syndromes in multiple sclerosis. *Neurology* **38**, 1830–1830 (1988).
66. Babita Ghai, M., Dipika Bansal, M. & Raju Kanukula, M. High Prevalence of Hypovitaminosis D in Indian Chronic Low Back Patients. *Pain physician* **18**, E853–E862 (2015).
67. Kuru, P., Akyuz, G., Yagci, I. & Giray, E. Hypovitaminosis D in widespread pain: its effect on pain perception, quality of life and nerve conduction studies. *Rheumatology international* **35**, 315–322 (2015).
68. Sedighi, M. & Haghnegahdar, A. Role of vitamin D3 in Treatment of Lumbar Disc Herniation—Pain and Sensory Aspects: Study Protocol for a Randomized Controlled Trial. *Trials* **15**, (2014).
69. Tae-Hwan, K. *et al.* Prevalence of vitamin D deficiency in patients with lumbar spinal stenosis and its relationship with pain. *Pain Physician* **16**, 165–176 (2012).
70. Rosanoff, A., Weaver, C. M. & Rude, R. K. Suboptimal magnesium status in the United States: are the health consequences underestimated? *Nutrition Reviews* **70**, 153–164 (2012).
71. Mauro, G. L., Martorana, U., Cataldo, P., Brancato, G. & Letizia, G. Vitamin B12 in low back pain: a randomised, double-blind, placebo-controlled study. *Eur Rev Med Pharmacol Sci* **4**, 53–58 (2000).
72. W, W. & S, W. Methylcobalamin as an adjuvant medication in conservative treatment of lumbar spinal stenosis. *J Med Assoc Thai* **83**, 825–831 (2000).
73. Sturmer, T. Pain and high sensitivity C reactive protein in patients with chronic low back pain and acute sciatic pain. *Annals of the Rheumatic Diseases* **64**, 921–925 (2005).
74. Pedersen, L. M., Schistad, E., Jacobsen, L. M., Røe, C. & Gjerstad, J. Serum levels of the pro-inflammatory interleukins 6 (IL-6) and -8 (IL-8) in patients with lumbar radicular pain due to disc herniation: A 12-month prospective study. *Brain, Behavior, and Immunity* **46**, 132–136 (2015).
75. Wang, K. *et al.* A cohort study comparing the serum levels of pro- or anti-inflammatory cytokines in patients with lumbar radicular pain and healthy subjects. *Eur Spine J* **25**, 1428–1434 (2016).
76. Mylona, E., Samarkos, M., Kakalou, E., Fanourgiakis, P. & Skoutelis, A. Pyogenic vertebral osteomyelitis: a systematic review of clinical characteristics. in *Seminars in arthritis and rheumatism* **39**, 10–17 (2009).
77. Colmenero, J. *et al.* Pyogenic, tuberculous, and brucellar vertebral osteomyelitis: a descriptive and comparative study of 219 cases. *Annals of the rheumatic diseases* **56**, 709–715 (1997).
78. Tsiodras, S. & Falagas, M. E. Clinical assessment and medical treatment of spine infections. *Clinical orthopaedics and related research* **444**, 38–50 (2006).
79. Mete, B. *et al.* Vertebral osteomyelitis: eight years' experience of 100 cases. *Rheumatology international* **32**, 3591–3597 (2012).
80. An, H. S. & Seldomridge, J. A. Spinal infections: diagnostic tests and imaging studies. *Clinical orthopaedics and related research* **444**, 27–33 (2006).
81. Trager, R. *Lumbosacral radiculopathy: Causes and mimics of sciatica and low back nerve root disorders.* (CreateSpace Independent Publishing Platform, 2015).

Chapter 7 The prognosis of sciatica

Key points

- The prognosis of sciatica depends on its cause, baseline health status, treatments utilized, and many other individual and lifestyle factors
- Three-quarters of patients with discogenic sciatica improve significantly by three months by staying active and taking basic over-the-counter medications

Natural history of sciatica

The largest improvements in sciatic pain, paresthesia, and lower extremity weakness occur in the first **three months**, then slowly after that.[1] One study found that at three months, 75% of patients were completely recovered or much better; these patients were given advice to stay active and take pain medications if necessary.[2] At one year, 82% of patients report at least some improvement of sciatica.[3]

Most cases of discogenic sciatica will recover completely without **residual symptoms**. About 18% of patients have no change or worsening of symptoms after 1 year.[3] About 17% of patients will have ongoing sciatic pain lasting two years.[1] Only about 8% of patients have chronic ongoing symptoms for at least five years.[4]

Sciatica caused by **lumbar stenosis** has a worse prognosis than discogenic sciatica.[5,6] Only 9% of patients report having a "good response" at six month follow up with minimal conservative treatment.[5] Lumbar stenosis is not necessarily permanent, and conservative, manual therapy and rehabilitative techniques can significantly improve the prognosis compared to its natural history.

Age does not affect prognosis of sciatica.[7,8] A lumbar disc herniation (LDH) in a younger patient has more nucleus pulposus tissue which takes longer to dehydrate and resorb.[9] However, older patients have weaker degradation of disc fragments due to less immune and vascular responses.[10] The factors of younger and older age balance out to have a net zero effect on prognosis of sciatica.

Social and demographic variables influence the prognosis of sciatica. Those that **drive over two hours per day**,[11] have a job involving **heavy labor,**[5,11] are **obese**,[7,12] or have a compensation claim[6] are expected to have a slower recovery from sciatica. **Smokers** have two times the odds of having ongoing sciatica after 1 year compared to non-smokers.[13,14]

A baseline of better **general health** helps speed recovery from sciatica.[15] Those with fewer subjective health complaints,[15] or those that **exercise** vigorously or regularly several times per week (including heavy gardening or housework) improve faster.[6] The prognosis of sciatica is worse in those with a history of chronic back pain over 1 year[3] or those with prior episodes of sciatica.[15]

Chronic sciatica correlates with poor overall health status and worrying and anxiety about pain.[6] Those with more comorbid subjective health complaints tend to recover slower from sciatica.[3] Those with **fear avoidance** beliefs,[6] **kinesiophobia** (fear of movement),[3,13] and those that perform light or no exercise[6] recover slower from sciatica.

Symptoms and prognosis

The sciatic pain severity does not affect prognosis.[8,13] Pain severity is not a reliable marker for nerve damage or source of symptoms in sciatica. Other factors such as **neurological deficits** and **neural tension signs** are more reliable predictors of prognosis.

The prognosis is worse the further the pain radiates in the lower extremity. Those with sciatic pain proximal to the knee have a greater likelihood of long-term recovery than those with pain **distal to the knee** at six months[16] and fourteen months after onset.[17]

The level of LDH has no influence over prognosis in sciatica.[8] What matters more is the amount of inflammation, compression or overall damage to the nerve root. Discogenic back pain with nerve root compression is more likely to radiate distal to the knee while absence of nerve root compression is more likely to radiate proximal to the knee.[18] The more a nerve is injured the further its symptom distribution will be.

Examination findings and prognosis

Centralization of sciatic pain (retreat from distal to proximal) predicts a faster recovery from sciatica. Those that experience centralization with a directional preference have a faster recovery from discogenic sciatica.[19] One study found that patients that did not centralize were more likely to undergo low back surgery.[19]

The presence of **neurological deficits** indicates a worse prognosis of discogenic sciatica. Those with muscular weakness,[13] reduced sensation,[1] and/or a reduced tendon reflex[13] have greater odds of having sciatica for at least one year.

Those with multiple **neural tension** signs have a slightly worse prognosis. A positive Bragard's test,[4,14] crossed straight leg raise,[14] or straight leg raise less than 60 degrees[3] are associated with slower recovery. A positive SLR also increases the likelihood of longer lasting motor weakness.[20]

Palpation findings of at least eight of the classic fibromyalgia tender points,[6] or **diffuse tenderness**[6] worsens the prognosis for sciatica.

Advanced imaging and prognosis

Nerve root compression increases pain and disability in the short-term but speeds recovery in the long-term. Compression of nerve roots increases the odds that pain travels distal to the knee,[18] and increases the odds of neurological deficits.[18,21] However, those with nerve compression have much greater odds of recovering by one year compared to those that do not.[22] Sciatica with nerve compression involves more symptoms initially but results in a better long-term prognosis.

Large disc herniations increase pain and disability in the short-term but have a similar prognosis to small LDHs. Disc herniations over three millimeters in anterior to posterior dimension are more likely to cause pain distal to the knee, severe pain over 7/10, and inability to work.[23] Some studies indicate large herniations resorb faster than small ones.[24] In most cases, the size of LDHs generally does not influence long-term (1 year) outcome.[25]

The type of disc impairment affects prognosis. **Sequestrations** and **extrusions** with a greater degree of disc migration heal the fastest and have the best prognosis.[9,10] Disc bulges have the worst prognosis.[27]

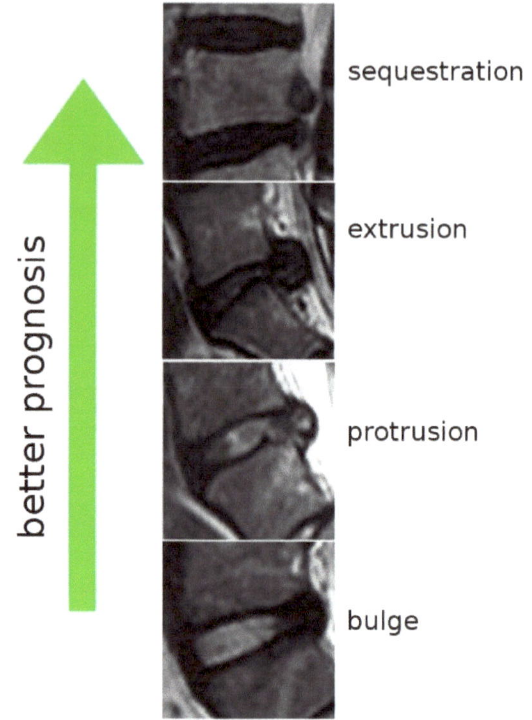

Figure 187: Disc impairment and prognosis. Sciatica prognosis is worst with disc bulges and best with extrusions and sequestrations. Image modified from Zhang et al,[26] CC-BY-4.0 license.

Spontaneous Regression

Spontaneous regression, also called **spontaneous resorption** or **spontaneous resolution** of an LDH describes its rapid reduction in size, usually within the first year of onset of symptoms. The speed at which LDHs resorb is highly variable and depends on multiple factors. Most lumbar LDHs reduce in size over the first year of symptoms, with 88% reducing at least 50% in size between 3-12 months.[9] The probability of spontaneous regression is highest for disc **sequestrations** at 96%, followed by extrusions (70%), focal protrusions (41%), and is lowest for disc bulges (13%).[24]

Symptomatic improvement does not always correlate with radiographic evidence of resorption of disc material.[24] Those with fast resorption of 40% within two months have faster relief of leg pain.[10] However, the majority of disc herniations take longer than two months to resorb. Pain relief also typically occurs long before the LDH is fully resorbed. Sciatic pain usually improves even in those without any resorption.[28] In those with spontaneous resorption, symptoms improve in a matter of 1-3 months while the disc usually does not resorb for about 9 or more months.[29] Resorption of disc material may help but is not necessary to begin recovering from sciatica.

Regression is thought to occur by any of three mechanisms: **Retraction**, **dehydration**, and **phagocytosis**.[24] Retraction describes the disc material returning to its original position. Dehydration is a loss of water that shrinks the LDH material. Phagocytosis is the breakdown of LDH material by the immune system. One or more mechanisms may be involved in a single patient.

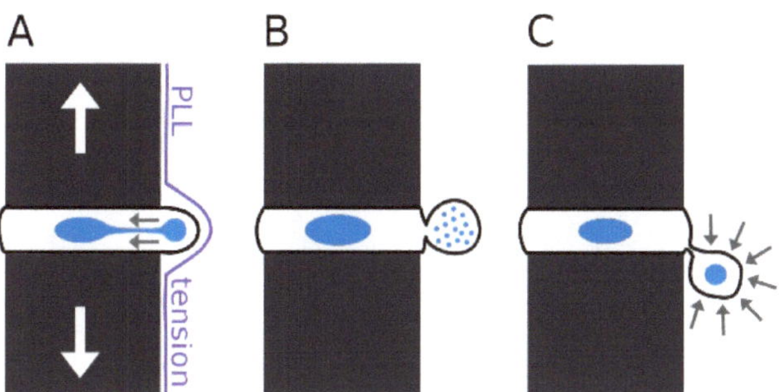

Figure 188: The mechanisms of LDH regression: retraction (A), dehydration (B), and phagocytosis (C). Image by Robert Trager, DC.

Retraction is a mechanical resorption of disc bulges and protrusions through an annular tear aided by posterior ligament tension and reduction in disc pressure. Retraction describes LDH material going back into the disc through an **annular tear**, the same passage from which it herniated.[30] This may account for improvement of bulges and protrusions[24] which have a strong connection to the parent disc, as opposed to extrusions and sequestrations. Tension of the **posterior longitudinal ligament** may help with retraction by pushing anteriorly on the disc material.[31,32] Lumbar traction[32] and directional preference exercises[33] may aid in retraction of disc material by reducing **intra-discal pressure**.

Discs herniations with more **water content**, shown by a **hyperintense T2 signal** on MRI, resorb at a faster rate.[28,31,34] Disc herniation material with more water is thought to have a greater capacity to dehydrate. It is thought that dehydration may shrink the LDH but cannot completely resolve it.[35] Disc herniations that are brighter on T2 MRI resorb faster, probably due to dehydration.

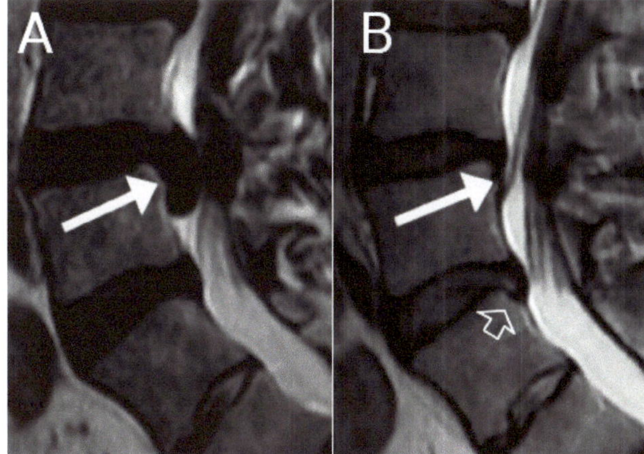

Figure 189: Regression of a large disc herniation at L4-5 (solid arrows) over three years. A: Initial MRI, B: Three-years later. A new disc lesion is evident at L5-S1 on the follow-up (transparent arrow) MRI. Image Creative Commons Attribution License from Hakan, 2016 - Spontaneous Regression of Herniated Lumbar Disc with New Disc Protrusion in the Adjacent Level

Phagocytosis of LDH material depends on the ability of the immune system to access it. Phagocytosis occurs faster with **detachment** and **migration**, which occur if the LDH disconnects from the parent disc, moves away, forming a sequestration.[34] As a result, there is more surface area for macrophages to degrade the disc material.[35] Sequestrated herniations resorb faster due to greater immune-mediated degradation.

Phagocytosis relies on exposure of disc material to blood vessels. When a disc herniates, its outer rim undergoes **neovascularization**, the formation of new capillaries within it.[36] These new capillaries deliver monocytes that turn into macrophages which break down the disc material.[36] Sequestrations are phagocytosed fastest because they are exposed to epidural blood vessels, and also have a larger free margin that can be invaded by new capillaries.[37]

Guarding

Muscle activity

Those with low back pain (LBP) and sciatica have increased activity of the **global stability** and decreased activity of the **local stability**. The global muscles, also called tonic muscles, are more superficial and prone towards tightness and shortness. The local muscles, also called phasic muscles are deeper muscles predisposed to weakness or inhibition. The pain-spasm-pain cycle, pain-adaptation, and excessive bracing against movement or **guarding** may explain the alteration in muscle tone. Initially these patterns are protective but may become problematic when they persist beyond the cause of sciatica.

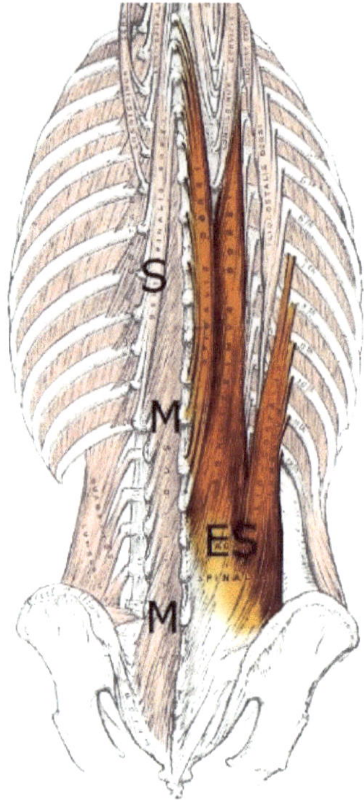

Figure 190: Local vs. global stability of the lumbar spine. Local stability muscles (left) include the semispinalis (S). multifidus (M), and rotatores (not shown). The global stability muscles (right) are the erector spinae (ES). Image modified from Gray's anatomy (public domain) by Robert Trager DC

The global stability muscles of the spine are the erector spinae, which generate force to initiate and control large motions of the spine. The local spinal stability muscles are the smaller, deeper transversospinal muscles which help with spine stiffness and posture. In LBP and sciatica, the **thoracolumbar erector spinae** muscles increase in tone while the **transversospinal muscles** decrease in tone.

The global **erector spinae** consist of the iliocostalis, longissimus, and spinalis muscles. The erector muscles primarily extend the spine but also become active in lateral flexion and rotation.[38] The local stability transversospinal muscles include the semispinalis, multifidus, and rotatores. Of these, **multifidus** is the largest and most important in the low back. The multifidus, especially its dep fibers, stabilize the spine and protect it against excessive unwanted **torsion** and **shearing**.[38]

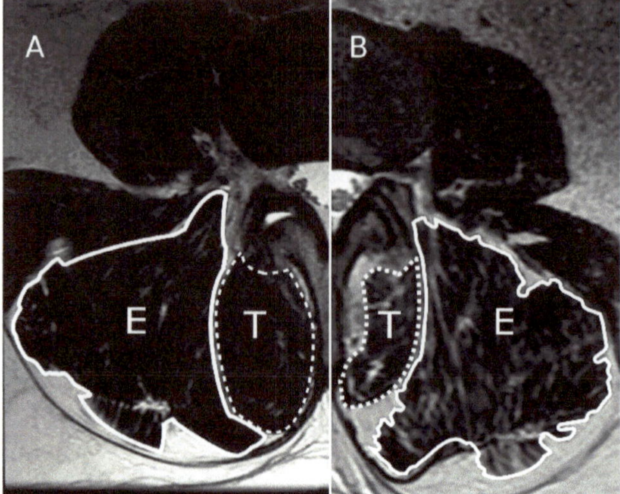

Figure 191: Erector spinae (E) and transversospinalis (T) muscles: normal vs. atrophy. Axial T2-weighted MRI at L3-4 of two patients with sciatica. A normal transversospinalis muscle group (A) is contrasted with moderate atrophy and fat deposition within and around the transversospinalis group (B). Images shared with patients' permission from Robert Trager DC.

Those with LBP and sciatica have increased activation of the erector spinae during movements including walking,[39] bending,[40] prone hip extension,[41] and even while sitting or standing.[42] In healthy people the lumbar erectors relax at the end range of lumbar flexion. This normal response is the **flexion-relaxation phenomenon**.

Those with LBP have **increased erector activity**, rather than reduced, during flexion.[40] In some cases the lumbar erectors are excessively tight for at least six months following an episode of discogenic sciatica.[43] The increase in erector tightness reduces spinal range of motion (ROM), shearing, and torsional forces.

Other examples of increased global or tonic muscle tone in sciatica include the **rectus abdominis** and **hamstrings**. The hamstrings are thought to increase in tone to help stabilize the **sacroiliac joint** (SIJ) via their connection through the sacrotuberous ligament.[41] The rectus abdominis increases in tone which helps stabilize the spine.[39] In extreme cases of discogenic sciatica people cannot even passively flex the lumbar spine or hips due to erector and hamstring tightness, this is called the **board sign.**[44]

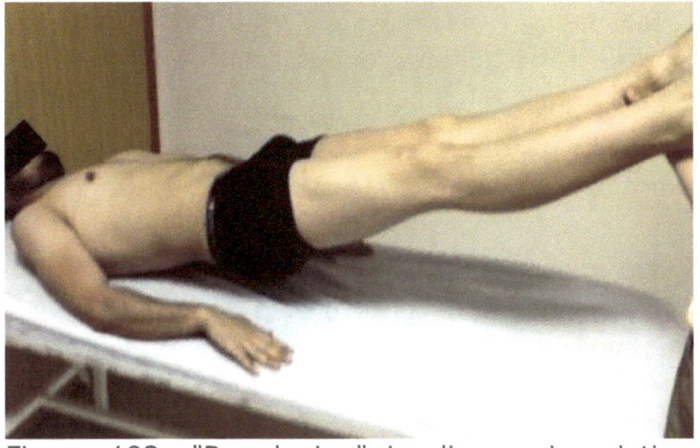

Figure 192: "Board sign" in discogenic sciatica. Spasms in the lumbar erectors and hamstrings cause the patient's body to also lift when the examiner raises both of the patient's legs. Image modified from Kurt et al[44] using CC-BY 4.0 license.

Increased global or tonic muscle activity can have neurological and psychological causes. The **pain-spasm-pain cycle** proposes that pain causes muscle spasms, which in turn leads to more pain. Any spinal injury including a LDH may stimulate the nociceptive (pain-sensing) neurons which in turn reflexively stimulate the motor neurons of the spinal cord, causing spasm.[45]

The **pain-adaptation model** states that in a state of pain muscles become more active when they are acting as antagonists.[45] For example, when flexing the spine, the erectors (which extend the spine) become active, which limits movement. Another explanation for increased abnormal **cognitive** and **emotional** influences. Those suffering from stress or anxiety[39] and are fearful of movement[46] are more likely to have abnormal increases in paraspinal muscle tone.

Increased erector spinae tone may be an adaptive, protective mechanism to compensate for a loss of **spinal stability**.[40] Persistent tightness of the erectors during trunk flexion may protect injured or damaged spinal structures.[40]

Global muscle tone may be a **compensation** for local weakness in those with sciatica.[41] For example, the erector spinae may become tight to stabilize the spine when the multifidus becomes weak or atrophied. The rectus abdominus may tighten in response to transversus abdominis weakness, and the hamstrings may tighten to compensate for gluteal weakness. The body sacrifices normal ROM and biomechanics to preserve stability.

Table 30: Compensations in sciatica

Weak muscle	Compensatory increase in tone
Multifidus	Erector spinae
Transversus abdominis	Rectus abdominus
Gluteal muscles	Hamstrings

Chronic guarding

Those with acutely inflamed intervertebral discs (IVDs) or nerve roots may benefit from an increase in global stability, however this pattern may be unnecessary and even detrimental in the long-term. The favoring of erector spinae over multifidus activity leads to a pattern of spinal compression and a loss of deep stability. Guarding that becomes chronic does not necessarily serve a purpose and may delay recovery due to increased inflammation, altered biomechanics, and increased spinal loading.

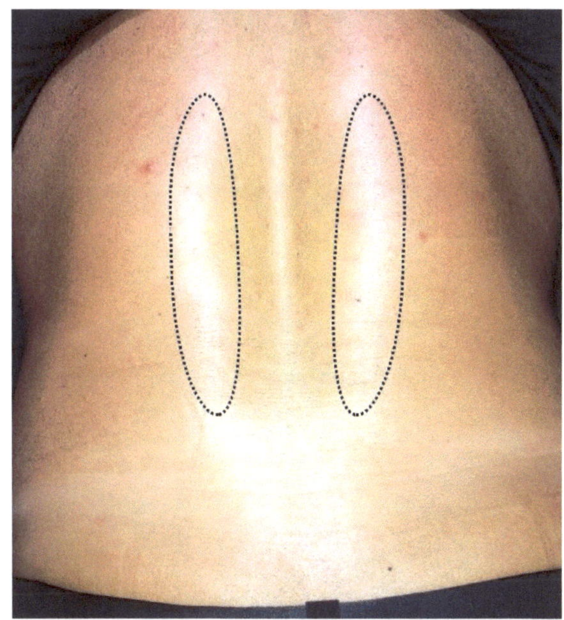

Figure 193: Hypertonic thoracolumbar erector spinae (dotted lines) in a 35-year-old man with a 3-year history of discogenic radicular sciatica. These muscles remain active despite the patient lying face-down in a relaxed position.

Increased lumbar erector tone may interfere with blood flow and promote accumulation of inflammatory and acidic substances.[45] The combination of inflammation and altered movement patterns in those with LBP promotes **lumbar subcutaneous edema**[47] that can be felt[48] and seen[49] using MRI. The chronic increase in erector tone is thought to contribute to an ongoing cycle of ischemia, inflammation, swelling, and venous congestion.[50] Some of these inflammatory substances include bradykinin, lactate, and substance P.[50] The trapping of inflammatory mediators may perpetuate the pain-spasm-pain cycle and lead to chronicity of sciatic pain.

Chronic increased paraspinal muscle tone adversely increases **spinal loading**. Persistent tension of the erectors is thought to increase axial loading on the IVDs and raise **intra-discal pressure**.[51] In a 99 kilogram (kg) adult the psoas can add 40-70 kg compressive force, while the erector spinae can add 15 kg.[52] Gunn hypothesized that shortening of the paraspinal muscles can compress the disc, leading to nerve root impingement.[53] Over time the compensatory increase in erector spinae activity may increase the risk of re-aggravation of discogenic sciatica due to abnormal and persistent loading of the spine.

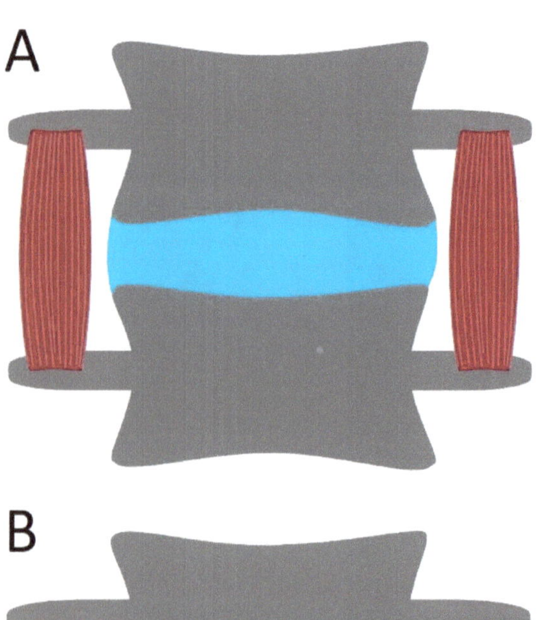

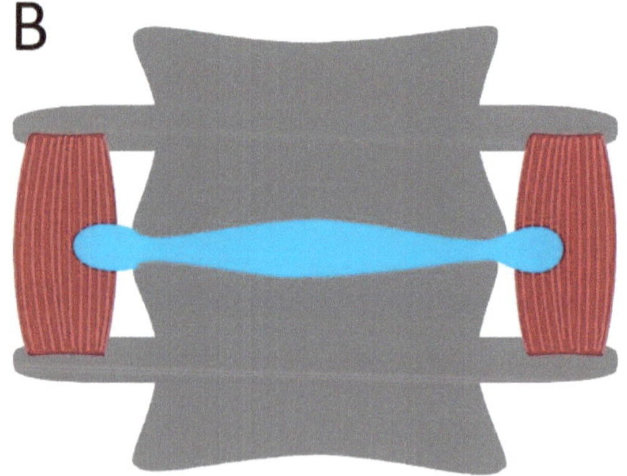

Figure 194: Shortening of the paraspinal muscles and the effect on the lumbar disc. Image A is a normal disc, B is a compressed disc due to shortened paraspinal muscles. This image highlights the overlap of myofascial disorders and lumbar disc disease. Image by Robert Trager, DC, adapted from the work of Chan Gunn, MD.

In discogenic sciatica, the erector spinae are more resistant to atrophy than the multifidi which creates a **muscle imbalance**. The erectors are less prone to atrophy because they are stimulated in the guarding response and because they have a **polysegmental innervation** (multiple nerve roots).[54] Each segment of multifidus is innervated by only one nerve root,[54] which is why this this muscle rapidly weakens in a radiculopathy. Those with discogenic sciatica have more severe atrophy and fatty infiltration of the multifidus compared to the erector spinae.[55,56] The erector spinae stay active during sciatica and nerve root injury while the multifidi weaken and atrophy.

Those with greater amounts of **fear-avoidance** beliefs have increased lumbar erector tone[46] and a longer duration of sciatica.[6] Fear-avoidance is a fear and anxiety about experiencing pain that leads to avoidance of activities. Fear, distress, and anxiety about moving the lower back can increase erector tone which stiffens the spine and prevents movement.[51] For example a patient with discogenic sciatica may avoid bending for months even after the disc has begun to heal. The fear-avoidance response alters movement and delays the rehabilitation of the multifidus. Fear avoidance increases erector tone which delays recovery from sciatic pain.

References

1. Grøvle, L., Haugen, A. J., Natvig, B., Brox, J. I. & Grotle, M. The prognosis of self-reported paresthesia and weakness in disc-related sciatica. *European Spine Journal* **22**, 2488–2495 (2013).
2. Vroomen, P. C. A. J., Krom, M. C. T. F. M. de & Knottnerus, J. A. Predicting the outcome of sciatica at short-term follow-up. *British Journal of General Practice* **52**, 119–123 (2002).
3. Haugen, A. J. *et al.* Estimates of success in patients with sciatica due to lumbar disc herniation depend upon outcome measure. *European Spine Journal* **20**, 1669–1675 (2011).
4. Lequin, M. B. *et al.* Surgery versus prolonged conservative treatment for sciatica: 5-year results of a randomised controlled trial. *BMJ Open* **3**, e002534–e002534 (2013).
5. Bejia, I., Younes, M., Zrour, S., Touzi, M. & Bergaoui, N. Factors predicting outcomes of mechanical sciatica: a review of 1092 cases. *Joint Bone Spine* **71**, 567–571 (2004).
6. Jensen, O. K., Nielsen, C. V. & Stengaard-Pedersen, K. One-year prognosis in sick-listed low back pain patients with and without radiculopathy. Prognostic factors influencing pain and disability. *The Spine Journal* **10**, 659–675 (2010).
7. Ashworth, J., Konstantinou, K. & Dunn, K. M. Prognostic factors in non-surgically treated sciatica: A systematic review. *BMC Musculoskelet Disord* **12**, 208 (2011).
8. Verwoerd, A. *et al.* Systematic review of prognostic factors predicting outcome in non-surgically treated patients with sciatica. *European Journal of Pain* **17**, 1126–1137 (2013).
9. Takada, E., Takahashi, M. & Shimada, K. Natural history of lumbar disc hernia with radicular leg pain: Spontaneous MRI changes of the herniated mass and correlation with clinical outcome. *Journal of orthopaedic surgery (Hong Kong)* **9**, 1 (2001).
10. Autio, R. A. *et al.* Determinants of spontaneous resorption of intervertebral disc herniations. *Spine* **31**, 1247–1252 (2006).
11. Tubach, F., Beauté, J. & Leclerc, A. Natural history and prognostic indicators of sciatica. *Journal of Clinical Epidemiology* **57**, 174–179 (2004).

12. Rihn, J. A. *et al.* The Influence of Obesity on the Outcome of Treatment of Lumbar Disc Herniation: Analysis of the Spine Patient Outcomes Research Trial (SPORT). *The Journal of Bone and Joint Surgery (American)* **95**, 1 (2013).
13. Haugen, A. J. *et al.* Prognostic factors for non-success in patients with sciatica and disc herniation. *BMC musculoskeletal disorders* **13**, 183 (2012).
14. Peul, W. C., Brand, R., Thomeer, R. T. & Koes, B. W. Influence of gender and other prognostic factors on outcome of sciatica. *Pain* **138**, 180–191 (2008).
15. Grøvle, L. *et al.* Prognostic factors for return to work in patients with sciatica. *The Spine Journal* **13**, 1849–1857 (2013).
16. Hill, J. C. *et al.* Clinical Outcomes Among Low Back Pain Consulters With Referred Leg Pain in Primary Care. *Spine December 01, 2011* **36**, 2168–2175 (2011).
17. Atlas, S. J. *et al.* The Quebec Task Force classification for Spinal Disorders and the severity, treatment, and outcomes of sciatica and lumbar spinal stenosis. *Spine* **21**, 2885–2892 (1996).
18. Beattie, P. F., Meyers, S. P., Stratford, P., Millard, R. W. & Hollenberg, G. M. Associations between patient report of symptoms and anatomic impairment visible on lumbar magnetic resonance imaging. *Spine* **25**, 819–828 (2000).
19. Skytte, L. P., May, S. & Petersen, P. Centralization: Its Prognostic Value in Patients With Referred Symptoms and Sciatica. *Spine June 1, 2005* **30**, (2005).
20. Suri, P., Rainville, J. & Gellhorn, A. Predictors of Patient-Reported Recovery From Motor or Sensory Deficits Two Years After Acute Symptomatic Lumbar Disk Herniation. *PM&R* **4**, 936-944.e1 (2012).
21. Thapa, S. S., Lakhey, R. B., Sharma, P. & Pokhrel, R. K. Correlation between Clinical Features and Magnetic Resonance Imaging Findings in Lumbar Disc Prolapse. *J Nepal Health Res Counc* **14**, 85–88 (2016).
22. Barzouhi, A. el *et al.* Influence of Low Back Pain and Prognostic Value of MRI in Sciatica Patients in Relation to Back Pain. *PLOS ONE* **9**, e90800 (2014).
23. Pantelinac, S. & Devecerski, G. Functional disability and MRI findings in lumbar disc herniation. *HealthMED* 676 (2013).
24. Chiu, C.-C. *et al.* The probability of spontaneous regression of lumbar herniated disc: a systematic review. *Clinical rehabilitation* **29**, 184–195 (2015).
25. el Barzouhi, A. *et al.* Prognostic value of magnetic resonance imaging findings in patients with sciatica. *Journal of Neurosurgery: Spine* **24**, 978–985 (2016).
26. Zhang, J. *et al.* Identification of lumbar disc disease hallmarks: a large cross-sectional study. *Springerplus* **5**, (2016).
27. Jensen, T. S., Albert, H. B., Sorensen, J. S., Manniche, C. & Leboeuf-Yde, C. Magnetic Resonance Imaging Findings as Predictors of Clinical Outcome in Patients With Sciatica Receiving Active Conservative Treatment. *Journal of Manipulative & Physiological Therapeutics* **30**, 98–108 (2007).
28. Iwabuchi, M., Murakami, K., Ara, F., Otani, K. & Kikuchi, S.-I. The predictive factors for the resorption of a lumbar disc herniation on plain MRI. *Fukushima journal of medical science* **56**, 91–97 (2010).
29. Macki, M. *et al.* Spontaneous regression of sequestrated lumbar disc herniations: Literature review. *Clinical Neurology and Neurosurgery* **120**, 136–141 (2014).
30. Teplick, J. G. & Haskin, M. E. Spontaneous regression of herniated nucleus pulposus. *American journal of roentgenology* **145**, 371–375 (1985).
31. Henmi, T. *et al.* Natural history of extruded lumbar intervertebral disc herniation. *J. Med. Invest.* **49**, 40–43 (2002).
32. Sarı, H., Akarırmak, Ü., Karacan, I. & Akman, H. Computed tomographic evaluation of lumbar spinal structures during traction. *Physiotherapy Theory and Practice* **21**, 3–11 (2005).
33. McKenzie, R. A. & May, S. *The Lumbar Spine: Mechanical Diagnosis & Therapy, 2 Vol Set.* (Orthopedic Physical Therapy Products, 2003).
34. Splendiani, A. *et al.* Spontaneous resolution of lumbar disk herniation: predictive signs for prognostic evaluation. *Neuroradiology* **46**, 916–922 (2004).
35. Kim, E. S., Oladunjoye, A. O., Li, J. A. & Kim, K. D. Spontaneous regression of herniated lumbar discs. *Journal of Clinical Neuroscience* **21**, 909–913 (2014).
36. Kobayashi, S. *et al.* Ultrastructural analysis on lumbar disc herniation using surgical specimens: role of neovascularization and macrophages in hernias. *Spine* **34**, 655–662 (2009).
37. Löhr, M. *et al.* Gadolinium enhancement in newly diagnosed patients with lumbar disc herniations are associated with inflammatory peridiscal tissue reactions – Evidence of fragment degradation? *Clinical Neurology and Neurosurgery* **119**, 28–34 (2014).
38. MacDonald, D. A., Moseley, G. L. & Hodges, P. W. The lumbar multifidus: does the evidence support clinical beliefs? *Manual therapy* **11**, 254–263 (2006).
39. van der Hulst, M., Vollenbroek-Hutten, M. M., Rietman, J. S. & Hermens, H. J. Lumbar and abdominal muscle activity during walking in subjects with chronic low back pain: support of the "guarding" hypothesis? *Journal of Electromyography and Kinesiology* **20**, 31–38 (2010).
40. Colloca, C. J. & Hinrichs, R. N. The Biomechanical and Clinical Significance of the Lumbar Erector Spinae Flexion-Relaxation Phenomenon: A Review of Literature. *Journal of Manipulative and Physiological Therapeutics* **28**, 623–631 (2005).
41. Arab, A. M., Ghamkhar, L., Emami, M. & Nourbakhsh, M. R. Altered muscular activation during prone hip extension in women with and without low back pain. *Chiropractic & Manual Therapies* **19**, 18 (2011).
42. Arena, J. G., Sherman, R. A., Bruno, G. M. & Young, T. R. Electromyographic recordings of low back pain subjects and non-pain controls in six different positions: effect of pain levels. *Pain* **45**, 23–28 (1991).
43. Sánchez-Zuriaga, D., López-Pascual, J., Garrido-Jaén, D. & García-Mas, M. A. A Comparison of Lumbopelvic Motion Patterns and Erector Spinae Behavior Between Asymptomatic Subjects and Patients With Recurrent Low Back Pain During Pain-Free Periods. *Journal of Manipulative and Physiological Therapeutics* **38**, 130–137 (2015).
44. Kurt, E. E., Büyükturan, Ö., Tuncay, F. & Erdem, H. R. Tight Hamstring Syndrome Related Lumbar Disc Herniation and Its Rehabilitation Program to Two Case Reports. *British Journal of Medicine & Medical Research* **17**, 1–9 (2016).
45. van Dieën, J. H., Selen, L. P. & Cholewicki, J. Trunk muscle activation in low-back pain patients, an analysis of the literature. *Journal of Electromyography and Kinesiology* **13**, 333–351 (2003).
46. Watson, P. J., Booker, C. K. & Main, C. J. Evidence for the role of psychological factors in abnormal paraspinal activity in patients with chronic low back pain. *Journal of Musculoskeletal Pain* **5**, 41–56 (1997).
47. Langevin, H. M. *et al.* Ultrasound evidence of altered lumbar connective tissue structure in human subjects with chronic low back pain. *BMC Musculoskeletal Disorders* **10**, 151 (2009).
48. Cooper, M., Hacking, J. C. & Dixon, A. K. Sacral edema: Computed tomographic and anatomical observations. *Clin. Anat.* **8**, 56–60 (1995).
49. Quattrocchi, C. C. *et al.* Lumbar subcutaneous edema and degenerative spinal disease in patients with low back pain: a retrospective MRI study. *Musculoskelet Surg* **99**, 159–163 (2015).
50. Mense, S. Nociception from skeletal muscle in relation to clinical muscle pain. *Pain* **54**, 241–289 (1993).
51. Hodges, P. W. & Moseley, G. L. Pain and motor control of the lumbopelvic region: effect and possible mechanisms. *Journal of Electromyography and Kinesiology* **13**, 361–370 (2003).
52. Nachemson, A. The possible importance of the psoas muscle for stabilization of the lumbar spine. *Acta Orthopaedica Scandinavica* **39**, 47–57 (1968).
53. Gunn, C. C. Radiculopathic Pain: Diagnosis and Treatment of Segmental Irritation or Sensitization. *Journal of Musculoskeletal Pain* **5**, 119–134 (1997).
54. Kottlors, M. & Glocker, F. X. Polysegmental innervation of the medial paraspinal lumbar muscles. *Eur Spine J* **17**, 300–306 (2008).
55. Battié, M. C., Niemelainen, R., Gibbons, L. E. & Dhillon, S. Is level- and side-specific multifidus asymmetry a marker for lumbar disc pathology? *The Spine Journal* **12**, 932–939 (2012).
56. Bouche, K. G. *et al.* Computed tomographic analysis of the quality of trunk muscles in asymptomatic and symptomatic lumbar discectomy patients. *BMC Musculoskeletal Disorders* **12**, 65 (2011).

Chapter 8 The treatment of sciatica

Key points

- The treatment of sciatica differs according to its cause
- Most cases warrant a trial of conservative treatment
- Integrated programs including manual therapies and exercise may be superior to any single therapy
- Surgery is indicated in the presence of red flags and/or a lack of response to conservative treatment

Triage

The first part of treatment in sciatica is the referral of patients with red flags who require emergent or **urgent medical treatment**. Red flags can occur in the form of medical history, symptoms, examination findings, imaging findings, other tests, or an overall diagnostic impression. Clinicians should send these patients to an emergency department in case imaging and/or surgery is necessary.

Acute discogenic **cauda equina syndrome** (CES) is the most common medical emergency in those with sciatica and is found in about 0.5%[i] of patients.[1] Cauda equina syndrome is diagnosed when one or more features are present in conjunction with sciatic pain: (1) reduced sensation in the saddle area, (2) sexual dysfunction, with possible neurologic deficit in the lower extremity (motor or sensory loss or reflex change), or (3) bladder and/or bowel dysfunction.[2] The most common cause of CES is lumbar disc herniation (LDH), followed by tumor, infection, lumbar spinal stenosis (LSS), inflammation, hematoma, and vascular disorders and other more rare conditions.[2]

Less than 1% of those with sciatica have **serious pathology**. One large study of patients with sciatica identified serious pathology such as **cancer**, **tumors**, **spinal cord compression**, and avascular necrosis in 0.8% of patients.[1] Another large study of patients undergoing MRI for evaluation of low back pain (LBP) and/or sciatica identified infection or an unknown malignancy in a combined 0.8% of patients.[3] Other rare but serious causes of sciatica include **aortic dissection** and **fracture**, including pathologic fractures or those causing significant nerve damage.

Non-surgical healthcare practitioners may help with the triage process for those with sciatic pain. One systematic review found that a triage process involving **physiotherapists**, **nurse practitioners**, and/or **chiropractors** was able to shorten wait times, improve access to effective care, improve health outcomes, reduce cost, and reduce the use of unnecessary imaging and medical consultant time.[4] Another study found that patients with low back and leg pain who presented to a non-surgical multidisciplinary clinic required fewer referrals to a surgeon.[5]

Choosing the best treatment

The ability to effectively treat sciatica correlates with the ability to accurately diagnose its source. When a specific cause of sciatica cannot be determined, it should be classified or categorized to the extent possible to guide treatment. For example, classification of **intraspinal** versus **extraspinal** sciatica helps determine if treatment will include spinal manipulative therapy (SMT), traction, and directional preference exercises.

Conservative and manual therapies may be effective for multiple types of sciatica. Needling therapies are effective for intraspinal conditions such as discogenic sciatica,[7] and extraspinal conditions including deep gluteal syndrome (DGS).[8] Passive physiotherapy such as instrument assisted soft tissue manipulation, cupping, and taping may be used in intra- and extraspinal sciatica. Education and advice may also have broad applications.

Clinical prediction rules help determine which treatments will help the most. These rules identify cases for which SMT, traction, stability exercises, or directional preference exercises are most appropriate and/or effective. The choice to perform other conservative treatments is guided by research, clinical experience, and/or preference of the patient. For example, needling therapies work best in those that have a dysfunctional multifidus or high score on a low back dysfunction questionnaire,[9] but should be avoided in those that faint at the sight of a needle.

---

[i] Konstantinou's study had 3 cases in their series of 614 patients with sciatica (0.49%)

Table 31: Prediction rules in treatment of sciatica

SMT:[10] 4/5 variables present:
• Duration of symptoms <16 days • FABQ work subscale score <19 • ≥1 hip with >35° of internal rotation • Hypomobility in the L/S • No symptoms distal to knee
Spinal traction:[11]
• Leg symptoms • Signs of nerve root compression including a positive SLR (symptoms <45°) or neurological deficit • Either peripheralization with extension movements or a crossed SLR
Stabilization[12]
• Age < 40 • Greater flexibility (e.g. SLR ROM >91°) • Instability catch or aberrant movements during L/S flexion or extension • Positive prone instability test • For patients who are postpartum: Positive posterior pelvic pain provocation (P4), and ASLR and modified Trendelenburg tests, & pain provocation with palpation of the long dorsal sacroiliac ligament or pubic symphysis
Specific exercise of extension[12]
• Symptoms distal to buttock • Symptoms centralize with L/S extension • Symptoms peripheralize with L/S flexion • DP of extension
Specific exercise of flexion[12]
• Age > 50 • DP for flexion • Imaging evidence of LSS
Specific exercise of lateral shift[12]
• Frontal plane deviation of the shoulders relative to pelvis • DP for lateral translation of pelvis
Directional preference (DP), spinal manipulative therapy (SMT), lumbar (L/S), straight leg raise (SLR), lumbar spinal stenosis (LSS)

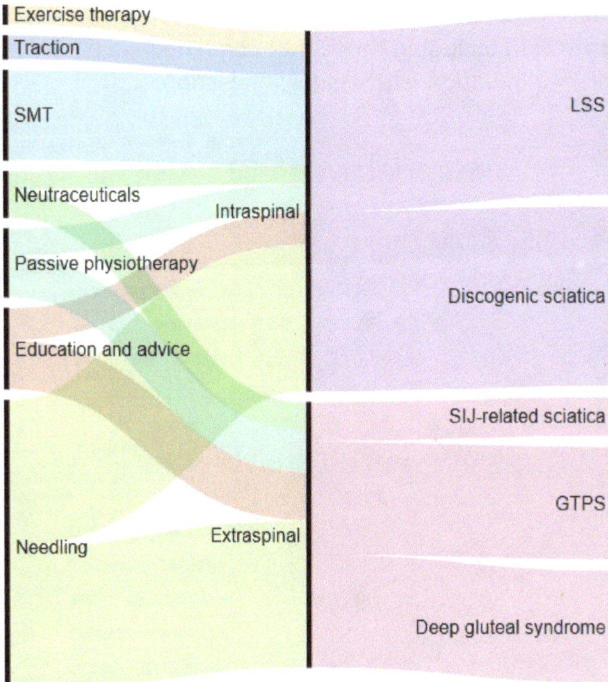

Figure 195: Overview of conservative and manual treatment effectiveness for the five most common causes of sciatica. Data adapted from Lewis.[6] Odds ratio for global effect corresponds with the thickness of each treatment row. Spinal stability, directional preference, and neural mobilization exercises were considered to be exercise therapy. Needling includes dry needling and acupuncture. Treatments were categorized according to the conditions they are typically used for and/or have evidence supporting efficacy. Abbreviations: Spinal manipulative therapy (SMT), greater trochanteric pain syndrome (GTPS), lumbar spinal stenosis (LSS), sacroiliac joint (SIJ).

Cost effectiveness

When cost is a factor in deciding which treatment or treatments to use for sciatica, a step-by-step approach may be best. This approach takes advantage of the favorable prognosis of most cases of sciatica, with most patients improving significantly during the first three months.[14] A large economic review of treatments for sciatica found that a **stepped approach** was most cost effective, which included initial treatment with either NSAIDs, education and advice, activity restriction, and non-opioids or opioids before moving to other treatment options.[13]

This economic review also predicted the most cost-effective conservative and non-medical treatment strategies for sciatica to be a combination of **education and advice** with **acupuncture**, **manipulation**, **traction**, and/or **physiotherapy**.[13] The combination of education and advice with either acupuncture or manipulation was predicted to be more cost-effective than disc surgery.[13] Many **integrated treatments** were predicted to have a high utility gain (cost effectiveness) including those that combined acupuncture or manipulation with epidural injection.

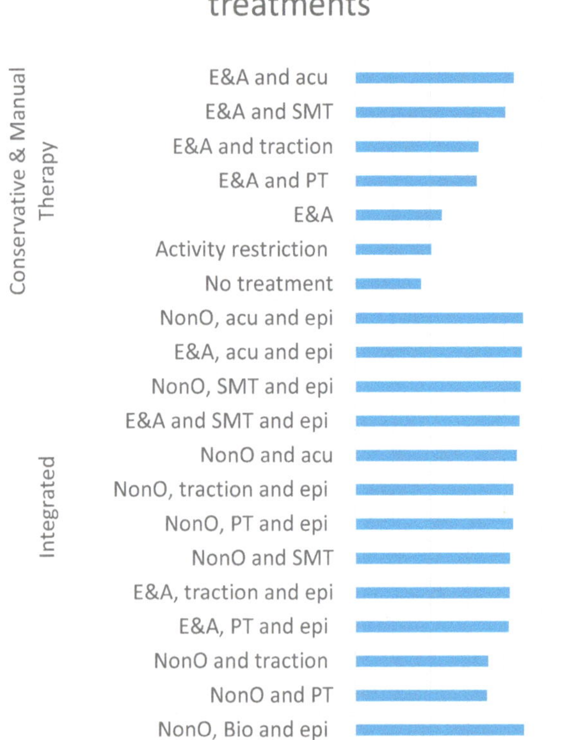

Figure 196: Treatment success and cost. Data adapted from Fitzsimmons.[13] Exercise and advice (EA), active and passive physical therapy (PT) had similar utility gain and were listed together here. Biologicals (Bio) are biological agents such as adalimumab. Other abbreviations: epidurals (epi), acupuncture (acu), nonopioids (NonO), and spinal manipulative therapy (SMT)

The cost-effectiveness study found that **no treatment** was less cost-effective than most other treatment options, but still greater than usual care and consultations with or without NSAIDs.[13] Sciatica has a relatively good prognosis, so no treatment is an option for those with less severe symptoms and no red flags, who are willing to allow symptoms to gradually improve. No treatment is a poor choice for those with severe sciatica, neurological damage, or indications for surgery.

Phases of care

One approach for sciatica or lumbosacral radiculopathy is to work through phases of care one at a time. A typical treatment plan begins with (1) **pain control**, followed by treatments for (2) **flexibility and strength**, then (3) **normalization of biomechanics**.[15] This treatment approach meshes with the cost-effective stepped approach, but may not be ideal for all patients. The drawbacks of the phases of care model are a delay in rehabilitation, potential to atrophy, and slower recovery. While a phased approach may be required for some patients that are immobilized by severe pain, more often patients benefit from treatments of all three phases simultaneously.

Pain control may begin with conservative treatments including acupuncture and manipulation.[13] Acupuncture is one of the most effective tools to reduce sciatic pain, and reduces pain by 25 points on a 100 point scale compared to no treatment.[6] Acupuncture is the second-best pain-relieving agent for sciatica overall, second only to biological agents. The next best conservative options for pain relief are manipulation and traction.[6]

Flexibility and rehabilitative goals can likewise be started early in the treatment of sciatica. Strengthening is important to prevent **atrophy** and instability. Flexibility and functional exercises are important to prevent abnormal biomechanics and prolonged muscle guarding. If rehabilitative phases of care are delayed until pain is reduced, patients may suffer sequelae of sciatica including atrophy, instability, and chronic muscle tightness and guarding.

Integrated treatment approach

Studies have found that treatments that combine different therapies have a greater probability of success for alleviating sciatica. These approaches are called **multimodal**, **integrated**, or **multidisciplinary**. One study found that patients with sciatica improved the most when they received a combination of treatments including SMT, traction, exercises, and/or a back brace.[16] Most treatments for sciatica are synergistic.

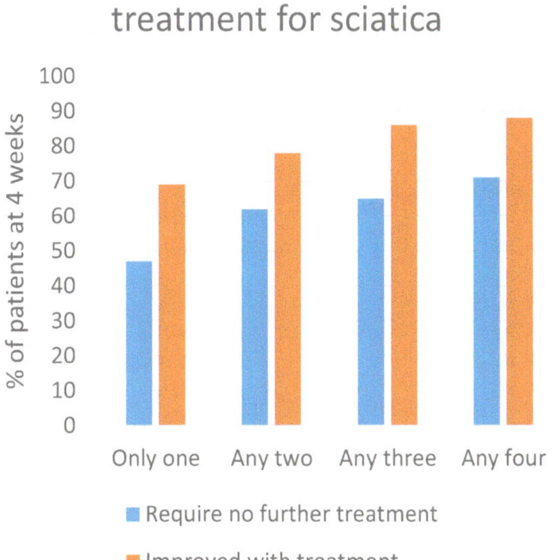

Figure 197: Multimodal treatment programs outperform single treatments. A large study of 322 patients with sciatica were assigned to groups with one or multiple types of treatment including traction, manipulation, exercises, and/or back brace. Patients with a greater number of treatment types subjectively improved to a greater degree as well as did not seek further treatment compared to those with fewer types of treatment. Data adapted from Coxhead.[16]

Combined treatments for sciatica may be superior because they address different components of pathology simultaneously. These include inflammation, neural tension, soft tissue restriction, joint restriction, circulation, movement patterns, and psychological components of pain.

Studies have found that joint **manipulation** and **mobilization** work better when integrated with **exercise** therapies. A large study of patients with sciatica found that the combined treatments of joint mobilization and exercise led to better overall improvement than exercise alone.[17] Another study found that the combination of SMT and home exercises reduced back-related leg pain more than either therapy in isolation.[18]

A cost-effectiveness model predicted that conservative and **manual therapy** treatments such as acupuncture, manipulation, traction, and physical therapy had a greater probability of success when integrated with **medications** or **epidurals**.[13] None of these treatment options were predicted to be worse when combined with a medical approach. Independent trials also support the success of integrated treatments.

One trial found that the combination of **acupuncture** and **nerve root block** worked better than either therapy in isolation.[19] A systematic review concluded that the combination of acupuncture and medication was more effective in treating sciatica than medication alone.[20]

Trial of care

A conservative and nonoperative trial of one to two months is appropriate for those with discogenic sciatica and no red flags or absolute indications for surgery. One international survey of surgeons identified that 46% preferred a minimum **4-8 weeks of conservative treatment**, 23% preferred 8-12 weeks, 11% preferred more than 12 weeks, and 20% performed surgery within 4 weeks of conservative treatment. One study found that patients had 3.5 times the odds of crossing over from a nonoperative to operative treatment if they did not improve between 2 and 8 weeks of care.[21] Patients without absolute indications for surgery are warranted a trial of care for up to two months during which time they are monitored for improvement.

Those with **lumbar stenosis** can be treated conservatively for months. In the absence of red flags or absolute indications for surgery, surgical referral is usually not as urgent compared to LDHs. There is generally a lower incidence of severe motor weakness (5% have grade 3/5 or worse),[22] and there is no consensus on superiority of surgery versus nonoperative treatment.[23]

The appropriate duration of a trial of care for **extraspinal sciatica** is less clear. Multiple studies on piriformis syndrome reported using a **three-month** trial of conservative treatment before deciding to perform surgery.[24–26] In many cases DGS and piriformis syndrome is misdiagnosed, leading to an unintentionally long time between symptom onset and surgery.

Surgery

Chiropractors, physical therapists, and other hands-on practitioners may encounter a patient with severe sciatica that does not improve or even worsens despite treatment. These providers should be aware of the patients most likely to undergo surgery and the general indications for surgery, so they can refer patients to medical personnel for evaluation and treatment.

Patients with **cauda equina syndrome** (CES) and/or red flags may require **emergent surgery** whereas those with relative indications for surgery may trial a conservative treatment approach. Those with discogenic CES who are operated within 24-48 hours have better outcomes compared to those who delay surgery.[27] A systematic review identified that lumbar disc surgeries were more beneficial if performed within six months' onset of symptoms.[28]

Surgery leads to more **rapid recovery** of those with lumbar discogenic sciatica, but after 1-2 years outcomes are similar for both treatments.[29] A systematic review comparing surgical and nonsurgical treatment for LSS found that no conclusion could be made regarding which type of treatment was superior.[23]

Frequency of surgical intervention

Less than a quarter of those with **discogenic sciatica** undergo surgery. One large study of 2026 patients referred to a neurosurgical center for lumbar discogenic radiculopathy found that only 4.9% of patients underwent surgery.[30] Other similar studies have reported surgical rates of 17%[31] and 19.4% of patients.[32]

The surgical rate for **lumbar stenosis** is higher than that of discogenic sciatica; about 1 to 2 out of three patients will have surgery. One center reported performing surgery on 31% of those with LSS[33], another reported 44%.[34] and another 66%.[35]

Surgery is not commonly performed on those with deep gluteal or **piriformis syndrome**. One study reported a 5% surgical rate for piriformis syndrome,[24] another reported 6%[25], another 12%,[26] while another reported 35%.[38]

Indications for surgery

The decision to perform surgery is guided by the level of disability, pain, response to conservative treatment, presence of red flags, and **shared decision making** of the patient and surgeon.[39–41] There are few absolute indications for surgery including CES and red flag signs, symptoms, and diseases. Any clinical finding should also correlate with imaging findings before considering surgery.[42,43]

Absolute indications for surgery for sciatica include the presence of **cauda equina syndrome** and/or acute, progressive, and severe motor deficits. Any sign or symptom of CES, including altered **bladder function** should also prompt a surgical referral. **Less than grade three** strength (Medical Research Council, MRC grades 0 to 5) of functionally important muscles of the hip, thigh, and/or leg is an absolute indication for surgery[41] whereas isolated 0-2/5 weakness of the toe muscles is not.[44] Referral is also indicated when motor deficits progress despite an adequate trial of care.[45]

Relative indications for surgery include **persistent pain** despite a trial of care or pain that affects quality of life.[41] A large survey found that surgeons considered the most important indications for surgery to be the **severity of pain** or disability, followed by **failure of conservative treatment**, neurological deficit, and duration of complaints.[46] One review concluded that the main indicator for early surgery is to "shorten the period of suffering."[47] The Clinical Reasoning in Spine Pain protocols recommends the 3/5 rule, meaning that a surgical referral is initiated when strength is 3/5 or less, even though surgery may not be performed.[45] Some authors consider **persistent 4/5 strength** despite conservative treatment,[48] and hyperalgesic sciatica (extreme sensitivity to pain) that is resistant to morphine as another indicator for surgery.[44]

Table 32: Prevalence and interpretation of weakness in discogenic sciatica. The Medical Research Council grading is used for the strength level. The table includes multiple references due to some studies excluding those with weakness <3/5 and no study that included both LDH and LSS. Strength grading is according to the Medical Research Council (MRC) grades 0 to 5 (normal)

Strength (muscle testing)	Incidence LDH	Incidence LSS	Surgical indication
≤2/5	4%[36]		Absolute
3/5	28%[37]	5% (≤3/5)[22]	Relative
4/5	32%[37]	18%[22]	Relative
5/5	40%[37]	77%[22]	Elective

A survey of surgeons found that the preference to operate increased with greater **severity of motor weakness**. For a hypothetical scenario of a patient with an LDH causing pain, foot drop, and 0/5 weakness, 84% of surgeons said they would operate within 24 hours. For grade 1-2/5 weakness 79% stated they would operate, for grade 3/5 – 52%, and grade 4/5 – 29% would operate within 24 hours.[49]

Elective indications for surgery are based on a lack of response to treatment and the patient's preferences. One study found that the patient's preference for disc surgery significantly influenced their ultimate choice to undergo surgery or conservative treatment.[47] One review concluded that the decision to undergo surgery should be influenced by the preferences of the **well-informed patient**.[42]

One trial comparing disc surgery with nonoperative treatment found that patients were more likely to elect to have surgery if they felt the natural course of **recovery was too slow**, were **unable to cope** with leg pain, or wanted to minimize the time to recovery.[50] Patients whose pain was satisfactorily controlled were more likely to postpone surgery.[50] Another study found that those with LSS were more likely to undergo surgery if they were dissatisfied with their symptoms or felt their symptoms were getting worse.[35]

Surgical indications for **extraspinal sciatica** are like those of spine-related sciatica. Patients with piriformis syndrome are more likely to undergo surgery if they fail to improve with conservative treatment[24–26,38] or have neurological deficits.[38] A trial of conservative care is indicated for most cases of extraspinal sciatica considering there are no red flags.

Predicting the need for surgery

Medical history

Patients who have a greater amount of **cigarette smoking pack-years**,[51] or **prior episodes** of LBP are more likely to undergo disc surgery.[31] Those with better **mental health status**, **shorter duration of symptoms** and **younger age** are more likely to have a positive postoperative outcome.[52] Those that score higher on depression and fear-avoidance questionnaires,[53] or have a long duration of **sick leave** or a **worker's compensation** claim[52] are more likely to have a negative postoperative outcome.

Symptoms

Patients with **severe symptoms** including the level of sciatic pain and disability are more likely to undergo disc surgery. Patients with LDH[54] or LSS[55] with higher levels **disability** as measured by questionnaire scores are more likely to have surgery. Studies have found that both LDH[47] and LSS[55] patients higher **pain levels** were more likely to elect to have surgery. Another found that patients that with **sciatica increased by sitting** were more likely to benefit from early surgery.[56]

Despite worse symptoms correlating with early surgery, patients with greater **baseline severity of symptoms** and more severe leg pain are more likely to have a negative postoperative disc surgery outcome.[52] Those with greater amounts of LBP also have a worse outcome with surgery.[57] Although patients with severe pain are more likely to opt for early surgery, they do not necessarily have better outcomes by doing so.

Clinical features

Isolated examination findings do not reliably predict the need for lumbar disc surgery.[54] Common examination findings such as sensory loss, reflex loss, and motor loss do not correlate well with a surgical outcome for LDHs.[52,54] The only examination finding that correlates with increased likelihood of disc surgery is the **straight leg raise**. One review found that patients with a positive **straight leg raise** had over four times the odds of having disc surgery (OR 4.38).[31]

Lumbar stenosis patients with **motor deficit** have 10 times the odds of having surgery compared to those without.[33] This may be the case for LDHs as well, however many studies evaluating the likelihood of surgery have excluded patients with severe weakness or motor strength less than 3/5.[32,47,50,58] This process creates a selection bias towards patients with similar motor strength and may result in less of a difference between groups.

Imaging findings

The likelihood of undergoing surgery increases with LDHs **further from the midline** and **closer to the intervertebral foramen**.[32] Those with central LDHs are least likely to undergo surgery.[32] One study found that those with **extraforaminal** LDHs (far lateral) had 2.7 times the risk of undergoing surgery.[59] Further lateral LDHs have more severe radicular leg pain,[60] which may explain the increased surgical rate.

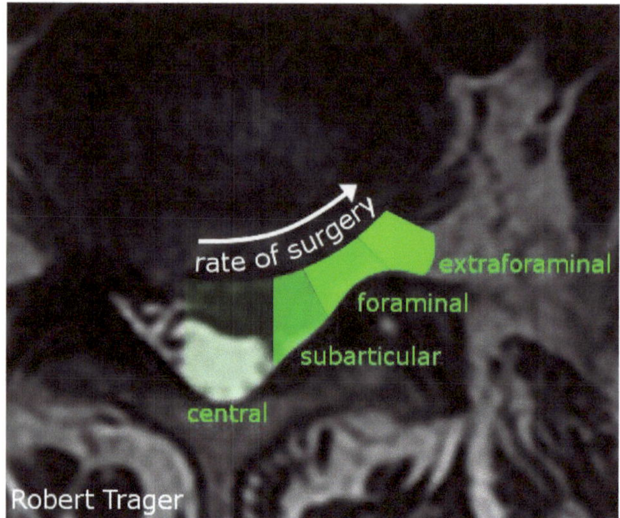

Figure 198: The rate of surgery increases with LDH further from the midline. The opacity of each zone is shaded with the surgical rate from Motiei-Langroudi et al.[32] of 13% for central LDHs, 52% for subarticular, 75% for foraminal, and 100% for extraforaminal. The study only included one extraforaminal herniation, but this data is corroborated by Ha[59] who identified a surgical risk ratio of 2.67 for far lateral compared to posterolateral herniations.

The type of **disc morphology** (shape) may guide the decision to have surgery. The progression from disc protrusion to extrusion to sequestration correlates with increasing motor deficit,[61] likelihood of disc regression or resorption,[62] and prognosis without surgery.[63] According to these principles, some of the worst-appearing and most symptomatic LDHs have the best prognosis.

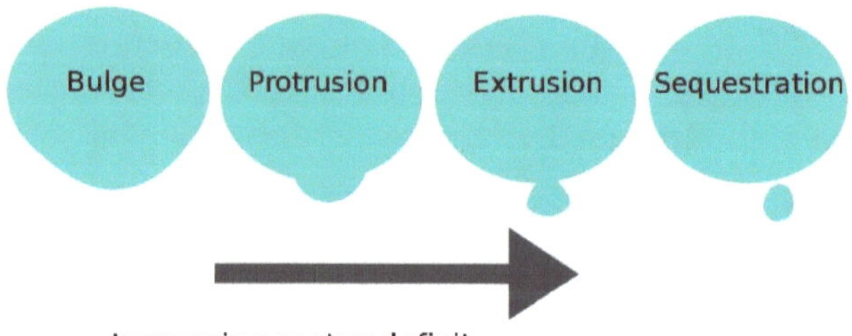

Figure 199: All other factors being equal, worse clinical symptoms but better prognosis and likelihood of spontaneous regression correspond with disc lesions that are more sequestrated, e.g. from bulge to protrusion, extrusion, to sequestration. Image by Robert Trager, DC.

Disc bulges have the lowest association with radicular symptoms[64] and worst prognosis.[65] Those with transligamentous, uncontained LDHs such as **sequestrations** have more severe initial symptoms but a greater likelihood of resorption, therefore a better prognosis.[48] One study recommended a minimum of two months of conservative treatment for uncontained or sequestered LDHs to allow for resorption to occur.[66]

Patients with a higher grade of disc morphology are more likely to undergo surgery despite the better prognosis and increased likelihood of disc resorption. One study found that **uncontained**[ii] extrusions and sequestrations had a higher surgical rate within one month of symptom onset (56% compared to 21% for contained herniations).[66] Another study found the lowest surgical rate among disc bulges (3%), higher among protrusions (29%), and highest for extrusions 69% (this study had no sequestrations).[32] The discrepancy between prognosis and surgical rate may be explained by the symptom severity and shared decision making of the surgeon and patient.

The likelihood of surgery correlates with increasing **AP dimension** of LDH.[32] One study found a mean AP diameter of 5.2 mm in those undergoing conservative treatment compared to 7.7 mm in those undergoing surgery.[32]

Degenerative deformities increase the likelihood of undergoing surgery for those with LSS. Those with LSS having a greater degree of lumbar coronal **Cobb angle** are more likely to undergo surgery.[55] Those with degenerative spondylolisthesis are also more likely to have surgery. Conversely, patients without **degenerative spondylolisthesis** (≤5% slippage) or scoliosis (≥10° curvature) have greater odds of improving with nonsurgical treatment (OR 2.5).[34]

Those with a greater **severity of lumbar stenosis** are more likely to undergo surgery.[33] One study found that those with the most severe grade of LSS had 3.5 times the odds of having surgery compared to those with the least severe grade.[33]

Directional preference management

Directional preference management (DPM), also called **mechanical diagnosis and therapy** (MDT), the McKenzie method, or directional preference (DP)

[ii] Uncontained means not bound by the posterior longitudinal ligament or annulus fibrosus[67]

exercises involve **static positions** and **dynamic repeated movements** that aim to centralize radiating spinal pain. Centralization is the process of reducing or abolishing radiating pain and/or moving it from distal to proximal. This chapter gives a brief overview of the utility of DPM. Readers can find in-depth training and textbooks about DPM through the McKenzie Institute

Directional preference management is effective in treating **low back related leg pain**.[68] Some studies show it helps discogenic sciatica,[37,69,70] but there is less evidence regarding LSS and other specific conditions. Mechanical diagnosis and therapy has been found to improve the degree of straight leg raising,[37] lumbar ROM,[71] reduce **kinesiophobia**,[70] and reduce resting muscle tone in the erector spinae.[72] This treatment system helps reduce pain as well as restore function.

Patients with sciatica respond best to DP exercises if they have **centralization** with motion testing, peripheralization of pain with the opposite motion, and a strong preference for sitting or walking.[12] Even though symptoms or imaging findings may give clues to a directional preference, the only way to know is to perform the movements. Those that experience centralization have greater odds (OR 2.7) of long-term success with treatment lasting over 6 months.[73]

A patient with sciatica may perform their DP exercises in a static position or repeatedly. The patient may hold a static posture or use the help of a table, a prop, or therapist. Dynamic or repeated movements can be active or passive.

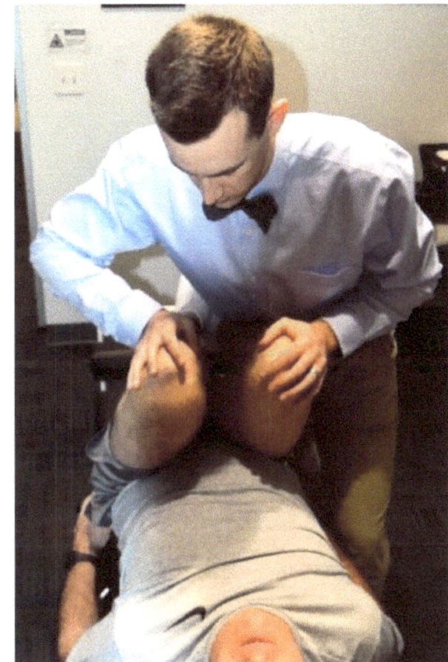

Figure 200: Treating lumbar flexion directional preference with a passive knee-to-chest maneuver

Although DPM is movement-guided and not necessarily condition-based, research has shown it to help those with **intervertebral disc (IVD) disorders**. Studies have shown DP exercises reduce pain related to disc bulges, protrusions, extrusions, sequestrations, and high-intensity zones.[69,70,74,75] Those with discogenic pain are most likely to centralize in extension, extension with hips off center, or side-gliding forces before extension.[74,76]

The morphology (e.g. protrusion versus extrusion) of disc lesions does not affect the effectiveness of MDT in those with sciatica. The annulus fibrosus does not need to be intact in order for these exercises to give benefit.[69] In addition, short-term symptomatic improvement does not correlate with improvement of disc on MRI.[77] When a patient rapidly improves with MDT, this usually does not mean the disc lesion has retracted, resorbed, or resolved.[77] Directional preference exercises evidently works via mechanisms other than changing the shape of disc lesions.

The **prone press-up** exercise is a commonly used technique for those with a DP of extension, however there are numerous other exercises which may be customized to each patient. Patients may perform lumbar extension exercises while standing, or may use a lumbar roll while lying supine[78] or sitting to increase lumbar extension.[79]

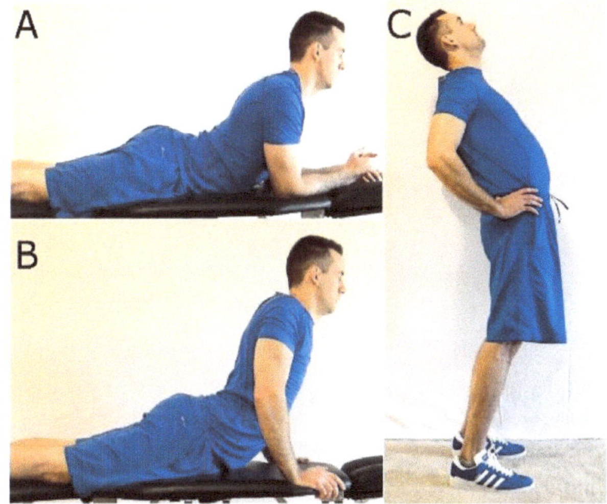

Figure 201: Examples of exercises for a patient with a directional preference of extension. These exercises may follow a progression from (A) static prone position to a (B) repeated end-range press up, and (C) extension while standing.

Those with symptomatic **lumbar spinal stenosis** most often improve with flexion-based exercises. One study found about 70% of LSS patients centralized with flexion, 19% extension, and 11% did not have a DP.[80] Flexion is often beneficial for LSS because it widens the lumbar spinal canal and gives the cauda equina more space. Patients with LSS are usually older and less likely to have an acute LDH.

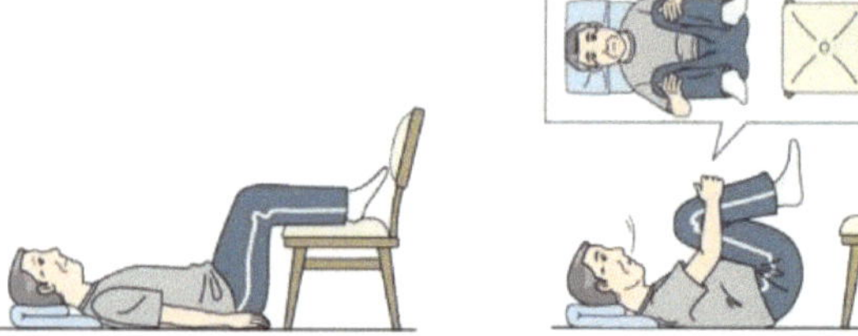

Figure 202: Double knee-to-chest exercises. A chair allows for rest between repetitions. Image from Oka,[81] CC-BY-4.0 license, no changes.

Patients can perform **double knee-to-chest** exercises while lying supine, flex the spine while standing, perform rotation in flexion while lying supine, or perform flexion while sitting. Practitioners can aid with these movements while in the clinic. For older patients or those with limited hip mobility, **single-knee-to-chest** exercises may suffice to encourage lumbar flexion. **Flexion in step-standing** is another variation useful for those that prefer to be standing.

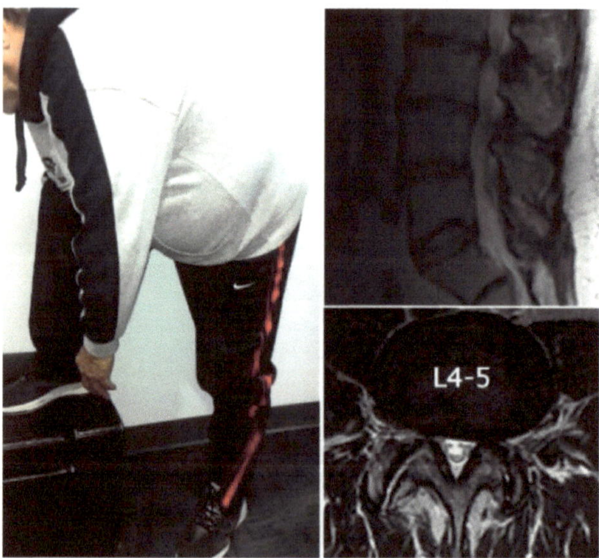

Figure 203: Flexion in step standing. A 64-year-old man presented with chronic LBP radiating to the posterior thighs and legs, BL lower extremity weakness, left foot drop, and used an ankle-foot orthosis to walk. MRI revealed multilevel degenerative and congenital LSS. This exercise and regular use of a stationary bike reduced his pain to mild/occasional and he was able to resume playing golf, although the foot drop remained. Case shared with patient's permission by Robert Trager, DC.

Multimodal treatment programs may be more effective when they incorporate DPM. Studies have shown benefit when combined with **neural mobility**[74] and **core stability exercises**.[70,82] Integrated treatment programs including other exercises may have greater benefit than DPM alone.

Rehabilitative exercises should agree with the patient's directional preference. Uphill or **inclined treadmill walking** and **cycling** can flex the lumbar spine and benefit those with a DP of flexion, typically those with LSS.[83] Flexion-based exercises may aggravate symptoms in those with an extension preference, typically discogenic sciatica. Patients with discogenic sciatica may prefer **core stability exercises** in which the lumbar spine is neutral.

Those with sciatica may perform directional preference exercises throughout the day. Common protocols include 10 repetitions every waking hour,[74] 10-15 repetitions every 1-2 hours,[76] or 10 repetitions every 2 to 3 waking hours.[84] Patients with LSS may benefit from rest periods of flexion during walking to alleviate neurogenic claudication.

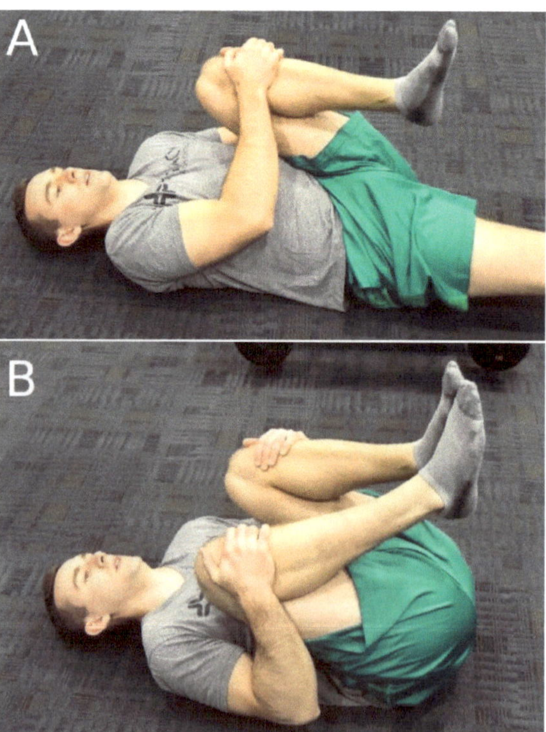

Figure 204: Variations of knee-to-chest exercises using a single knee (A) and double knee (B)

Lumbar stabilization exercises

The goals of exercise programs in sciatica are to improve **strength**, normalize **biomechanics**, improve **spinal stability**, and re-establish **proprioception**. Improvement of function and strength of the multifidus, psoas, diaphragm, transversus abdominus, and pelvic floor leads to better stabilization of the spine when confronted with axial loads, shearing, or torsional forces. Rehabilitation of these muscles and restoration of spinal stability reduces the risk of disc and nerve injury or irritation.

In 1937, Paul Williams, MD, designed the first formal exercise program for lumbar IVD-related sciatica. The focus of his program was to obtain a neutral posture and alleviate sciatic pain. He recommended abdominal curl-ups, gluteal bridges, knee-to chest supine stretches, and a lunging hip flexor stretch.[85]

Lumbar spine stabilization exercises have been shown to significantly reduce pain in those with sciatica caused by LDH or nerve root damage.[82,86,87] These exercise programs also improve the degree of straight leg raising,[82,87] strength,[82] sensation,[82] lumbar flexion ROM,[87] and reduce the overall level of disability.[86] Lumbar stabilization exercise programs give better outcomes for LDH and sciatica than generic exercise programs that aim to increase circulation.[82,86]

Exercise versus rest

Those with sciatica should avoid **strict bed-rest** but may perform short periods of structured positions for relief. Regular spinal loading is necessary to keep the IVDs healthy, while excessive rest is detrimental to the health of the spine, discs, and core musculature. Disuse leads to **atrophy** of the spine and pelvis which could delay recovery from sciatica.

Ancient physicians recommended that sciatic patients stay active. Hippocrates (c. 400 BCE) recommended "**frequent moving** to prevent ankylosis."[88] Paulus Aegineta (c. 625-690 CE) recommended exercise by walking, frequent bending of the body, leaping, and running.[89] A temple statue in Thailand from around the year zero depicts a yoga pose for sciatica.[90]

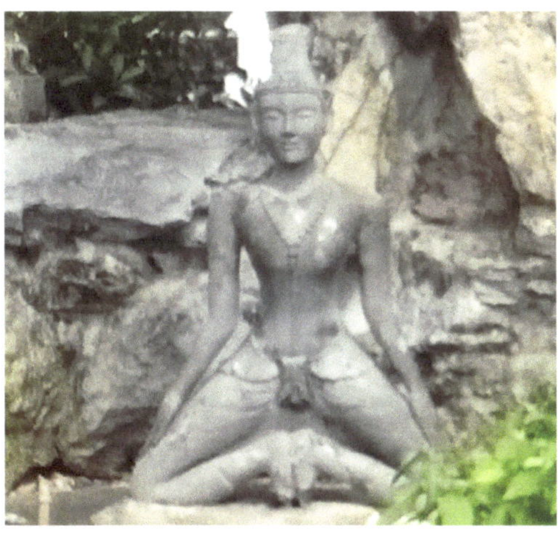

Figure 205: Statue of a yoga position at the Wat Pho temple in Thailand dating to around the year zero. The inscription states that the position is for sciatica.[90] Photo by Ovedc, Creative Commons Attribution-Share Alike 4.0 International License.

Strict bed-rest only became popular for treating sciatica in the early 1900s. Bed-rest became less popular after a study in 1986 that found patients with LBP recovered faster if they rested only two days as opposed to one week.[91]

Brief periods of strategic rest throughout the day or evening may be beneficial for those with acute and severe sciatic pain. Lying on the back or side with the knees bent may give significant relief for those with increased **neural tension** and/or **acute discogenic sciatica**. Patients may hold these positions for 5-15 minutes multiple times interspersed through the day.

One beneficial position is the **static opener** described by Shacklock.[92] This is a side-lying position designed to widen the spinal canal and **intervertebral foramina** on the uppermost side. The patient lies with the side of sciatic pain facing up and the non-painful side down, placing a bolster under their lumbar spine. This position causes lumbar lateral flexion away from the side of pain. If lying on an elevated surface such as a table or bed, the patient may increase lateral flexion by slowly hanging one then both legs off of the surface.

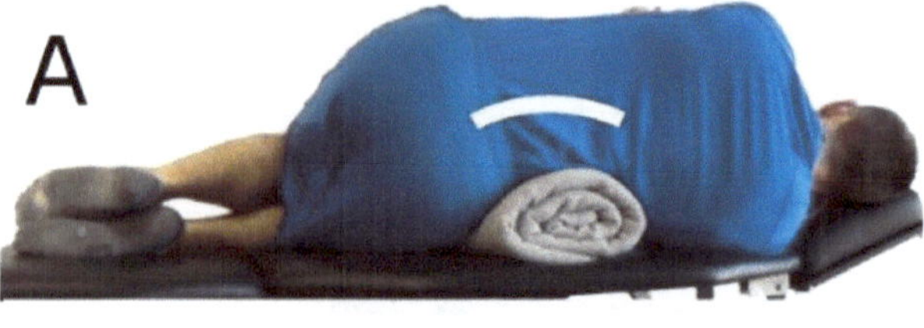

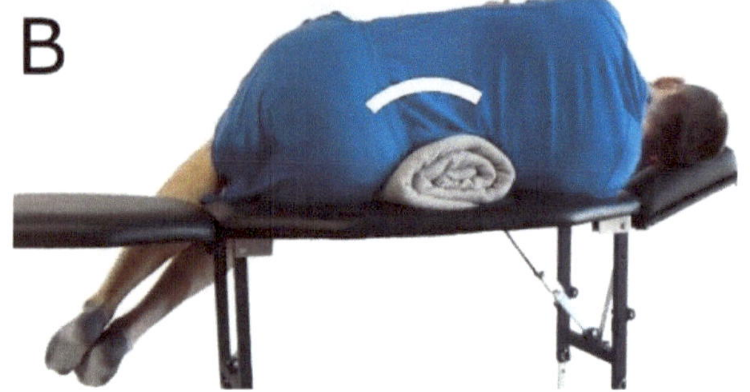

Figure 206: Lumbar static opener. Image A shows the starting position; B shows increased lateral flexion

The **semi-traction position** as described by Liebenson[93] is useful for those with acute discogenic sciatic pain. This position is obtained by lying supine and placing a bolster under the knees with the knees bent.

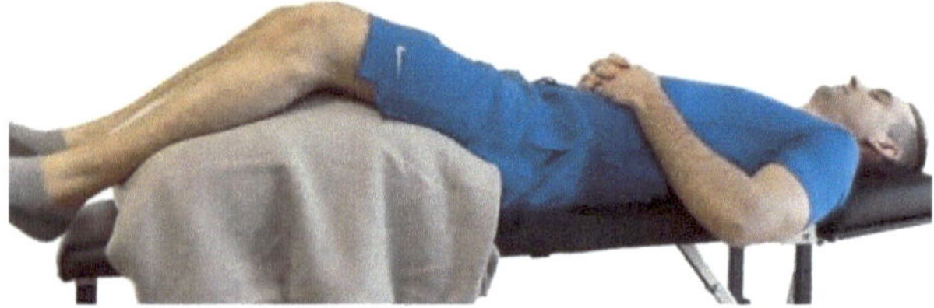

Figure 207: Semi-traction position

Strict rest is detrimental to the IVDs. Discs become **dehydrated** after extended periods of prolonged bed-rest or weightlessness. One study found that discs lost 6-7% of their hydration following a 60-day period of horizontal bed-rest. Astronauts who live for prolonged periods without gravity may have detrimental effects caused by the lack of forces on the discs. Astronauts have a higher risk of LDH than the general population.[94] Total rest or absence of gravity causes the IVDs to eventually lose water and possibly make them more susceptible to herniation.

Research supports advice to stay active and perform structured exercise rather than bed-rest for sciatica. Large systematic reviews have found that bed rest gives little or no benefit for treating sciatica.[6,95] Patients with sciatica should be directed towards activities and exercises that are appropriate for their specific condition.

Rest causes **deconditioning** of the structure and function of the lumbar spine and pelvis. Prolonged **immobilization** leads to decreased production of **glycosaminoglycans** in the IVDs.[96] Research on astronauts shows that seven days in a weightless environment reduces the ability of our nervous system to stimulate muscle contraction.[97] Bed rest causes atrophy in the lumbar multifidus within the first two days.[98] Prolonged bed rest causes weakness in the spine and muscles and makes it more difficult to recover from sciatica.

Exercise targeting deep lumbar **stability muscles** protects against sciatic pain. Those that exercise vigorously several times per week prior to developing sciatica have a better prognosis for recovery.[99] Those who do not exercise vigorously may have weak spinal stability muscles and are more likely to develop sciatica. One study found that middle-aged people with severe fatty infiltration of the multifidus had more than double the odds of developing sciatica.[100] Weakness of the deep stabilizing muscles is a risk factor for chronic sciatica while strength of these muscles protects against it.

Exercise programs for sciatica that do not worsen lower extremity symptoms or disc pathology should be safe even in the acute phase or first 6-8 weeks. Lumbar spine stability programs have been used successfully in those with LDH,[86,87,101] positive straight leg raise <60°,[101] and EMG evidence of lumbar or sacral nerve root damage.[101]

Exercise may strengthen the IVD. Animal studies have shown that exercise in the long-term increases **collagen** and **proteoglycan** production in the disc.[96] The discs also become better at imbibition (absorbing water).[102] These positive effects of exercise on the disc are thought to be partly due to improved **nutrient supply**. This includes increased transport of sulphate and improved uptake of oxygen, glycogen, and glucose.[96] The disc cells are also thought to undergo adaptation and shift towards an **anabolic** (building) state.

Not all types of exercise have a beneficial effect on the disc. **Axial loading** is preferred over loading at end ranges of flexion or rotation.[96] Slow to moderate speed exercise is preferred over explosive movements.[96] **Dynamic loading** is preferred over static loading,[96] which inhibits diffusion of nutrients into the IVD.[103] The most beneficial pattern of exercise is to incorporate rest between periods of exercise, which allows the discs to resorb water.[96]

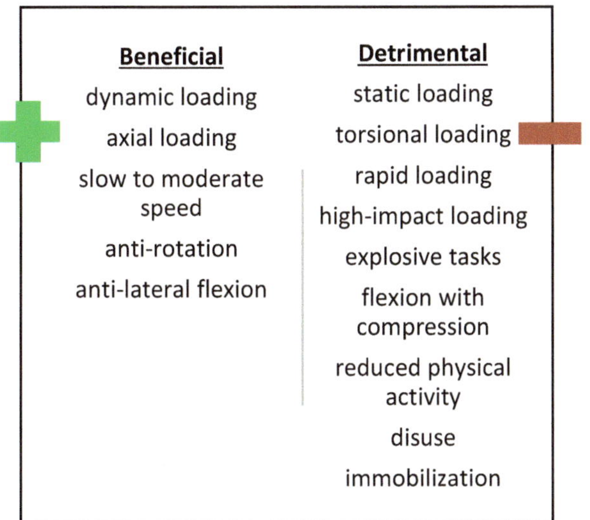

Figure 208: Types of exercise that benefit or damage the IVD, adapted from Belavy[96]

Patient selection

Lumbar spine stabilization exercises work best for those with a high degree of straight leg raising, younger age, and aberrant movement or presence of lumbar instability. One study found that if two or more of the following four variables were present, the odds of improvement with stabilization increased by a factor of 6.3: Age less than 40 years, straight leg raising over 91 degrees, aberrant movement present, and a positive prone instability test.[104] Despite this prediction rule seeming to select young healthy patients, even those with severe discogenic sciatica may improve with a lumbar spine stabilization exercise program.

Lumbar stabilization exercise programs have been used successfully in sciatic patients with LDH,[86,87,101] positive straight leg raise <60°,[101] and EMG evidence of lumbar or sacral nerve root damage.[101] While these patients may require extra caution, they are still capable of showing improvement.

Exercise progression

Each person with sciatica should perform a customized exercise program. All sciatic patients should be monitored during their exercise program to make sure signs and symptoms show improvement and are not worsening. Patients should be brought through exercise progressions slowly and advanced only when they can tolerate exercises without **peripheralization** of sciatic pain and without increases in neurological **deficits** (e.g. numbness, weakness). While exercises should not peripheralize sciatic pain they may aggravate local LBP.

Lumbar spine stabilization exercises may work better when performed in conjunction with **directional preference** exercises. Stabilization exercises can be modified so that they correspond with the patient's directional preference. For example, curl-ups and dead bugs may be more appropriate for those who cannot tolerate lumbar extension. Glute bridges may be better for those who prefer lumbar extension.

The initial phase of exercise for acute severe sciatica includes basic **supine**, **prone**, or **quadruped** exercises that have a **broad** and **fixed base of support** and are in the **sagittal plane**. These exercises are gentle on the spine and are less likely to aggravate acute discogenic sciatica. Those with discogenic sciatica and a positive **Valsalva test** may initially avoid exercises that require too much demand with bracing the core and instead focus on directional preference or diaphragmatic breathing before completing other basic stabilization exercises.

Table 33: Exercise progressions

Basic stabilization	• Diaphragmatic breathing • Bracing • Curl-ups • Dead bugs • Directional preference
Advanced stabilization	• Bird-dog progressions • Gluteal bridges • Straight leg lowering • Side bridges • Anti-rotational press
Functional integration	• Lunges • Single leg step-downs • Cardiovascular / endurance • Sport-specific drills

Advanced stabilization exercises can begin upon completion of the basic stabilization program, when pain has reduced from severe to moderate, and/or has begun to centralize from the lower extremity into the gluteal region or low back. Advanced exercises involve quadruped movements with a reduced base of support and greater strength requirements. They also include those not only the sagittal plane but the **coronal plane** (side bridges) and **transverse plane** (anti-rotational press).

Diaphragmatic breathing

Training the diaphragm is necessary to rehabilitate low-back related sciatic pain because these patients have a decreased ability to contract the respiratory diaphragm.[105] Diaphragmatic breathing in conjunction with the deep abdominal muscles helps establish **intra-abdominal pressure**, which in turn stabilizes and protects the lumbar spine and SIJs.

Clinicians may give the patient cues to help them properly activate the diaphragm. One internal cue is to place either the clinician's or patient's hands on the patient's abdomen and say, "breathe into your belly" then ask the patient to feel the belly rise with inspiration. Palpating the edge of the diaphragm may also help the patient become aware of its presence and achieve a stronger diaphragm contraction.

Resisted inspiration is an exercise to improve breathing mechanics. It is performed by placing a 3-5 lb. object on the abdomen and having the patient raise it with inspiration and let it sink with expiration.

A

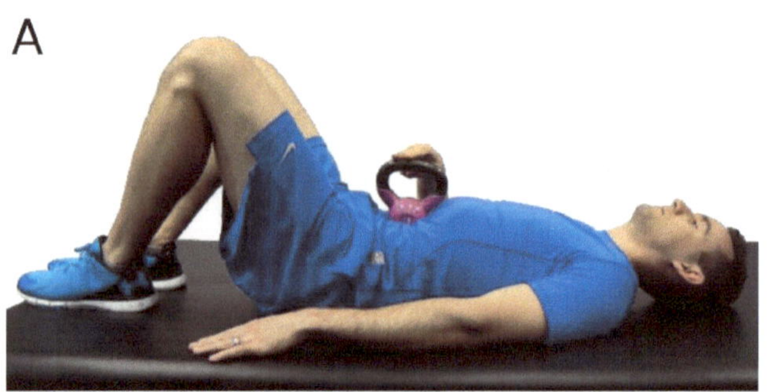

B

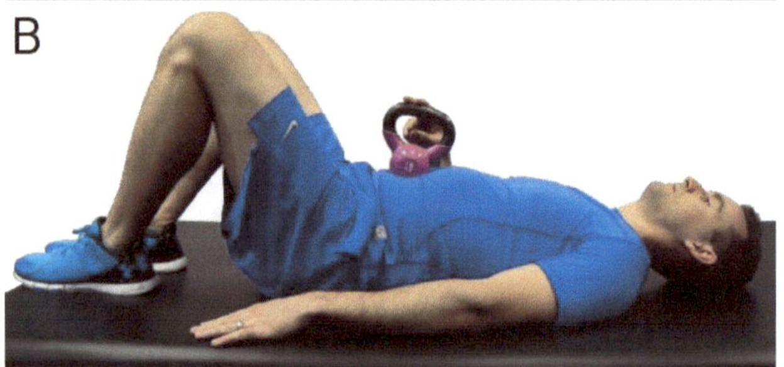

Figure 209: Resisted inspiration exercise. Expiration (A) and inspiration (B).

When a patient is able to perform supine diaphragmatic breathing, they can progress to breathing in more challenging positions. These include the **supine 90-90** and dead-bug. Once a patient breathes properly, they can progress to bracing, then integrate these concepts with other lumbar stabilization exercises.

Bracing

Bracing is a coordinated contraction of the **abdominal wall** muscles. This maneuver increases intra-abdominal pressure, which helps stabilize the lumbar spine and SIJs. Bracing stabilizes more effectively than drawing-in or hollowing exercises that isolate the transversus abdominus.[106] Bracing should be started as soon as symptoms permit. Those with a positive Valsalva's test may have peripheralization of sciatic pain with bracing, which is a contraindication for this exercise.

Variations include bracing alone, with heel slides, leg lifts, or bridging; or while standing, walking, or doing rows while standing.[104] Bracing should be integrated with advanced and functional exercises such as side planks, anti-rotational presses, and straight leg lowering.

Supine progressions

Basic supine stability exercises include curl-ups and dying bugs. Both exercises maintain a neutral lumbar spine and minimize forces across the lumbar discs.[107] These are good beginner exercises even for those with acute severe sciatic pain because they are less likely to exacerbate symptoms.

Curl ups combine bracing with abdominal muscle strengthening. Curl-ups have been used successfully as part of lumbar spine stabilization exercise program for people with LDH.[86,101] To perform this exercise the patient lies flat on their back with one knee flexed and one straight. The side of the flexed knee alternates each set. Both hands are placed under the lumbar lordosis to support the spine. The trunk is flexed just enough to lift the shoulder blades off the ground and held in an isometric contraction for 5 seconds.[107]

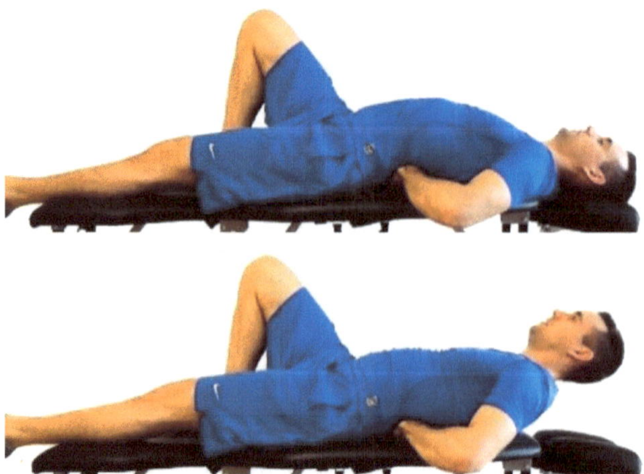

Figure 210: Curl-ups

Dying bugs, also called dead bugs, combine bracing with a coordinated crawling or marching of the upper and lower limbs. This exercise is performed by simultaneously flexing the ipsilateral shoulder and hip, while extending the other arm and hip, then alternating these repeatedly.

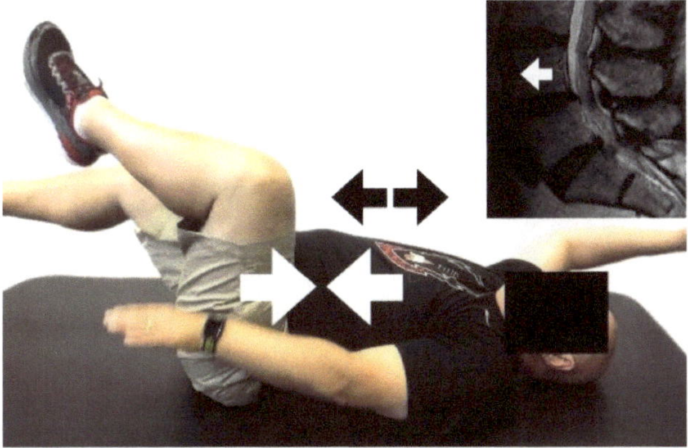

Figure 211: Dying bugs in a 61-year-old man with left S1 radicular sciatic pain related to degenerative LSS. Arms are moved in opposing movements simultaneously with hips. This exercise was used due to signs of instability including an L4 anterolisthesis (small arrow) and because it did not increase symptoms. Case shared with permission from patient by Robert Trager, DC.

Quadruped progressions

Quadruped exercises are meant to minimize loads across the lumbar spine while allowing for rehabilitation of the lumbar extensor muscles. The multifidus and erector spinae are the primary muscle groups involved in these exercises.[104] Quadruped exercises are performed with both hands and knees on the ground with the spine in a neutral position and the abdomen braced.

These exercises are started by raising just one limb off the ground at a time -- either an arm or a leg. The next progression is the **bird-dog**, which is performed by alternating diagonal arm and leg movements. The bird-dog develops bracing, lumbar stabilization, and proprioception. The bird-dog has been used successfully as part of a lumbar spine stabilization exercise program for discogenic sciatica.[86,87]

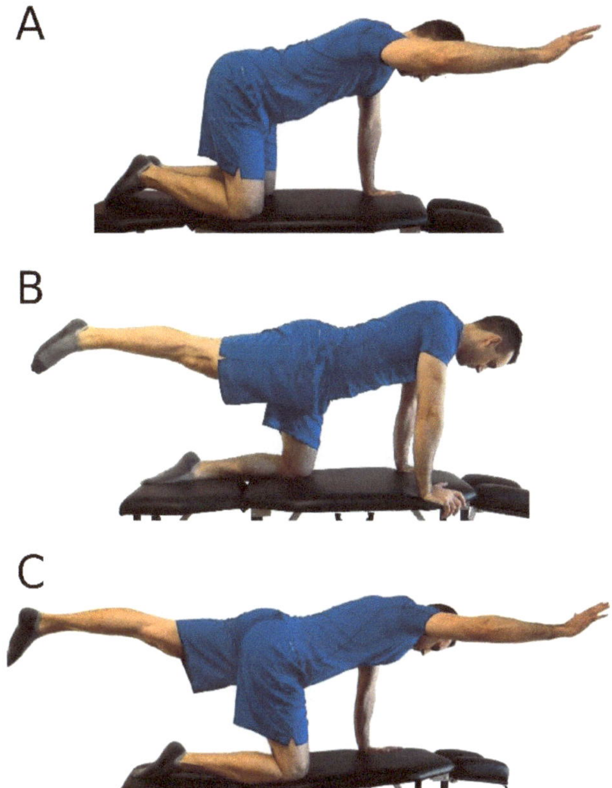

Figure 212: Bird-dog progressions. Start with one arm (A), then one leg (B), then combine contralateral movements (C).

Anti-rotation and lateral flexion

Anti-rotational and anti-lateral flexion exercises improve the ability of the deep local spinal stabilizing muscles to prevent unwanted torsion and lateral flexion. In these exercises the spine is kept in a neutral position and the rotational or lateral flexion forces are resisted using the core muscles.

The Pallof press or **antirotational press** is performed with an exercise band pulling the body at a rotational vector. The patient presses the band in front of them and back again, slowly, while resisting the rotational vector. This exercise is typically performed standing but can be performed in a lunge.

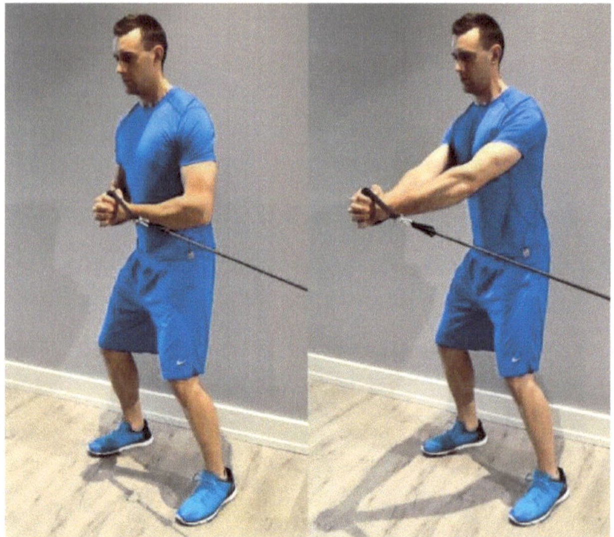

Figure 213: The Pallof or antirotational press.

Patients may perform **side planks** or **side bridges** in a side-lying position with one base of support at the elbow and forearm and the other base at the knees or feet. The patient lifts the pelvis and spine simultaneously upwards while bracing and maintaining a neutral spine. This exercise challenges the quadratus lumborum and oblique abdominals.[104] Side planks have been used successfully as part of a lumbar spine stabilization exercise program for discogenic sciatica.[86]

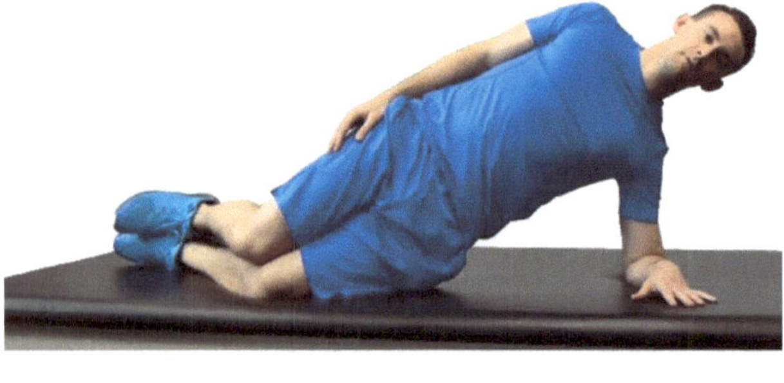

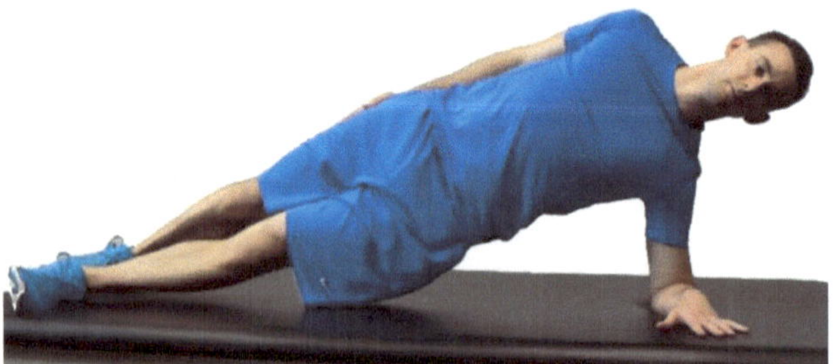

Figure 214: Side plank progressions

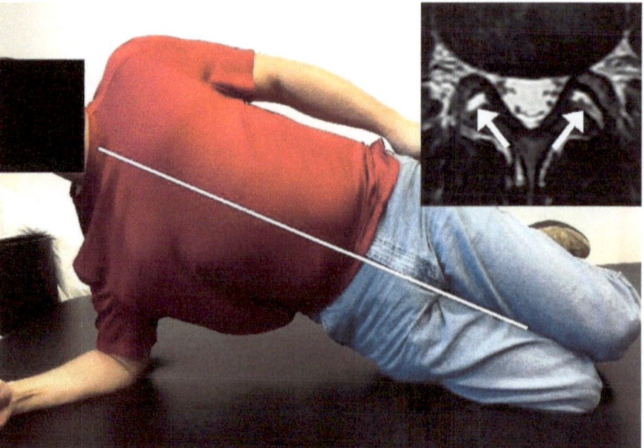

Figure 215: Side planks in a 47-year-old man with a L sided L5 and S1 radiculopathy related to a disc bulge and instability of L4 on L5. The facet joint effusion seen on MRI was over 3 mm bilaterally (arrows), a sign of instability and sign of a favorable response to stability training. The patient should be instructed to keep the torso in line with the thighs (line). Case shared with permission from patient by Robert Trager, DC.

Functional integration

The final phase of rehabilitation includes advanced cardiovascular or endurance exercises, single-leg stability and strengthening, and sport-specific drills. These exercises help return the patient to their normal activities of daily living and/or sports.

Clinicians and patients may wait until there is significant improvement to perform functional exercises. This includes the centralization of pain to the proximal extremity or spine, return of motor strength to at least to 4/5, normalization of Valsalva's test. These requirements should help prevent accidents such as valgus knee collapse during lunging or running, or re-aggravation of discogenic sciatica during cycling or sports.

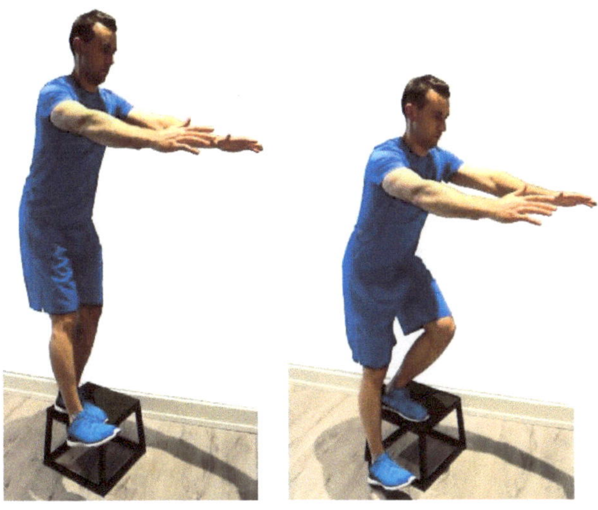

Figure 216: Single-leg step downs. Image by Robert Trager DC

Lunges, swimming, bicycling, and running have all been used successfully in the final phases of rehabilitation for those with discogenic sciatica.[101] Other exercises that can be used are single leg squats or step-downs, lunge variations, and drills specific to the patient's respective normal activities or sports.

Spinal manipulation and mobilization

Spinal manipulation is an assisted passive motion applied to the spinal or SIJs.[108] Manipulation usually refers to a **high-velocity, low-amplitude** (HVLA) thrust that moves a joint just beyond its normal active ROM whereas mobilization refers to **low-velocity** movements within or up to the limit of joint range.[108] Spinal manipulation can be used for sciatic pain originating from the lumbar discs, apophyseal joints, and SIJs.

Patients with sciatica that receive SMT have **4.9 times greater odds** of improving compared to no treatment at all.[6] The success rate of SMT when appropriately used for sciatica with no contraindications to treatment ranges from 60% to 77% over a span of 1 to 3 months depending on the severity and condition of the patient.[109,110]

Therapists have been manipulating the spine for thousands of years.[111] For centuries this profession was called **bonesetting** until it was organized into osteopathy and then chiropractic. One example of bonesetting for sciatica was recorded by Captain James Cook, who was treated by the King of Tahiti's team of physicians for sciatica in 1777:[112]

> *...as many of [the physicians] as could get around me, began to squeeze me with both hands, from head to foot, but more particularly on the parts where the pain was lodged, till they made my bones crack... the operation gave me immediate relief... [they] repeated their prescription the next morning... and again in the evening... I found the pains entirely removed. (Senn p. 141)*

Langworthy, Smith, and Paxson, who published the first chiropractic textbook in 1906,[113] described manipulation of the SIJ to treat sciatica.[114] Medical doctors also manipulated the SIJ to alleviate sciatica in the early 1900s.[115–118] Joel Ernest Goldthwait of Massachusetts General Hospital popularized this practice and claimed that positional corrections of the SIJ alleviated irritation of the nearby nerves.[116]

Mechanisms and clinical effects

Spinal manipulation may help discogenic sciatica by altering spinal **biomechanics** and **physiology** rather than spinal position or the size and shape of LDHs. Studies using lumbar MRI have found that the size and shape of LDHs are not changed by multiple sessions of SMT.[119–121] Even when a patient obtains dramatic relief following SMT for discogenic sciatica there is no significant change in the size of the LDH.[119]

Many studies examining HVLA manipulation for discogenic sciatica have found that it reduces sciatic pain.[109,119,121,122] Manipulation is thought to block nociceptive (pain) impulses[108,122] by stimulating the **mechanoreceptors** in the spinal joints.[108] This mechanism can be explained by the gate control theory, which proposes that non-painful stimuli suppress painful stimuli at the spinal cord level.

Improvements in **ROM** and improved **muscle function** may explain the reduction in pain offered by SMT.[120] Studies of HVLA manipulation for discogenic sciatica often report an improved lumbar ROM following treatment.[119,123] This improved motion could be caused by relaxation of hypertonic (tight) muscles[108,122] to enable better spinal motion.[119]

Spinal manipulation is thought to release **adhesions** surrounding LDHs or facet joints.[108,124] This adhesive tissue can limit sliding of the nerve roots as well as spine and extremity movement. Studies of HVLA manipulation for discogenic sciatica often report an improved degree of straight-leg raising following treatment.[119,120,123] This improved mobility may result from freeing the nerve roots from adhesive tissue.

Spinal manipulation may help discogenic sciatica by improving **cerebrospinal fluid flow** to the spinal nerve roots. Magnetic resonance myelography after three weeks of SMT shows an increase in nerve sleeve diameter.[121] This is thought to represent an improved filling of cerebrospinal fluid around the nerve root.[121] Improved fluid circulation around the nerve may help sciatic pain by allowing for the outflow of chemical irritants such as the inflammatory mediators released by the nucleus pulposus.

Side posture manipulation

Side posture manipulations are a common HVLA treatment for LBP and have been shown to benefit **discogenic sciatica**[109,110,124] as well as **SIJ syndromes**.[108] The facet joints limit lumbar rotation to a total of 2-3° during this technique, which is thought to protect against excess torsion on the IVD.[125]

Despite the relative safety of this treatment, certain patients rarely will worsen. Worsening of symptoms can be from treatment itself or due to acceleration of an already progressing LDH. Any side posture HVLA manipulation should be avoided in patients with severe sciatic pain, multiple neurological deficits, and/or pain that radiates beyond the knee.

In a side posture manipulation the side of sciatic pain is positioned upwards in order to gap the intervertebral foramen on the side of herniation and reduce disc and nerve pressure.[124] The patient's top knee is bent and the therapist contacts the posterior superior iliac spine (for sacroiliac manipulations) or the mamillary process of the lumbar spine depending on which joint is being manipulated. The therapist delivers a thrust anteriorly with the contact hand and at the same time drops with their body after reaching end-range with the contacted joint.

Side posture manipulation can be used to treat radiating pain from the SIJ. One study comparing injections, physiotherapy exercises, and SIJ manipulation for SIJ-related sciatica found that manipulation was the most effective treatment, with a success rate of 72%.[126] Patients with inflammatory arthritis of the SIJ were not studied and thus data is lacking as to whether manipulation would be of benefit in these cases.

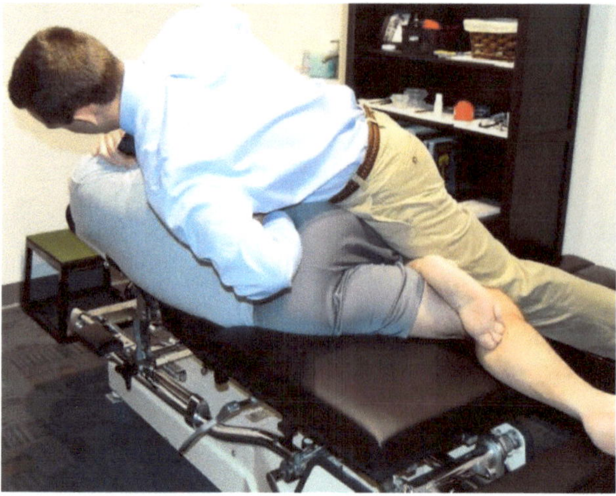

Figure 217: Side posture manipulation of the SIJ and lumbar spine. Similar or identical manipulations were used in multiple studies that showed benefit in cases of discogenic sciatica.[109,110,124] Image by Robert Trager, DC.

Flexion-distraction

Flexion-distraction is a **low velocity non-thrust** technique with components of manipulation, mobilization, and traction that is often used for LBP. The flexion component alleviates LSS by temporarily widening the lumbar spinal canal.[127] This technique is also thought to create a **negative intradiscal pressure** to help decompress damaged discs.[127] Flexion distraction triggers the **flexion-relaxation response** which relaxes the frequently tight erector spinae muscles.[127] There is some evidence that flexion-distraction is useful for discogenic LBP and sciatica.[128]

Flexion-distraction has been used successfully and safely in patients with ongoing discogenic sciatica following lower back surgeries (e.g. microdiscectomies, decompression laminectomies).[128] For this reason, it could be safer or at least more appropriate for disc-related sciatica.

To perform flexion distraction the therapist uses one hand to stabilize the lumbar spine while the other hand moves the lower part of a customized table, which holds the patient's lower body. The lower part of the table is separated slightly from the upper part which provides a mild **traction**. The therapist can move the lower part of the table in **rhythmic oscillations** of flexion and extension, lateral flexion, and/or rotation. These movements enhance the traction force on the lower back, especially if the legs strapped to the table.

The treatment and directions of movement should be tailored to the patient's tolerance as recommended in the Cox flexion-distraction course. Treatment can be as gentle as needed depending on the setup of the table and should not increase or peripheralize radiating pain.

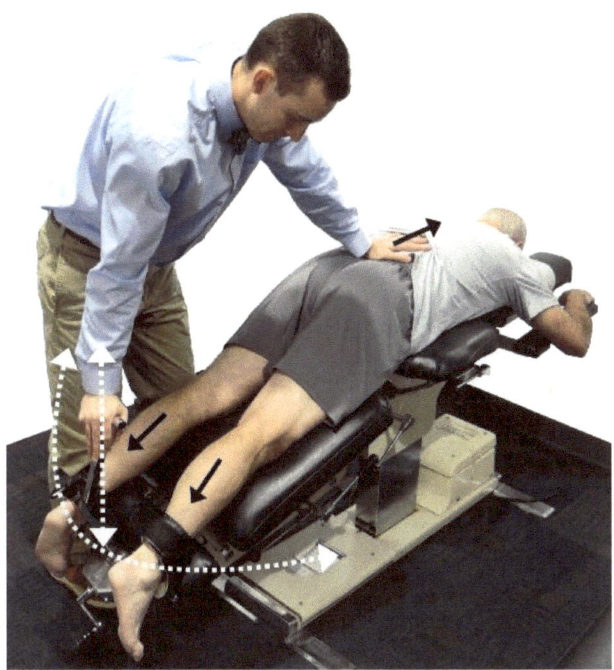

Figure 218: Flexion distraction. The therapist moves the table in a range that is comfortable for the patient. The table has a hinge just above the pelvis that permits flexion, extension, lateral flexion and rotation

Feng's manipulation

Feng's manipulation for LDHs involves a seated rotational HVLA manipulation. This technique was developed in the 1970s from Traditional Chinese Tuina (bonesetting).[119] Multiple studies have shown benefit of Feng's manipulation in discogenic sciatica.[119–121] As with side posture manipulations, Feng's manipulation should be avoided in patients with severe sciatic pain, multiple neurological deficits, and/or pain that radiates beyond the knee.

To perform Feng's manipulation, the practitioner rotates the patient's trunk steadily to end range then quickly loads the spinous process of the affected vertebral level to induce more torsion.[129]

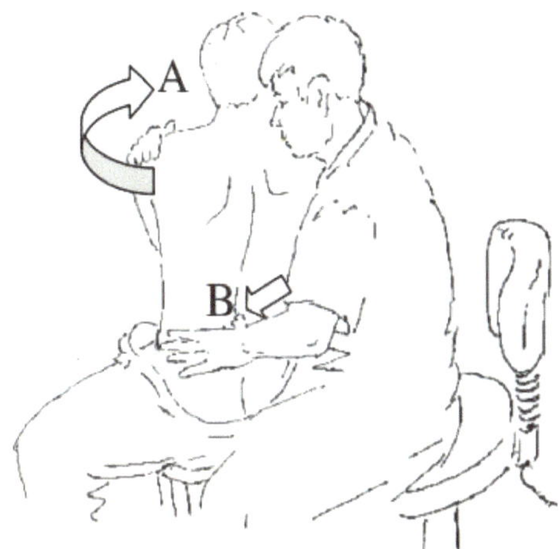

Figure 219: Feng's SMT for a LDH. Image from Han,[129] CC BY 4.0 license

Spinal mobilization

Thoracic mobilization can be used to increase thoracic spine extension. One study found that rhythmic posterior to anterior mid-thoracic mobilization along with William's lumbar flexion exercises, pelvic tilt exercises, and neck stretches was beneficial in treating back and leg pain associated with lumbar spondylolisthesis.[130] This may be because improving thoracic extension mobility reduces the need for lumbar mobility in an already damaged and hypermobile lumbar spine.

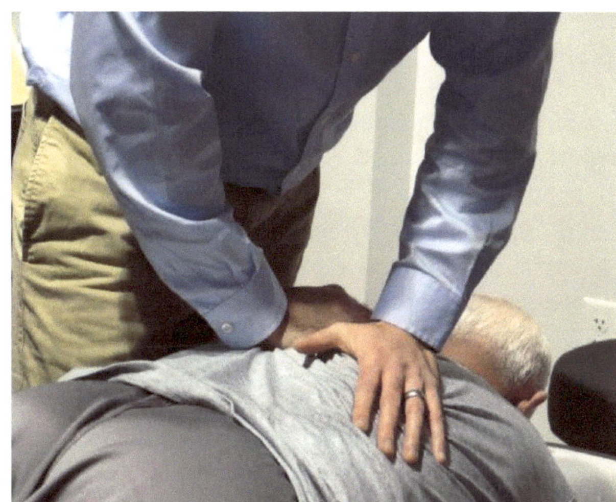

Figure 220: Thoracic spine mobilization.

Rhythmic oscillation is a joint and soft-tissue mobilization technique. It is a low-velocity, low-force, non-thrust technique involving **small amplitude** movements. Sustained rhythmic oscillation at 1-2 cycles per second is thought to stimulate the proprioceptive input of the spine, which in turn helps muscles relax and promotes joint health.[131]

A type of rhythmic oscillation called **Pulsation Oscillation Long Duration** or POLD has been shown to help centralize discogenic sciatica.[132] This technique uses transverse rhythmic mobilization of the lumbar spine and incorporates aspects of manual therapy to the paravertebral muscles and manual decompression.[132] A randomized study found that a total of three 45 to 60-minute sessions of POLD per week over 3 weeks significantly reduced gluteal pain, thigh pain, and leg pain, and improved lumbar forward flexion.[132]

Spinal mobilization with leg movements (SMWLM) is a lower back mobilization combined with sciatic nerve tensioning. The intention of this maneuver is to restore normal motion to the zygapophyseal joints, which in turn may alleviate strain on the discs and help sciatic pain.[133] One trial showed this technique was successful in alleviating sciatic pain in patients with LDH.[134]

To perform SMWLM for sciatica the patient lies on their side, with the side of limited straight leg raise up. One therapist pushes the spinous process of the affected vertebral level medially, while second therapist brings the patient's leg into a straight leg raise.[133] The technique should be repeated slowly three times on the first day of treatment and increased to include more repetitions at further visits. It should not be so aggressive that it increases sciatic pain.

Patient selection and safety

The success of SMT decreases with increasing neurological deficits[108] and radiation of pain distal to (beyond) the knee.[10,108] Spinal manipulation should not be performed on those with major neurological deficits such as **cauda equina syndrome** or rapidly progressing deficits. This includes patients with deficits spanning multiple nerve root distributions (e.g. L4, L5, S1), bilateral deficits, S3 or S4 nerve root signs, and perineal numbness or genitourinary problems. Spinal manipulation can still be successful, however, with minor deficits that trace to a single nerve root.[109,110,124] Neurological deficits in discogenic sciatica are a **precaution** but not a contraindication to SMT.

Spinal manipulation works best as part of an integrated treatment program, for example in combination with traction and core stability exercises. If a patient is not a suitable candidate for SMT, other treatments can be performed initially, and SMT can be reconsidered after symptoms improve.

High-velocity, low-amplitude, short lever manipulation is safe for discogenic sciatica provided it is not used in cases with severe or progressing neurological deficits. Aside from an initial temporary discomfort following SMT,[108] the risks of true adverse reactions are low. Spinal manipulation rarely may worsen pre-existing LDHs. The risk of a manipulation causing cauda equina syndrome is less than 1 in 3.7 million.[125] In trials of SMT for discogenic sciatica 2% of patients were slightly worse or worse following 1-3 months of treatment.[124,136] Other trials reported no adverse events.[18,110,122] Spinal manipulation is safe and effective for sciatica in an adequately selected patient.

Table 34: Patient selection and precautions for spinal manipulative therapy (SMT) in sciatica

More likely to respond to SMT	• Sciatic pain proximal to knee • Few or no neurological deficits[108,135] • Treatment combined with home exercise program[18] • Straight leg raise more than 60°[135] • At least one hip with internal ROM >35°[10] • Treatment is combined with traction, exercises, or back brace[16] • Disc sequestration[110] (compared to other disc lesions)
Less likely to respond to SMT	• Pain radiates distal to knee[10,108] • Multiple neurological deficits • Lumbar instability (i.e. movement) on dynamic lateral radiograph[108] • Previous low back surgery[109,123]

Neurodynamic treatment

Neurodynamic treatment, also called **neural mobilization**, neuromobilization, and neural manual therapy, can help reduce sciatic pain and improve nerve function. This therapy can target any part of the sciatic nerve from spine to foot as well as its connections up through the spinal cord. Neurodynamic treatment consists of tension maneuvers, also called **tensioners** that strain (stretch) the sciatic nerve and sliding or gliding maneuvers, also called **sliders** which cause nerve excursion (gliding).

In 1872, the Austrian surgeon Theodor Billroth reportedly cured a patient from sciatica by surgically opening the thigh and stretching the sciatic nerve.[137] This led to the popularization of neurectasy, the process of surgically stretching and freeing the sciatic nerve from suspected adhesions. At the time, one surgeon claimed that 60 out of 70 sciatica sufferers were either cured or greatly relieved by the procedure.[138]

Practitioners of neurectasy noticed the sciatic nerve became longer and separated from adhesions to surrounding tissue.[139] Often there was a temporary reduction in sensation of the sciatic nerve distribution afterwards. Some surgeons felt that the benefits obtained were due to tearing of the **nervi nervorum**, the small nerves that provide sensation to the sciatic nerve sheath.[140]

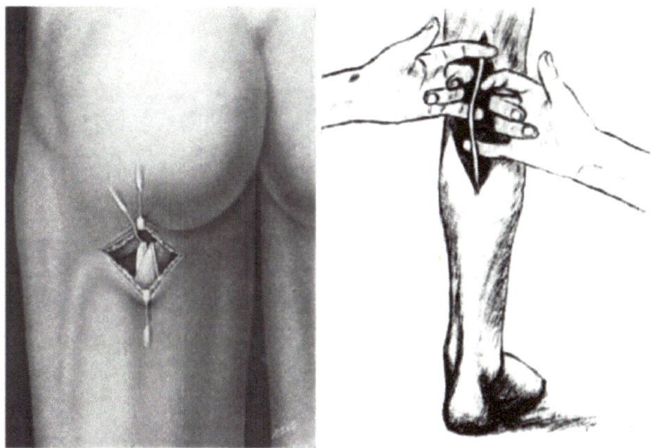

Figure 221: Left - Exposure of the sciatic nerve for neurectasy. From "Surgery: Its Principles and Practice," Da Costa, 1919. Right - Nerve stretching in the popliteal fossa, from "Surgery, Gynecology and Obstetrics, volume 4, 1907."

Despite the widespread interest and success, there were reports of adverse events including problems with wound healing, iatrogenic neurologic deficits, and even death in cases of aggressive neurectasy.

Due to the drawbacks of neurectasy another procedure was developed called **subcutaneous nerve stretching** in which the patient's hamstrings and calf muscles were stretched vigorously, typically performed with the patient anesthetized. Unfortunately, this was reported to have the risk of traction injury to the spinal cord.

Neural mobilization techniques may reduce sciatic nerve or nerve root **swelling**. Repeated dorsiflexion alternating with plantarflexion of the ankle has been shown to help fluid disperse along the tibial nerve in the leg.[141]

These repeated movements may create a **pumping mechanism** through the nerve.[141] An alternate explanation is that the effects of gravity during neural mobilization with the leg elevated helps drain swelling from the sciatic nerve.[142]

This therapy is thought to remove **acidic substances** and **inflammatory mediators** present in cases of nerve swelling.[142] A study using an animal model for sciatic nerve injury showed that sciatic nerve mobilization reduces mediators of nerve pain, pain sensitivity, and improves recovery from sciatic nerve injury.[143] When inflammation and swelling are reduced within the nerve then abnormal and often painful discharges along the nerve are also reduced.

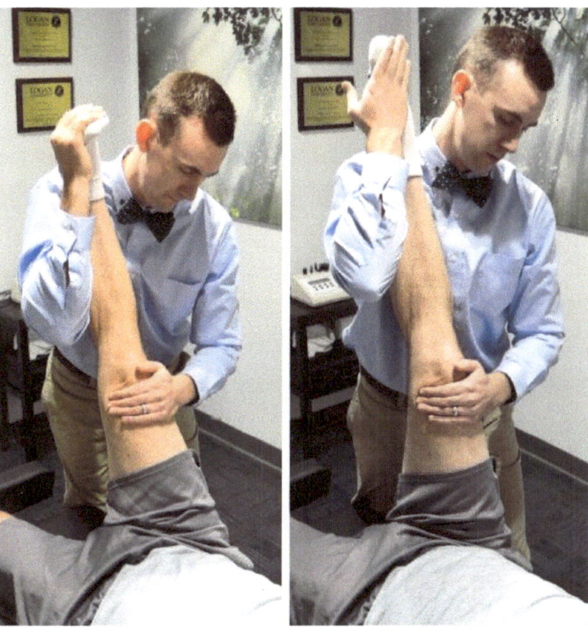

Figure 222: Distal sciatic nerve gliding technique. Emphasis is placed on the tibial nerve portion. First the patient is brought to the maximal SLR2 position just before pain onset, then the ankle is dorsiflexed, and leg raised higher. The neck can also be extended for this to allow greater SLR degree.

Neural mobilization may help the sciatic nerve glide and lengthen.[142] It may remove **neural fibrosis** either directly[142] or as a byproduct of removing swelling in the nerves.[141] which is important in combating adhesions that restrict normal movement. The sciatic nerve and its roots may glide better when swelling is reduced due to having less contact with surrounding structures.

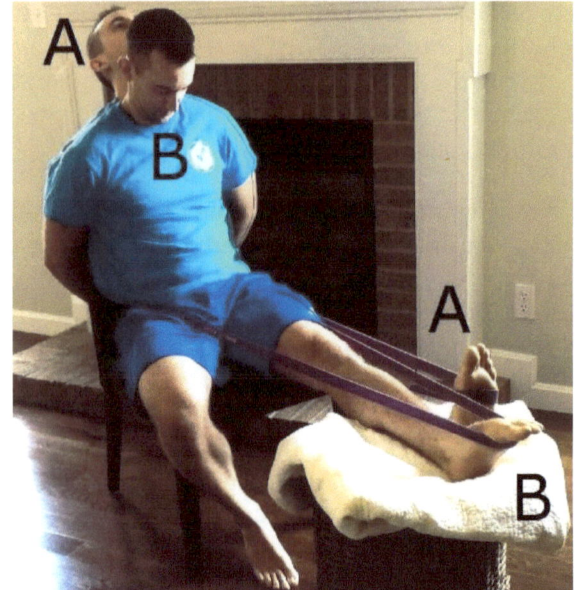

Figure 223: Distal sciatic nerve gliding "gas pedal" with exercise band. The neck and ankle simultaneously flex then extend. Neck extension reduces sciatic nerve tension while ankle dorsiflexion increases tension. Ankle plantarflexion reduces tension while neck flexion increases it. The actions cancel one another out leading to constant tension across the sciatic nerve, while movement enhances neural mobility. Image by Robert Trager, DC.

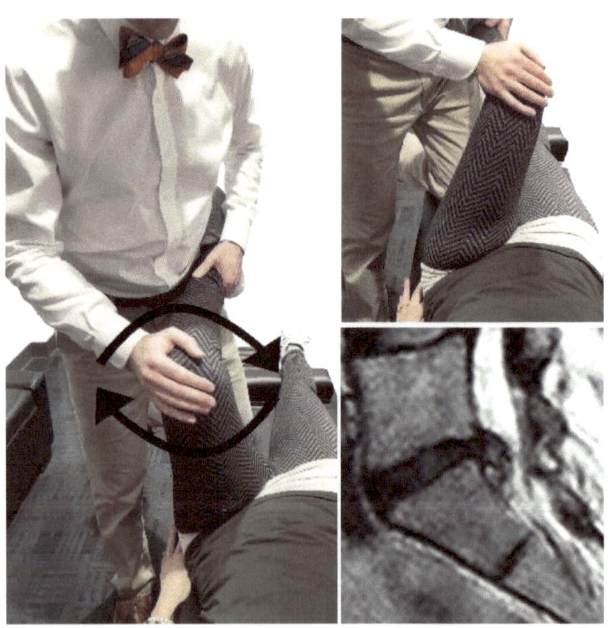

Figure 224: Sciatic nerve mobilization using hip circumduction. This 57-year-old woman presented with severe L S1 radicular sciatica related to LDH at L5-S1. The patient's ROM was taken to her tolerance level. Any increase in knee extension caused severe pain. Gentle sciatic nerve mobilization helped reduce pain and improve gait. Case shared with patient's permission by Robert Trager, DC.

Patients with normal strength, sensation, and reflexes benefit the most from nerve mobilization.[144] One study identified that patients with **neurological deficits**, neuropathic pain, or musculoskeletal pain do not respond as well to neural mobilization.[144] Another study found that neurodynamic treatments following lumbar spinal surgery (discectomy, fusion, laminectomy) did not improve outcomes when added to a regimen of standard physiotherapy exercises.[145]

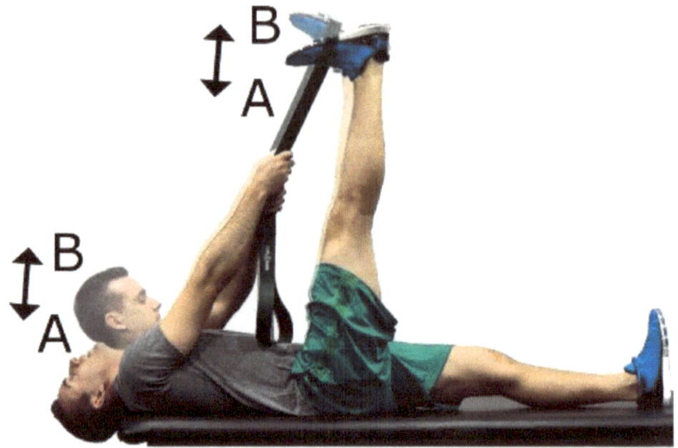

Figure 225: At-home sciatic nerve flossing "gas pedal" technique using a band to aid with simultaneous flexion/extension at ankle and neck. Alternatively, a belt can be used, but this method allows for the foot to be passively dorsiflexed.

Table 35: Patient selection for sciatic nerve mobilization

More likely to respond	**Less likely to respond**
• Normal strength, sensation, and reflexes[144] • Tender sciatic nerve[144] • Positive straight leg raise[144] • Peripheral nerve sensitization[144]	• Post-surgical[145] • Multiple neurological deficits[144] • Denervation[144] • Neuropathic pain[144] • Musculoskeletal pain[144]

Tensioners

Sciatic nerve tensioning techniques, also called tensioners, cause **strain** and **elongation** of the sciatic nerve. The nerve path is elongated from both ends.[146] These techniques do not necessarily cause sliding or excursion of the sciatic nerve. Tensioners are more aggressive than other neural mobilizations and can provoke sciatic symptoms.[142]

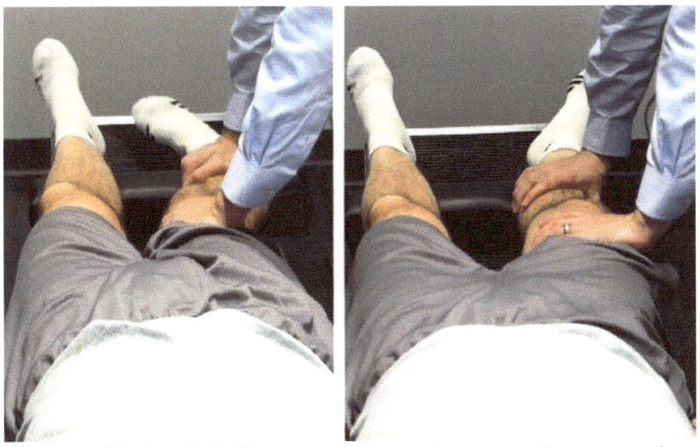

Figure 226: Sciatic nerve tensioner using passive internal hip rotation. Movements can be performed repetitively and gently back and forth.

Sciatic nerve tensioners have been found to help centralize discogenic sciatic pain and reduce the level of disability when added to a physical therapy program consisting of spinal mobilization and exercise.[147]

Sliders

Sciatic nerve sliders or sliding, also called **flossing**, cause **gliding** and **elongation** of the sciatic nerve while minimizing the strain placed on the nerve. The nerve path is elongated at one end and shortened or kept in the same position at the other end. Sliders cause more sciatic nerve excursion and less strain compared to tensioners. Sciatic nerve sliders have been shown to reduce pain and improve ROM in cases of acute discogenic sciatica.[148]

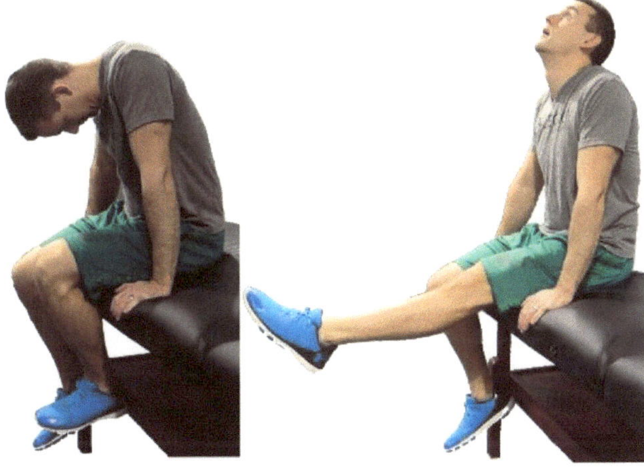

Figure 227: Seated slider. Left and right positions are alternated. Knee flexion reduces sciatic nerve tension while neck flexion increases it. The opposing effects cancel one another out to keep sciatic tension constant while enhancing neural mobility. Image by Robert Trager, DC.

Sliding techniques may be better for those with severe sciatic pain or nerve **mechanosensitivity** because they avoid aggressive stretching of the nerve.[142] Despite being safer there still is some risk of exacerbating symtpoms.[149] The patient's response must be monitored through the day following treatment to determine if a greater or lesser degree of flossing is indicated.[149]

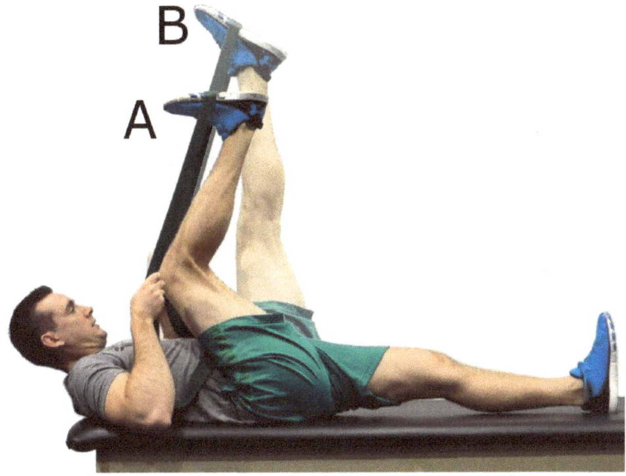

Figure 228: Supine sciatic nerve gliding with exercise band. There is simultaneous flexion at the ankle (dorsiflexion increases sciatic nerve tension), knee (reduces tension) and hip (increases tension) then simultaneous extension performed at the highest comfortable degree of straight leg raising. The opposing effects cancel one another out to keep sciatic tension constant while enhancing neural mobility. Image by Robert Trager, DC.

Interface treatment

Interface treatments for sciatica involve soft tissue or joint manipulation along the nerve pathway.[142] These treatments are meant to mobilize adhesions or improve joint mobility in order to optimize nerve function. Manipulation of the fascia in the gluteal region, the hamstrings, and soleus muscle could all be considered interface treatment as the sciatic nerve passes through these regions. Joint manipulation at the hip and fibular head are also forms of interface treatment.

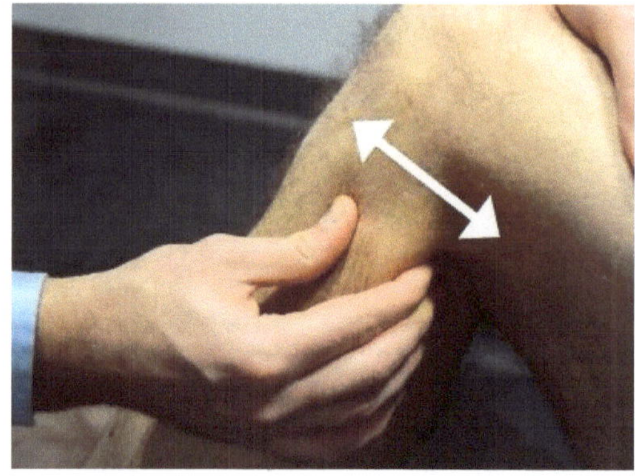

Figure 229: Mobilization of the fibular head, an example of interface treatment. This can be used with peroneal nerve-distribution sciatica. Mobilization of the fibular head may affect the common peroneal nerve which passes nearby.

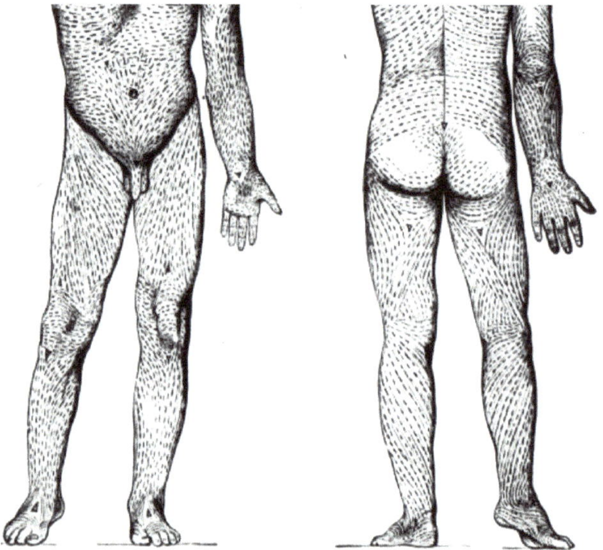

Figure 230: Langer's lines. These lines correspond with the distribution of Ruffini's corpuscles. Public domain from Toldt, 1919

Dermoneuromodulation

Dermoneuromodulation (DNM) is any method of helping change the nervous system by affecting the skin. **Skin stretch** can mobilize entrapped cutaneous nerves and desensitize sites of secondary hyperalgesia from a proximal lesion. Dermoneuromodulation targets the nerve-skin interface[150] rather than deeper structures such as muscles, joints, or deep fascia. It is performed gently, to maximize non-painful mechanoreceptive neural input while minimizing nociceptive input.

In 1912 Wetterwald of France recognized the "neurodermal" effects of manual therapy of the skin.[151] He hypothesized that sciatica was related to cellulitis (inflamed subcutaneous tissue) surrounding the sciatic cutaneous nerve branches.[152] Wetterwald recommended elongating the sciatic nerve in a straight leg raise position while lifting and pinching the skin at the points of sciatic nerve cutaneous branches.[152]

Modern DNM stems from the work of Diane Jacobs who recognized the importance of touching the skin to provide mechanoreception through its cutaneous nerves. She innovated the use of **directional skin stretch** to maximally stimulate Ruffini's corpuscles and superficial nerves in their ligamentous subcutaneous tunnels.[150]

Mechanoreceptive signals from skin stretch may alleviate pain by reducing nociceptive signaling in the spinal cord. **Ruffini corpuscles** are mechanoreceptors found in the dermis that respond slowly to sustained skin stretching. These receptors convey mechanoreceptive stretch information via large diameter myelinated type Aβ nerve fibers to the brain. Along the way, they give off collateral branches that effect other ascending pathways in the dorsal horn of the spinal cord.[150] It is thought that mechanoreceptive input from Ruffini corpuscles inhibits ascending nociceptive (pain) pathways (C and Aδ fibers).[150]

Ruffini corpuscles respond to stretching parallel to the skin surface. They attach to and sense movement of long collagen fibrils in the dermis.[153] These collagen fibrils are organized in patterns called **Langer's lines** or **tension lines** which are parallel to the long axis of limbs and transverse around the torso. The pattern of distribution of Ruffini corpuscles matches that of Langer's lines.[153,154] Skin stretch along Langer's lines may best stimulate Ruffini corpuscles and offer greater therapeutic mechanoreceptive neural input.

Superficial nerves pass from the subcutaneous tissue to the skin through specialized tunnels called **retinacula cutis** or **skin ligaments**.[155] Nerves pass through deep fascia to superficial fascia via the retinacula cutis profundis, and to the dermis via the retinacula cutis superficialis. Lines of adhesion are areas where skin is less mobile due to a greater density of skin ligaments.[156]

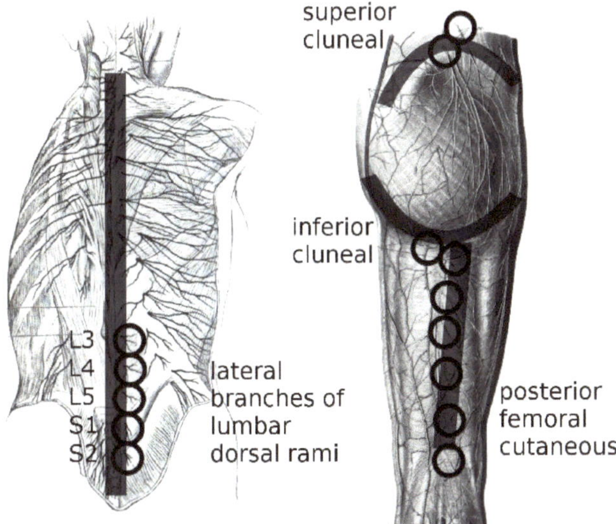

Figure 231: Overlap between skin adhesion lines (shaded areas) and skin ligaments (circles). Skin adhesion lines are drawn after Stecco[156] while lumbar lateral branch and cluneal nerve information comes from Loukas.[155] Left image is public domain from Henle, Right is public domain from Sobotta, both images are modified by Robert Trager, DC.

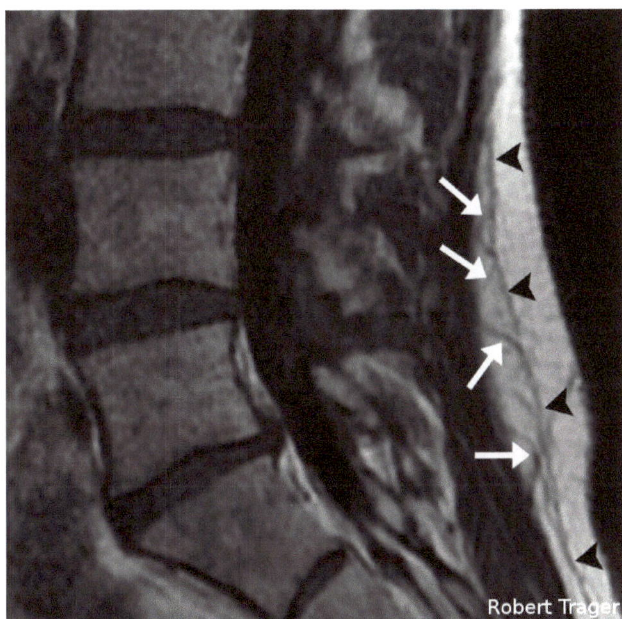

Figure 232: Sagittal T1-weighted MRI showing skin ligaments / retinacula cutis profundis (arrows) and superficial fascia (arrowheads) of the low back. Skin ligaments contain cutaneous nerve branches from the nerves (highlighted yellow), which are branches of the dorsal primary ramus. These cutaneous nerves then enter and traverse the superficial fascia. Image by Robert Trager, DC.

Manual therapy directed at areas of skin ligaments may reduce pain by stimulating the cutaneous nerves that pass through them.[150,157] Retinacula cutis are highly innervated with free nerve endings and mechanoreceptors.[156] Manual therapy that directionally stretches skin along Langer's lines stimulates the Ruffini's corpuscles in skin ligaments. Therapy directed to the sciatic cutaneous nerve branches may help inhibit nociceptive signals entering the cord at their respective segmental levels.

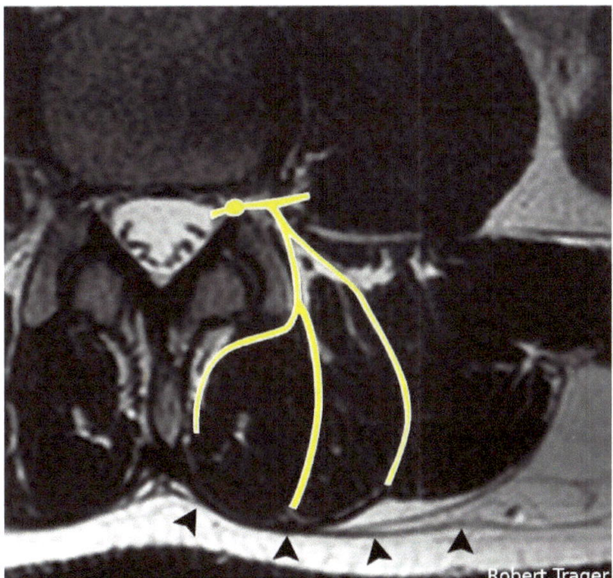

Figure 233: Axial T1-weighted MRI showing nerve branches from the dorsal primary ramus (highlighted) which give off additional cutaneous branches that enter and traverse the superficial fascial layer (arrowheads). Image by Robert Trager, DC.

Taping

Taping carries minimal risk and is an easy-to-perform method of alleviating sciatic pain. Different methods of taping for sciatica include both elastic (kinesio tape) and inelastic tape. There is some evidence that kinesio taping improves ROM and improves recovery in those with chronic LBP.[158] Kinesio taping the lumbar spine reduces the need for analgesics in those with LDH.[159] It has also been found to reduce pain and improve hip ROM in those with piriformis syndrome.[160]

Kinesio taping can alleviate sciatica by unloading inflamed and sensitive neural tissue.[161] This technique involves stretching the skin proximally along the involved dermatome or region of radiating pain to reduce neural tension. Taping causes movement of the **superficial fascia** and **skin ligaments** [162] which contain cutaneous nerves.[163] The skin can be used as an access point to reduce neural tension along the sciatic distribution. Taping to create a proximal shortening of superficial fascia will also slacken the rami of cutaneous nerves in their skin ligaments. Kinesio taping may help sciatica by reducing the neural tension in the cutaneous branches of the sciatic nerve distribution.

Some evidence suggests that **inelastic tape** applied to the lumbar spine alters and improves **movement patterns**.[164,165] Taping along the paraspinal muscles has been shown to limit lumbar flexion and increase movement of the hips and knees during lifting.[165] This method of taping may work by providing tactile cues and sensory feedback.[164,165]

Skin and subcutaneous tissue can either be lengthened or shortened depending on how the tape is applied.[162,166] According to Fukui, the recoil effect can be avoided and skin can be guided in the direction of tape application. To guide skin in the direction of taping, the tape is applied **incrementally** as the tape is stretched, instead of being applied all at once.[166] Guiding the skin stretch in the plantar foot **towards the heel**, in the low back **towards the lumbar spinous processes**, and in the posterior thigh **towards the buttocks** guides the skin and its underlying cutaneous nerves proximally and may reduce sciatic pain by unloading cutaneous nerves in these regions.

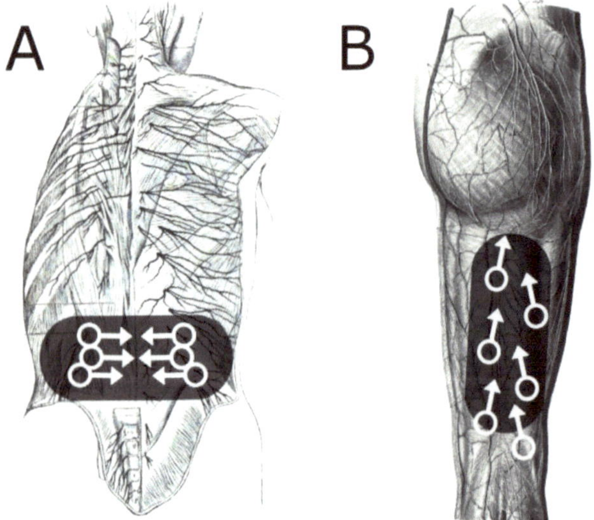

Figure 234: Kinesio taping patterns for sciatica involving the back and thigh. A - Skin stretch towards lumbar spinous processes stimulates the lateral branches of the dorsal primary rami. B – Skin stretch superiorly in the posterior thigh stimulates the posterior femoral cutaneous nerve. Images modified by author from public domain images (A) Morris' Human Anatomy (1907) and (B) Sobotta's 1922 atlas.

Kinesio taping in specific patterns along the sciatic nerve path may improve **neural mobility** and **ROM**. Kinesio taping along the sciatic nerve in the thigh has been shown to improve the degree of **straight-leg-raise** in those with sciatica.[167] Taping from the base of the toes to the heel has also been shown to improve the degree of straight-leg-raising.[166] Taping towards the lumbar spinous processes improves lumbar flexion ROM.[166]

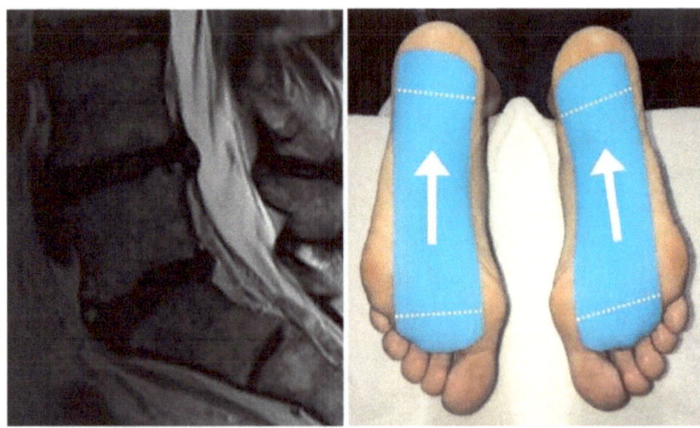

Figure 235: Skin taping to stimulate plantar nerves. Left - T2 weighted sagittal lumbar MRI. Right - Direction of skin taping. This 52-year-old woman presented with acute bilateral severe radiating pain in the posterolateral thighs, burning pain in the plantar feet, and L5 and S1 deficits. MRI revealed disc bulges at L4-5 and L5-S1. Foot pain was immediately eliminated using Fukui's taping method shown.

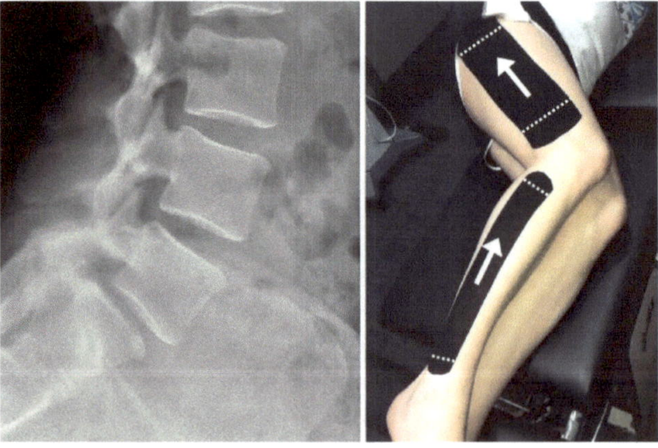

Figure 236: Kinesio taping for a right sided L5 radiculopathy (along L5 dermatome) related to a degenerative anterolisthesis at L5 on S1 in a 40-year-old female. The clinician applied kinesio tape in the cranial direction along the L5 dermatome and pain radiation. Taping and flexion-distraction alleviated symptoms over a 2-month span. Case shared with patient's permission by Robert Trager, DC.

Taping may work best when it runs in the same direction as the lines of force of fascia.[156] These lines run **longitudinally along the limbs** and **transversely along the torso**, and have a similar pattern to Langer's skin tension lines, the pattern of Ruffini corpuscles,[153,154] and dermatomes. Taping in this pattern stretches skin in a manner that is best perceived by the Ruffini corpuscles. The skin stretch generated by taping provides mechanoreceptive input that reduces nociceptive signals.

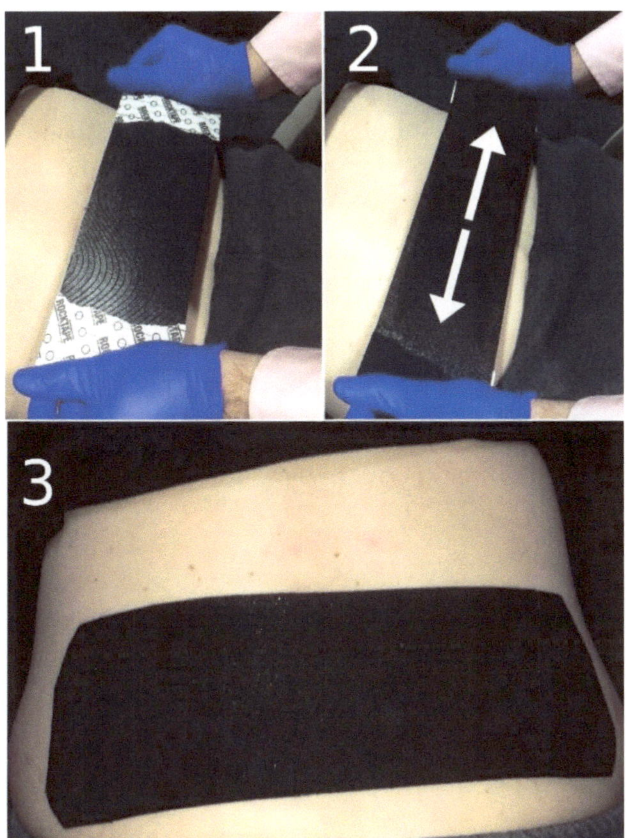

Figure 237: Kinesio taping to stimulate the lumbar dorsal primary rami. (1) Center of tape removed. (2) Tape stretched to 125% (3) Tape is applied which will then recoil towards spinous processes, pulling skin, superficial fascia, and nerves with it.

An alternative method for intraspinal sciatica that does not take advantage of the lines of force is to apply tape parallel to the spine bilaterally. This method is useful in helping maintain lumbar extension in patients with an extension directional preference. The tape gives proprioceptive feedback which helps avoid lumbar flexion and provides mechanoreception to inhibit pain.

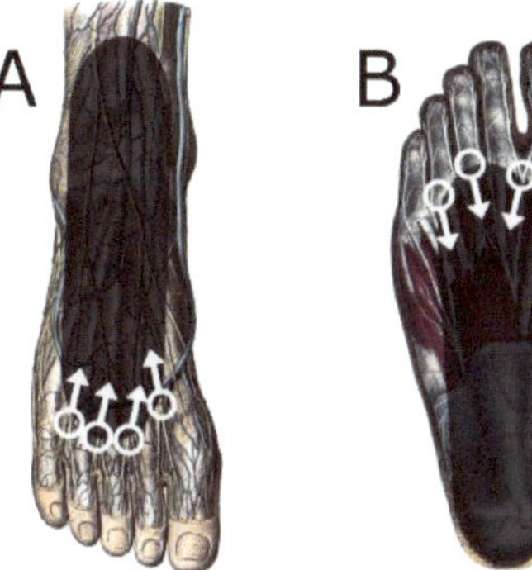

Figure 238: Kinesio taping for sciatica involving the feet. A - skin stretch cranially, unloading the superficial peroneal nerve. B – skin stretch towards the heel, unloading the plantar nerves. Images modified by author from Hirschfeld & Léveillé's 1866 Névrologie et esthésiologie, public domain images.

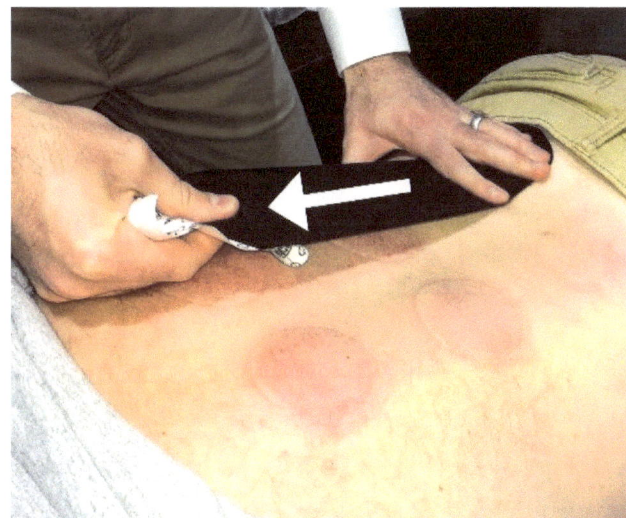

Figure 239: Method of kinesio taping parallel to the spine, which is applied on both sides of the spine (only one shown). Image by Robert Trager, DC.

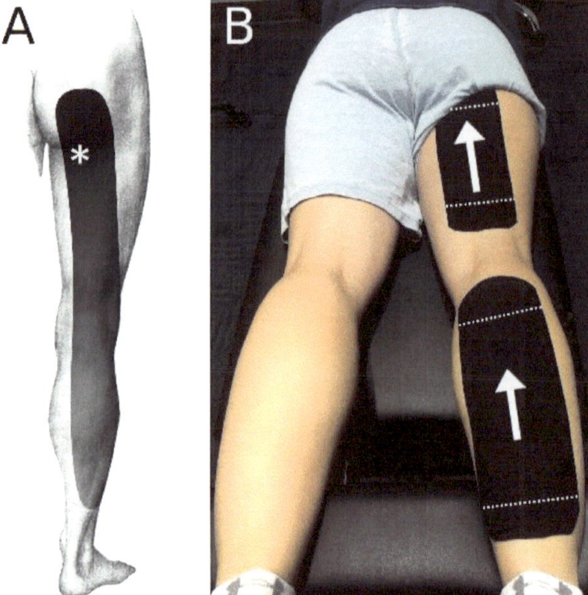

Figure 240: Kinesio taping in proximal hamstring syndrome. This 46-year-old woman presented with a 2-month history of radiating pain (A) from the proximal hamstring caused by a slip on ice. Her pain pattern, site of maximal tenderness (*), and positive active-30° hamstring test were supported sciatic nerve entrapment related to a hamstring strain. Taping and hamstring strengthening alleviated symptoms over a six week span. Case shared with patient's permission by Robert Trager, DC.

Traction

Lumbar traction is the method of using a pulling force to help separate the joints of the lower back. Clinicians can apply traction using specialized tables, while patients may self-administer traction using gravity at home. Traction can be purely axial or biased towards flexion, extension, rotation, or lateral flexion. Patients with sciatica that receive lumbar traction have 1.3 times greater odds of improving compared to no treatment.[6] Lumbar traction is effective for treating **discogenic sciatica**.[168-171]

Traction is one of the oldest treatments for spinal problems. The first known mention of its use is the Indian epic *Srimad Bhagwat Mahapuranam* written circa 3500-1800 BCE.[172] Hippocrates (c. 400 BCE) hung patients upside-down by their legs and used a mechanical axial traction device to treat spinal problems.[173] Traction was also popularized in Europe and the Near East by Albucasis[174] circa 1000 CE and later by Şerafeddin Sabuncuoğlu (1385-1468 CE).[175]

Mechanisms of traction

One theory is that traction lowers the **intra-discal pressure** and creates a suction force that draws displaced disc material inwards.[170] It has been suggested that traction works best for **disc bulges** and **protrusions**, which are best able to retract into their parent disc.[62] Traction also can reduce the appearance of high-intensity zones,[176] which are thought to represent annular tears.

One study using real-time MRI found that LDHs may reduce by 18% in anterior-posterior dimension during 30 minutes of traction.[176] Another study found a significant reduction in the size of LDHs using multiple sessions of traction over three weeks.[168]

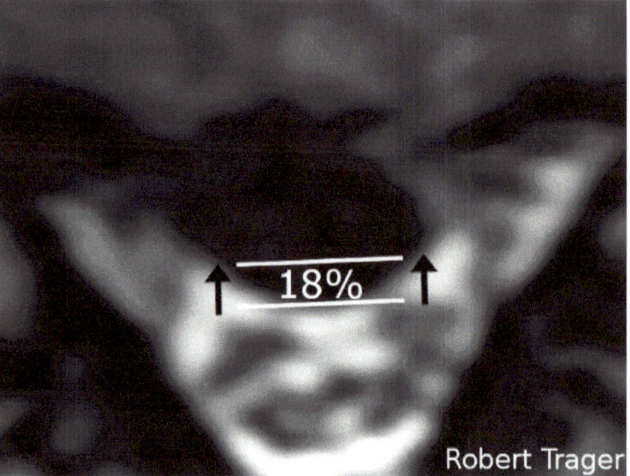

Figure 241: Effects of traction on disc AP diameter. During traction the anterior to posterior dimension of an LDH reduces by about 18%.[177]

Traction increases **IVD height**. One study using real-time MRI during traction found the most prominent effects at the posterior disc of L3-4, L4-5, and L5-S1.[177] This study found that a 30 minute session of axial horizontal traction at 42% of body weight increased the posterior part of the lower lumbar discs by an average of over 7%.[177] The central and anterior portions of the disc increased by about 4%.[177]

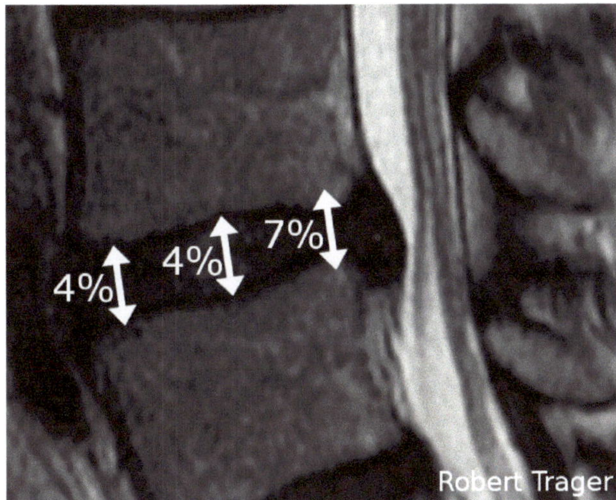

Figure 242: Effects of traction on disc height. During traction the IVD height increases posteriorly by 7% and centrally and anteriorly by 4%.[176]

Traction may reduce disc lesions by enhancing **water absorption** in the disc. The nucleus pulposus is rich in **proteoglycans** such as keratan and chondroitin sulfate. These molecules are **hydrophilic** and attract water. Traction force enhances this hydrophilic effect, and speeds the rate of water diffusion into the nucleus pulposus.[178] The bulk of water entering the disc may increase disc height and subsequently reduce disc bulging or herniation.

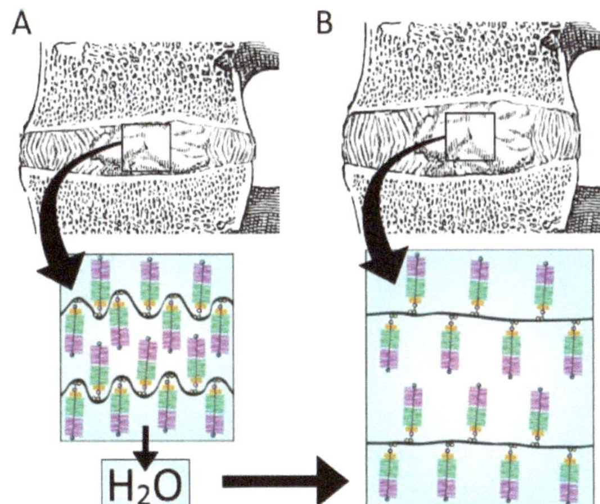

Figure 243: Traction force increases water absorption into the disc. (A) During prolonged standing or sitting the disc becomes compressed and loses water. (B) Traction force enhances the ability of hydrophilic proteoglycans to absorb water. Proteoglycans adapted from Roughley CC-BY-4.0, with changes.[182]

The ligaments surrounding the disc are pulled taut which may help retract displaced disc material inwards.[179] It is thought that traction tenses the **posterior longitudinal ligament** (PLL) which pushes displaced disc material back into the intervertebral space.[180,181]

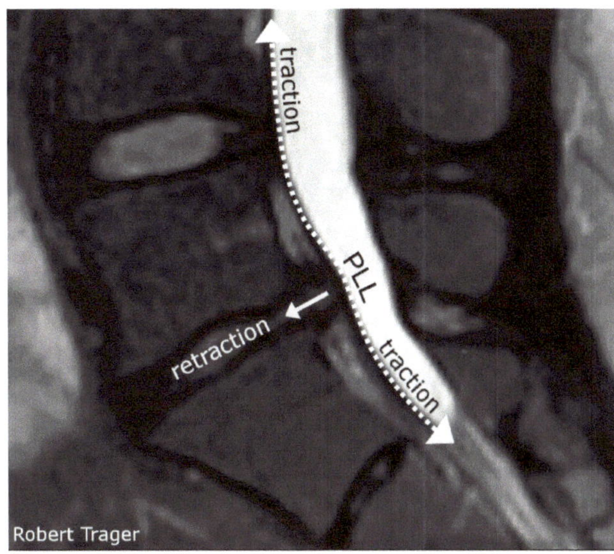

Figure 244: Effect of traction on the PLL and disc protrusion. The traction force pulls the PLL (dotted line) taut which helps push disc material anteriorly into the intervertebral space. This 28-year-old patient with L S1 discogenic radiculopathy responded well to hanging and inversion table forms of traction. Image shared with patient's permission by Robert Trager DC.

The **ventromedial ligaments** of Trolard may also help retract disc material. This mechanism should work best for **subligamentous disc herniations**, also called "contained disc herniations," which have not passed beyond the PLL.

Traction reduces the **lumbar lordosis**. One study found that 30 minutes of 42% body weight axial traction reduced the lumbar lordosis by almost 5°.[177] This may be helpful for sciatic patients with hyperlordosis as a result of hip flexion contracture.

Traction improves **neural mobility**. One study of patients with discogenic sciatica found that multiple sessions of traction increased the degree of **straight leg raising** by an average of 12°.[183] This effect may relate to the ability of traction to reduce the size of LDHs, which restrict nerve root sliding.

Traction reduces **paraspinal muscle tightness**. Studies using electromyography have shown that paraspinal muscle activity is reduced during traction.[168,184] This is helpful for patients with chronic spasms and/or guarding of the erector spinae muscles. This effect may be secondary to the effect of traction on the IVD. Paraspinal spasms are a neurological reflex induced by discogenic pain. When traction force reduces the size of a LDH, the reflexive spasms may resolve.

Traction has effects apart from the disc that contribute to its ability to improve sciatica. Traction widens the intervertebral foramina[176] and facet joints,[176] and may mobilize the hip and SIJs.

Traction techniques

A traction range of **30-60% of body weight** is optimal for discogenic sciatica.[183] Forms of traction involving friction on a table may require the higher end of the weight range while those without friction such as gravity-assisted traction may be better at the lower end of the range.

Traction sessions may be beneficial from 30 seconds multiple times per day[169] to 30 minutes performed once per day.[171] The exact parameters differ depending on what equipment is being used, individual patient tolerance, and the percent body weight used. Traction aided by gravity can use up to 50% of body weight and is typically applied in short durations and performed multiple times per day. Mechanical traction is tolerable for longer periods and sessions range from 5 to 30 minutes.[171,183]

Mechanical traction uses a harness around the pelvis and/or thoracic section to distract the lower back. The clinician may place the spine in a neutral, flexed, or extended position. One study found that a thirty minute session of traction force ranging from 50-95 lbs. significantly reduced discogenic sciatic pain and disability.[171]

Gravitational traction involves hanging with the aid of gravity either partially upside-down, completely upside-down, or upright. One can hang upright with an upper body harness or simply hang by the arms, or hang upside down using an **inversion table** or chair. Lying with the lower body elevated may also have a slight traction effect. Hanging from a **pull-up bar** causes about 50% of body weight to traction the lumbar spine.

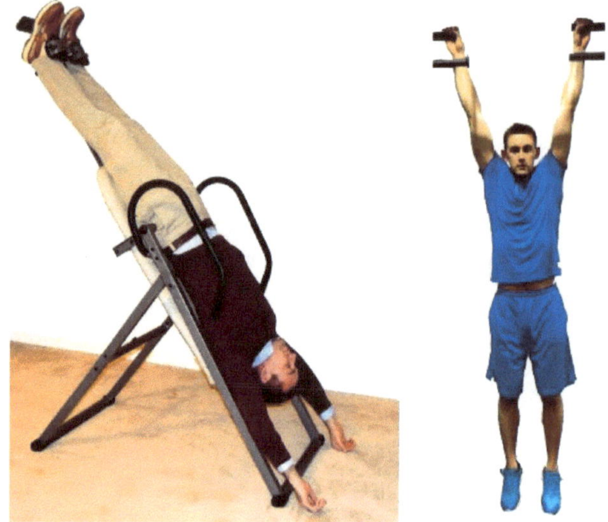

Figure 245: Gravitational traction. Left - inversion table. Right - Hanging from a pull-up bar. Image by Robert Trager, DC.

One study found a significant reduction in discogenic sciatic pain using a protocol of hanging from a pull-up bar for twenty sets of 30 seconds per day for two months.[169] One randomized trial examined the effect on discogenic sciatica of six two-minute inversion table sessions three times per week for four weeks on discogenic sciatica and found a significant reduction in the need for discectomy compared to patients that did not receive this therapy.[170]

Patient selection

Traction works best for those with no neurological deficits, those over 30 years old, those with low fear-avoidance scores, and those that do not work in a career of manual labor.[185] It is possible that traction may benefit certain types of disc lesions better than others, such as disc bulges and protrusions contained by the PLL.

Lumbar traction should be used with certain precautions. A few case reports have described worsening of LDHs during traction.[186,187] Traction may be uncomfortable for some patients when it exceeds 60% of body weight.[188] Mechanical traction harnesses may make breathing more difficult.[188] Inversion therapy may cause anxiety when performed for longer than a couple of minutes[170] and can elevate systolic blood pressure.[188] Although inversion tables can be balanced according to height, some people may require help returning to upright. Contraindications to traction are listed below.

Table 36: Contraindications to traction, adapted from Moret et al[189]

Symptoms	•	Problems with urination (cauda equina syndrome)
	•	Tightness of the chest with exertion or at night
Medical history	•	Abnormality of the trunk or trunk obesity
	•	Disorders of the heart, lungs, liver, or pancreas
	•	Lower back surgery within the past 6 months
	•	Malignancy
	•	Pregnancy
	•	Severe disorders of the blood
	•	Severe trauma
Medications	•	Anticoagulants

Lumbosacral orthoses (braces)

Lumbosacral orthoses (LSOs), also called **lumbar supports** and **abdominal belts**, are medical devices used to stiffen the trunk and treat LBP.[190] Clinicians and patients should avoid prolonged use of orthoses which may lead to deconditioning. Orthoses are useful in a subset of patients with low-back related sciatica.

Indigenous peoples used lumbosacral orthoses for sciatica. Natives of Scotland wore a sealskin girdle around the waist to treat sciatica.[191] People in England in the 1600s CE used wraps of wool or animal skin.[192] Modern folk medicine practices in multiple countries recommend corsets with herbs or topical analgesics.[193] Medical lumbar orthoses for sciatica became popular in the early 1900s when clinicians believed sciatica was caused by a displacement of the SIJ.[116]

Two recent trials in 2014 and 2015 found that non-extensible LSOs improved outcomes in those with **LBP**.[194,195] A meta-analysis regarding treatment of **spondylolysis** and grade 1 **spondylolisthesis** in children and young adults found that using an orthosis (compared to no orthosis) increased the success rate by 3% (from 86% to 89%), which was not statistically significant.[196] Orthoses are still used for spondylolysis and spondylolisthesis, but this practice is mostly supported by consensus.[197]

Lumbosacral orthoses range from flexible to stiff. Materials such as neoprene, rubber, and/or Lycra make up **extensible** LSOs. These allow for the most flexibility of the trunk[190] and may improve **proprioception** when worn.[198] **Non-extensible** LSOs incorporate canvas, polyester, and/or nylon. These materials increase trunk stiffness by 14% when worn,[190] and have been found to be effective in treating LBP.[194,195] **Rigid** LSOs contain molded hard plastic. These limit ROM the most and are best for cases of fracture and spinal instability.

The primary effect of LSOs is to limit **trunk ROM**, especially flexion, extension, and lateral bending.[199] Braces do this by increasing **passive trunk stiffness**. Non-extensible and rigid LSOs significantly increase trunk stiffness while extensible LSOs do not.[190]

Lumbosacral orthoses prevent global ROM but do not prevent **intervertebral translation**.[200] Therefore, rest and/or rehabilitation may be required to ensure that spinal instability heals while the brace is used. Athletes wearing a non-extensible LSO may expect to begin to return to play after 4-6 weeks, and should wear the LSO during rehabilitation and sport-specific exercise.[201]

Lumbosacral orthoses do not cause trunk muscle atrophy in the short-term but may do so in the long-term. One study found that LSOs do not adversely affect strength when used for **three-weeks**.[202] Another study found that the **lumbar multifidus** and lateral abdominal muscles reduced in cross-sectional area after **eight-weeks** daytime use of an extensible LSO.[205] To prevent muscle atrophy LSOs should be used for three weeks or less, or only worn part of the day.

Patients with skin conditions aggravated by bracing should avoid LSOs. Pregnant patients may be able to use only soft, extensible back supports. Patients with unstable fractures that are surgical candidates may not benefit from bracing.

Needling therapies

Minimally invasive needling therapies for sciatica include acupuncture and dry needling. Acupuncture is the practice of using thin metallic needles to penetrate the skin at specific **acupuncture points**, while dry needling targets **myofascial trigger points** or areas of nerve-related pain. Practitioners should be certified in acupuncture or dry needling to use either technique and know their indications, contraindications, risks, and precautions. This chapter serves as an overview of the mechanisms and utility of needling therapies for sciatica and does not replace a training course.

A review in 2015 found that acupuncture gives 7.9 times greater odds for success in alleviating sciatica compared to no treatment.[6] Another review found that acupuncture gave a small but significant advantage for sciatic pain relief compared to ibuprofen.[206]

People may have used forms of needling to treat sciatica for thousands of years. The mummy Ötzi "The Iceman" dating to 3,300 BCE found in the Alps at the Austria-Italy border may have received acupuncture treatment for sciatica. Ötzi had degenerative changes of the spine and SIJ pointing to possible sciatica.[207] He also had tattoos along the calves and ankles corresponding to potential treatment sites.[208]

The classic traditional Chinese medical text, *The Huangdi Neijing* from 100 BCE described acupuncture treatments for back pain and possibly discogenic sciatica.[209] The text advised bloodletting for those with LBP and what we would call today a positive Valsalva test.[iii]

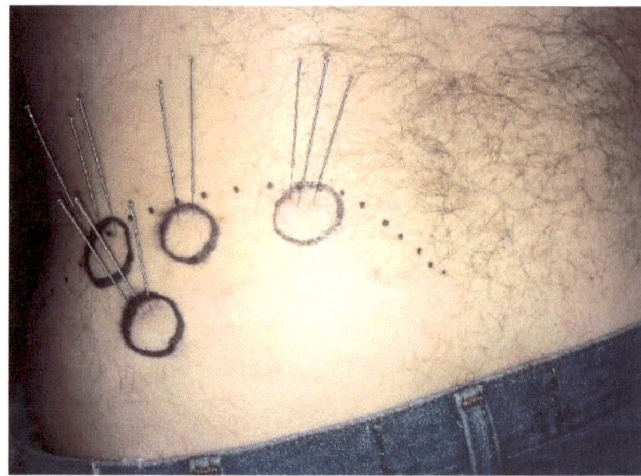

Figure 246: Dry needling of soft tissue surrounding the cluneal nerves. Needles are placed according to the location of tender points along the iliac crest, with the intention of reducing cluneal entrapment. Case shared with permission of Legacy Medical Centers and patient.

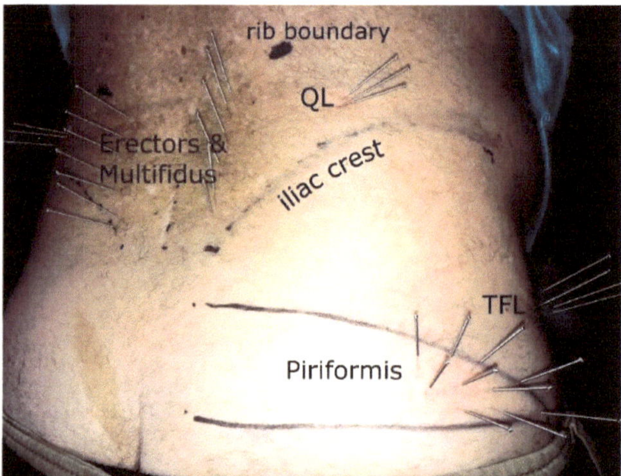

Figure 247: Dry needling for a patient with L4-5 LSS and right sided hip arthritis causing a right sided L5 radiculopathy with associated gluteal trigger points. This is also called hip-spine syndrome. Markings are shown of the rib boundaries, iliac crests, and piriformis boundaries, which guide needle placement. Case shared with permission of Legacy Medical Centers and patient.

S1 radicular sciatica is a common example of the neuro-anatomical correlation of needling points. This condition often causes trigger points along the hamstring and soleus, and pain along the sciatic trunk and posterior femoral cutaneous nerve distribution. Needling along these trigger points, the cutaneous nerve pain distribution, or dermatome may have equal benefit to the patient.

[iii] *When it is the vessel of the flesh structures that lets a person's lower back ache, then the patient cannot cough.¶ When he coughs, the sinews shrink and become tense.¶ Pierce the vessel of the flesh structures – generate two wounds – at a location outside the major yang vessel and behind the severed bone of the minor yang vessel.*[209]

The specific points used for sciatica depend on the patient's diagnosis and pain pattern. Needling for sciatica is usually performed within the L4, L5, S1, or S2 **segmental levels**. It can be performed along a **sensory nerve** pathway, acupuncture **meridian** or channel, or chain of trigger points depending on the diagnosis or technique being used. For example, those with L5 radicular pain may benefit most from gallbladder acupoints, needling along the lateral femoral cutaneous nerve, and tensor fascia latae.

Those with discogenic sciatica may benefit most from lumbar **paraspinal needling**.[211] Paraspinal dry needling or acupuncture points[212] may work by stimulating the **medial branch** of the **lumbar dorsal primary rami** (DPR). A medial branch of the DPR passes through the intermuscular space between the multifidus and longissimus.[210] Stimulation of the DPR branches may aid in pain relief and benefit the multifidus muscle which it innervates.

Table 37: Corresponding trigger points and cutaneous nerves in sciatica, adapted from Dorsher[203,204]

Segment	Trigger points	Sensory nerves
L4	Vastus lateralis, tibialis anterior, extensor digitorum brevis	Superficial and deep peroneal
L5	Tensor fascia latae, peroneus longus, peroneus brevis, gluteus minimus anterior fibers	Lateral femoral cutaneous, lateral sural cutaneous, superficial peroneal
S1	Gluteus minimus medial fibers, lateral gastrocnemius, tibialis posterior, abductor digiti minimi, hamstring, popliteus, upper soleus, lower soleus	Posterior femoral cutaneous, lateral sural cutaneous, lateral plantar
S2	Medial gastrocnemius, distal medial soleus, abductor hallucis	Posterior femoral cutaneous, medial sural cutaneous, medial plantar

Needling therapies may benefit sciatica by **neuromodulation**, the process of engaging with neural pathways to diminish pain.[212] Acupuncture provides mechano-receptive input that inhibits nociceptive (pain) signaling in the dorsal horn of the spinal cord.[213] Needling within the same dermatome or nerve distribution as sciatic pain may maximize these anti-nociceptive benefits,[204] because the mechanoreceptive signals dampen nociceptive signals within the same cord segment.

Needling of paraspinal points may improve **muscle function** in the lumbar spine. It is thought that needling releases shortened paraspinal muscles that compress the IVD.[214] In those with LBP, needling can also stimulate the **multifidus** and improve its ability to contract.[215,216] A properly functioning multifidus protects the spine from instability. Needling may benefit intraspinal sciatica by normalizing muscle tone and improving the function of the deep stabilizing muscles.

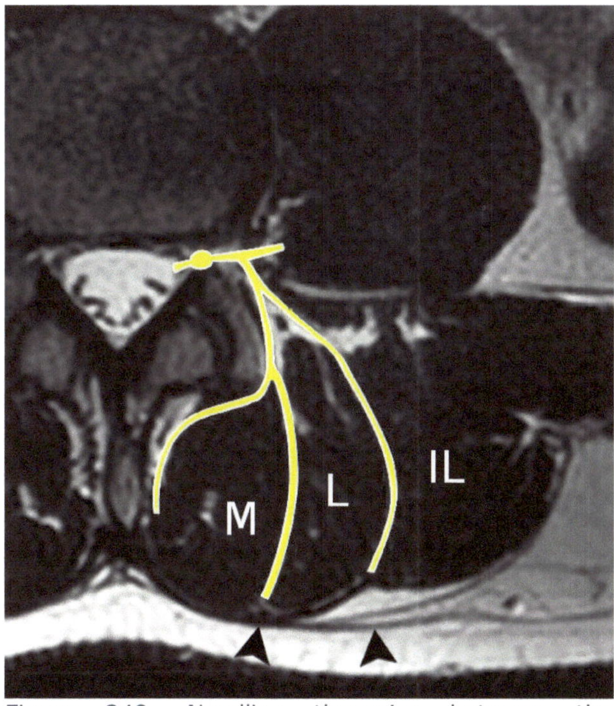

Figure 248: Needling therapies between the multifidus (M) and longissimus (L) may stimulate the cutaneous nerve from the medial branch of the DPR (arrowhead). Needling this point may offer pain relief through neuromodulation as well as stimulation of the multifidus. The nerve between the longissimus and iliocostalis (IL) is the intermediate branch of the DPR.[210] The intermediate branch may also be stimulated by needling. Image by Robert Trager, DC.

Table 38: Dry needling areas commonly used for sciatica: Trigger points and their associated cutaneous nerves.

Trigger points	Superficial nerves
Erector spinae	Lumbar dorsal primary rami[212]
Erector spinae	L2 dorsal primary ramus[212]
Erector spinae and transversospinalis[217]	L4 dorsal primary ramus[217]
Biceps femoris and semitendinosus[212]	Posterior femoral cutaneous [212]
Gastrocnemius, plantaris[212]	Posterior femoral cutaneous, medial sural cutaneous[212]
Gluteus maximus and medius, piriformis[212]	Superior and middle cluneal[212]
Tensor fascia latae, gluteus medius and minimus[212]	Lateral femoral cutaneous[212]
Gluteus maximus and piriformis[212]	Inferior cluneal[212]
Vastus lateralis[212]	Lateral femoral cutaneous[212]
Peroneus longus[218]	Lateral sural cutaneous[212]
Peroneus longus and brevis	Lateral sural cutaneous[212]
Flexor hallucis longus[212]	Saphenous[212]

Needling may help sciatica by improving **vasodilation** and **blood flow**. Needling is thought to stimulate a neurological reflex[219] that reverses the sympathetic-mediated vasoconstriction[220] often found in sciatic patients. One study found that acupuncture at the paraspinal EX B2 points increased sciatic nerve blood flow.[219] Another study found that dry needling of the gluteus minimus increased temperature of the thigh and calf of those with sciatica.[220]

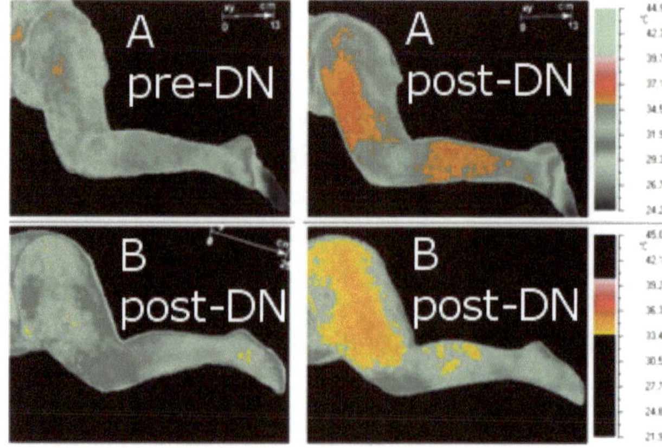

Figure 249: Effects of gluteus medius dry needling (DN) on two patients (patient A and patient B) with sciatica and trigger points in this muscle. Thermography scans show an increase in skin temperature 6 minutes following DN of over 1°C. From Skorupska et al,[220] Creative Commons Attribution License 4.0.

When needling therapies are used as part of an integrated treatment program, caution should be taken to avoid spreading traces of blood from the needling site. For this reason, it is most sanitary to use manual therapies such as gua sha, IASTM, and cupping prior to needling therapies as opposed to afterwards.

Cupping

Cupping is the technique of using cups with a **vacuum** suction force on the body surface. In **dry cupping**, only the cup is used, and blood is not removed from the body although it may come to the skin surface. In wet cupping a small cut is made then a vacuum is created over the area to remove blood. Cupping can also be used to mobilize soft tissue and help with manual therapy.

A systematic review found evidence that cupping is beneficial for short-term **pain relief**.[221] One study found that dry cupping reduced sciatic pain with 5 treatments spread out over 15 days.[222] Another study found that cupping was effective for treating LDH.[223] Cupping has also been shown to increase the degree of **straight leg raising**, increase lumbar flexion ROM, and reduce paraspinal tenderness in those with local LBP.[224]

Cupping is thought to help the body excrete **inflammatory cytokines** (messenger proteins) through the skin.[225] The vacuum effect of cupping brings blood and interstitial fluids to the surface along with inflammatory cytokines. It is thought that excretion of these proteins through the skin helps clear the blood of inflammation. Cupping has been shown to lower blood levels of inflammatory markers including the **erythrocyte sedimentation rate,**[225-227] **C-reactive protein,**[225,226] **and substance P,**[228] when these substances are elevated.

Cupping improves **blood flow** in the treated area. Doppler ultrasound and blood perfusion imaging studies have shown that cupping on the lower back improves local blood flow.[229,230] The **negative pressure** generated by the cup reduces vascular resistance and increases blood flow.[229] The increase in local blood flow is thought to help clear inflammatory and pain- generating substances,[225] stimulate healing,[224,227] and increase mobility of tight muscles.[227]

Silicone cups are ideal for dry cupping. They are inexpensive, hygienic, easy to sterilize, do not require the use of a flame, and do not require puncturing the skin as done in wet cupping. The cupping strength and skin color response can be monitored during treatment because silicone cups are transparent.

Cupping for sciatica is typically performed along the origin and course of the sciatic nerve in the low back, gluteal region, thigh, and calf.[227] In the low back **paraspinal points** are used alongside the spinous processes.[231] Common cupping points for sciatica include the acupoints corresponding to the **second sacral foramen**, the **piriformis,**[227] and the **mid-calf.**[232]

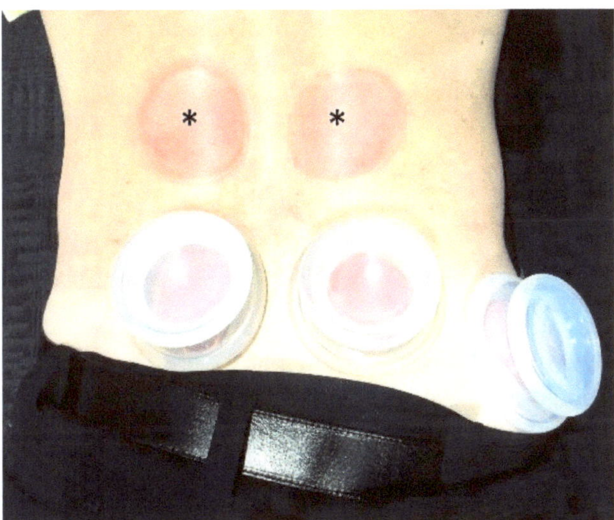

Figure 250: Cupping of the lower back and gluteal region. This 38-year-old man presented with R L4 and L5 distribution sensory symptoms related to an L4-5 anterolisthesis and disc bulge. There is a lasting increase in perfusion in the region where the cups were removed (*) Case shared with permission from patient, by Robert Trager, DC.

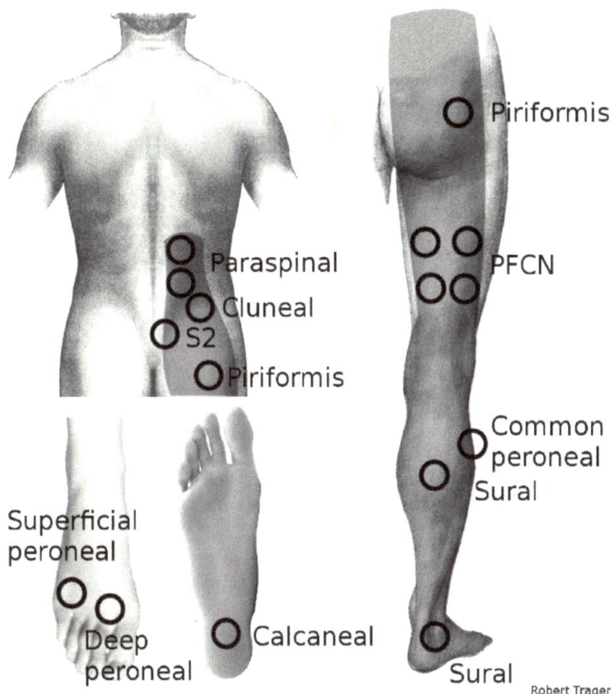

Figure 251: Cupping points for sciatica, including those over nerves and soft tissue. Image of leg modified from Andrea Allen (CC by 2.0), Plantar surface of foot modified from Pixel AddIct CC BY 2.0. Other background images public domain from Gray's Anatomy.

Cupping may be used to target cutaneous nerves to reduce pain via mechanoreceptive input. The superior **cluneal nerves** are easily cupped where they emerge at the iliac crest. The **posterior femoral cutaneous nerve** provides a broad area to stimulate in the posterior thigh. The region between the 4th and 5th toes has been used since at least 700 CE[233] and corresponds with the **superficial peroneal nerve**. Cupping on the heel has been used for sciatica since the 900s CE[234] and may stimulate the **medial calcaneal nerves**.

Cupping for sciatica can be performed from 3 to 20 minutes.[222,227] This treatment should be done for only 3 minutes on the first visit[227,235] to determine the patient's skin discoloration response. Cupping for sciatica can be performed every 2 days[232] and up to 3 times per week.[227]

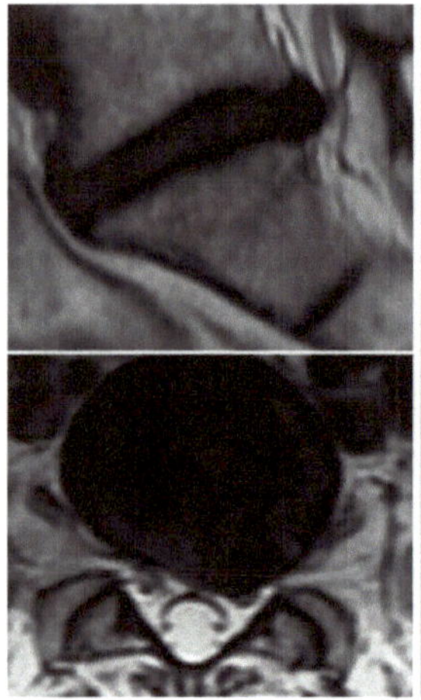
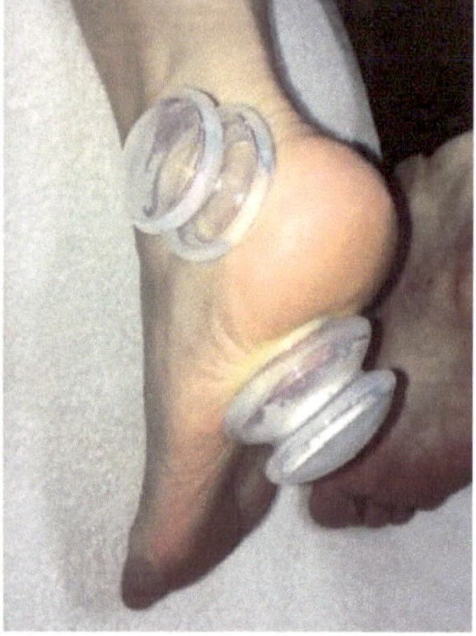

Figure 252: Cupping over the sural and plantar nerves in a patient with discogenic left S1 radiculopathy and neural mechanosensitivity to pressure in these regions. Image shared with permission from patient by Robert Trager DC.

Strong suction may be required in order to mobilize blood flow and have a therapeutic benefit.[227] This level of suction will raise the skin into the cup, which can be seen through transparent silicone cups. Strong cupping should be avoided on the first visit in preference for light or medium strength cupping. Cupping typically creates a red circle in the skin and at this point may be stopped to avoid bruising.[235]

Table 39: Contraindications to cupping, adapted from Jam[235] and Ilkay[227]

Assessment	• Bleeding injuries • Burns • Dermatitis • Fracture • Grade III sprain or strain • Infection • Open wounds • Severe edema • Varicose veins – avoid cupping over
Medical history	• Bleeding disorders e.g. hemophilia
Medications	• Anticoagulants

One should be cautious in cupping in patients with sciatic nerve mechanosensitivity. Cupping directly over the sciatic nerve could exacerbate symptoms.[235]

Cupping should not be performed in the groin. Cupping can be used lightly only in the first six months of pregnancy, and not near the abdomen.

Cupping has been related to bloodletting throughout history. Wet cupping and bloodletting have become less popular in modern-day due to the need to handle potentially infectious materials and to sterilize the cupping apparatus. Bloodletting for sciatica began as early as 1200 BCE as mentioned in the Indian text the Sushruta Samhita[236] and persisted into the early 1900s in Europe and America.[237,238] The same bleeding points are used to perform less invasive therapies including dry cupping, acupressure, and reflexology. Blood does not have to be drawn to have a therapeutic effect.

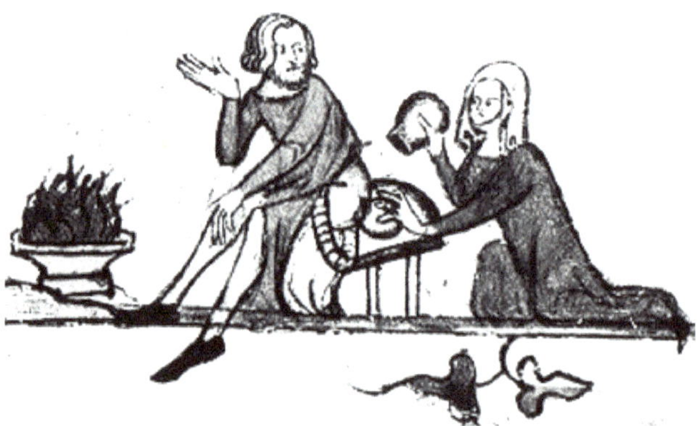

Figure 253: Flash cupping with fire on the hip, possibly at the piriformis point. Image is from an early 14th century illuminated manuscript, Wellcome Images, Creative Commons License 4.0

Hippocrates' (c. 400 BCE) wrote that Iranian nomads developed sciatica from frequent horseback riding, and treated their sciatica by venesection behind the ear.[iv] Galen of Pergamon[v] (c. 129-216 CE) and Paulus Aegineta[241] (625-690 CE) recommended bloodletting in the arm or leg for sciatica. The medical school of Salerno, Italy, recommended bloodletting from the sciatic vein in the leg in the 13th century CE. [242]

Ancient Near eastern physicians thought cupping and bloodletting helped sciatica by draining out an overabundance of humors from vessels.[234] From the 9th to 10th Centuries CE, practitioners mainly described using the sciatic vein,[233] which we know today as the **small saphenous vein**.[233] In Iranian medicine sciatica is called irq-al-nasa or ergho-nasaa. The

[iv] *"...when the disease is commencing, they open the vein behind either ear.... for whenever men ride much and very frequently on horseback, then many are affected with rheums in the joints, sciatica, and gout..."[239]*

[v] *"Sciatica... is quickly cured, if you cut around the popliteal or ankle veins... especially for the reason of abundance of humors coming out..." (Author's translation)[240]*

term nasaa describes a vein which historically was thought to collect fluid from the hip, increase in diameter, and cause symptoms of sciatica.[243] Proponents such as Mesue[233] (777-857 CE) treated sciatica by bloodletting or cupping from the foot to help eliminate excess fluid from the nasaa vein.[243]

Counter-irritants

A counter-irritant or **rubefacient** (causing skin redness) is a substance applied to the skin that causes a local inflammation to relieve inflammation in deeper or underlying tissues. When a counter-irritant is applied to the skin there is a local release of inflammatory mediators including substance P.[244] Blood vessels beneath the skin become dilated and the skin becomes reddened.

Indigenous people and ancient physicians around the world used counter-irritants to treat sciatica for thousands of years. Popular counter-irritants included chili peppers, a type of cacti called *Euphorbium*,[89,245] and mustard.[241,246,247] The Spanish physician Francisco Hernández observed the native Aztecs use of a salve made with chilis for sciatica in the 1570s:[248]

> *...[chilis] mixed with green tomatoes, returns and empties the phlegmatic humors wherever they are, especially those that occupy the hip joint, which will be the cause of sciatica... (Author's translation, Hernández p. 72)*

Counter-irritants may work by **desensitization**. Those with sciatica have a heightened pain response to **capsaicin** (the active component of chili peppers) in both the leg affected by sciatica and the other leg.[249] This is thought to be caused by the pain wind-up phenomenon in the spinal cord leading to increased perception of long-standing pain.[249] While the initial response to capsaicin is amplified pain, successive exposures to capsaicin cause less and less pain.[250] The **increased pain tolerance** with repeated counter-irritation is thought to be due to changes in neural synapses.[250] This process can be likened to the increased tolerance one gradually acquires to eating spicy food.

Another explanation as to why counter-irritants relieve pain is the depletion of inflammatory mediators in the sciatic nerve pathway.[251] This is often called **substance P depletion**. When capsaicin is applied to the skin, it triggers the release of substance P at nerve terminals. Substance P is found in the sciatic trunk and all of its branches.[252] Counter-irritants create an inflammatory reaction in the periphery which depletes inflammatory mediators, including substance P, from the sciatic nerve and reduces the nerve's ability to transmit pain.

Counter-irritants may also alleviate pain by stimulating the production of **somatostatin**. When capsaicin is applied to the skin it triggers a dramatic increase in somatostatin in the blood, which is thought to block pain signals at the spinal cord level.[253]

Capsaicin is the molecule within chili peppers that causes a burning sensation in the mouth when eaten or upon contact with the skin. A large review found that capsaicin has moderate to poor efficacy for treating chronic musculoskeletal or neuropathic pain.[254] One small study found that an 8% capsaicin patch was effective in lowering radicular pain related to failed back surgery.[255] Capsaicin is only moderately effective as an isolated treatment; however, it may help as part of a multi-modal treatment program.

Methyl salicylate is the main active ingredient in wintergreen oil. It contains **salicylic acid** like that found in acetylsalicylic acid (aspirin). One milliliter of 25% wintergreen oil contains as much salicylate as one 325 mg aspirin tablet. A systematic review found that counter-irritants containing salicylates have moderate to poor efficacy in treating musculoskeletal and arthritic pain.[256]

Mint plants have been used for sciatica for centuries. Dioscorides wrote that *Calamintha* (lesser calamint) "is applied to sciatica... to eliminate waste or morbid matter, burning the outward skin."[246] The plant was also taken as a drink mixed with honey and vinegar.[89] Mint plants contain **menthol**, a terpene alcohol. It gives a cooling and sometimes irritating sensation to the skin by blocking ion channels.[257] Menthol may alleviate pain via desensitization like capsaicin.

Combination therapies including capsaicin, menthol, and wintergreen and peppermint oils may work better than any individual agent.[100,244] One study found a significant reduction in LBP using a topical application of methylsalycylate (and other salicylates), camphor, menthol, and capsaicin.[244] Combination therapy also allows less of each ingredient to be used, which lessens the adverse effect of skin irritation especially from capsaicin.[100]

Myofascial techniques

Myofascial treatments are beneficial for intraspinal and extraspinal causes of sciatica. These techniques reduce pain and muscle spasm and may have beneficial effects on circulation, swelling, inflammation, and densification of fascia.

Myofascial techniques have been used to treat sciatica for thousands of years. Babylonian tablets dating to 668 BCE recommend **massaging** the feet and hands with oil for sciatica.[258] The Charaka Saṃhitā, an ayurvedic text (c. 300 BCE), also recommended massage with oil.[259] Hildegard of Bingen, Germany recommended dry brush massage for sciatica circa 1150 CE.[260]

Myofascial techniques may help sciatica by improving the function and mobility of the **thoracolumbar fascia**. One study found that Fascial Manipulation® directed at the deep lumbar fascia significantly reduced pain in those with chronic LBP and sciatica.[261] Deep friction may restore normal gliding and reduce stiffness in the lumbar fascia.[261]

Myofascial techniques may help with sciatica by dispersing **lumbar subcutaneous edema** and its associated inflammatory mediators. Removal of these inflammatory substances with myofascial techniques may lessen sciatic pain. Techniques including gua sha are thought to eliminate toxins and promote circulation to the treated areas.[262]

Releasing shortened muscles and fibrotic tissue in the lower back may alleviate impingement of nerves that exit the spine.[214] For example, manual therapy directed at the **quadratus lumborum** may help L5 spinal nerve entrapment. This nerve can be compressed while passing through a myofascial canal (lumbosacral tunnel syndrome) that is structurally connected to the QL. Lengthening the QL and reducing fibrotic tissue within it may allow its associated myofascial tunnel to open.

Manual techniques may improve sciatic nerve mobility by releasing **adhesions** between the epimysium and fascia of the thigh and sciatic nerve paraneural sheath. Restoration of sciatic nerve sliding can reduce sciatic tension signs and overall sciatica symptoms.

Gua sha

Gua sha or guasha is a type of **press-stroking**, also called **scraping**, that has been practiced as part of traditional East Asian medicine for centuries.[263] Gua sha is the predecessor to modern instrument-assisted soft tissue manipulation (IASTM) techniques which target fascia, muscles, and areas of nerve entrapment. Gua sha was initially designed to work with acupoints, channels, and Qi, however its benefits may also relate to its effects on fascia.[263]

Gua sha increases **circulation** and temporarily increases temperature in the treated area.[264,265] One study found gua sha increases **superficial blood flow** by 400% for over seven minutes, which then slowly tapers for over 25 minutes.[264] This increase in circulation could help remove inflammation such as lumbar subcutaneous edema that is often found in those with discogenic radiculopathy and LSS.

It is thought that gua sha benefits LDHs by removing **inflammatory mediators** and toxins from the surrounding tissue.[262] One study using an animal model for LDH found that serum levels of the inflammatory **interleukin-1** were reduced following gua sha.[262] The increased blood flow caused by gua sha may help eliminate inflammatory toxins.[262]

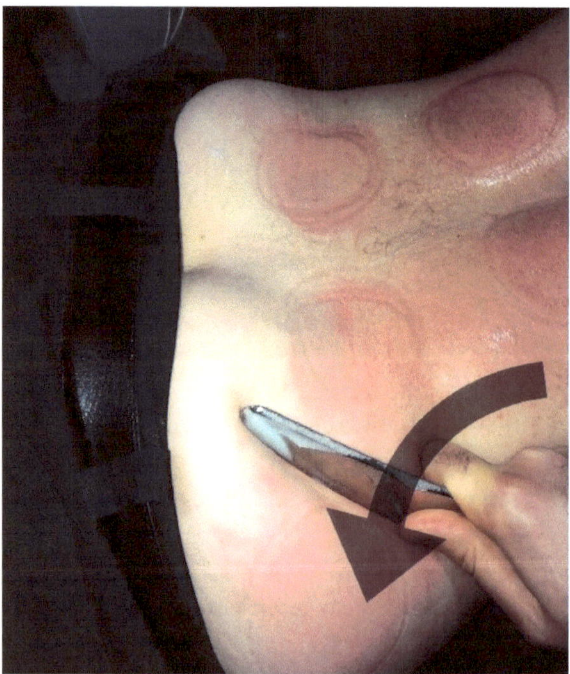

Figure 254: Gua sha over a region previously cupped. The direction of the stroke followed the curved arrow. This patient had radicular sciatica related to an L4 isthmic spondylolisthesis and L4-5 disc bulge. Shared with permission from patient, by Robert Trager, DC.

Gua sha is more effective in treating LBP when **petechiae** (small red spots) form on the skin, and less effective when petechiae do not appear.[266] The petechiae are thought to represent an increase in **vasodilation** and **extravasation** of blood cells from capillaries,[264] but could also represent a removal of inflammatory mediators from deeper structures.

The best evidence for gua sha in treating musculoskeletal disorders is for local neck[267] and back pain.[268] There is some evidence that gua sha is effective in reducing discogenic back pain and sciatica. Two studies that examined this found that the gua sha was about as effective as acupuncture[269] and more effective than traditional Chinese Tuina SMT.[269,270]

Technique

To perform gua sha one press-strokes a lubricated body surface with a smooth-edged tool. Modern gua sha or IASTM tools are made of stainless steel which can be easily disinfected. The technique is typically performed until petechiae form on the skin, these are also called skin eruptions, blemishes, or **sha**. Strokes performed in one direction help express the sha and achieve therapeutic benefit. For sciatica, strokes are typically in either a superior-inferior or inferior-superior direction.

Gua sha should be performed along the path of sciatic pain and superior and inferior to the area of most pain. One study found that gua sha was more effective in treating localized back pain when it was performed along the urinary bladder meridian, which corresponds with the **erector spinae** muscles.[266] Lateral strokes inferior to the ribcage can also be used to target the quadratus lumborum.[263]

For an S1 and S2 radiculopathy or sciatica along the posterior lower extremity, gua sha is applied along the erector spinae, gluteal region, posterior thigh, and calf. For an L5 radicular sciatica gua sha should be performed along the gallbladder meridian which spans the **iliotibial band** and lateral leg.

Gua sha may also be used to target scar tissue and fibrous adhesions that cause sciatica. One case noted improvement of a deep DGS related to a gluteal scar.[263] Gua sha can be used to treat **cluneal nerve entrapment** at the iliac crest. Patients that have had prior surgeries around the hip, sciatic nerve entrapment caused by chronic proximal hamstring injuries, scars from back surgeries, and peripheral nerve entrapments may all benefit from gua sha.

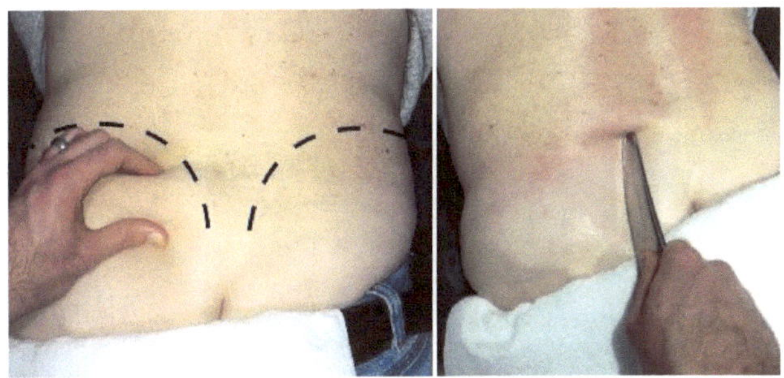

Figure 255: Left gluteal cellulalgia. This middle-aged male construction worker presented with a 3-day history of signs and symptoms of discogenic left S1 radiculopathy after lifting a heavy steel beam at work. He had left sciatic pain into the calf and left gluteal and hamstring weakness. The left gluteal region had multiple hard areas of fascial thickening that were tender but non-radiating (left). The patient's pain centralized with prone press-ups as well as gua sha at the gluteal region/iliac crest (right). Image shared with patient's permission by Robert Trager, DC.

Localized pressure

Localized pressure may target trigger points and acupoints involved in sciatica. **Ischemic compression** is performed by locating a painful trigger point or nodule that exacerbates sciatic pain, and holding pressure for 8 seconds up to 1 minute maximum.[271,272] One study found a highly significant reduction in back-related leg pain in patients who received **acupressure** compared to those who received a combination of physical therapy exercises and modalities.[273]

Patients may perform ischemic compression at home with a small moderately firm ball, for example a lacrosse ball. The ball can be used to target the gluteus medius, gluteus minumus, and piriformis. Light pressure can be used against a wall or more firm pressure against the ground. The ball is moved very slowly, about 1 inch every 10 seconds. The ball should not be placed directly on the sciatic nerve itself, which can trigger tingling and below the knee.

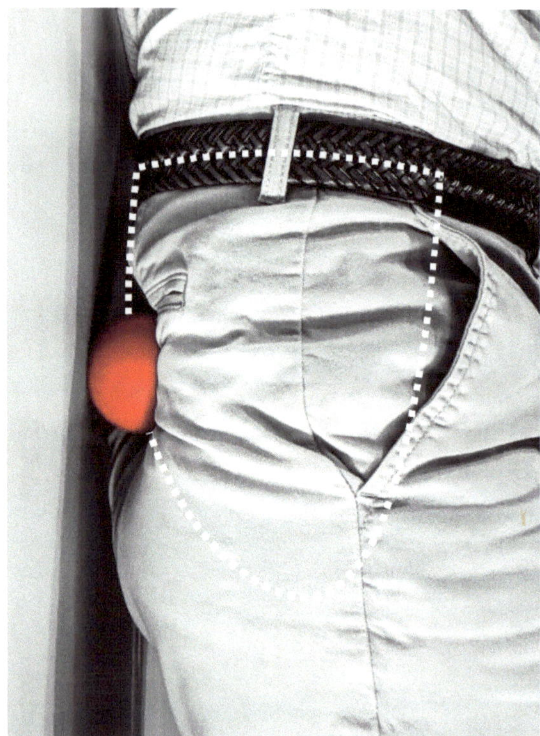

Figure 256: Self-treatment of gluteal muscles using a lacrosse ball. Pressure may be applied gently using a wall and lacrosse ball in the boundary shown (dotted line). Image by Robert Trager, DC.

Localized pressure can be used to target the hamstrings while sitting. A ball is placed under the hamstrings alongside the sciatic nerve and moved every few minutes further distally. This maneuver should not increase radiating sciatic pain but reduce it. Pressure should be gentle.

Manual nerve techniques

Manual techniques include various passive, hands-on nerve mobilizations that aim to desensitize and mobilize the sciatic nerve. These techniques can reduce spontaneous pain and improve longitudinal and medial glide of the sciatic nerve. Sliding dysfunction can originate at the spinal nerve root level but also at muscular and osteofibrous interfaces through the pelvis and in the lower extremity. Manual nerve techniques may encourage movement at the interface between the muscular epimysium formed by the biceps femoris, semimembranosus, adductor magnus and the sciatic nerve paraneural sheath.

Manual nerve techniques should be gentle. They should centralize sciatic pain rather than peripheralizing and aggravating sciatic symptoms. Small movements, pressures, or repetitions of these techniques are most appropriate.

Sciatic nerve mobilization techniques combine manual compression at sciatic nerve entrapment points with flossing or sliding neural mobilization. Examples include Barral's sciatic nerve release, techniques found in the Active Release Technique system, and Abelson's Motion Specific Release for the sciatic nerve. Common entrapment points include the piriformis muscle, hamstrings, and soleus.

Diaphragm techniques

The diaphragm has myofascial connections to the back and front of the body that affect its function. It acts as a bridge between the posterior **thoracolumbar fascia**, psoas, and quadratus lumborum and the anterior **deep abdominal muscles**.[274,275] Normally the quadratus lumborum assists the contraction of the diaphragm by stabilizing the spine and the lower ribs, and the transversus abdominus helps generate intra-abdominal pressure. Dysfunction of any part of this connected chain may interrupt the ability of the diaphragm to generate **intra-abdominal pressure** and stabilize the spine.

Tactile feedback can be used to optimize diaphragmatic excursion. The practitioner places their hands along the anterior and lateral abdominal wall and asks the patient to "breathe into the hands."[276] This provides **sensory awareness** and allows the patient to feel the outward expansion of the abdominal wall caused by maximum contraction of the diaphragm.[276]

Another method of manual therapy involves using light pressure to release tension in the **costal attachments** of the diaphragm.[277] This technique may help increase diaphragmatic excursion in those with a poor ability to contract the diaphragm. Manual therapy directed along all of the attachment points of the diaphragm anteriorly and posteriorly including the thoracolumbar fascia may also help with mobility of the diaphragm.[277]

Education and advice

A systematic review and meta-analysis in 2015 found that clinicians providing patient education and advice had 1.75 times greater odds for success in alleviating sciatica compared to no treatment.[6]

Educational material prior to the late 1990s focused on biomechanical advice[278] while newer programs incorporate the **biopsychosocial approach (BPS)**.[279] The BPS approach incorporates biological, psychological, and social components of pain. Therapeutic

neuroscience education (TNE) and pain neuroscience education (PNE), are BPS-based educational interventions that teach patients neuro-biological and neuro-physiological explanations of pain instead of anatomical or biomechanical ones.[280,281]

The **functional disturbance** or **non-injury model** are similar models which emphasize that LBP is often caused by abnormal **muscle activation** rather than disc degeneration, and does not lead to permanent damage.[282] Another model, the **process approach**, emphasizes the patient's active self-care and recovery process, as opposed to passive care.[283]

The **biomedical model**, also called the structural or anatomical model, is a traditional treatment approach for sciatica in which pain is explained using anatomy, pathology, and biomechanics. The biomedical model may have side effects including increased fear, anxiety, and feeling of vulnerability.[280,284] One study found that clinicians using pathological and anatomical terms with LBP patients created negative thoughts and disengagement from care.[285]

Studies have shown that neuroscience-based education programs improve **neural mobility**. A therapeutic neuroscience program has been shown to improve the degree of **straight leg raising** in patients with lumbar radiculopathy,[280] and chronic LBP.[286] One study that compared a neuroplasticity versus mechanical explanation for LBP found that the neuroplasticity patients were 7.2 times more likely to improve their SLR.[281] This group had a 5° improvement in SLR.[281] Improvement in neural mobility is thought to relate to the patient allowing the clinician to push them further,[280] reduced muscle tone,[281,286] improved blood flow,[281] or other unknown mechanisms.[286]

Therapeutic neuroscience education programs improve forward bending **ROM**. TNE has been shown to improve forward bending flexibility in those with chronic LBP[286,287] and radiculopathy[280] as measured by the fingertip-to-floor test. Improvements in forward bending are thought to relate to the patient pushing themselves further due to reconceptualization of the injury[280] and reduced paraspinal muscle tone.[286]

One study found that patients educated in a "**functional-disturbance**" model of LBP were more likely to report to work after a period of LBP, have higher levels of work ability, be bothered to a lesser degree by pain, and experience lower levels of sadness and depression.[282]

Patient selection

Patients with chronic (long-lasting) sciatica or risk factors for chronic symptoms may be ideal candidates for TNE. Patients with acute symptoms may still benefit from an education program, however those with serious pathology such as red flags or cauda equina syndrome should be identified prior to starting TNE as they may urgently require other treatment options.[288,289]

Those with **psychosocial risk factors** for chronicity, also called **yellow flags** or **barriers to recovery** are thought to be ideal patients for TNE.[288] Patients with greater worrying and anxiety about pain,[99] fear avoidance beliefs,[99] a compensation claim,[99], or kinesiophobia (fear of movement)[290,291] have a worse prognosis for sciatic pain.

Those with **central sensitization** are also thought to be good candidates for TNE.[288] Central sensitization should be strongly suspected in those with low-back related leg pain with **disproportionate**, **non-mechanical**, and **unpredictable** patterns of pain provocation in response to multiple non-specific aggravating or easing factors.[292]

Table 40: Examples of education for sciatica

Diagnosis • "[R]ed flags help identify rare serious from frequent 'normal' back conditions"[282] • Serious pathology is found in less than 1% of patients[1,3] • Degenerative discs are common and not always painful*
Anatomy • "The back [is] the strongest structure in the body"[282] • The sciatic nerve is the thickest nerve in the body... its upper part is protected by a layer of fat*[300] • The body naturally breaks down herniated disc material over time*[301]
Pain • "In some patients, following an injury, surgery, emotional period... the alarm system does not calm down... leaving them with an extra sensitive alarm system"[284] • "The brain can misinterpret signals from the body[282] • "Pain is not necessarily a sign of [injury]..."[282] • "When we have pain, move less... the brain areas are not exercised... and... become blurred"[281] • Abnormal muscle activation, as part of a pain-spasm-pain cycle, can create pain*
Treatment • "Treatments... are a... means for temporary symptom [relief]... to resume light activity and return to normal movement patterns"[282] • "I am going to do some manual treatments to your back... to help your brain sharpen its maps"[281] • Light activity will not further injure the discs[278]
Prognosis • 75% of patients will be much better or recovered by three months.[14] • "[A] disc herniation [does not mean] a weakened and disabled back for life..."[282] • "Only 5 to 10% of patients [with sciatica] require surgery"[302]
**quotes with an asterisk are original from this text, referenced within this or other chapters*

Patients with **chronic pain** may benefit from TNE.[284,293,294] Patients with chronic pain often have central sensitization.[293] One study found that LBP spreading to the upper back increased the odds of chronic pain.[295] In the case of sciatica, chronic symptoms may be defined as those lasting longer than three months. Patients with chronic sciatica may be good candidates for TNE.

It may be more appropriate to emphasize the biomedical or anatomical explanations for patients with **acute nociceptive pain**.[288,293,296] Patients with nociceptive pain are recognized by having localized proportionate pain with aggravating and alleviating factors, and the absence of night pain and other factors.[297] For example, an acute discogenic radicular sciatic pain patient with antalgia would classify as nociceptive. The TNE approach should also be used in these patients but less emphasis is placed on it.[293]

Education and advice programs

An education program for sciatica should include a review of pain science, anatomy, and an explanation of the diagnosis, prognosis, and treatment(s) that will be provided. These goals are in accordance with what patients with sciatica want: A clear **diagnosis**, **explanation of pain**, and a **prognosis** or at least reassurance that the cause is not serious.[298,299]

A neuroscience education program includes education of pain science. Clinicians can describe the purpose of pain as an **alarm system** and use visual images of axon potentials to help.[280] Clinicians may describe the anatomy and physiology of neurons, and explain how the brain interprets or produces pain.[286,294] Visual images of the brain can be used to help explain the brain's somatosensory cortex (map of the body) and how it becomes **blurred** during pain.[284]

Clinicians can explain **peripheral nerve sensitization** and **central sensitization** to patients with the aid of visual images of action potentials.[280] Peripheral sensitization can be explained as increased nerve sensitivity rather than tissue damage,[280] while central sensitization can be explained as increased responsiveness of central nervous system neurons.

Education of the **anatomy** of the lower back or sciatic nerve distribution should be paired with neurophysiology material.[286,289] In accordance with the biopsychosocial model, components of biology should not be completely left out or ignored.[289] In this sense, structural components of the spine can be explained.

De-education

Much of the neuroscience education for sciatica is geared towards changing **faulty beliefs** related to pain. Patients may be unnecessarily fearful of moving in a way that triggers pain because they associate pain with worsening structural damage.[303] Multiple studies have identified that those with **kinesiophobia** (fear of movement) have a slower recovery from sciatica.[291,304–306] Clinicians should avoid promoting faulty beliefs, because patients often derive beliefs regarding pain from their clinicians.[307]

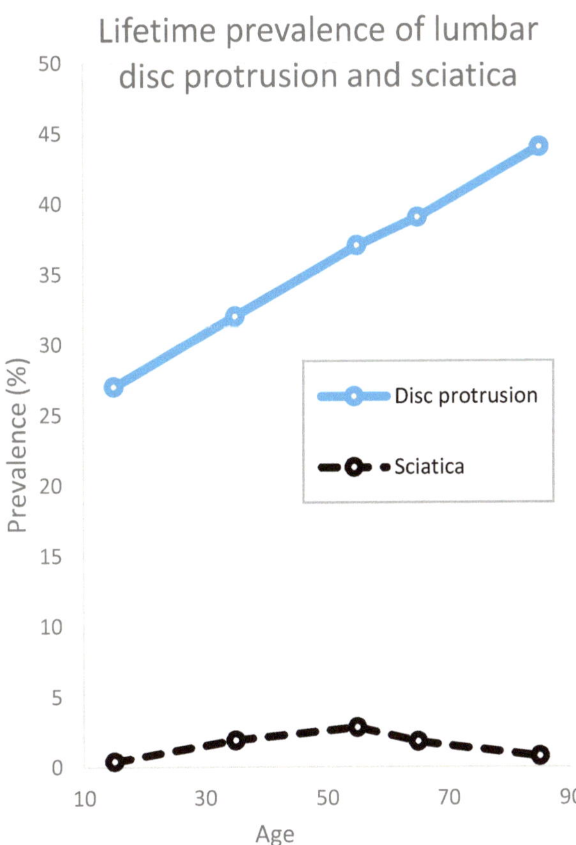

Figure 257: Lifetime prevalence of disc protrusion compared to that of sciatica. LDHs increase over time compared to sciatic pain which is most prevalent in the 6th decade of life. Data adapted from sources Savettieri[310] for sciatica, and from Brinjikji[309] for LDHs.

The notion that "**pain equals tissue damage**" or "hurt equals harm" is not true in the case of LBP or sciatica.[279,294,296] This concept is unfortunately propagated by nearly half of publicly available online education for LBP.[279] The severity of sciatic pain (e.g. on a scale of 0 to 10) has no correlation with its prognosis,[291,308] and does not indicate the source of pain (e.g. disc, stenosis, piriformis syndrome). Conversely, degenerative spinal conditions such as disc bulges are often asymptomatic.[309] Pain levels in a complex condition such as sciatica do not necessarily reflect tissue damage.

Clinicians, friends, or family may warn those with sciatica to "**let pain be your guide**" or "stop if you feel pain." These messages may increase fear-avoidance if patients follow them strictly. One review concluded there was ample evidence that phrases such as these were counterproductive to recovery.[311] More appropriate strategies may be to monitor signs that correlate better with recovery such as centralization and changes to muscle strength or and sensation. One study included advice to "stay active but reduce activity if leg pain is increased."[82] Clinicians should give patients clear instructions regarding what activities patients can do at each phase of recovery rather than a general statement to avoid pain.

The belief that "**I'm just getting old**" does not explain why sciatica occurs. Radicular sciatica is most common in the 6th decade,[310,312] whereas degenerative spinal changes, including disc protrusions, increase gradually through life.[309] One review found that common degenerative changes including disc bulges, annular fissures, and endplate changes did not increase the odds of having radicular pain.[64] By age 40, half of asymptomatic people have disc bulges and 68% have disc degeneration.[309] Sciatica does not correlate with normal-for-age degenerative spinal changes.

Patients with LBP often believe that their back is **fragile**, vulnerable, and needs protection.[303] This may be because pain often is triggered by a trivial event.[313] This view may also stem from negative beliefs relating to diagnostic imaging. Over half of those that receive an imaging study state that the results influence their activity levels.[314] Clinicians may also unintentionally promote the concept of fragility by having patients rest excessively or rely on passive over active care.

Language used by chiropractic and osteopathic models has historically focused on a "**bone out of place**" model. Some of this language has spilled into the lay language – patients often describe LBP in mechanical terms such as "out," "moved," and "slipped." [307] The notion that vertebrae can subluxate (go out of place) and be corrected by practitioners with hands-on techniques is not supported by evidence.[315] Patients being taught this model may be fearful that they could suffer severe damage such as paralysis with a trivial injury.[313] Some authors suspect that this model may encourage patients to depend on passive care, a "fix", or maintenance treatments rather than relying on active self-care.[293,316]

While it is tempting for manual therapists to explain that they are directly altering their patient's structure, there is not much evidence to support this. Traction has been shown to reduce the dimension of LDHs,[176] but these effects may revert once the patient stands. Directional preference exercises can improve radicular sciatic signs and symptoms without affecting the size of LDHs.[77] It may be more appropriate to explain manual therapy in terms of activation of the patient's endogenous pain-relief system,[284,317] or providing mechanical signals that block nociceptive (alarm) signals.[293]

Some patients may lament that "**I'll have this the rest of my life**" or "it can only get worse."[318,319] They may be pleasantly surprised to find out that only about 8% of cases of sciatica last five years or more.[320] Also, the prevalence of sciatica decreases after the 6th decade. An effective treatment plan incorporating active care and reassurance could reduce the percentage of people with chronic sciatica even more. Clinicians should reinforce to patients that most cases are not permanent.

Positive beliefs

One goal of an education program for sciatica is to reinforce **positive beliefs**, when appropriate. One study of patients with LBP found that positive beliefs correlated with an improved treatment outcome and lowered perceived disability.[321] These patients were more likely to believe that they were going to get better and were more confident that they could cope with their condition.[321]

Reviewing diagnostic imaging with patients

Clinicians often borrow terminology from radiology reports to explain pain to patients.[307] Unfortunately, language often used in radiology[307] regarding "**degenerative changes**" invokes the most negative thoughts in patients.[307,319] Some clinicians replace degenerative terminology with "wear and tear" when explaining pain, however this invokes a similar negative response.[307,319] Clinicians should be cautious when explaining insignificant findings so patients do not think they have serious pathology.

Patients that read their diagnostic imaging reports may misinterpret the medical jargon and have an unpleasant reaction. **Rewording** the medical language may help avoid this response. In the case of sciatica, a reworded report would qualify that disc degeneration normal for the patient's age is probably unrelated to their symptoms. One study of upper extremity MRI reports found that 70% of patients preferred a reworded report.[322]

A brief **spinal imaging education program** may change the way patients think about back pain.[314] A spinal imaging education program may include a visual aid showing the prevalence of age-relevant degenerative changes in people without pain, an explanation that imaging findings do not explain the day-to-day fluctuation of pain and do not correlate with clinical improvements.[314,323] Such a program may also highlight positive or normal imaging findings, and involve an explanation that muscles and joints require movement.[314,323]

Enhanced imaging reports include the prevalence of common degenerative findings for the patient's age. One study found that an enhanced imaging report helped improve back-related beliefs.[314] These reports may help both clinicians and patients navigate which findings are relatively normal or common for the patient's age.

Communication

Communication is important for conveying a sense of empowerment rather than disempowerment. Language can be used to improve the patient's **trust** and **confidence** in diagnosis and treatment.[285] Clinicians should be careful to avoid medical jargon that triggers a negative emotional response.

Patients want to have their diagnosis explained. This gives an understanding of goals of treatment, greater confidence in the treatment plan, and conveys a sense of empowerment.[285] One study found that patients who felt they were given a **carefully considered explanation** felt more confidence and value with the treatment plan.[285] Patients given a rushed or "production line" explanation, or were told "it... sounds pretty bad, but don't worry about it" had a negative view of the treatment.[285] A personalized approach to patient communication helps form a

therapeutic alliance between the doctor and patient.

Patients can become frustrated and anxious with diagnostic uncertainty,[303] and providers can become uncomfortable.[324] In addition, half of patients with back pain presenting to a medical doctor feel that imaging is necessary.[325] A systematic review identified that if an **adequate examination** was performed, patients' perceived need for imaging was reduced.[298] If the clinician performs a thorough examination, there will be a greater confidence in the diagnosis and treatment plan.

Some of the best understood terms are "**muscle spasm**," "**sensation**," "**manipulation**," "**mobilization**," "**soft tissue technique**," and "**rehabilitation**."[319] Most people do not have an accurate understanding of sciatica, LSS, LDH, nerve root pain, and other technical descriptions of sciatica.[319] Providers should communicate in a way that patients understand. If clinicians mention a complicated diagnosis, they should describe its (1) prevalence in the normal population, (2) prognosis, and (3) treatment. It is always appropriate for clinicians to ask patients if they comprehend the topics of conversation.

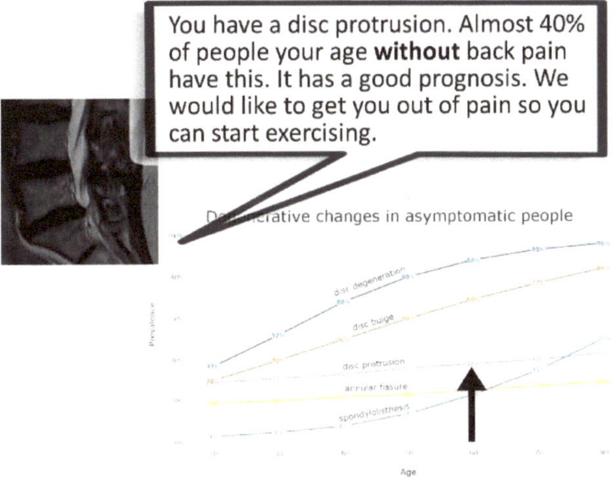

Figure 258: Example of communication of MRI findings to a patient with the aid of the graph at the beginning of chapter 3. Image shared with permission from patient by Robert Trager, DC.

Much of the clinical encounter can focus on using empowering language. This includes describing the features that are normal in any given patient, for example – "Your muscle strength is good," "those that exercise regularly tend to recover faster." It may also be helpful to give positive messages regarding active care, for example – " Keeping flexible, active, and strong will help keep your back healthy and reduce the pain."[293]

Medical **metaphors** are interpretations that patients feel are useful for communicating and remembering what is wrong with them.[285] Some biomedical or structural metaphors may be less helpful – "She was talking about a donut with jam in between... but didn't help me work out a way to fix it"[285] or "My vertebra is twisted out of place... it will probably never stay in."[293] In comparison, neuroscience explanations may have a more empowering connotation – "**Your lower back has a sort of memory and is overreacting**..."[285] Clinicians should be aware that metaphors may have a positive or negative connotation.

Jargon is specialized language or terms used by practitioners and not understood by patients. One study of taped interviews of patients with general practitioners, chiropractors, physical therapists, and osteopaths identified that patients misunderstood many back-pain related terms.[319]

The term "**neurological involvement**" is one of the least understood terms and causes some patients to feel alarmed. The term "**chronic**," may be misinterpreted as indicating a severe or incurable condition.[319] The term "**arthritis**" can be misinterpreted as a progressively worsening, incurable condition.[319] One study found that patients explaining their pain with degenerative terms such as "**wear and tear**," "**aging**" or "**damage**" felt they had a poor prognosis.[307] Another study found that degenerative terms provoked feelings of anxiety and a lack of control.[285]

Nocebo effects are unintentional negative effects caused by expectations of increased pain. Clinicians' can transfer their fear-avoidance beliefs to their patients.[316] For example, providers using a biomedical model are more likely to recommend limiting physical activity.[303] Terminology can also create a nocebo effect. Patients hearing they have "**degeneration**" or "**disc space loss**" have a poorer perception of their prognosis.[307]

Sensorimotor retraining

The goals of sensory and motor retraining for sciatica are to reverse the **central nervous system** changes related to chronic pain and to improve movement.[326,327] This approach involves sensory acuity training, visual feedback, movement, and other types of feedback or cues in various combinations. Evidence is growing that hands-on manual therapies performed in conjunction with feedback also influence the central nervous system.[296,328] A systematic review found a combined sensorimotor treatment approach reduced pain and disability in those with chronic LBP.[329] Sensorimotor training aims to create positive **neuroplastic changes** that reduce pain and improve function.

Some evidence suggests that sensorimotor interventions help normalize brain function in those with chronic LBP.[330] Sensorimotor training such as visual feedback[331], tactile feedback[296,332], and graded motor imagery[333] have been suggested to normalize or remap dysfunctional areas of brain cortex. **Cortical remapping** is in turn thought to improve proprioception and reduce pain.[296,332]

Sensorimotor retraining is thought to restore **sensory-motor congruence**, which is the agreement between actual and intended movement.[334,335] It is thought that a mismatch between predicted and actual sensory feedback creates an error in information processing that leads to pain.[335] Tactile training, mirror therapy, and graded motor imagery may create better sensory-motor congruence by improving cortical maps.[334] Sensorimotor training is thought to improve the body schema and create better agreement between sensory feedback and motor control.[335]

Visual feedback may strengthen **body awareness** and reduce nociceptive signals. It has been hypothesized that seeing ones' normal-appearing lower back creates a discrepancy between pain signals and visual cues.[332,335] This causes the nervous system to **reject nociceptive signals** that contradict the visual information of seeing a normal low back.[332,335] In addition, visual cues may help reduce the enlarged representation of the low back in the brain of LBP sufferers.[331] Visual cues may enhance ones' perception of their lower back and signals that would otherwise lead to pain.

Sensorimotor retraining may cause a **distraction** from pain.[331,335] For example, tasks such as graded motor imagery training requires **attention** and central nervous system processing.[334] This may also be true for sensory discrimination training and motor training exercises. It has been suggested that the analgesic effect of visual feedback may be caused by a change in brain activity into a **sensory-perceptual processing mode**.[331] Sensorimotor retraining causes a shift in focus towards normal sensations and movements and away from pain.

Sensory training may improve **motor control** by improving cortical sensory maps.[335] There is some evidence that tactile acuity correlates positively with improved lumbopelvic control.[336] It has been suggested that, due to this correlation, sensory training may improve lumbar motor control.[336] Sensorimotor training has been suggested to improve control over low back movements and lead to better biomechanical loading.[337]

Patient selection

Some authors suggest that sensory training works best on patients with an **expanded** pattern of sensory dissociation.[338] Patients that perceive the painful area as smaller may not respond as well. Most research of sensorimotor retraining has focused on those in chronic pain;[334] however, it has been hypothesized to also be useful in those with acute symptoms with the goal of preventing chronic pain and CNS changes.[333]

Sensory discrimination training

Tactile acuity training involves stimulating the body over a predetermined area and asking the patient where the stimulation occurs. One case series showed that tactile sensory training over the back over an evenly spaced nine-block grid significantly reduced LBP and improved forward flexion ROM.[281] In this study the authors used the dull end of a pen, while another study used the sharp end of a paper clip.[333] Other sensory modalities may work for training, such as pallesthesia (vibration). Each sensory tool may stimulate slightly different mechanoreceptors and different depths of tissue.

In **two-point discrimination training** the clinician asks the patient to distinguish between touch from one or two points of a caliper. The clinician repeatedly touches either a single point or two points, then shows the patient if they are correct or not. One study found that practice with this technique at with increasingly greater difficulty reduced LBP and improved two-point discrimination.[332]

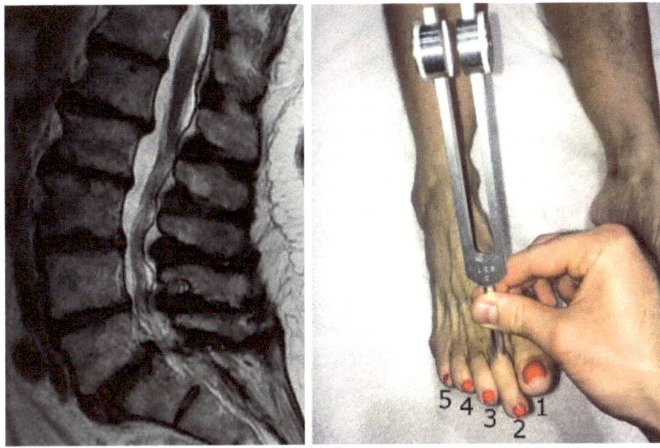

Figure 259: Pallesthesia training. This 69-year-old woman presented with chronic LBP radiating to the R>L lower extremities, with paresthesia along the R shin and foot dorsum and segmental deficits corresponding with an L5 radiculopathy caused by LSS. She had a poor accuracy when distinguishing vibration sense between the 2nd, 3rd, and 4th toes. Training of vibration sense in these toes improved her localization accuracy, and along with a larger program of flexion-distraction, gua sha, and lumbar stabilization exercises, helped alleviate symptoms. Case shared with permission from patient by Robert Trager, DC.

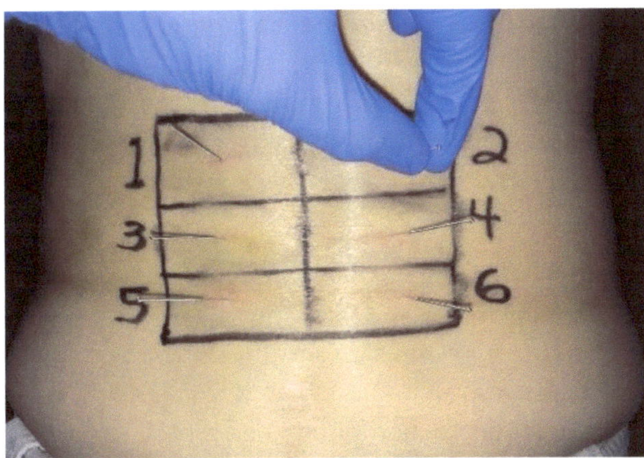

Figure 260: Sensory discrimination training in a patient with lumbar spinal stenosis. Training was begun with simple touch then progressed to needles. Six 1" needles were inserted into the paraspinal muscles and numbered 1-6. Each needle was gently manipulated for 3 seconds, and the patient was asked to guess which number needle was being manipulated. If wrong, the patient was corrected. The patient progressed the following week to a 9-box grid. Case shared with permission of patient and Legacy Medical Centers. This method is based on the work of Wand.[337]

Graphesthesia training involves practicing the ability to recognize writing on the skin. One study used **numbers** between 0 and 9, the first five **letters** of the alphabet, A, B, C, D, and E, in capitals and non-capital form (a, b, c, d, e).[333] Another study used letters and **three letter words**.[327] Both studies found that graphesthesia training on the lower back reduced LBP.[326,327]

Needling therapies may be adapted for sensory training. One study found that **acupuncture** was more effective in reducing LBP when paired with sensory discrimination training.[337] In this study the clinician inserted seven paired lumbar acupuncture needles and numbered them 1 through 14. The clinician then rotated one needle at a time for three seconds and asked the patient to identify which needle was being manipulated and corrected the patient if they made an error. It appears that the effect of needling is enhanced when it is used as a form of active sensory training.

The difficulty of sensory training can be modified to keep up with a patient's **localization accuracy**. One study increased the difficulty level when patients achieved an 80% accuracy.[327] For example, when working with localization over grids or points, the number of grids/points can be increased when a patient achieves a high accuracy level. Some patients may start with a grid of 4 blocks or 4 needles, progress to 6, then 9 and so on, as their sensory discrimination improves.

Visual feedback

Visual feedback training involves allowing the patient to see themselves during motor or sensory exercises. One study found that exercises in which patients visualized their back with a **mirror** were more effective in reducing LBP compared to exercises without a mirror.[335] Another study had patients lie prone on a table while watching a **real-time video** of their back for 1 minute. The study found that this intervention alone was able to reduce LBP intensity.[331] It is possible that visual feedback could be paired with other manual therapies and exercises to enhance their effectiveness.

Manual therapies

Manipulation and **manual therapy** may aid sensorimotor retraining when paired with feedback. One author hypothesized that constant verbalization and tactile feedback during manual therapy could improve cortical maps.[296] Examples of this include the practitioner telling the patient what their hand (or tool/instrument) is touching, and asking the patient how the treatment feels.[296]

Taping may provide tactile cues that alter movement patterns. One study found that the application of strapping tape along the paraspinal regions helped redistribute movement from the lower back to the hips and knees during a lifting task.[165] Taping could be used in conjunction with motor control to normalize biomechanics in those with sciatica.

Nutraceuticals

Vitamin D

Vitamin D is a hormone produced in the skin when exposed to ultraviolet-B radiation. It has widespread effects in the nervous and musculoskeletal systems, including lowering inflammation, protecting against nerve damage, and supporting normal muscle function.[339] Vitamin D deficiency is common in the united states with 42% of the population below 20 ng/mL.[340] Deficiency of vitamin D causes increased pain and muscle and nerve **hypersensitivity**.[339,341]

Vitamin D receptors are found in the spinal cord, spinal nerve roots, dorsal root ganglia, and glial cells.[339] These receptors are also thought to be involved in cartilage cell growth and **connective tissue production** in the IVD.[342] Genetic variation in vitamin D receptors has been hypothesized to explain the hereditary aspect of spinal degeneration.[343]

Sciatic pain is more common in those deficient in vitamin D. One study of people with low-back pain found that **radicular pain** was more common in those with low vitamin D levels.[344] Another similar study corroborated these findings, and found that those with LBP and low vitamin D were more likely to have **back-related leg pain**. Patients deficient in vitamin D (<20 ng/ml) had 3.6 times greater odds of having severe leg pain compared to those with normal vitamin D levels (>30 ng/ml).[345]

Vitamin D may reduce back and radicular pain in patients with chronic pain following **failed back surgery syndrome** (FBSS). One study of post-surgical patients found that raising vitamin D to normal levels with a dose of 20,000 IU/day for 10 days then maintenance at 600 IU/day reduced pain significantly.[346] Another case series of FBSS showed that taking 2,000-5,000 IU/day significantly reduced pain within a time frame of 3-6 weeks.[347]

Sulfur

Sulfur (sulphur) is the third most abundant mineral in the body. It is required for normal function of **connective tissue** in the IVD and production of the antioxidant **glutathione**. It is mostly obtained through consumption of sulfur-containing proteins, and a small amount comes from other sources like garlic, onion, broccoli, and mineral water.[348] Dietary deficiency of sulfur may be common especially among the elderly and in those that do not eat enough protein.[348]

Sulfur-containing connective tissue **proteoglycans** (proteins with attached sugars) help the IVDs to retain water by osmosis.[349] Water is what gives the discs their gelatinous and flexible properties. The amount of sulfate in the anulus fibrosus (the outer part of the disc) decreases with disc degeneration and aging.[350] Those with less sulfated proteoglycans in the disc are at a greater risk of disc degeneration.[342] Lower production of sulfated proteoglycans increases the likelihood of seeing a dark nucleus pulposus on T2-weighted MRI.[351] Sulfur is required for a healthy well-functioning disc.

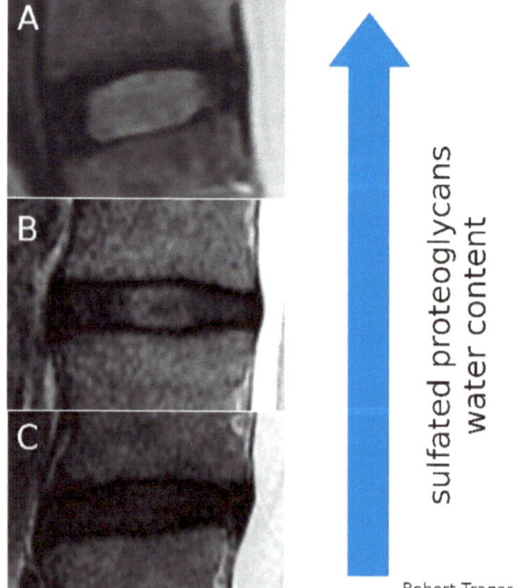

Figure 261: Correlation of sulfated proteoglycans with water retention and T2-weighted imaging appearance of nucleus pulposus. Normal disc (A), blurred disc (B), and "black" disc (C). The IVD nucleus normally has a bright white appearance which indicates high water content but becomes dark in degenerated discs due to dehydration. Dehydration correlates with a reduction of sulfated proteoglycans. Images from Robert Trager with permission from patients.

Chondroitin sulfate is a sulfur-containing **glycosaminoglycan** (GAG), an important connective tissue component of the IVD. Oral supplementation with this substance is thought to help rebuild the sulfated GAGs within degenerated discs.[349] One case study found that supplementation for two years with glucosamine, chondroitin sulfate (800-1,200 mg/day), and manganese helped reverse degenerative disc changes and alleviate discogenic sciatica and LBP.[349] Studies using labeled sulfate have found that it incorporates into the **nucleus pulposus** and **anulus fibrosus** of the IVD.[352] Chondroitin sulfate may help discogenic sciatica by supporting normal IVD connective tissue structure and function.

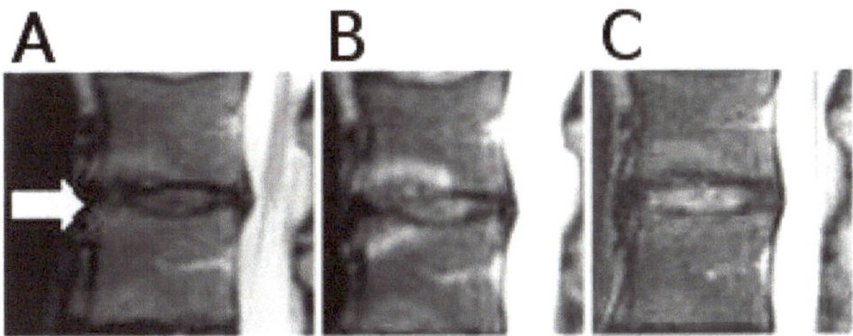

Figure 262: Improved disc hydration in a 56-year-old man over a 2-year span by taking glucosamine, chondroitin sulfate, and manganese ascorbate. Image A: Initial, B: 1 year post, and C: 2-years post. The water signal of the nucleus pulposus (arrow) transitions from dark to bright indicating greater hydration over time. Image 2003 van Blitterswijk et al; licensee BioMed Central Ltd. Image is open access: verbatim copying and redistribution is permitted in all media for any purpose (https://www.ncbi.nlm.nih.gov/pmc/articles/PMC165439/)

Dimethyl sulfoxide (**DMSO**) is a sulfur-containing liquid solvent rapidly absorbed through the skin. It reduces pain by slowing the conduction velocity of c-fibers, a type of nerve fiber involved in sciatic nerve pain.[353] DMSO helps protect neurons[354] by inhibiting the **NMDA receptor**[355] and scavenging free radicals.[356] One case series showed benefit of DSMO for back pain with radiation to the hips, buttocks, and legs at a dose of 10 to 15 mL of 90% DMSO applied topically two to three times daily.[357] At this concentration DMSO can cause a rash or unpleasant odor, however a weaker 50% solution may be more tolerable.[358] It is applied to the area of pain and gently spread and allowed to absorb. Dimethyl sulfoxide may help sciatica by reducing excessive sciatic nerve transmission and inflammation.

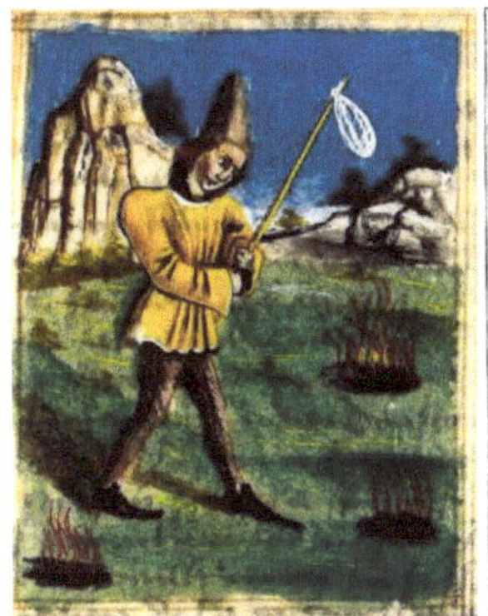
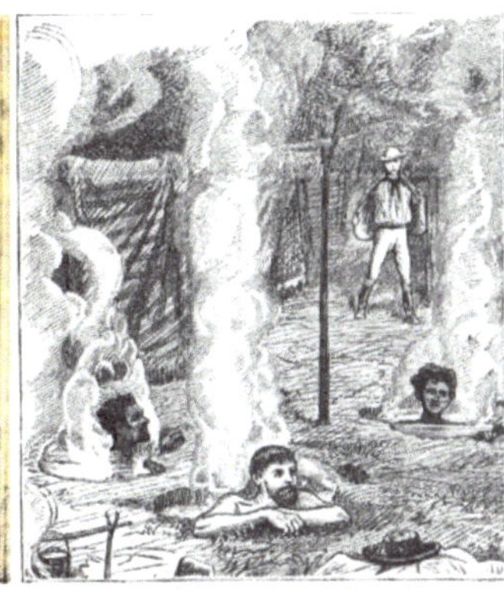

Figure 263: Left: Collecting sulphur, by Matthaeus Platearius of the medical school of Salerno, Italy, circa 1480-1500 CE, CC BY 4.0 License, Wellcome Images. Right: Bathing in the hot lakes, Brett's handy guide to New Zealand, 1890, Public domain

Indigenous and ancient peoples bathed in hot sulphur springs to treat sciatica. In the 1600's, early British explorers observed this practice of the native Māori in New Zealand.[360,361] Americans learned this from Native Americans who used the hot springs in Byron, California for sciatica.[362] Other examples include the peat and sulphur mud baths of Austria,[363] the hot springs of Hammam 'Ali, Yemen,[364] the Marienbad springs of the Czech Republic,[365] the Kissingen springs of Germany,[366] the hot thermal springs of Ischia, Italy,[367] and the Epsom springs[368,369] and hot sulphur springs of Bath, England.[370]

A medical text from 1782 described the use of sulphur-rich water of Bath for sciatica:[371]

> *"The waters of this spring, drunk and used as baths, and also pumped on the affected part, have performed distinguished cures in... chronic rheumatisms and sciatica..." (Black, p. 265)*

Many ancient medicines for sciatica included sulfur for example those of Aurelianus,[241] Paulus Aegineta,[89] and Galen.[372] Aegineta (c. 625-290 CE) recommended baths with euphorbium (resin of *Euphorbia*), adarce (a mineral sediment), black hellebore, castor, *Anacyclus pyrethrum* (pellitory), pepper, and dried wild grape.[89] He advised applying dried pine pitch, sulphur, and pepper sprinkled on the skin, and all covered with paper immediately after the bath.[89] British medical doctors briefly revived this treatment in the mid-1800s[373] and again in the early 1900s.[374] Some doctors have used dried sulfur to cover the leg affected by sciatica as was done in ancient times.[375]

Magnesium

Magnesium is a mineral that acts as an enzyme co-factor in reactions involving adenosine triphosphate (ATP), the energy currency of our cells. Over 300 enzyme systems use magnesium including those involved in nerve transmission, muscle contraction, and metabolism. Almost half of the United States population (48%) consumes less than the recommended amount of magnesium in the diet.[376] Magnesium deficiency causes **inflammation**, **muscle spasms** and cramps, weakness, and difficulty sleeping, all of which may be worsened by sciatica.

Magnesium has been successfully used to lower inflammation[377] and neuropathic pain.[378] It has shown benefit in trials for fibromyalgia[379] and migraine at a dose of 600 mg/day.[380] Animal studies have shown that magnesium protects the sciatic nerve from injury and helps it regenerate following injury.[381,382]

Magnesium is thought to help neurological conditions by **blocking the N-methyl-D-aspartate receptor** (**NMDAR**).[383] The NMDAR is a channel found in the cell membrane of neurons that contributes to spinal cord hyperexcitability and neuropathic pain.[384] When glutamate or glycine bind to it, it allows calcium to enter the neuron, which stimulates depolarization and transmission of nerve signals. Magnesium may reduce sciatic pain signals by preventing entry of calcium into neurons of the sciatic nerve.

Ancient physicians used magnesium to treat sciatica. Caelius Aurelianus (c. 450 CE) recommended using a topical application of *glebae calcis* (a mixture of calcium and magnesium), sulphur, mustard and water with a covering of soft wool soaked in hot sweet oil.[241] Dioscorides[246] (40-90 CE) and Galen[372] (c. 129-216 CE) of Turkey and Paulus Aegineta[89] (c. 625-290 CE) of Greece recommended using *adarces,* a salt product from the magnesium-rich salt lakes in Turkey, for sciatica.[391] Dioscorides wrote it "draw[s] fluids from depths, and it is good for sciatica."[246] Pliny (23-79 CE) recommended using salt "burnt at a white heat" (probably magnesium)[vi] taken internally or applied in bags for sciatica.[392]

Epsom salts are a therapeutic bath salt made of **magnesium sulfate**. This treatment is named after the springs in Epsom, England, which have a naturally high concentration of magnesium sulfate (2 grams per liter).[393] Medical literature recommending ingestion of Epsom salts for sciatica appeared through the 1800s[368,369] and bathing with the salts became more popular in the 1900s.

Ancient and indigenous peoples used natural mineral waters and geothermal springs to treat sciatica. The bodies of water they used are high in magnesium and/or sulfur. The human body is capable of absorbing magnesium and sulfur transdermally (through the skin). Research has shown that taking a bath in Epsom Salt raises plasma concentration of magnesium and sulfur.[394]

Table 41: Natural waters historically used for sciatica (with minerals in mg/L): Magnesium (Mg)

Spring	Mg	Sulfate
Epsom, England[385]	286	1,860
Ischia, italy[386]	127	553
Marienbad, Czech Republic[387]	125	4,049
Kissingen, Germany[387]	123	782
Byron, California[387]	81	1,285
Wildbad lavaredo, Germany[388]	75	848
Bath, England[389]	57	1,015
Te Aroha, New Zealand[390]	4	390

Water soluble vitamins

Vitamin B12 participates in DNA regulation, metabolism, and stimulates production of **myelin**, the insulating material around nerves. **Methylcobalamin**, a form of B12, has been shown to increase the distance that patients with LSS can walk before sciatic symptoms begin, at a dose of 0.5mg/day.[395] Another study showed that intramuscular injections of B12 reduced LBP and sciatic pain.[396] Vitamin B12 is thought to help sciatica by increasing production of proteins and myelin required to regenerate the injured nerve.[396]

Enzymes need adequate **Vitamin C**, also called L-ascorbic acid or ascorbate, to produce **collagen**. Collagen is the major protein of IVDs and connective tissue throughout the body. Vitamin C also has anti-inflammatory properties and suppresses C-reactive protein which is often elevated in sciatica.[397] Those

[vi] *Magnesium burns pure white, has therapeutic value, and is more abundant in nature than titanium which also burns white.*

deficient in vitamin C have greater odds of developing back pain with radiating pain below the knee.[398] One study of a patient with scurvy-related sciatica (and other problems) was relieved of his symptoms in three weeks using a total daily dose of 300 mg/day.[399] Vitamin C deficiency has been suggested to be a cause of disc degeneration and sciatica due to its importance in suppression of inflammation and its role in collagen production in the discs.[397]

Other supplements

Palmitoylethanolamide (PEA) is a naturally occurring lipid found in our body. It inhibits mast cells, which are often responsible for inflammation along the sciatic nerve pathway.[400–402] It also acts upon cannabinoid receptors which helps reduce inflammation and pain.[401–403] Multiple studies have shown that it reduces sciatic pain and improves function. The typical dose is 600 mg per day.[400–404]

Lipoic acid, also called **α-lipoic acid** (alpha lipoic acid) and **thioctic acid**, is a naturally occurring sulfur-containing compound. Lipoic acid acts as an antioxidant, increases glutathione production, and increases vasodilation and blood flow.[405] It is best known as a therapy for diabetic neuropathy, but new research shows that it is effective in treating discogenic sciatica with a dose of 600mg/day.[406,407] It is thought that lipoic acid helps sciatica by increasing blood flow to the small blood vessels of the injured sciatic nerve roots.[407]

Acetyl-L-carnitine is an amino acid derivative that is produced by the human body. It allows the cellular energy-producing centers in the body, the mitochondria, to function properly. Acetyl-L-carnitine is best known for reducing pain, improving sensory perception, and helping nerve fibers regenerate in diabetic neuropathy.[408] One study showed that it aids in recovery from discogenic sciatica at a dose of 1,180 mg/day.[406] Acetyl-L-carnitine may help sciatica due to its benefits on neuronal mitochondria.

Omega-3 (ω-3) fatty acids are part of cell membranes including neurons.[409] These are found in fish oil products and some vegan sources including marine algae. It is thought that modern diets include more omega-6 fatty acids than omega-3s and this imbalance promotes inflammation.[409] Degenerative disc changes are slightly less common in those with a high dietary intake of fish.[410]

Docosahexaenoic acid (DHA) and eicosapentaeneoic acid (EPA) are types of omega-3s that suppress inflammation and support the formation of myelin (the insulating nerve sheath).[409] A meta-analysis including 823 patients found that omega-3 fatty acids were effective in treating inflammatory joint pain.[411] One study found that 1,200 grams omega-3 DHA and EPA total per day improved discogenic pain in 60% of 125 patients.[412] Another study showed that DHA and EPA reduced symptoms in those with neuropathic pain and radiculopathy.[413] Omega-3 fatty acids may help sciatica by reducing inflammation and supporting normal integrity of the nerve sheath.

Melatonin is a hormone best-known for its role in sleep; however, it also affects the IVD. Melatonin stimulates NP cells to produce aggregan,[414] a water-binding proteoglycan that helps the disc stay hydrated. Animal studies suggest that damage to the pineal gland leads to disc degeneration.[415] Research in humans has found a correlation between pineal gland calcification and disc degeneration. When the pineal gland is calcified it produces less melatonin.[416] However, evidence is lacking regarding treatment of sciatica with melatonin.

References

1. Konstantinou, K. *et al.* Characteristics of patients with low back and leg pain seeking treatment in primary care: baseline results from the ATLAS cohort study. *BMC musculo-skeletal disorders* **16**, 332 (2015).
2. Fraser, S., Roberts, L. & Murphy, E. Cauda equina syndrome: a literature review of its definition and clinical presentation. *Archives of physical medicine and rehabilitation* **90**, 1964–1968 (2009).
3. Lingawi, S. S. How often is low back pain or sciatica not due to lumbar disc disease? *Neurosciences (Riyadh)* **9**, 94–97 (2004).
4. McEvoy, C., Wiles, L., Bernhardsson, S. & Grimmer, K. Triage for Patients with Spinal Complaints: A Systematic Review of the Literature. *Physiotherapy Research International* **22**, e1639 (2017).
5. Kindrachuk, D. R. & Fourney, D. R. Spine surgery referrals redirected through a multi-disciplinary care pathway: effects of nonsurgeon triage including MRI utilization. *Journal of Neurosurgery: Spine* **20**, 87–92 (2013).
6. Lewis, R. A. *et al.* Comparative clinical effectiveness of management strategies for sciatica: systematic review and network meta-analyses. *Spine J* **15**, 1461–1477 (2015).
7. Tang, S., Mo, Z. & Zhang, R. Acupuncture for lumbar disc herniation: a systematic review and meta-analysis. *Acupuncture in Medicine* **36**, 62–70 (2018).
8. Zou, Z. Fifty-two Cases of the Piriformis Syndrome Treated by Centro-square Needling. *Journal of Traditional Chinese Medicine* **29**, 11–12 (2009).
9. Sherman, K. J. *et al.* Characteristics of patients with chronic back pain who benefit from acupuncture. *BMC Musculoskeletal Disorders* **10**, 114 (2009).
10. Flynn, T. *et al.* A clinical prediction rule for classifying patients with low back pain who demonstrate short-term improvement with spinal manipulation. *Spine* **27**, 2835–2843 (2002).
11. Fritz, J. M. *et al.* Is there a subgroup of patients with low back pain likely to benefit from mechanical traction?: Results of a randomized clinical trial and subgrouping analysis. *Spine* **32**, E793–E800 (2007).
12. Fritz, J. M., Cleland, J. A. & Childs, J. D. Subgrouping patients with low back pain: evolution of a classification approach to physical therapy. *journal of orthopaedic & sports physical therapy* **37**, 290–302 (2007).
13. Fitzsimmons, D. *et al.* Cost-effectiveness of different strategies to manage patients with sciatica. *PAIN®* **155**, 1318–1327 (2014).

14. Vroomen, P. C. A. J., Krom, M. C. T. F. M. de & Knottnerus, J. A. Predicting the outcome of sciatica at short-term follow-up. *British Journal of General Practice* **52**, 119–123 (2002).
15. Kennedy, D. J. & Noh, M. Y. The role of core stabilization in lumbosacral radiculopathy. *Physical medicine and rehabilitation clinics of North America* **22**, 91–103 (2011).
16. Coxhead, C., Meade, T., Inskip, H., North, W. & Troup, J. Multicentre trial of physiotherapy in the management of sciatic symptoms. *The Lancet* **317**, 1065–1068 (1981).
17. Jewell, D. V. & Riddle, D. L. Interventions That Increase or Decrease the Likelihood of a Meaningful Improvement in Physical Health in Patients With Sciatica. *Phys Ther* **85**, 1139–1150 (2005).
18. Bronfort, G. *et al.* Spinal manipulation and home exercise with advice for subacute and chronic back-related leg pain: a trial with adaptive allocation. *Annals of internal medicine* **161**, 381–391 (2014).
19. Qu, M., Ding, X. N., Liu, H. B. & Liu, Y. Q. [Clinical observation on acupuncture combined with nerve block for treatment of lumbar disc herniation]. *Zhongguo Zhen Jiu* **30**, 633–636 (2010).
20. Qin, Z., Liu, X., Wu, J., Zhai, Y. & Liu, Z. Effectiveness of acupuncture for treating sciatica: a systematic review and meta-analysis. *Evidence-Based Complementary and Alternative Medicine* **2015**, (2015).
21. Ramakrishnan, A., Webb, K. M. & Cowperthwaite, M. C. One-year outcomes of early-crossover patients in a cohort receiving nonoperative care for lumbar disc herniation. *Journal of Neurosurgery: Spine* **27**, 391–396 (2017).
22. Amundsen, T. *et al.* Lumbar Spinal Stenosis: Clinical and Radiologic Features. *Spine* **20**, 1178 (1995).
23. Zaina, F., Tomkins-Lane, C., Carragee, E. & Negrini, S. Surgical versus non-surgical treatment for lumbar spinal stenosis. *Cochrane Database Syst Rev* **12**, (2012).
24. Han, S. K., Kim, Y. S., Kim, T. H. & Kang, S. H. Surgical Treatment of Piriformis Syndrome. *Clinics in orthopedic surgery* **9**, 136–144 (2017).
25. Michel, F. *et al.* Piriformis muscle syndrome: Diagnostic criteria and treatment of a monocentric series of 250 patients. *Annals of Physical and Rehabilitation Medicine* **56**, 371–383 (2013).
26. Fishman, L. M. *et al.* Piriformis syndrome: diagnosis, treatment, and outcome—a 10-year study. *Archives of physical medicine and rehabilitation* **83**, 295–301 (2002).
27. Thakur, J. D. *et al.* Early intervention in cauda equina syndrome associated with better outcomes: a myth or reality? Insights from the Nationwide Inpatient Sample database (2005–2011). *The Spine Journal* **17**, 1435–1448 (2017).
28. Schoenfeld, A. J. & Bono, C. M. Does Surgical Timing Influence Functional Recovery After Lumbar Discectomy? A Systematic Review. *Clin Orthop Relat Res* **473**, 1963–1970 (2015).
29. Jacobs, W. C. *et al.* Surgery versus conservative management of sciatica due to a lumbar herniated disc: a systematic review. *European Spine Journal* **20**, 513–522 (2011).
30. Mahmood, T. S. *et al.* Clinical Results of 30 years surgery on 2026 patients with lumbar disc herniation. *World Spin Column J* **3**, 80–6 (2012).
31. Suri, P., Carlson, J. & Rainville, J. Nonoperative treatment for lumbosacral radiculopathy: what factors predict treatment failure?, Nonoperative Treatment for Lumbosacral Radiculopathy: What Factors Predict Treatment Failure? *Clin Orthop Relat Res* **473, 473**, 1931, 1931–1939 (2015).
32. Motiei-Langroudi, R., Sadeghian, H. & Seddighi, A. S. Clinical and magnetic resonance imaging factors which may predict the need for surgery in lumbar disc herniation. *Asian spine journal* **8**, 446–452 (2014).
33. Kim, H.-J. *et al.* Factors influencing the surgical decision for the treatment of degenerative lumbar stenosis in a preference-based shared decision-making process. *Eur Spine J* **24**, 339–347 (2015).
34. Matsudaira, K. *et al.* Predictive Factors for Subjective Improvement in Lumbar Spinal Stenosis Patients with Nonsurgical Treatment: A 3-Year Prospective Cohort Study. *PLOS ONE* **11**, e0148584 (2016).
35. Kurd, M. F. *et al.* Predictors of treatment choice in lumbar spinal stenosis: a spine patient outcomes research trial study. *Spine* **37**, 1702–1707 (2012).
36. Buttermann, G. R. Treatment of Lumbar Disc Herniation: Epidural Steroid Injection Compared with Discectomy: A Prospective, Randomized Study. *JBJS* **86**, 670–679 (2004).
37. Brötz, D. *et al.* A prospective trial of mechanical physiotherapy for lumbar disk prolapse. *J Neurol* **250**, 746–749 (2003).
38. Jawish, R. M., Assoum, H. A., Khamis, C. F. & others. Anatomical, clinical and electrical observations in piriformis syndrome. *J Orthop Surg Res* **5**, 3 (2010).
39. Delitto, A., Piva, S. R., Moore, C. G. & Welch, W. C. Surgery versus nonsurgical treatment of lumbar spinal stenosis. *Ann Intern Med* **163**, 397–8 (2015).
40. Fernandez, M. *et al.* Surgery or physical activity in the management of sciatica: a systematic review and meta-analysis. *European Spine Journal* **25**, 3495–3512 (2016).
41. Sabnis, A. B. & Diwan, A. D. The timing of surgery in lumbar disc prolapse: A systematic review. *Indian journal of orthopaedics* **48**, 127 (2014).
42. Arts, M. P. & Peul, W. C. Timing and minimal access surgery for sciatica: a summary of two randomized trials. *Acta Neurochirurgica* **153**, 967–974 (2011).
43. Hadžić, E., Dizdarević, K., Hajdarpašić, E., Džurlić, A. & Ahmetspahić, A. Low back and lumbar radicular syndrome: comparative study of the operative and non-operative treatment. *Medicinski Glasnik* **10**, (2013).
44. Sedighi, M. & Haghnegahdar, A. Lumbar Disk Herniation Surgery: Outcome and Predictors. *Global Spine Journal* **4**, 233–243 (2014).
45. Murphy, D. D. R. *Clinical Reasoning in Spine Pain. Volume I: Primary Management of Low Back Disorders Using the CRISP Protocols*. (Donald R. Murphy, 2013).
46. Gadjradj, P. S. *et al.* Management of symptomatic lumbar disk herniation: an international perspective. *Spine* **42**, 1826–1834 (2017).
47. Peul, W. C., Brand, R., Thomeer, R. T. W. M. & Koes, B. W. Improving prediction of "inevitable" surgery during non-surgical treatment of sciatica. *PAIN* **138**, 571–576 (2008).
48. Folman, Y., Shabat, S., Catz, A. & Gepstein, R. Late results of surgery for herniated lumbar disk as related to duration of preoperative symptoms and type of herniation. *Surgical Neurology* **70**, 398–401 (2008).
49. Arts, M. P., Peul, W. C., Koes, B. W. & Thomeer, R. T. W. M. Management of sciatica due to lumbar disc herniation in the Netherlands: a survey among spine surgeons. *Journal of Neurosurgery: Spine* **9**, 32–39 (2008).
50. Peul, W. C. *et al.* Surgery versus Prolonged Conservative Treatment for Sciatica. *New England Journal of Medicine* **356**, 2245–2256 (2007).
51. Chiang, S.-L. *et al.* Cigarette smoking dose as a predictor of need for surgical intervention in patients with lumbar disk herniation. *Journal of Medical Sciences* **34**, 23 (2014).
52. Wilson, C. A., Roffey, D. M., Chow, D., Alkherayf, F. & Wai, E. K. A systematic review of preoperative predictors for postoperative clinical outcomes following lumbar discectomy. *The Spine Journal* **16**, 1413–1422 (2016).
53. Alodaibi, F. A., Fritz, J. M., Thackeray, A., Koppenhaver, S. L. & Hebert, J. J. The Fear Avoidance Model predicts short-term pain and disability following lumbar disc surgery. *PLOS ONE* **13**, e0193566 (2018).
54. White, A. P., Harrop, J. & Dettori, J. R. Can clinical and radiological findings predict surgery for lumbar disc herniation? A systematic literature review. *Evid Based Spine Care J* **3**, 45–52 (2012).
55. Neuman, B. J. *et al.* Patient Factors That Influence Decision Making: Randomization versus Observational Nonoperative versus Observational Operative Treatment for Adult Symptomatic Lumbar Scoliosis (ASLS). *Spine (Phila Pa 1976)* **41**, E349–E358 (2016).
56. Peul, W. C., Arts, M. P., Brand, R. & Koes, B. W. Timing of surgery for sciatica: subgroup analysis alongside a randomized trial. *Eur Spine J* **18**, 538–545 (2009).
57. Kleinstueck, F. *et al.* The outcome of decompression surgery for lumbar herniated disc is influenced by the level of concomitant preoperative low back pain. *European Spine Journal* **20**, 1166–1173 (2011).
58. el Barzouhi, A. *et al.* Prognostic value of magnetic resonance imaging findings in patients with sciatica. *Journal of Neurosurgery: Spine* **24**, 978–985 (2016).
59. Ha, D. H., Shim, D. M., Kim, T. K., Oh, S. K. & Kim, J. Relative Risk of Operation between Lumbar Far Lateral Disc Herniation and Posterolateral Disc Herniation: A Retrospective Cohort Study. *Journal of the Korean Orthopaedic Association* **52**, 442–447 (2017).
60. Park, H. W. *et al.* The Comparisons of Surgical Outcomes and Clinical Characteristics between the Far Lateral Lumbar Disc Herniations and the Paramedian Lumbar Disc Herniations. *Korean J Spine* **10**, 155–159 (2013).
61. Krishnan, V., Rajasekaran, S., Aiyer, S. N., Kanna, R. & Shetty, A. P. Clinical and radiological factors related to the presence of motor deficit in lumbar disc prolapse: a prospective analysis of 70 consecutive cases with neurological deficit. *Eur Spine J* **26**, 2642–2649 (2017).
62. Chiu, C.-C. *et al.* The probability of spontaneous regression of lumbar herniated disc: a systematic review. *Clinical rehabilitation* **29**, 184–195 (2015).
63. Takada, E., Takahashi, M. & Shimada, K. Natural history of lumbar disc hernia with radicular leg pain: Spontaneous MRI changes of the herniated mass and correlation with clinical outcome. *Journal of orthopaedic surgery (Hong Kong)* **9**, 1 (2001).
64. Suri, P., Boyko, E. J., Goldberg, J., Forsberg, C. W. & Jarvik, J. G. Longitudinal associations between incident lumbar spine MRI findings and chronic low back pain or radicular symptoms: retrospective analysis of data from the longitudinal assessment of imaging and disability of the back (LAIDBACK). *BMC musculoskeletal disorders* **15**, 1 (2014).
65. Jensen, T. S., Albert, H. B., Sorensen, J. S., Manniche, C. & Leboeuf-Yde, C. Magnetic Resonance Imaging Findings as Predictors of Clinical Outcome in Patients With Sciatica Receiving Active Conservative Treatment. *Journal of Manipulative & Physiological Therapeutics* **30**, 98–108 (2007).
66. Ito, T., Takano, Y. & Yuasa, N. Types of lumbar herniated disc and clinical course. *Spine* **26**, 648–651 (2001).
67. Fardon, D. F. *et al.* Lumbar disc nomenclature: version 2.0: Recommendations of the combined task forces of the North American Spine Society, the American Society of Spine Radiology and the American Society of Neuroradiology. *The Spine Journal* **14**, 2525–2545 (2014).
68. Surkitt, L. D., Ford, J. J., Hahne, A. J., Pizzari, T. & McMeeken, J. M. Efficacy of directional preference management for low back pain: a systematic review. *Physical therapy* **92**, 652–665 (2012).

69. Albert, H. B., Hauge, E. & Manniche, C. Centralization in patients with sciatica: are pain responses to repeated movement and positioning associated with outcome or types of disc lesions? *Eur Spine J* **21**, 630–636 (2012).
70. Svensson, G. L., Wendt, G. K. & Thomeé, R. A structured physiotherapy treatment model can provide rapid relief to patients who qualify for lumbar disc surgery: a prospective cohort study. *Journal of rehabilitation medicine* **46**, 233–240 (2014).
71. Bybee, R. F., Olsen, D. L., Cantu-Boncser, G., Allen, H. C. & Byars, A. Centralization of symptoms and lumbar range of motion in patients with low back pain. *Physiotherapy theory and practice* **25**, 257–267 (2009).
72. Hagovska, M., Takáč, P. & Petrovičová, J. Changes in the Muscle Tension of Erector Spinae after the Application of the McKenzie Method in Patients with Chronic Low Back Pain. *Phys Med Rehab Kuror* **24**, 133–140 (2014).
73. May, S., Gardiner, E., Young, S. & Klaber-Moffett, J. Predictor Variables for a Positive Long-Term Functional Outcome in Patients with Acute and Chronic Neck and Back Pain Treated with a McKenzie Approach: A Secondary Analysis. *J Man Manip Ther* **16**, 155–160 (2008).
74. Broetz, D., Burkard, S. & Weller, M. A prospective study of mechanical physiotherapy for lumbar disk prolapse: Five year follow-up and final report. *NeuroRehabilitation* **26**, 155–158 (2010).
75. Kilpikoski, S., Laslett, M., Airaksinen, O. & Kankaanpää, M. Pain centralization and lumbar disc MRI findings in chronic low back pain patients. *International Journal of Mechanical Diagnosis and Therapy* **6**, 3–11 (2011).
76. Kilpikoski, S. *The McKenzie method in assessing, classifying and treating non-specific low back pain in adults with special reference to the centralization phenomenon*. (University of Jyväskylä, 2010).
77. Broetz, D. *et al.* Lumbar disk prolapse: Response to mechanical physiotherapy in the absence of changes in magnetic resonance imaging. Report of 11 cases. *NeuroRehabilitation* **23**, 289–294 (2008).
78. Bohen, S., Ramey, A., Rudolph, K., Sinn, E. & Tooley, D. Pain centralization and lumbar disc mri findings in chronic low back pain patients. *International Journal of Mechanical Diagnosis and Therapy* **6**, (2011).
79. Machado, L. A. C. Bs. (Honours), de Souza, M. von S. Bs. (Honours), Ferreira, P. H. & Ferreira, M. L. The McKenzie Method for Low Back Pain: A Systematic Review of the Literature With a Meta-Analysis Approach. *Spine April 20, 2006* **31**, (2006).
80. Longtin, C. *et al.* Systematic flexion-based approach for patients with radiological signs of lumbar spinal stenosis: Myth or reality? A retrospective study. *Annals of Physical and Rehabilitation Medicine* doi:10.1016/j.rehab.2017.03.005
81. Oka, H. *et al.* A comparative study of three conservative treatments in patients with lumbar spinal stenosis: lumbar spinal stenosis with acupuncture and physical therapy study (LAP study). *BMC complementary and alternative medicine* **18**, 19 (2018).
82. Albert, H. B. & Manniche, C. The efficacy of systematic active conservative treatment for patients with severe sciatica: a single-blind, randomized, clinical, controlled trial. *Spine* **37**, 531–542 (2012).
83. Backstrom, K. M., Whitman, J. M. & Flynn, T. W. Lumbar spinal stenosis-diagnosis and management of the aging spine. *Manual Therapy* **16**, 308–317 (2011).
84. Browder, D. A., Childs, J. D., Cleland, J. A. & Fritz, J. M. Effectiveness of an extension-oriented treatment approach in a subgroup of subjects with low back pain: a randomized clinical trial. *Physical therapy* **87**, 1608–1618 (2007).
85. Williams, P. C. Lesions of the Lumbosacral Spine. *J Bone Joint Surg Am* **19**, 690–703 (1937).
86. Ye, C. *et al.* Comparison of lumbar spine stabilization exercise versus general exercise in young male patients with lumbar disc herniation after 1 year of follow-up. *Int J Clin Exp Med* **8**, 9869–9875 (2015).
87. Bakhtiary, A. H., Safavi-Farokhi, Z. & Rezasoltani, A. Lumbar stabilizing exercises improve activities of daily living in patients with lumbar disc herniation. *Journal of Back and musculoskeletal Rehabilitation* **18**, 55–60 (2005).
88. Hippocrates, Coxe, J. R. & Galen. *The writings of Hippocrates and Galen*. (Philadelphia : Lindsay and Blakiston, 1846).
89. Aegineta, P. *The Seven Books of Paulus Ægineta*. (Sydenham Society, 1844).
90. Salguero, C. P. *The Spiritual Healing of Traditional Thailand*. (Findhorn Press, 2006).
91. Deyo, R. A., Diehl, A. K. & Rosenthal, M. How many days of bed rest for acute low back pain? *New England Journal of Medicine* **315**, 1064–1070 (1986).
92. Shacklock, M. *Clinical Neurodynamics: A New System of Neuromusculoskeletal Treatment, 1e*. (Butterworth-Heinemann, 2005).
93. Liebenson, C. *Rehabilitation Of The Spine: A Practitioner's Manual*. (Lippincott Williams & Wilkins, 2007).
94. Johnston, S. L., Campbell, M. R., Scheuring, R. & Feiveson, A. H. Risk of Herniated Nucleus Pulposus Among U.S. Astronauts. *Aviation, Space, and Environmental Medicine* **81**, 566–574 (2010).
95. Hagen, K. are B., Jamtvedt, G., Hilde, G. & Winnem, M. F. The updated Cochrane review of bed rest for low back pain and sciatica. *Spine* **30**, 542–546 (2005).
96. Belavý, D. L., Albracht, K., Bruggemann, G.-P., Vergroesen, P.-P. A. & Dieën, J. H. van. Can Exercise Positively Influence the Intervertebral Disc? *Sports Med* **46**, 473–485 (2016).
97. Stuempfle, K. & Drury, D. The Physiological Consequences of Bed Rest. *Journal of Exercise Physiology* (2007).
98. Belavý, D. L., Gast, U. & Felsenberg, D. Exercise and transversus abdominis muscle atrophy after 60-d bed rest. *Medicine and science in sports and exercise* **49**, 238–246 (2017).
99. Jensen, O. K., Nielsen, C. V. & Stengaard-Pedersen, K. One-year prognosis in sick-listed low back pain patients with and without radiculopathy. Prognostic factors influencing pain and disability. *The Spine Journal* **10**, 659–675 (2010).
100. Hebert, P. R., Barice, E. J. & Hennekens, C. H. Treatment of Low Back Pain: The Potential Clinical and Public Health Benefits of Topical Herbal Remedies. *J Altern Complement Med* **20**, 219–220 (2014).
101. Saal, J. A. & Saal, J. S. Nonoperative treatment of herniated lumbar intervertebral disc with radiculopathy: an outcome study. *Spine* **14**, 431–437 (1989).
102. Neufeld, J. H. Induced narrowing and back adaptation of lumbar intervertebral discs in biomechanically stressed rats. *Spine* **17**, 811–816 (1992).
103. Arun, R. *et al.* 2009 ISSLS Prize Winner: What influence does sustained mechanical load have on diffusion in the human intervertebral disc?: an in vivo study using serial postcontrast magnetic resonance imaging. *Spine* **34**, 2324–2337 (2009).
104. Hicks, G. E., Fritz, J. M., Delitto, A. & McGill, S. M. Preliminary Development of a Clinical Prediction Rule for Determining Which Patients With Low Back Pain Will Respond to a Stabilization Exercise Program. *Archives of Physical Medicine and Rehabilitation* **86**, 1753–1762 (2005).
105. Vostatek, P., Novak, D., Rychnovský, T. & Rychnovská, Š. Diaphragm postural function analysis using magnetic resonance imaging. *PloS one* **8**, e56724 (2013).
106. Vera-Garcia, F. J., Elvira, J. L. L., Brown, S. H. M. & McGill, S. M. Effects of abdominal stabilization maneuvers on the control of spine motion and stability against sudden trunk perturbations. *J Electromyogr Kinesiol* **17**, 556–567 (2007).
107. McGill, S. M. & Karpowicz, A. Exercises for spine stabilization: motion/motor patterns, stability progressions, and clinical technique. *Archives of physical medicine and rehabilitation* **90**, 118–126 (2009).
108. Kirkaldy-Willis, W. H. & Cassidy, J. D. Spinal manipulation in the treatment of low-back pain. *Canadian Family Physician* **31**, 535 (1985).
109. McMorland, G., Suter, E., Casha, S., du Plessis, S. J. & Hurlbert, R. J. Manipulation or Microdiskectomy for Sciatica? A Prospective Randomized Clinical Study. *Journal of Manipulative and Physiological Therapeutics* **33**, 576–584 (2010).
110. Ehrler, M. *et al.* Symptomatic, MRI Confirmed, Lumbar Disc Herniations: A Comparison of Outcomes Depending on the Type and Anatomical Axial Location of the Hernia in Patients Treated With High-Velocity, Low-Amplitude Spinal Manipulation. *Journal of Manipulative & Physiological Therapeutics* **39**, 192–199 (2016).
111. Oths, K. S. & Hinojosa, S. Z. *Healing by Hand: Manual Medicine and Bonesetting in Global Perspective*. (Rowman Altamira, 2004).
112. Senn, N. *Tahiti: The Island Paradise*. (W. B. Conkey, 1906).
113. Leach, R. A. *The Chiropractic Theories: A Textbook of Scientific Research*. (Lippincott Williams & Wilkins, 2004).
114. Smith, O. G., Langworthy, S. M. & Paxson, M. C. *A Text Book, Modernized Chiropractic*. (Laurance Press Company, 1906).
115. Morris, J. Sciatica. *The Alabama Medical Journal* **18**, (1905).
116. Goldthwait, J. E., Osgood, R. B. & Painter, C. F. *Diseases of the Bones and Joints: Clinical Studies*. (Leonard, 1909).
117. Magunson, P. B. Backache--Some disputed points in the mechanics thereof. *International Clinics* **4**, (1916).
118. Fiske, E. Mechanical influences in sciatica. *Am J Orthop surg* **19**, 563 (1921).
119. Zhang, W. *et al.* Therapeutic effects of Chinese osteopathy in patients with lumbar disc herniation. *The American journal of Chinese medicine* **41**, 983–994 (2013).
120. Feng, W., Wang, F., Bi, Y., Xu, K. & Wang, S. Clinical study on the treatment of sequestrated lumbar disk herniation by feng's spinal manipulation. *Int J Clin Exp Med* **9**, 18698–18706 (2016).
121. Feng, Y., Gao, Y., Yang, W. & Feng, T. Reduction in nerve root compression by the nucleus pulposus after Feng's Spinal Manipulation. *Neural Regen Res* **8**, 1139–1145 (2013).
122. Santilli, V., Beghi, E. & Finucci, S. Chiropractic manipulation in the treatment of acute back pain and sciatica with disc protrusion: a randomized double-blind clinical trial of active and simulated spinal manipulations. *The Spine Journal* **6**, 131–137 (2006).
123. Stern, P. J., Cote, P. & Cassidy, J. D. A series of consecutive cases of low back pain with radiating leg pain treated by chiropractors. *Journal of manipulative and physiological therapeutics* **18**, 335–342 (1994).
124. Leemann, S., Peterson, C. K., Schmid, C., Anklin, B. & Humphreys, B. K. Outcomes of Acute and Chronic Patients With Magnetic Resonance Imaging–Confirmed Symptomatic Lumbar Disc Herniations Receiving High-Velocity, Low-Amplitude, Spinal Manipulative Therapy: A Prospective Observational Cohort Study With One-Year Follow-Up. *Journal of Manipulative & Physiological Therapeutics* **37**, 155–163 (2014).
125. Oliphant, D. Safety of spinal manipulation in the treatment of lumbar disk herniations: a systematic review and risk assessment. *Journal of Manipulative and Physiological Therapeutics* **27**, 197–210 (2004).

126. Visser, L. H. *et al.* Treatment of the sacroiliac joint in patients with leg pain: a randomized-controlled trial. *Eur Spine J* **22**, 2310–2317 (2013).
127. Gay, R. E., Bronfort, G. & Evans, R. L. Distraction manipulation of the lumbar spine: a review of the literature. *Journal of manipulative and physiological therapeutics* **28**, 266–273 (2005).
128. Gudavalli, M. R., Olding, K., Joachim, G. & Cox, J. M. Chiropractic Distraction Spinal Manipulation on Postsurgical Continued Low Back and Radicular Pain Patients: A Retrospective Case Series. *Journal of Chiropractic Medicine* (2016).
129. Han, L. *et al.* Short-term study on risk-benefit outcomes of two spinal manipulative therapies in the treatment of acute radiculopathy caused by lumbar disc herniation: study protocol for a randomized controlled trial. *Trials* **16**, (2015).
130. Mohanty, P. P. & Pattnaik, M. Mobilisation of the thoracic spine in the management of spondylolisthesis. *J Bodyw Mov Ther* **20**, 598–603 (2016).
131. Juan López Díaz. *POLD CONCEPT - ENGLISH PRESENTATION.*
132. López-Díaz, J. V., Arias-Buría, J. L., Lopez-Gordo, E., Lopez Gordo, S. & Aros Oyarzún, A. P. Effectiveness of continuous vertebral resonant oscillation using the POLD method in the treatment of lumbar disc hernia". A randomized controlled pilot study. *Manual Therapy* **20**, 481–486 (2015).
133. Mulligan, B. R. *Manual Therapy: Nags, Snags, MWMs, etc - 6th Edition.* (Orthopedic Physical Therapy Products, 2010).
134. Yadav, S., Nijhawan, M. A. & Panda, P. Effectiveness of spinal mobilization with leg movement (SMWLM) in patients with lumbar radiculopathy (L5/S1 nerve root) in lumbar disc herniation. *Int J Physiother Res* **2**, 712–18 (2014).
135. Morrison, M. The best back to manipulate? *Annals of the Royal College of Surgeons of England* **66**, 52 (1984).
136. Peterson, C. K. *et al.* Symptomatic Magnetic Resonance Imaging–Confirmed Lumbar Disk Herniation Patients: A Comparative Effectiveness Prospective Observational Study of 2 Age- and Sex-Matched Cohorts Treated With Either High-Velocity, Low-Amplitude Spinal Manipulative Therapy or Imaging-Guided Lumbar Nerve Root Injections. *Journal of Manipulative and Physiological Therapeutics* **36**, 218–225 (2013).
137. Keane, J. R. Neurectasy The short history of therapeutic nerve stretching and suspension. *Neurology* **40**, 829–829 (1990).
138. Bryant, T. *A Manual for the practice of surgery.* (H.C. Lea, 1885).
139. Halley, G. The Surgical Treatment of Sciatica. *Scottish Medical and Surgical Journal* **10**, (1902).
140. Marshall, J. Neurectasy; or Nerve-Stretching for the Relief or Cure of Pain. (1887).
141. Brown, C. L. *et al.* The effects of neurodynamic mobilization on fluid dispersion within the tibial nerve at the ankle: an unembalmed cadaveric study. *Journal of Manual & Manipulative Therapy* **19**, 26–34 (2011).
142. Ridehalgh, C. Straight leg raise treatment for individuals with spinally referred leg pain: exploring characteristics that influence outcome. (University of Brighton, 2014).
143. Santos, F. M. *et al.* Neural mobilization reverses behavioral and cellular changes that characterize neuropathic pain in rats. *Mol Pain* **8**, 57 (2012).
144. Schäfer, A., Hall, T., Müller, G. & Briffa, K. Outcomes differ between subgroups of patients with low back and leg pain following neural manual therapy: a prospective cohort study. *European Spine Journal* **20**, 482–490 (2011).
145. Scrimshaw, S. V. & Maher, C. G. Randomized controlled trial of neural mobilization after spinal surgery. *Spine* **26**, 2647–2652 (2001).
146. Ellis, R. F. Neurodynamic evaluation of the sciatic nerve during neural mobilisation: ultrasound imaging assessment of sciatic nerve movement and the clinical implications for treatment. (Auckland University of Technology, 2011).
147. Adel, S. M. Efficacy of neural mobilization in treatment of low back dysfunctions. *Journal of American Science* **7**, 566–573 (2011).
148. Anikwe, E., Tella, B., Aiyegbusi, A. & Chukwu, S. Influence of Nerve Flossing Technique on acute sciatica and hip range of motion. *International Journal of Medicine and Biomedical Research* **4**, 91–99 (2015).
149. McGill, S. *Low Back Disorders, 3E.* (Human Kinetics, 2016).
150. Jacobs, D. *Dermo Neuro Modulating: Manual Treatment for Peripheral Nerves and Especially Cutaneous Nerves.* (Diane Jacobs, 2016).
151. Wetterwald, F. (Dr). Le rôle thérapeutique du mouvement. Notions générales. in *Manuel pratique de kinésithérapie* (F. Alcan, 1912).
152. Wetterwald, F. (Dr). *Traitement manuel dans les maladies de la nutrition. Les Névralgies...* (1910).
153. Halata, Z. & Munger, B. L. Identification of the Ruffini corpuscle in human hairy skin. *Cell and tissue research* **219**, 437–440 (1981).
154. Chambers, M. R., Andres, K. H., Duering, M. v. & Iggo, A. The Structure and Function of the Slowly Adapting Type Ii Mechanoreceptor in Hairy Skin. *Exp Physiol* **57**, 417–445 (1972).
155. Loukas, M. *et al.* Iliolumbar membrane, a newly recognised structure in the back. *Folia morphologica* **65**, 15 (2006).
156. Stecco, C. *Functional Atlas of the Human Fascial System E-Book.* (Elsevier Health Sciences, 2014).
157. Ishida, T. *et al.* Anatomical structure of the subcutaneous tissue on the anterior surface of human thigh. *Okajimas Folia Anat Jpn* **92**, 1–6 (2015).
158. Nelson, N. L. Kinesio taping for chronic low back pain: A systematic review. *Journal of Bodywork and Movement Therapies* **20**, 672–681 (2016).
159. Keles, B. Y., Yalcinkaya, E. Y., Gunduz, B., Bardak, A. N. & Erhan, B. Kinesio Taping in patients with lumbar disc herniation: A randomised, controlled, double-blind study. *Journal of Back and Musculoskeletal Rehabilitation* **30**, 543–550 (2017).
160. Hashemirad, F., Karimi, N. & Keshavarz, R. The effect of Kinesio taping technique on trigger points of the piriformis muscle. *Journal of Bodywork and Movement Therapies* **20**, 807–814 (2016).
161. McConnell, J. Recalcitrant chronic low back and leg pain—a new theory and different approach to management. *Manual Therapy* **7**, 183–192 (2002).
162. Pamuk, U. & Yucesoy, C. A. MRI analyses show that kinesio taping affects much more than just the targeted superficial tissues and causes heterogeneous deformations within the whole limb. *Journal of Biomechanics* **48**, 4262–4270 (2015).
163. Nash, L. G., Phillips, M. N., Nicholson, H., Barnett, R. & Zhang, M. Skin ligaments: *Clin. Anat.* **17**, 287–293 (2004).
164. Beaudette, S. M., Pinto, B. L. & Brown, S. H. M. Tactile Feedback can be Used to Redistribute Flexion Motion Across Spine Motion Segments. *Ann Biomed Eng* **46**, 789–800 (2018).
165. Pinto, B. L., Beaudette, S. M. & Brown, S. H. M. Tactile cues can change movement: An example using tape to redistribute flexion from the lumbar spine to the hips and knees during lifting. *Human Movement Science* **60**, 32–39 (2018).
166. Tsutomu Fukui. *Skin Taping - Skin Kinesiology and Its Clinical Application.* (2015).
167. Rauscher, C., Korn, K. von & Richter, M. Untersuchung der Wirksamkeit eines im Verlauf des N. ischiadicus angebrachten Kinesiotapes auf Neurodynamik und Schmerz bei unilateraler offensichtlich-auffälliger neurodynamischer Reaktion. *manuelletherapie* **20**, 129–136 (2016).
168. Kang, J.-I., Jeong, D.-K. & Choi, H. Effect of spinal decompression on the lumbar muscle activity and disk height in patients with herniated intervertebral disk. *J Phys Ther Sci* **28**, 3125–3130 (2016).
169. Khani, M. & Jahanbin, S. A Randomized Controlled Trial on the Effect of Repeated Lumbar Traction By A Door-mounted Pull-up Bar on the Size and Symptoms of Herniated Lumbar Disk: *Neurosurgery Quarterly* **25**, 508–512 (2015).
170. Prasad, K. M. *et al.* Inversion therapy in patients with pure single level lumbar discogenic disease: a pilot randomized trial. *Disability and rehabilitation* **34**, 1473–1480 (2012).
171. Sherry, E., Kitchener, P. & Smart, R. A prospective randomized controlled study of VAX-D and TENS for the treatment of chronic low back pain. *Neurological research* (2013).
172. Naderi, S., Andalkar, N. & Benzel, E. C. HISTORY OF SPINE BIOMECHANICS: PART I—THE PRE-GRECO-ROMAN, GRECO-ROMAN, AND MEDIEVAL ROOTS OF SPINE BIOMECHANICS. *Neurosurgery* **60**, 382–391 (2007).
173. Vasiliadis, E. S., Grivas, T. B. & Kaspiris, A. Historical overview of spinal deformities in ancient Greece. *Scoliosis* **4**, 6 (2009).
174. al-Zahrawi, A. al-Q. K. I. A. *Albucasis on Surgery and Instruments.* (University of California Press, 1973).
175. Bademci, G., Batay, F. & Sabuncuoglu, H. First detailed description of axial traction techniques by Serefeddin Sabuncuoglu in the 15th century. *European Spine Journal* **14**, 810–812 (2005).
176. Chung, T.-S., Yang, H.-E., Ahn, S. J. & Park, J. H. Herniated Lumbar Disks: Real-time MR Imaging Evaluation during Continuous Traction. *Radiology* **275**, 755–762 (2015).
177. Chow, D. H., Yuen, E. M., Xiao, L. & Leung, M. C. Mechanical effects of traction on lumbar intervertebral discs: A magnetic resonance imaging study. *Musculoskeletal Science and Practice* **29**, 78–83 (2017).
178. Mitchell, U. H., Beattie, P. F., Bowden, J., Larson, R. & Wang, H. Age-related differences in the response of the L5-S1 intervertebral disc to spinal traction. *Musculoskeletal Science and Practice* **31**, 1–8 (2017).
179. Tekeoglu, I., Adak, B., Bozkurt, M. & Gürbüzoglu, N. Distraction of lumbar vertebrae in gravitational traction. *Spine* **23**, 1061–1063 (1998).
180. Henmi, T. *et al.* Natural history of extruded lumbar intervertebral disc herniation. *J. Med. Invest.* **49**, 40–43 (2002).
181. Sarı, H., Akarırmak, Ü., Karacan, I. & Akman, H. Computed tomographic evaluation of lumbar spinal structures during traction. *Physiotherapy Theory and Practice* **21**, 3–11 (2005).
182. Roughley, P. J. & Mort, J. S. The role of aggrecan in normal and osteoarthritic cartilage. *Journal of experimental orthopaedics* **1**, 8 (2014).
183. Meszaros, T. F., Olson, R., Kulig, K., Creighton, D. & Czarnecki, E. Effect of 10%, 30%, and 60% body weight traction on the straight leg raise test of symptomatic patients with low back pain. *Journal of Orthopaedic & Sports Physical Therapy* **30**, 595–601 (2000).
184. Vernon, H., Meschino, J. & Naiman, J. Inversion therapy: a study of physiological effects. *The Journal of the Canadian Chiropractic Association* **29**, 135 (1985).
185. Cai, C., Pua, Y. H. & Lim, K. C. A clinical prediction rule for classifying patients with low back pain who demonstrate short-term improvement with mechanical lumbar traction. *European spine journal* **18**, 554–561 (2009).
186. Donaldson, G. A., Donaldson-Hugh, M. E. A. & Chumas, P. D. Cauda equina syndrome following traction for acute sciatica. *British Journal of Neurosurgery* **16**, 370–372 (2002).

187. Deen, H. G., Rizzo, T. D. & Fenton, D. S. Sudden Progression of Lumbar Disk Protrusion During Vertebral Axial Decompression Traction Therapy. *Mayo Clinic Proceedings* **78**, 1554–1556 (2003).
188. Wegner, I. *et al.* Traction for low-back pain with or without sciatica. *The Cochrane Library* (2013).
189. Moret, N. C., Stap, M. van der, Hagmeijer, R., Molenaar, A. & Koes, B. W. Design and feasibility of a randomized clinical trial to evaluate the effect of vertical traction in patients with a lumbar radicular syndrome. *Manual Therapy* **3**, 203–211 (1998).
190. Cholewicki, J., Lee, A. S., Reeves, N. P. & Morrisette, D. C. Comparison of trunk stiffness provided by different design characteristics of lumbosacral orthoses. *Clin Biomech (Bristol, Avon)* **25**, 110–114 (2010).
191. Black, G. F. *Scottish Charms and Amulets.* (Neill and Company, 1894).
192. Culpeper, N. *The English Physitian Enlarged: With Three Hundred, Sixty and Nine Medicines, Made of English Herbs that Were Not in Any Impression Untill This, Being an Astrologo-physical Discourse of the Vulgar Herbs of this Nation ...* (John Streater, 1666).
193. Cilingir, D., Hintistan, S., Yigitbas, C. & Nural, N. Nonmedical methods to relieve low back pain caused by lumbar disc herniation: a descriptive study in northeastern Turkey. *Pain Management Nursing* **15**, 449–457 (2014).
194. Kawchuk, G. N., Edgecombe, T. L., Wong, A. Y. L., Cojocaru, A. & Prasad, N. A non-randomized clinical trial to assess the impact of nonrigid, inelastic corsets on spine function in low back pain participants and asymptomatic controls. *The Spine Journal* **15**, 2222–2227 (2015).
195. Morrisette, D. C. *et al.* A randomized clinical trial comparing extensible and inextensible lumbosacral orthoses and standard care alone in the management of lower back pain. *Spine* **39**, 1733 (2014).
196. Klein, G., Mehlman, C. T. & McCarty, M. Nonoperative Treatment of Spondylolysis and Grade I Spondylolisthesis in Children and Young Adults: A Meta-analysis of Observational Studies. *Journal of Pediatric Orthopaedics* **29**, 146–156 (2009).
197. Garet, M., Reiman, M. P., Mathers, J. & Sylvain, J. Nonoperative Treatment in Lumbar Spondylolysis and Spondylolisthesis. *Sports Health* **5**, 225–232 (2013).
198. Cholewicki, J., Shah, K. R. & McGill, K. C. The effects of a 3-week use of lumbosacral orthoses on proprioception in the lumbar spine. *Journal of orthopaedic & sports physical therapy* **36**, 225–231 (2006).
199. van Poppel, M. N., de Looze, M. P., Koes, B. W., Smid, T. & Bouter, L. M. Mechanisms of action of lumbar supports: a systematic review. *Spine* **25**, 2103–2113 (2000).
200. Axelsson, P., Johnsson, R. & Strömqvist, B. Effect of lumbar orthosis on intervertebral mobility: a roentgen stereophotogrammetric analysis. *Spine* **17**, 678–681 (1992).
201. Terai, T. *et al.* Effectiveness of three types of lumbar orthosis for restricting extension motion. *Eur J Orthop Surg Traumatol* **24**, 239–243 (2014).
202. Fayolle-Minon, I. & Calmels, P. Effect of wearing a lumbar orthosis on trunk muscles: Study of the muscle strength after 21days of use on healthy subjects. *Joint Bone Spine* **75**, 58–63 (2008).
203. Dorsher, P. T. Myofascial Referred-Pain Data Provide Physiologic Evidence of Acupuncture Meridians. *The Journal of Pain* **10**, 723–731 (2009).
204. Dorsher, P. T. Neuroembryology of the Acupuncture Principal Meridians: Part 1. The Extremities. *Medical Acupuncture* **29**, 10–19 (2017).
205. Rostami, M., Noormohammadpour, P., Sadeghian, A. H., Mansournia, M. A. & Kordi, R. The Effect of Lumbar Support on the Ultrasound Measurements of Trunk Muscles: A Single-Blinded Randomized Controlled Trial. *PM&R* **6**, 302–308 (2014).
206. Ji, M. *et al.* The efficacy of acupuncture for the treatment of sciatica: a systematic review. *management* **99**, 461–473 (2007).
207. Kean, W. F., Tocchio, S., Kean, M. & Rainsford, K. D. The musculoskeletal abnormalities of the Similaun Iceman ("ÖTZI"): clues to chronic pain and possible treatments. *Inflammopharmacology* **21**, 11–20 (2013).
208. Dorfer, L. *et al.* A medical report from the stone age? *The Lancet* **354**, 1023–1025 (1999).
209. Unschuld, P. U. & Tessenow, H. *Huang Di Nei Jing Su Wen: An Annotated Translation of Huang Di's Inner Classic – Basic Questions, 2 Volumes, Volumes of the Huang Di Nei Jing Su Wen Project. Paul U. Unschuld, General Editor.* (University of California Press, 2011).
210. Saito, T. *et al.* Analysis of the Posterior Ramus of the Lumbar Spinal NerveThe Structure of the Posterior Ramus of the Spinal Nerve. *Anesthes* **118**, 88–94 (2013).
211. LI, L. *et al.* Acupuncture Jiaji Treatment on Lumbar Disc Herniation Systematic Review in Clinical Randomized Controlled Trials [J]. *Chinese Archives of Traditional Chinese Medicine* **6**, 006 (2011).
212. Robinson, N. G. *Interactive Medical Acupuncture Anatomy.* (CRC Press, 2016).
213. Lund, I. & Lundeberg, T. Mechanisms of acupuncture. *Acupuncture and Related Therapies* **4**, 26–30 (2016).
214. Gunn, C. C. Radiculopathic Pain: Diagnosis and Treatment of Segmental Irritation or Sensitization. *Journal of Musculoskeletal Pain* **5**, 119–134 (1997).
215. Koppenhaver, S. L. *et al.* Changes in lumbar multifidus muscle function and nociceptive sensitivity in low back pain patient responders versus non-responders after dry needling treatment. *Manual therapy* **20**, 769–776 (2015).
216. Koppenhaver, S. L. *et al.* The association between dry needling-induced twitch response and change in pain and muscle function in patients with low back pain: a quasi-experimental study. *Physiotherapy* **103**, 131–137 (2017).
217. Groenemeyer, D. H. W., Zhang, L., Schirp, S. & Baier, J. Localization of acupuncture points BL25 and BL26 using computed tomography. *J Altern Complement Med* **15**, 1285–1291 (2009).
218. Xia, Y., Cao, X., Wu, G.-C. & Cheng, J. *Acupuncture therapy for neurological diseases: a neurobiological view.* (Springer, 2010).
219. Inoue, M. *et al.* Acupuncture treatment for low back pain and lower limb symptoms—the relation between acupuncture or electroacupuncture stimulation and sciatic nerve blood flow. *Evidence-Based Complementary and Alternative Medicine* **5**, 133–143 (2008).
220. Skorupska, E., Rychlik, M., Pawelec, W., Bednarek, A. & Samborski, W. Trigger point-related sympathetic nerve activity in chronic sciatic leg pain: a case study. *Acupuncture in Medicine* **32**, 418–422 (2014).
221. Cao, H. *et al.* Cupping therapy for acute and chronic pain management: a systematic review of randomized clinical trials. *Journal of Traditional Chinese Medical Sciences* **1**, 49–61 (2014).
222. Sheeraz, M., Quamari, M. A. & Ahmed, Z. A comparative clinical study on the effects of Mehjama Nariya and Hijamat Bila Shart in Irqunnasa (Sciatica). *Spatula DD-Peer Reviewed Journal on Complementary Medicine and Drug Discovery* **3**, 161–166 (2013).
223. Fu, D. & Chang, X. Efficacy of Cupping with Pain-relieving plaster for lumbar disc herniation pain. *JOURNAL OF TRADITIONAL CHINESE MEDICINE UNIVERSITY OF HUNAN* **28**, 66–67 (2008).
224. Markowski, A. *et al.* A Pilot Study Analyzing the Effects of Chinese Cupping as an Adjunct Treatment for Patients with Subacute Low Back Pain on Relieving Pain, Improving Range of Motion, and Improving Function. *The Journal of Alternative and Complementary Medicine* **20**, 113–117 (2013).
225. Baghdadi, H. *et al.* Ameliorating role exerted by Al-Hijamah in autoimmune diseases: effect on serum autoantibodies and inflammatory mediators. *International journal of health sciences* **9**, 207 (2015).
226. Ahmed, S. M., Madbouly, N. H., Maklad, S. S. & Abu-Shady, E. A. Immunomodulatory effects of blood letting cupping therapy in patients with rheumatoid arthritis. *The Egyptian journal of immunology* **12**, 39–51 (2004).
227. Chirali, I. *Traditional Chinese Medicine Cupping Therapy, 3e.* (Churchill Livingstone, 2014).
228. H, T. *et al.* [Impacts of bleeding and cupping therapy on serum P substance in patients of postherpetic neuralgia]. *Zhongguo Zhen Jiu* **33**, 678–681 (2013).
229. X, T., Xh, X. & Gq, Z. [Effect of cupping on hemodynamic levels in the regional sucked tissues in patients with lumbago]. *Zhen Ci Yan Jiu* **37**, 390–393 (2012).
230. Liu, W., Piao, S., Meng, X. & Wei, L. Effects of cupping on blood flow under skin of back in healthy human. *World Journal of Acupuncture - Moxibustion* **23**, 50–52 (2013).
231. Kim, H., Jeon, J. & Kim, Y. Clinical Effect of Acupotomy Combined with Korean Medicine: A Case Series of a Herniated Intervertebral Disc. *Journal of acupuncture and meridian studies* **9**, 31–41 (2016).
232. Bamfarahnak, H., Azizi, A., Noorafshan, A. & Mohagheghzadeh, A. A tale of Persian cupping therapy: 1001 potential applications and avenues for research. *Complementary Medicine Research* **21**, 42–47 (2014).
233. Missori, P., Domenicucci, M. & Currà, A. Bloodletting from the Ankle Vein to Treat Sciatic Pain. *Pain Med* **16**, 30–36 (2015).
234. Abu-Asab, M., Amri, H. & Micozzi, M. *Avicenna's Medicine: A New Translation of the 11th-Century Canon with Practical Applications for Integrative Health Care.* (Inner Traditions / Bear & Co, 2013).
235. Jam, B. Tissue Distraction Release with Movement (TDR-WM): A Novel Method of Soft-tissue Release. (2016).
236. Bhishagratna, K. L. & others. *An English translation of the Sushruta Samhita based on original Sanskrit text.* **1**, (Wilkin's Press, 1907).
237. Collins, J. *The Treatment of diseases of the nervous system.* (W. Wood and Company, 1900).
238. Forchheimer, F. & Irons, E. E. *Forchheimer's therapeusis of internal disease.* (D. Appleton and Co., 1915).
239. Heraclitus, of E. *et al. Hippocrates.* (Heinemann, 1923).
240. Galenus, C. & identificato, T. non. *Galeni Opera ex octaua Iuntarum editione. Quae, quid superioribus praestet, pagina versa ostendit. Ad amplissimum Venetorum medicorum Collegium: Galeni librorum quinta classis eam medicinae partem, quae ad pharmaciam spectat, exponens; simplicium medicamentorum, substitorum, purgantium, antidotorum, componendorum tam per locos quam per genera medicamentorum, ponderum denique, ac mensurarum doctrinam comprehendit.* (apud Iuntas, 1609).
241. Caelius Aurelianus. *Caelii Aureliani Siccensis, ...De acutis morbis. lib.3. De diuturnis. lib.5. Ad fidem exemplaris manuscripti castigati, & annotationibus illustrati. Cum indice copiosissimo, ac locupletissimo.* (apud Guliel. Rouillium, sub scuto Veneto, 1566).
242. Salerno school. Regimen Sanitatis Salernitanum with commentary, Harley MS 3706. (15th century).
243. Hashemi, M., Halabchi, F. & others. Changing Concept of Sciatica: A Historical Overview. *Iranian Red Crescent Medical Journal* **18**, (2016).

244. Ginsberg, F. & Famaey, J. A Double-Blind Study of Topical Massage with Rado-Salil® Ointment in Mechanical Low-Back Pain. *Journal of international medical research* **15**, 148–153 (1987).
245. Musto, C. J. The Ancient and Medieval Pharmaceutical Treatments for Arthritis, Gout, and Sciatica. (NC State University, 2009).
246. Osbaldeston, T. A. *Dioscorides, De Materia Medica*. (Ibidis press, 2000).
247. Rhazes & Meyerhof. *Thirty-Three Clinical Observations*. **23**, (Isis, 1935).
248. Hernández, F. *Quatro libros De la naturaleza, y virtudes de las plantas, y animales que estan receuidos en el vso de medicina en la Nueua España, y la methodo, y correccion, y preparacion, que para administrallas se requiere con lo que el Doctor Francisco Hernandez escriuio en lengua Latina...* (en casa de la viuda de Diego Lopez Daualos, 1615).
249. Aykanat, V. *et al.* Intradermal capsaicin as a neuropathic pain model in patients with unilateral sciatica. *British journal of clinical pharmacology* **73**, 37–45 (2012).
250. Bonin, R. P. & De Koninck, Y. A Spinal Analogue of Memory Reconsolidation Enables Reversal of Hyperalgesia. *Nat Neurosci* **17**, 1043–1045 (2014).
251. *Capsaicin as a Therapeutic Molecule*. (Springer, 2014).
252. Brimijoin, S., Lundberg, J. M., Brodin, E., Ho, T. & others. Axonal transport of substance P in the vagus and sciatic nerves of the guinea pig. *Brain research* **191**, 443–457 (1980).
253. Horváth, K. *et al.* Analgesic topical capsaicinoid therapy increases somatostatin-like immunoreactivity in the human plasma. *Neuropeptides* **48**, 371–378 (2014).
254. Mason, L., Moore, R. A., Derry, S., Edwards, J. E. & McQuay, H. J. Systematic review of topical capsaicin for the treatment of chronic pain. *BMJ* **328**, 991 (2004).
255. Wagner, T., Poole, C. & Roth-Daniek, A. The Capsaicin 8% Patch for Neuropathic Pain in Clinical Practice: A Retrospective Analysis. *Pain Med* **14**, 1202–1211 (2013).
256. Mason, L. *et al.* Systematic review of efficacy of topical rubefacients containing salicylates for the treatment of acute and chronic pain. *BMJ* **328**, 995 (2004).
257. Patel, T., Ishiuji, Y. & Yosipovitch, G. Menthol: A refreshing look at this ancient compound. *Journal of the American Academy of Dermatology* **57**, 873–878 (2007).
258. Geller, M. J. *Renal and Rectal Disease Texts*. (Walter de Gruyter, 2005).
259. Sharma, P. V. *Caraka Samhita (Text With English Translation) 4 Volume Set*. (Chaukhambha Orientalia, 2005).
260. Strehlow, W. *Hildegard of Bingen's Spiritual Remedies*. (Inner Traditions / Bear & Co, 2002).
261. Branchini, M. *et al.* Fascial Manipulation® for chronic aspecific low back pain: a single blinded randomized controlled trial. *F1000Res* **4**, (2016).
262. Jiang, R. *et al.* Effect of scraping therapy on Interleukin-1 in serum of rats with lumbar disc herniation. *Journal of Traditional Chinese Medicine* **33**, 109–113 (2013).
263. Nielsen, A. *Gua sha: A Traditional Technique for Modern Practice, 2e*. (Churchill Livingstone, 2013).
264. Nielsen, A., Knoblauch, N. T. M., Dobos, G. J., Michalsen, A. & Kaptchuk, T. J. The effect of Gua Sha treatment on the microcirculation of surface tissue: a pilot study in healthy subjects. *Explore (NY)* **3**, 456–466 (2007).
265. Xu, Q.-Y. *et al.* The Effects of Scraping Therapy on Local Temperature and Blood Perfusion Volume in Healthy Subjects. *Evid Based Complement Alternat Med* **2012**, (2012).
266. Wang, Y. *et al.* Curative effect of scraping therapies on Lumbar Muscle Strain. *Journal of Traditional Chinese Medicine* **33**, 455–460 (2013).
267. Braun, M. *et al.* Effectiveness of traditional Chinese 'gua sha' therapy in patients with chronic neck pain: a randomized controlled trial. *Pain Med* **12**, 362–369 (2011).
268. Lauche, R. *et al.* Randomized Controlled Pilot Study: Pain Intensity and Pressure Pain Thresholds in Patients with Neck and Low Back Pain Before and After Traditional East Asian 'Gua Sha' Therapy. *Am. J. Chin. Med.* **40**, 905–917 (2012).
269. Wang, Z., Tao, Y., Wu, N. & others. The effect of coin scraping therapy for the treatment of lumbar disc herniation. *Zhongguo Zhongyi Gushangke Zazhi* **12**, 7–10 (2004).
270. Li Jie, X. Observation of Clinical Effects of Scraping Therapy for Treating Lumbar Intervertebral Disc Herniation. *Journal of Liaoning University of Traditional Chinese Medicine* (2013).
271. Chaitow, L. & DeLany, J. *Clinical Application of Neuromuscular Techniques, Volume 2: The Lower Body, 2e*. (Churchill Livingstone, 2011).
272. Travell, J. G. & Simons, D. G. *Myofascial Pain and Dysfunction: The Trigger Point Manual; Vol. 2., The Lower Extremities*. (Lippincott Williams & Wilkins, 1992).
273. Hsieh, L. L.-C. *et al.* Treatment of low back pain by acupressure and physical therapy: randomised controlled trial. *BMJ* **332**, 696–700 (2006).
274. Bordoni, B. & Zanier, E. Anatomic connections of the diaphragm: influence of respiration on the body system. *J Multidiscip Healthc* **6**, 281–291 (2013).
275. Bordoni, B. & Marelli, F. Failed back surgery syndrome: review and new hypotheses. *J Pain Res* **9**, 17–22 (2016).
276. Key, J. 'The core': Understanding it, and retraining its dysfunction. *Journal of Bodywork and Movement Therapies* **17**, 541–559 (2013).
277. Bordoni, B. & Zanier, E. The continuity of the body: hypothesis of treatment of the five diaphragms. *The Journal of Alternative and Complementary Medicine* **21**, 237–242 (2015).
278. Indahl, A., Haldorsen, E. H., Holm, S., Reikerås, O. & Ursin, H. Five-Year Follow-Up Study of a Controlled Clinical Trial Using Light Mobilization and an Informative Approach to Low Back Pain. *Spine* **23**, 2625 (1998).
279. Black, N., Sullivan, S. & Mani, R. A biopsychosocial understanding of lower back pain: Content analysis of online information. *European Journal of Pain* **22**, 728–744 (2018).
280. Louw, A., Diener, I. & Puentedura, E. J. The short term effects of preoperative neuroscience education for lumbar radiculopathy: A case series. *International journal of spine surgery* **9**, (2015).
281. Louw, A. *et al.* The effect of manual therapy and neuroplasticity education on chronic low back pain: a randomized clinical trial. *Journal of Manual & Manipulative Therapy* **25**, 227–234 (2017).
282. Frederiksen, P. *et al.* Can group-based reassuring information alter low back pain behavior? A cluster-randomized controlled trial. *PLOS ONE* **12**, e0172003 (2017).
283. Lederman, E. A process approach in osteopathy: beyond the structural model. *International Journal of Osteopathic Medicine* **23**, 22–35 (2017).
284. Louw, A., Nijs, J. & Puentedura, E. J. A clinical perspective on a pain neuroscience education approach to manual therapy. *Journal of Manual & Manipulative Therapy* **25**, 160–168 (2017).
285. Thomson, O. P. & Collyer, K. 'Talking a different language': a qualitative study of chronic low back pain patients' interpretation of the language used by student osteopaths. *International Journal of Osteopathic Medicine* **24**, 3–11 (2017).
286. Moseley, G. L. Evidence for a direct relationship between cognitive and physical change during an education intervention in people with chronic low back pain. *European Journal of Pain* **8**, 39–45 (2004).
287. Bodes Pardo, G. *et al.* Pain Neurophysiology Education and Therapeutic Exercise for Patients With Chronic Low Back Pain: A Single-Blind Randomized Controlled Trial. *Archives of Physical Medicine and Rehabilitation* **99**, 338–347 (2018).
288. Diener, I., Kargela, M. & Louw, A. Listening is therapy: Patient interviewing from a pain science perspective. *Physiotherapy theory and practice* **32**, 356–367 (2016).
289. Louw, A. *et al.* De-educate to re-educate: aging and low back pain. *Aging clinical and experimental research* **29**, 1261–1269 (2017).
290. Haugen, A. J. *et al.* Estimates of success in patients with sciatica due to lumbar disc herniation depend upon outcome measure. *European Spine Journal* **20**, 1669–1675 (2011).
291. Haugen, A. J. *et al.* Prognostic factors for non-success in patients with sciatica and disc herniation. *BMC musculoskeletal disorders* **13**, 183 (2012).
292. Smart, K. M., Blake, C., Staines, A., Thacker, M. & Doody, C. Mechanisms-based classifications of musculoskeletal pain: Part 1 of 3: Symptoms and signs of central sensitisation in patients with low back (±leg) pain. *Manual Therapy* **17**, 336–344 (2012).
293. Fryer, G. Integrating osteopathic approaches based on biopsychosocial therapeutic mechanisms. Part 2: Clinical approach. *International Journal of Osteopathic Medicine* **26**, 36–43 (2017).
294. Rufa, A., Beissner, K. & Dolphin, M. The use of pain neuroscience education in older adults with chronic back and/or lower extremity pain. *Physiotherapy theory and practice* 1–11 (2018).
295. Mehling, W. E., Ebell, M. H., Avins, A. L. & Hecht, F. M. Clinical decision rule for primary care patient with acute low back pain at risk of developing chronic pain. *The Spine Journal* **15**, 1577–1586 (2015).
296. Puentedura, E. J. & Flynn, T. Combining manual therapy with pain neuroscience education in the treatment of chronic low back pain: A narrative review of the literature. *Physiotherapy theory and practice* **32**, 408–414 (2016).
297. Smart, K. M., Blake, C., Staines, A., Thacker, M. & Doody, C. Mechanisms-based classifications of musculoskeletal pain: Part 3 of 3: Symptoms and signs of nociceptive pain in patients with low back (±leg) pain. *Manual Therapy* **17**, 352–357 (2012).
298. Hopayian, K. & Notley, C. A systematic review of low back pain and sciatica patients' expectations and experiences of health care. *The Spine Journal* **14**, 1769–1780 (2014).
299. Ong, B. N., Konstantinou, K., Corbett, M. & Hay, E. Patients' Own Accounts of Sciatica: A Qualitative Study. *Spine* **36**, 1251 (2011).
300. Moayeri, N. & Groen, G. J. Differences in Quantitative Architecture of Sciatic Nerve May Explain Differences in Potential Vulnerability to Nerve Injury, Onset Time, and Minimum Effective Anesthetic Volume. *Anesthes* **111**, 1128–1134 (2009).
301. Kim, E. S., Oladunjoye, A. O., Li, J. A. & Kim, K. D. Spontaneous regression of herniated lumbar discs. *Journal of Clinical Neuroscience* **21**, 909–913 (2014).
302. Deyo, R. A. Herniated Lumbar Intervertebral Disk. *Annals of Internal Medicine* **112**, 598 (1990).
303. Darlow, B. *et al.* Easy to harm, hard to heal: patient views about the back. *Spine* **40**, 842–850 (2015).
304. Haugen, A., Grøvle, L., Brox, J., Natvig, B. & Grotle, M. Pain-related fear and functional recovery in sciatica: results from a 2-year observational study. *J Pain Res* **9**, 925–931 (2016).
305. Verwoerd, A. J. H., Luijsterburg, P. A. J., Timman, R., Koes, B. W. & Verhagen, A. P. A single question was as predictive of outcome as the Tampa Scale for Kinesiophobia in people with sciatica: an observational study. *Journal of Physiotherapy* **58**, 249–254 (2012).

306. Verwoerd, A. J. H., Luijsterburg, P. A. J., Koes, B. W., el Barzouhi, A. & Verhagen, A. P. Does Kinesiophobia Modify the Effects of Physical Therapy on Outcomes in Patients With Sciatica in Primary Care? Subgroup Analysis From a Randomized Controlled Trial. *Phys Ther* **95**, 1217–1223 (2015).
307. Sloan, T. J. & Walsh, D. A. Explanatory and Diagnostic Labels and Perceived Prognosis in Chronic Low Back Pain. *Spine* **35**, E1120 (2010).
308. Verwoerd, A. *et al.* Systematic review of prognostic factors predicting outcome in non-surgically treated patients with sciatica. *European Journal of Pain* **17**, 1126–1137 (2013).
309. Brinjikji, W. *et al.* Systematic Literature Review of Imaging Features of Spinal Degeneration in Asymptomatic Populations. *American Journal of Neuroradiology* **36**, 811–816 (2015).
310. Savettieri, G. *et al.* Prevalence of lumbosacral radiculopathy in two Sicilian municipalities. *Acta Neurologica Scandinavica* **93**, 464–469 (2009).
311. McGregor, A. H., Burton, A. K., Sell, P. & Waddell, G. The development of an evidence-based patient booklet for patients undergoing lumbar discectomy and un-instrumented decompression. *Eur Spine J* **16**, 339–346 (2007).
312. Heliövaara, M., Mäkelä, M., Knekt, P., Impivaara, O. & Aromaa, A. Determinants of sciatica and low-back pain. *Spine* **16**, 608 (1991).
313. Darlow, B. Beliefs about back pain: the confluence of client, clinician and community. *International Journal of Osteopathic Medicine* **20**, 53–61 (2016).
314. Karran, E. L., Yau, Y.-H., Hillier, S. L. & Moseley, G. L. The reassuring potential of spinal imaging results: development and testing of a brief, psycho-education intervention for patients attending secondary care. *European Spine Journal* **27**, 101–108 (2018).
315. Mirtz, T. A., Morgan, L., Wyatt, L. H. & Greene, L. An epidemiological examination of the subluxation construct using Hill's criteria of causation. *Chiropractic & Osteopathy* **17**, 13 (2009).
316. Stilwell, P. & Harman, K. 'I didn't pay her to teach me how to fix my back': a focused ethnographic study exploring chiropractors' and chiropractic patients' experiences and beliefs regarding exercise adherence. *The Journal of the Canadian Chiropractic Association* **61**, 219 (2017).
317. Blickenstaff, C. & Pearson, N. Reconciling movement and exercise with pain neuroscience education: A case for consistent education. *Physiotherapy Theory and Practice* **32**, 396–407 (2016).
318. Siemonsma, P. C. *et al.* Cognitive Treatment of Illness Perceptions in Patients With Chronic Low Back Pain: A Randomized Controlled Trial. *Phys Ther* **93**, 435–448 (2013).
319. Barker, K. L., Reid, M. & Lowe, C. J. M. Divided by a lack of common language?-a qualitative study exploring the use of language by health professionals treating back pain. *BMC musculoskeletal disorders* **10**, 123 (2009).
320. Lequin, M. B. *et al.* Surgery versus prolonged conservative treatment for sciatica: 5-year results of a randomised controlled trial. *BMJ Open* **3**, e002534–e002534 (2013).
321. Wertli, M. M., Held, U., Lis, A., Campello, M. & Weiser, S. Both positive and negative beliefs are important in patients with spine pain: findings from the Occupational and Industrial Orthopaedic Center registry. *The Spine Journal* (2017). doi:10.1016/j.spinee.2017.07.166
322. Bossen, J. K. J., Hageman, M. G. J. S., King, J. D. & Ring, D. C. Does Rewording MRI Reports Improve Patient Understanding and Emotional Response to a Clinical Report? *Clin Orthop Relat Res* **471**, 3637–3644 (2013).
323. Karran, E. L., Medalian, Y., Hillier, S. L. & Moseley, G. L. The impact of choosing words carefully: an online investigation into imaging reporting strategies and best practice care for low back pain. *PeerJ* **5**, e4151 (2017).
324. Slade, S. C., Molloy, E. & Keating, J. L. The dilemma of diagnostic uncertainty when treating people with chronic low back pain: a qualitative study. *Clin Rehabil* **26**, 558–569 (2012).
325. Jenkins, H., Hancock, M., Maher, C., French, S. & Magnussen, J. Understanding patient beliefs regarding the use of imaging in the management of low back pain. *European Journal of Pain* **20**, 573–580 (2016).
326. Louw, A. *et al.* Immediate effects of sensory discrimination for chronic low back pain: a case series. *New Zealand Journal of Physiotherapy* **43**, 58–63 (2015).
327. Wälti, P., Kool, J. & Luomajoki, H. Short-term effect on pain and function of neurophysiological education and sensorimotor retraining compared to usual physiotherapy in patients with chronic or recurrent non-specific low back pain, a pilot randomized controlled trial. *BMC musculoskeletal disorders* **16**, 83 (2015).
328. Snodgrass, S. J. *et al.* Recognising neuroplasticity in musculoskeletal rehabilitation: A basis for greater collaboration between musculoskeletal and neurological physiotherapists. *Manual Therapy* **19**, 614–617 (2014).
329. Daffada, P. J., Walsh, N., McCabe, C. S. & Palmer, S. The impact of cortical remapping interventions on pain and disability in chronic low back pain: A systematic review. *Physiotherapy* **101**, 25–33 (2015).
330. Ng, S. K. *et al.* The Relationship Between Structural and Functional Brain Changes and Altered Emotion and Cognition in Chronic Low Back Pain Brain Changes. *The Clinical journal of pain* **34**, 237–261 (2018).
331. Diers, M., Löffler, A., Zieglgänsberger, W. & Trojan, J. Watching your pain site reduces pain intensity in chronic back pain patients. *European Journal of Pain* **20**, 581–585
332. Trapp, W. *et al.* A brief intervention utilising visual feedback reduces pain and enhances tactile acuity in CLBP patients. *Journal of back and musculoskeletal rehabilitation* **28**, 651–660 (2015).
333. Louw, A., Schmidt, S. G., Louw, C. & Puentedura, E. J. Moving without moving: immediate management following lumbar spine surgery using a graded motor imagery approach: a case report. *Physiotherapy theory and practice* **31**, 509–517 (2015).
334. Moseley, G. L. & Flor, H. Targeting cortical representations in the treatment of chronic pain: a review. *Neurorehabilitation and neural repair* **26**, 646–652 (2012).
335. Wand, B. M. *et al.* Seeing it helps: movement-related back pain is reduced by visualization of the back during movement. *The Clinical journal of pain* **28**, 602–608 (2012).
336. Luomajoki, H. & Moseley, G. L. Tactile acuity and lumbopelvic motor control in patients with back pain and healthy controls. *Br J Sports Med* **45**, 437–440 (2011).
337. Wand, B. M., Abbaszadeh, S., Smith, A. J., Catley, M. J. & Moseley, G. L. Acupuncture applied as a sensory discrimination training tool decreases movement-related pain in patients with chronic low back pain more than acupuncture alone: a randomised cross-over experiment. *Br J Sports Med* **47**, 1085–1089 (2013).
338. Adamczyk, W. M., Luedtke, K., Saulicz, O. & Saulicz, E. Sensory dissociation in chronic low back pain: Two case reports. *Physiotherapy theory and practice* 1–9 (2018).
339. Sedighi, M. & Haghnegahdar, A. Role of vitamin D3 in Treatment of Lumbar Disc Herniation—Pain and Sensory Aspects: Study Protocol for a Randomized Controlled Trial. *Trials* **15**, (2014).
340. Forrest, K. Y. Z. & Stuhldreher, W. L. Prevalence and correlates of vitamin D deficiency in US adults. *Nutr Res* **31**, 48–54 (2011).
341. Kuru, P., Akyuz, G., Yagci, I. & Giray, E. Hypovitaminosis D in widespread pain: its effect on pain perception, quality of life and nerve conduction studies. *Rheumatology international* **35**, 315–322 (2015).
342. Martirosyan, N. L. *et al.* Genetic Alterations in Intervertebral Disc Disease. *Front Surg* **3**, 59 (2016).
343. Kepler, C. K., Ponnappan, R. K., Tannoury, C. A., Risbud, M. V. & Anderson, D. G. The molecular basis of intervertebral disc degeneration. *The Spine Journal* **13**, 318–330 (2013).
344. Babita Ghai, M., Dipika Bansal, M. & Raju Kanukula, M. High Prevalence of Hypovitaminosis D in Indian Chronic Low Back Patients. *Pain physician* **18**, E853–E862 (2015).
345. Tae-Hwan, K. *et al.* Prevalence of vitamin D deficiency in patients with lumbar spinal stenosis and its relationship with pain. *Pain Physician* **16**, 165–176 (2012).
346. Waikakul, S. Serum 25-hydroxy-calciferol level and failed back surgery syndrome. *Journal of orthopaedic surgery* **20**, 18 (2012).
347. Schwalfenberg, G. Improvement of chronic back pain or failed back surgery with vitamin D repletion: a case series. *The Journal of the American Board of Family Medicine* **22**, 69–74 (2009).
348. Nimni, M. E., Han, B. & Cordoba, F. Are we getting enough sulfur in our diet? *Nutrition & Metabolism* **4**, 24 (2007).
349. van Blitterswijk, W. J., van de Nes, J. C. & Wuisman, P. I. Glucosamine and chondroitin sulfate supplementation to treat symptomatic disc degeneration: Biochemical rationale and case report. *BMC Complement Altern Med* **3**, 2 (2003).
350. Sztrolovics, R., Alini, M., Mort, J. S. & Roughley, P. J. Age-related changes in fibromodulin and lumican in human intervertebral discs. *Spine* **24**, 1765 (1999).
351. Solovieva, S. *et al.* Association between the aggrecan gene variable number of tandem repeats polymorphism and intervertebral disc degeneration. *Spine* **32**, 1700–1705 (2007).
352. Hansen, H.-J. & Ullberg, S. Uptake of S35 in the intervertebral discs after injection of S35-sulphate. An autoradiographic study. *Acta Orthopaedica Scandinavica* **30**, 84–90 (1961).
353. Evans, M. S., Reid, K. H. & Sharp, J. B. Dimethylsulfoxide (DMSO) blocks conduction in peripheral nerve C fibers: a possible mechanism of analgesia. *Neuroscience letters* **150**, 145–148 (1993).
354. Am, D. G. *et al.* Dimethyl sulfoxide provides neuroprotection in a traumatic brain injury model. *Restor Neurol Neurosci* **26**, 501–507 (2007).
355. Lu, C. & Mattson, M. P. Dimethyl Sulfoxide Suppresses NMDA- and AMPA-Induced Ion Currents and Calcium Influx and Protects against Excitotoxic Death in Hippocampal Neurons. *Experimental Neurology* **170**, 180–185 (2001).
356. Santos, N. C., Figueira-Coelho, J., Martins-Silva, J. & Saldanha, C. Multidisciplinary utilization of dimethyl sulfoxide: pharmacological, cellular, and molecular aspects. *Biochemical pharmacology* **65**, 1035–1041 (2003).
357. Blumenthal, L. S. & Fuchs, M. The clinical use of dimethyl sulfoxide on various headaches, musculoskeletal, and other general medical disorders. *Ann. N. Y. Acad. Sci.* **141**, 572–585 (1967).
358. Perez, R. *et al.* The treatment of complex regional pain syndrome type I with free radical scavengers: a randomized controlled study. *Pain* **102**, 297–307 (2003).
359. Jacob, S. W. & Appleton, J. *MSM the Definitive Guide: The Nutritional Breakthrough for Arthritis, Allergies and More.* (Freedom Press, 2015).
360. Bilbrough, E. E. *Brett's handy guide to New Zealand.* (H. Brett, 1890).

361. Cowan, J. *New Zealand: Or Ao-teä-roa (The Long Bright World): Its Wealth and Resources, Scenery, Travel-routes, Spas, and Sport.* (J. Mackay, government printer, 1908).
362. Jensen, C. A. *Byron Hot Springs.* (Arcadia Publishing, 2006).
363. Gutmann, E. *The Watering places and mineral springs of Germany, Austria, and Switzerland.* (Appleton, 1880).
364. Budge, E. A. W. *By Nile and Tigris: A Narrative of Journeys in Egypt and Mesopotamia on Behalf of the British Museum Between the Years 1886 and 1913.* (Murray, 1920).
365. Hirt, L. *The Diseases of the Nervous System: A Textbook for Physicians and Students.* (Appleton, 1893).
366. Diruf, O. *Kissingen. Its Baths and Mineral Springs: Written Principally for the Use of Visitors Taking the Waters.* (Stuber, 1887).
367. Jasolini, G. *De rimedi naturali che sono nell'isola di Pithecusa; hoggi detta Ischia. Libri due. Di Giulio Iasolino filosofo & medico in Napoli. ... Con due tauole copiose.* (appresso Giuseppe Cacchij, 1588).
368. Hale, E. M. *The Practice of Medicine.* (Gross and Delbridge, 1894).
369. M.D, R. R. *The Monthly Gazette of Health.* (1824).
370. Jones, T. E., Taylor & Ampère, L. *A new and universal geographical grammar: or, a complete systeme of geography, containing the ancient and present State of all the Empires, Kingdoms, States, and Republics, in the known world ...* (Printed for G. Robinson and T. Evans, 1772).
371. Black, W. *An Historical Sketch of Medicine and Surgery, from their origin to the present time ...* (J. Johnson, 1782).
372. Galen, Kühn, K. G. & Assmann, F. W. *Clavdii Galeni Opera omnia.* (prostat in officina libraria C. Cnoblochii, 1826).
373. Fuller, H. W. Sulphur Used Externally in Rheumatism. *Br Med J* **1**, 327–328 (1857).
374. McNutt Sr, W. Sulphur as a remedy for rheumatism. *California state journal of medicine* **15**, 30 (1917).
375. COWDEN, J. THE EXTERNAL APPLICATION OF SULPHUR IN SCIATIC NEURALGIA.: Read before the Illinois State Medical Society, at its Thirty-eighth Annual Meeting, in Rock Island, Ill., May 15, 1888. *Journal of the American Medical Association* **11**, 13–14 (1888).
376. Rosanoff, A., Weaver, C. M. & Rude, R. K. Suboptimal magnesium status in the United States: are the health consequences underestimated? *Nutrition Reviews* **70**, 153–164 (2012).
377. Simental-Mendía, L. E., Rodríguez-Morán, M. & Guerrero-Romero, F. Oral Magnesium Supplementation Decreases C-reactive Protein Levels in Subjects with Prediabetes and Hypomagnesemia: A Clinical Randomized Double-blind Placebo-controlled Trial. *Archives of Medical Research* **45**, 325–330 (2014).
378. Brill, S., Sedgwick, P. M., Hamann, W. & Vadi, P. P. di. Efficacy of intravenous magnesium in neuropathic pain. *Br. J. Anaesth.* **89**, 711–714 (2002).
379. Engen, D. J. *et al.* Effects of transdermal magnesium chloride on quality of life for patients with fibromyalgia: a feasibility study. *J Integr Med* **13**, 306–313 (2015).
380. Köseoglu, E., Talaslioglu, A., Gönül, A. S. & Kula, M. The effects of magnesium prophylaxis in migraine without aura. *Magnes Res* **21**, 101–108 (2008).
381. Pan, H.-C. *et al.* Magnesium supplement promotes sciatic nerve regeneration and downregulates inflammatory response. *Magnesium Research* **24**, 54–70 (2011).
382. Gougoulias, N., Hatzisotiriou, A., Kapoukranidou, D. & Albani, M. Magnesium administration provokes motor unit survival, after sciatic nerve injury in neonatal rats. *BMC Musculoskeletal Disorders* **5**, 33 (2004).
383. Rondón, L. J. *et al.* Magnesium attenuates chronic hypersensitivity and spinal cord NMDA receptor phosphorylation in a rat model of diabetic neuropathic pain. *The Journal of Physiology* **588**, 4205–4215 (2010).
384. Bourinet, E. *et al.* Calcium-Permeable Ion Channels in Pain Signaling. *Physiological Reviews* **94**, 81–140 (2014).
385. Malvern Waters, Malvern Springs and Wells. Available at: http://www.malvern-waters.co.uk/nationalparks.asp?search=yes&p=7&id=348. (Accessed: 17th January 2016)
386. Del Giudice, M. M. *et al.* Effectiveness of ischia thermal water nasal aerosol in children with seasonal allergic rhinitis: a randomized and controlled study. *International journal of immunopathology and pharmacology* **24**, 1103–1109 (2011).
387. Anderson, W. *Mineral Springs and Health Resorts of California: With a Complete Chemical Analysis of Every Important Mineral Water in the World ... A Prize Essay; Annual Prize of the Medical Society of the State of California, Awarded April 20, 1889.* (Bancroft Company, 1892).
388. South Tyrolean Water.
389. Bath - Hot Springs | Bathnes. Available at: http://www.bathnes.gov.uk/services/environment/bath-hot-springs. (Accessed: 17th January 2016)
390. The chemistry of waters of Te Aroha geothermal system. Available at: http://www.waikatoregion.govt.nz/tr201307/. (Accessed: 19th January 2016)
391. Karajian, H. A. *Mineral Resources of Armenia and Anatolia.* (Armen Technical Book Company, 1920).
392. Pliny, the E., Bostock, J. & Riley, H. T. (Henry T. *The natural history of Pliny.* (London, H. G. Bohn, 1856).
393. International Grotto Directory. Available at: http://www.thespasdirectory.com/profilego.asp?ref=2D3F34. (Accessed: 17th January 2016)
394. Waring, R. Report on Absorption of magnesium sulfate (Epsom salts) across the skin. *Analysis* 1–3 (2010).
395. W, W. & S, W. Methylcobalamin as an adjuvant medication in conservative treatment of lumbar spinal stenosis. *J Med Assoc Thai* **83**, 825–831 (2000).
396. Mauro, G. L., Martorana, U., Cataldo, P., Brancato, G. & Letizia, G. Vitamin B12 in low back pain: a randomised, double-blind, placebo-controlled study. *Eur Rev Med Pharmacol Sci* **4**, 53–58 (2000).
397. Smith, V. H. Vitamin C deficiency is an under-diagnosed contributor to degenerative disc disease in the elderly. *Medical hypotheses* **74**, 695–697 (2010).
398. Dionne, C. E. *et al.* Serum vitamin C and spinal pain: a nationwide study. *Pain* **157**, 2527–2535 (2016).
399. Allen, J. I., Naas, P. L. & Perri, R. T. Scurvy: bilateral lower extremity ecchymoses and paraparesis. *Annals of emergency medicine* **11**, 446–448 (1982).
400. Chirchiglia, D., Chirchiglia, P. & Signorelli, F. Nonsurgical lumbar radiculopathies treated with ultramicronized palmitoylethanolamide (umPEA): a series of 100 cases. *Neurologia i neurochirurgia polska* **52**, 44–47 (2018).
401. Keppel Hesselink, J. M. & Kopsky, D. J. Palmitoylethanolamide, a neutraceutical, in nerve compression syndromes: efficacy and safety in sciatic pain and carpal tunnel syndrome. *J Pain Res* **8**, 729–734 (2015).
402. Morera, C., Sabates, S. & Jaen, A. Sex differences in N-palmitoylethanolamide effectiveness in neuropathic pain associated with lumbosciatalgia. *Pain management* **5**, 81–87 (2015).
403. Domínguez, C. M. *et al.* N-palmitoylethanolamide in the treatment of neuropathic pain associated with lumbosciatica. *Pain management* **2**, 119–124 (2012).
404. Cruccu, G., Di, G. S., Marchettini, P. & Truini, A. Micronized Palmitoylethanolamide: A Post-Hoc Analysis of a Controlled Study in Over 600 Patients with Low Back Pain - Sciatica. *CNS Neurol Disord Drug Targets* (2019). doi:10.2174/1871527318666190703110036
405. Lipoic Acid. *Linus Pauling Institute* (2014). Available at: http://lpi.oregonstate.edu/mic/dietary-factors/lipoic-acid. (Accessed: 11th December 2016)
406. Memeo, A. & Loiero, M. Thioctic Acid and Acetyl-L-Carnitine in the Treatment of Sciatic Pain Caused by a Herniated Disc. *Clinical drug investigation* **28**, 495–500 (2008).
407. Ranieri, M. *et al.* The Use and Alpha-Lipoic Acid (ALA), Gamma Linolenic Acid (GLA) and Rehabilitation in the Treatment of Back Pain: Effect on Health-Related Quality of Life. *Int J Immunopathol Pharmacol* **22**, 45–50 (2009).
408. Sima, A. A. F., Calvani, M., Mehra, M. & Amato, A. Acetyl-l-Carnitine Improves Pain, Nerve Regeneration, and Vibratory Perception in Patients With Chronic Diabetic Neuropathy. *Diabetes Care* **28**, 89–94 (2005).
409. Dyall, S. C. & Michael-Titus, A. T. Neurological Benefits of Omega-3 Fatty Acids. *Neuromol Med* **10**, 219–235 (2008).
410. Seyithanoglu, H. *et al.* Association between nutritional status and Modic classification in degenerative disc disease. *J Phys Ther Sci* **28**, 1250–1254 (2016).
411. Goldberg, R. J. & Katz, J. A meta-analysis of the analgesic effects of omega-3 polyunsaturated fatty acid supplementation for inflammatory joint pain. *Pain* **129**, 210–223 (2007).
412. Maroon, J. C. & Bost, J. W. ω-3 Fatty acids (fish oil) as an anti-inflammatory: an alternative to nonsteroidal anti-inflammatory drugs for discogenic pain. *Surgical Neurology* **65**, 326–331 (2006).
413. Ko, G. D., Nowacki, N. B., Arseneau, L., Eitel, M. & Hum, A. Omega-3 fatty acids for neuropathic pain: case series. *The Clinical journal of pain* **26**, 168–172 (2010).
414. Li, Z. *et al.* Melatonin inhibits nucleus pulposus (NP) cell proliferation and extracellular matrix (ECM) remodeling via the melatonin membrane receptors mediated PI3K-Akt pathway. *Journal of Pineal Research* **63**, e12435 (2017).
415. Turgut, M., Başaloğlu, H. K., Yenisey, Ç. & Özsunar, Y. Surgical pinealectomy accelerates intervertebral disc degeneration process in chicken. *Eur Spine J* **15**, 605–612 (2006).
416. Turgut, A. T., Sönmez, I., Çakıt, B. D., Koşar, P. & Koşar, U. Pineal gland calcification, lumbar intervertebral disc degeneration and abdominal aorta calcifying atherosclerosis correlate in low back pain subjects: A cross-sectional observational CT study. *Pathophysiology* **15**, 31–39 (2008).

Index

www.ingramcontent.com/pod-product-compliance
Lightning Source LLC
Chambersburg PA
CBHW061134030426
42334CB00003B/38